NUTRITIONAL ASSESSMENT

SECOND EDITION

NUTRITIONAL ASSESSMENT

Robert D. Lee, DrPH, RD
Associate Professor
Central Michigan University

David C. Nieman, DrPH, FACSM
Professor
Appalachian State University

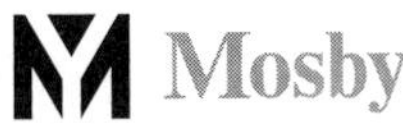

St. Louis Baltimore Boston Carlsbad Chicago Naples New York Philadelphia Portland
London Madrid Mexico City Singapore Sydney Tokyo Toronto Wiesbaden

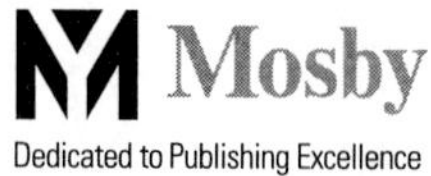

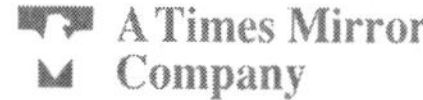

Vice President and Publisher: James M. Smith
Senior Acquisitions Editor: Vicki Malinee
Managing Editor: Janet R. Livingston
Assistant Editor: Jennifer L. Hartman
Project Manager: Mark Spann
Production Editors: Elizabeth Fathman, Julie Eddy
Designer: David Zielinski
Manufacturing Manager: Betty Richmond

SECOND EDITION

Printed in the United States of America
Composition by Wm. C. Brown
Printing/binding by Wm. C. Brown

Mosby-Year Book, Inc.
11830 Westline Industrial Drive
St. Louis, Missouri 63146

Library of Congress Cataloging in Publication Data

Lee, Robert D., 1952-
Nutritional assessment/Robert D. Lee and David C. Nieman. — 2nd ed.
p. cm.
Includes bibliographical references and index.
ISBN 0-8151-5319-8 (alk. paper)
1. Nutrition—Evaluation. I. Nieman, David C., 1950-
II. Title.
RC621.L43 1995
613.2—dc20

95-24647
CIP

95 96 97 98 99 / 9 8 7 6 5 4 3 2 1

Dedicated to my mother, Mary Z. Lee, whose love, patience, and faith give my life stability and meaning, and to the memory of my late father, Harry C. Lee, whose honesty, sincerity, and determination continue to be guiding principles in my life.

Robert D. Lee

To my loving wife, Cathy Nieman, MS, RD, for her insights, practical advice, and moral support.

David C. Nieman

PREFACE

Dietitians, health educators, nurses, physicians, and other health professionals often are challenged by their patients' and students' questions about the relationships between diet and health. How can I make sure that my diet gives me all of the important vitamins and minerals? How can I know if I am at risk of osteoporosis? Are Americans eating better than they did just 10 years ago? Are such programs as the National Cholesterol Education Program and the Special Supplemental Food Program for Women, Infants, and Children cost effective? Will the new food labels help me keep better track of my saturated fat intake? Which laboratory tests can best tell me if my iron status is adequate?

The second edition of *Nutritional Assessment* discusses these topics and many others, including computerized dietary analysis systems, national surveys of dietary intake and nutritional status, assessment techniques and standards for the hospitalized patient, nutritional assessment in the prevention of such diseases as coronary heart disease and diabetes, clinical assessment, and proper counseling techniques. This text builds on the strengths of its first edition and is primarily a textbook for students of dietetics and public health nutrition. It is also intended to be a valuable reference for health professionals who interact on a regular basis with patients who have diet-related medical problems.

ORGANIZATION

We recommend that study of *Nutritional Assessment* follow the progression of the 11 chapters in the order in which they are presented. Chapter 1 gives a thorough introduction to the topic of nutritional assessment, exploring various definitions and concepts. Chapter 2 reviews the wide assortment of standards for nutrient intake, such as the 1989 Recommended Dietary Allowances, the Food Exchange System, and the Food Guide Pyramid, and gives practical guidelines for their use.

Methods for measuring diet and the strengths and weaknesses of each technique are outlined in Chapter 3. Results from the Continuing Survey of Food Intakes by Individuals, the National Health and Nutrition Examination Survey (NHANES III), and other diet and nutrition surveys are interpreted in Chapter 4, and statistics on trends in the American diet are summarized. Eight computerized dietary analysis systems are reviewed in Chapter 5, with a complete discussion of their operating features, nutrient databases, and overall strengths and weaknesses.

Chapters 6 and 7 survey anthropometric techniques for both healthy and ill people, with complete descriptions of how to measure body skinfolds and circumferences and then make appropriate decisions on classification. Nutritional assessment, as it relates to prevention of coronary heart disease, hypertension, osteoporosis, and diabetes is reviewed in Chapter 8. Seventeen different laboratory tests are interpreted, and biochemical methods for assessing protein, iron, calcium, and other nutrient status are discussed in Chapter 9. Chapter 10 gives an overview of the clinical assessment of nutritional status. Chapter 11 reviews the major theories and techniques of both individual and group counseling methods.

FEATURES

Chapter Outline

Each chapter begins with an outline of the contents of the chapter. Reading this before beginning the chapter gives the student an idea of the material to be covered, and it is a useful review tool when the student is studying for exams.

Figures and Tables

There are more than 60 tables in the text, supplemented with 114 graphs, illustrations, and photographs. The photographs depict the exact procedures involved in skinfold measurement and other anthropometric techniques. All information is up-to-date, including the most current tables on nutrient standards from several different nations, food labeling criteria, anthropometric classifications, blood panel standards, and national survey results.

Summaries

A summary at the end of each chapter highlights all important chapter information and will be especially helpful when the student reviews for exams.

References

A complete list of up-to-date references is included at the end of each chapter. This list provides the student and instructor with extensive sources for continued study.

Assessment Activities

Most chapters end with two or three practical Assessment Activities to help the student better understand the concepts presented in the chapter. For example, activities are given for personal computerized dietary analysis, use of food composition tables, practice of anthropometry and one-on-one counseling, and interpretation of serum lipid and cholesterol results.

Appendixes

To make this textbook as practical as possible, a wide variety of questionnaires, checklists, and tables are given in the appendixes. Appendixes A, B, and C contain nutrient standards from the United Kingdom, Canada, and the United States. Various recording forms and questionnaires used in measurement of the diet are presented in Appendixes D through K. Appendix L is a nutrient breakdown of more than 650 different foods. Growth charts for children and adolescents are shown in Appendix M. A list of suppliers for nutritional assessment equipment and supplies is given in Appendix N. Various anthropometric standards are tabled in Appendixes O through R. Appendix S provides reference data for serum lipid and lipoprotein levels for children, adolescents, and adults. Appendix T contains a form for self-monitoring dietary intake, and Appendix U has a checklist for counseling competencies.

Glossary

Throughout the text, important terms are shown in boldface type. Concise definitions for these nearly 330 terms can be found in the glossary.

Acknowledgments

We would like to express our sincere gratitude to the Mosby editorial and production team for their continual encouragement and support. We are especially grateful to Jennifer Hartman, Liz Fathman, Janet Livingston, Terry Eynon, and Vicki Malinee who labored hard to see this project to completion. We would also like to express our appreciation to our colleagues at Central Michigan University and Appalachian State University for their support during the revision process. Special thanks goes to Dr. Saadia Saif, Chair of the Department of Human Environmental Studies at Central Michigan University, for her encouragement and support. We are particularly indebted to those professors who served as critical reviewers of the first edition. Their suggestions have been especially helpful, and we are grateful to each one for their contributions. They are:

Margaret Ann Bock, Ph.D., R.D., L.D., New Mexico State University
Nancy Cotugna, Dr.PH, R.D., University of Delaware
Jamie Dollahite, Ph.D., R.D., University of Arkansas
Sharon Hoerr, Ph.D., R.D., Michigan State University
Mary Lou Kiel, Ph.D., R.D., Pennsylvania State University
Paula Trumbo, Ph.D., Purdue University

Robert D. Lee
David C. Nieman

CONTENTS

ONE

INTRODUCTION TO NUTRITIONAL ASSESSMENT

OUTLINE

INTRODUCTION

Until about the middle of the twentieth century, infectious disease was the leading cause of death in developed countries, and nutritional deficiencies were common. Improved sanitation, vaccine development, improved health care, and increased quality and quantity of food now have virtually eliminated infectious disease as a major killer in developed countries, and nutrient deficiency is much less common.

However, with increased life expectancy, a higher living standard, and an abundance of food has come an epidemic of chronic diseases, many of which are related to excess consumption of high-fat foods and alcoholic beverages and inadequate consumption of foods high in complex carbohydrates and fiber. This situation, along with heightened public and professional interest in the role of nutrition in health and disease, has created an increased need for health professionals proficient in nutritional assessment. The ability to identify persons at nutritional risk and to effectively enhance their health status through improved nutrition has made nutritional assessment an important tool for health professionals concerned about making health care more cost effective.

GOOD NUTRITION ESSENTIAL FOR HEALTH

Good nutrition is critical for the well-being of any society and to each individual within that society. The variety, quality, and quantity of available food and the patterns of food consumption can profoundly affect health.

Scurvy, for example, was among the first diseases recognized as being caused by a nutritional deficiency. One of the earliest descriptions of scurvy was made in 1250 by the French writer Joinville, who observed it among the troops of Louis IX at the siege of Cairo. When Vasco da Gama sailed to the East Indies around the Cape of

Good Hope in 1497, more than 60% of his crew died of scurvy.[1] In 1747, James Lind, a British naval surgeon, conducted the first controlled human dietary experiment showing that consumption of citrus fruits cured scurvy.[2]

Deficiency Diseases Once Common

During the nineteenth century and the first half of the twentieth century, scurvy and other **deficiency diseases** such as **rickets, pellagra, beriberi, xerophthalmia**, and **goiter** (caused by inadequate dietary vitamin D, niacin, thiamin, vitamin A, and iodine, respectively) were commonly seen in the United States and throughout the world and posed a significant threat to human health (Figure 1-1).[3]

Nutritional deficiencies and **infectious disease** remain serious problems in many developing countries and even among certain population groups in the United States and other developed countries.[3] Sanitation measures, improved health care, vaccine development, and mass immunization programs have dramatically reduced the incidence of infectious disease in developed nations. An abundant food supply, **fortification** of some foods with important trace nutrients, **enrichment** to replace certain nutrients lost in food processing, and better methods of determining the nutrient content of foods have made nutrient deficiency diseases relatively uncommon in developed nations.[3] Among certain groups, however, deficiencies of certain nutrients remain a problem.[4]

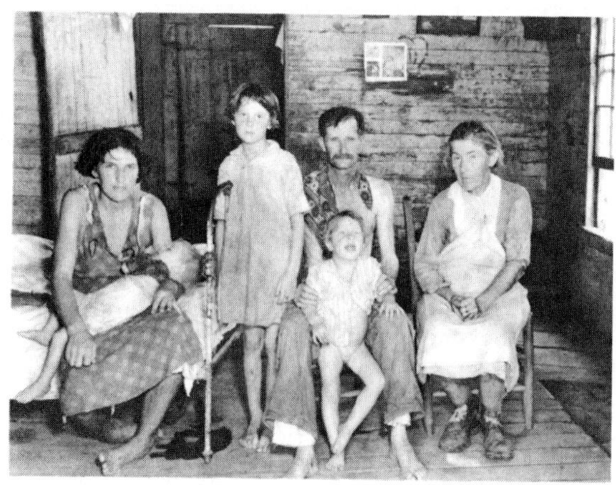

Figure 1-1 Poverty in America during the economic depression of the 1930s led to limited food choices and diets lacking essential nutrients. Nutritional deficiency diseases often resulted. Poverty among certain groups in America continues to prevent them from obtaining adequate nutrition and health care.

Chronic Diseases Now Epidemic

Despite the many advances of nutritional science, nutrition-related diseases not only continue to exist but result in a heavy toll of disease and death. In recent decades, however, they have taken a form different from the nutrient-deficiency diseases common in the early 1900s. Diseases of dietary excess and imbalance now rank among the leading causes of illness and death in America and play a prominent role in the epidemic of chronic disease that Western nations are currently experiencing.[5] In the 1988 *Surgeon General's Report on Nutrition and Health,* 5 of the 10 leading causes of death—**coronary heart disease** (heart attack), certain **cancers, stroke, diabetes mellitus**, and **atherosclerosis**—were linked with diet.[3] Table 1-1 ranks the 15 leading causes of death in 1993. Of these, five are linked with diet and four (accidents, suicide, homicide, and chronic liver disease and cirrhosis) are linked with excessive alcohol consumption.

The Surgeon General's Report on Nutrition and Health points out that although these diseases are caused by a combination of dietary and nondietary factors and that the exact proportion attributable to diet is uncertain, "it is now clear that diet contributes in substantial ways to the development of these diseases and that modification of diet can contribute to their prevention."[3] The report goes on to say that "for the two out of three adult Americans who do not smoke and do not drink excessively, one personal choice seems to influence long-term health prospects more than any other: what we eat."[3] The report's

TABLE 1-1 Estimated deaths and percent of total deaths for the 15 leading causes of death: United States, 1993

Rank	Cause of death	Number	Percent of total deaths
	All causes	2,268,000	100.0
1*	Diseases of the heart	739,860	32.6
2*	Malignant neoplasms	530,870	23.4
3*	Cerebrovascular disease	149,740	6.6
4	Chronic obstructive pulmonary disease	101,090	4.5
5†	Accidents and adverse effects	88,630	3.9
6	Pneumonia and influenza	81,730	3.6
7*	Diabetes mellitus	55,110	2.4
8	Human immunodeficiency virus infection	38,500	1.7
9†	Suicide	31,230	1.4
10†	Homicide and legal intervention	25,470	1.1
11†	Chronic liver disease and cirrhosis	24,730	1.1
12	Nephritis, nephrotic syndrome, and nephrosis	23,500	1.0
13	Septicemia	20,420	0.9
14*	Atherosclerosis	17,090	0.8
15	Certain conditions arising in the perinatal period	15,820	0.7
	All other causes	324,160	14.3

From the National Center for Health Statistics. 1994. *Monthly Vital Statistics Report* 42 (13).

*Causes of death in which diet plays a part.

†Causes of death in which excessive alcohol consumption plays a part.

main conclusion is that "overconsumption of certain dietary components is now a major concern for Americans. While many food factors are involved, chief among them is the disproportionate consumption of foods high in fats, often at the expense of foods high in complex carbohydrates and fiber that may be more conducive to health."[3]

The continuing presence of nutrition-related disease makes it essential that health professionals be able to determine the nutritional status of individuals. Both the American College of Physicians and the U.S. Preventive Services Task Force regard nutritional assessment and counseling as essential components of preventive services offered by physicians and other health professionals.[6] This will help identify persons who might benefit from nutritional intervention to improve their health and which interventions would be appropriate.

NUTRITIONAL SCREENING AND ASSESSMENT

Nutritional screening "is the process of identifying characteristics known to be associated with nutrition problems. Its purpose is to pinpoint individuals who are malnourished or at nutritional risk."[7] If nutritional screening identifies a person at nutritional risk, a more thorough evaluation of the individual's nutritional status can be performed. Nutritional screening can be done by any member of the health care team such as a dietitian, dietetic technician, dietary manager, nurse, or physician. Nutritional screening and how it fits into the nutritional care process are discussed in greater detail in Chapter 7, and examples of screening instruments are shown there.

Nutritional assessment is an evaluation of the nutritional status of individuals or populations through measurements of food and nutrient intake and evaluation of nutrition-related health indicators. The U.S. Department of Health and Human Services (DHHS) defines nutritional assessment as "the measurement of indicators of dietary status and nutrition-related health status to identify the possible occurrence, nature, and extent of impaired nutritional status," which can range from deficiency to toxicity.[4] The American Dietetic Association defines nutritional assessment as "a comprehensive approach, completed by a registered dietitian, to defining nutritional status that uses medical, nutrition, and medication histories; physical examination; anthropometric measurements; and laboratory data."[7] According to the World Health Organization (WHO), the ultimate purpose of nutritional assessment is to improve human health.[8]

Nutritional Assessment Methods

Four different methods are used to collect data used in assessing a person's nutritional status: anthropometric, biochemical or laboratory, clinical, and dietary (Figure 1-2). The mnemonic "ABCD" can help you remember these different methods. Each method will be explored in depth in later chapters.

Anthropometric Methods

Anthropometry is the measurement of the physical dimensions and gross composition of the body. Examples of anthropometry include measurements of height, weight, and head circumference and the use of measurements of **skinfold thickness, body density** (underwater weighing), and **bioelectrical impedance** to estimate the percentage of fat and lean tissue in the body. These results often are compared with standard values obtained from measurements of large numbers of subjects. Anthropometry will be covered in Chapters 6 and 8. At the end of most chapters are suggested exercises, called Assessment Activities, that allow you to apply the concepts covered. In the Assessment Activities of Chapter 6, you will try your hand at skinfold measurements to estimate percent body fat and compare several different methods of determining body composition.

Biochemical Methods

In nutritional assessment, biochemical or laboratory methods can include measuring a nutrient or its metabolite in blood, feces, or urine or measuring a variety of other components in blood and other tissues that have a relationship to nutritional status. The quantity of **albumin** and other **serum proteins** frequently is regarded as an indicator of the body's protein status, and **hemoglobin** levels in blood reflect iron status. Blood **cholesterol** levels, which are influenced by diet, reflect coronary heart disease risk.

Biochemical methods are covered in Chapters 7 through 9. An Assessment Activity in Chapter 8 suggests that you have your blood drawn and tested at a clinical laboratory and compare your results with recommended values. Assessment activities in Chapters 7 and 9 guide you through the application of key concepts as you evaluate biochemical and other data from patient records.

Clinical Methods

The medical history and physical examination are clinical methods used to detect **signs** and **symptoms** of **malnutrition**. Symptoms are disease manifestations that the patient is usually aware of and often complains about. Signs are observations made by a qualified examiner during physical examination. Painful cracks in the angles of the

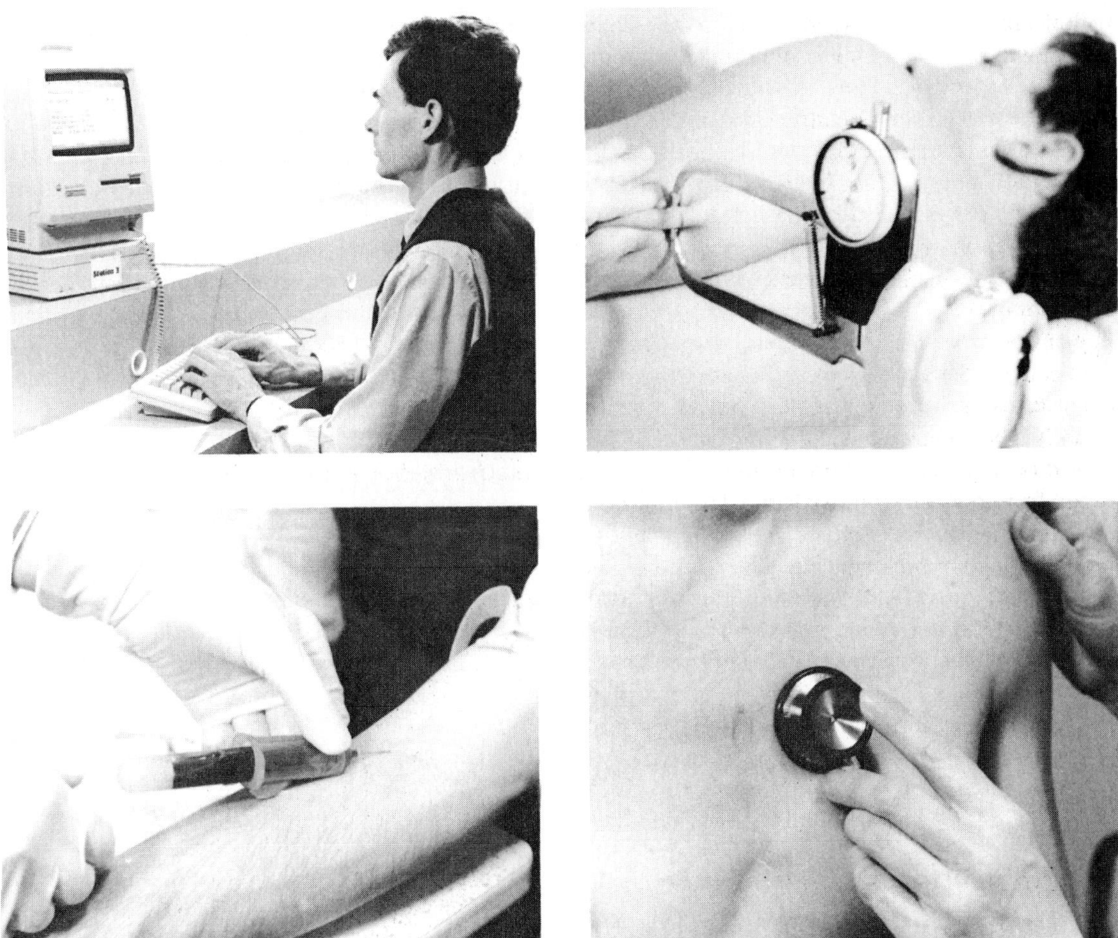

Figure 1-2 Examples of the four nutrition assessment methods include (clockwise from upper left) use of a personal computer and nutritional analysis software in diet analysis (dietary methods), skinfold measurements (anthropometric methods), blood tests (biochemical methods), and physical examination (clinical methods).

mouth, for example, may be symptomatic of riboflavin or niacin deficiency. Thyroid gland enlargement, sometimes caused by iodine deficiency, is a sign often first discovered by a physician during physical examination. Although the nutrition professional will not often collect this information, it is important to look for it in the medical record and have a keen eye to observe visible clinical signs. Such data may support and reinforce a suspected diagnosis of nutritional deficiency. Clinical signs and symptoms in nutritional assessment will be discussed in Chapter 10.

Dietary Methods

These generally involve surveys measuring the quantity of the individual foods consumed during the course of one to several days or assessing the pattern of food use during the previous several months. These can provide data on intake of nutrients or specific classes of foods. Chapters 2 through 4 cover dietary methods. One of the Assessment Activities in Chapter 3 involves collecting a 24-hour dietary recall from a classmate and analyzing his or her nutrient intake using food composition tables.

Included among dietary methods is the use of the computer to analyze dietary intake. A number of programs for personal computers are available that allow nutritionists and dietitians to quickly analyze the nutrient composition of dietary intake. These programs vary widely in price and certain features, such as the number and types of different foods and nutrients each program contains. Chapter 5 covers selection and use of nutritional analysis software. The Assessment Activity in Chapter 5 involves computerized analysis of the 24-hour recall and 3-day food record collected as part of the Assessment Activities in Chapter 3.

Importance of Nutritional Assessment

The use of nutritional assessment to identify diet-related disease has increased in importance in recent years because of our greater knowledge of the relationship between nutrition and health and our expanded ability to alter the nutritional state.[9]

Evidence related to the role of diet in maternal and child health indicates that well-nourished mothers produce healthier children.[10,11] Sufficient intake of energy and nutrients, including appropriate body weight before pregnancy and adequate weight gain during pregnancy, improves infant birth weight and reduces infant **morbidity** and **mortality**. Consequently, nutritional assessment has become an integral part of maternity care at the beginning of pregnancy and periodically throughout pregnancy and lactation.[3,10,11] Nutrition also can have a profound influence on health, affecting growth and development of infants, children, and adolescents; immunity against disease; morbidity and mortality from illness or surgery; and risk of such diseases as cancer, coronary heart disease, and diabetes.[3,12]

Interventions to alter a person's nutritional state can take many forms. In certain situations, nutrient mixes can be delivered into the esophagus, stomach, or small intestine through tubes **(enteral nutrition)** or administered directly into veins **(parenteral nutrition)** to improve nutritional status. Thus nutritional assessment is important in identifying persons at nutritional risk, in determining what type of nutrition intervention, if any, may be appropriate to alter nutritional status, and in monitoring the effects of nutrition intervention.

OPPORTUNITIES IN NUTRITIONAL ASSESSMENT

Numerous opportunities currently exist for applying nutritional assessment skills. As our understanding of the relationships between nutrition and health increases, these opportunities will also increase. Following are some examples of areas in which nutritional assessment can make a significant contribution to health care.

Meeting the Year 2000 Health Objectives

The Year 2000 Health Objectives are based on well-established diet-health relationships as well as information on subgroups within the U.S. population who are at risk for dietary excesses or deficiencies.[13] Dietitians and other health professionals proficient in nutritional assessment techniques will play a major role in implementing the National Health Promotion and Disease Prevention Objectives for the year 2000 developed by the U.S. DHHS.[14] Of the 300 health objectives to be met by the year 2000, 21 relate to nutrition. These are shown in Box 1-1.

For example, meeting objective 4 (reduce growth retardation among low-income children age 5 years and younger to less than 10%) requires health professionals skillful in anthropometry and able to intelligently use various standards

BOX 1-1

National Health Promotion and Disease Prevention Objectives for the Year 2000 Relating to Nutrition

Health status objectives

1. Reduce coronary heart disease deaths to no more than 100 per 100,000 people. (Age-adjusted baseline: 135 per 100,000 in 1987.)
2. Reverse the rise in cancer deaths to achieve a rate of no more than 130 per 100,000 people. (Age-adjusted baseline: 133 per 100,000 in 1987.)
3. Reduce overweight to a prevalence of no more than 20% among people age 20 years and older and no more than 15% among adolescents age 12 through 19 years. (Baseline: 26% for people age 20 through 74 in 1976–80, 24% for men and 27% for women, 15% for adolescents age 12 through 19 in 1976–80.)
4. Reduce growth retardation among low-income children age 5 years and younger to less than 10%. (Baseline: Up to 16% among low-income children in 1988, depending on age and race/ethnicity.)

Risk reduction objectives

5. Reduce dietary fat intake to an average of 30% of calories or less and average saturated fat intake to less than 10% of calories among people age 2 years and older. (Baseline: 36% of calories from total fat and 13% from saturated fat for people age 20 through 74 years in 1976–80; 36% of calories from total fat and 13% from saturated fat for women age 19 through 50 years in 1985.)
6. Increase complex carbohydrates and fiber-containing foods in the diets of adults to five or more daily servings for vegetables (including legumes) and fruits, and to six or more daily servings of grain products. (Baseline: Two and one half servings of vegetables and fruits and three servings of grain products for women age 19 through 50 years in 1985.)
7. Increase to at least 50% the proportion of overweight people age 12 years and older who have adopted sound dietary practices combined with regular physical activity to attain an appropriate body weight. (Baseline: 30% of overweight women and 25% of overweight men for people age 18 and older in 1985.)
8. Increase calcium intake so that at least 50% of youth age 12 through 24 years and 50% of pregnant and lactating women consume three or more servings daily of foods rich in calcium, and at least 50% of people age 25 years and older consume two or more servings daily. (Baseline: 7% of women and 14% of men age 19 through 24 years and 24% of pregnant and lactating women consumed three or more servings, and 15% of women and 23% of men age 25 through 50 years consumed two or more servings in 1985–86.)
9. Decrease salt and sodium intake so that at least 65% of home meal preparers prepare foods without adding salt, at least 80% of people avoid using salt at the table, and at least 40% of adults regularly purchase foods modified or lower in sodium. (Baseline: 54% of women age 19 through 50 years who served as the main meal preparer did not use salt in food preparation, and 68% of women age 19 through 50 years did not use salt at the table in 1985; 20% of all people age 18 years and older regularly purchased foods with reduced salt and sodium content in 1988.)

Continued

BOX 1-1

Cont'd

10. Reduce iron deficiency to less than 3% among children age 1 through 4 years and among women of childbearing age. (Baseline: 9% for children age 1 through 2 years, 4% for children age 3 through 4 years, and 5% for women age 20 through 44 years in 1976–80.)
11. Increase to at least 75% the proportion of mothers who breast-feed their babies in the early postpartum period and to at least 50% the proportion who continue breast-feeding until their babies are 5 to 6 months old. (Baseline: 54% at discharge from birth site and 21% at 5 to 6 months in 1988.)
12. Increase to at least 75% the proportion of parents and caregivers who use feeding practices that prevent baby bottle tooth decay.
13. Increase to at least 85% the proportion of people age 18 years and older who use food labels to make nutritious food selections. (Baseline: 74% use labels to make food selections in 1988.)

Services and protection objectives

14. Achieve useful and informative nutrition labeling for virtually all processed foods and at least 40% of fresh meats, poultry, fish, fruits, vegetables, baked goods, and ready-to-eat carry-away foods. (Baseline: 60% of sales of processed foods regulated by the FDA had nutrition labeling in 1988; baseline data on fresh and carry-away foods unavailable.)
15. Increase to at least 5000 brand items the availability of processed food products that are reduced in fat and saturated fat. (Baseline: 2500 items reduced in fat in 1986.)
16. Increase to at least 90% the proportion of restaurants and institutional food-service operations that offer identifiable low-fat, low-calorie food choices, consistent with the *Dietary Guidelines for Americans.* (Baseline: About 70% of fast foods and family restaurant chains with 350 or more units had at least one low-fat, low-calorie item on their menu in 1989.)
17. Increase to at least 90% the proportion of school lunch and breakfast services and child-care food services with menus that are consistent with the nutrition principles in the *Dietary Guide for Americans.*
18. Increase to at least 80% the receipt of home food services by people age 65 years and older who have difficulty in preparing their own meals or are otherwise in need of home-delivered meals.
19. Increase to at least 75% the proportion of the nation's schools that provide nutrition education from preschool through 12th grade, preferably as part of quality school health education.
20. Increase to at least 50% the proportion of work sites with 50 or more employees that offer nutrition education and/or weight management programs for employees. (Baseline: 17% offered nutrition education activities and 15% offered weight control activities in 1985.)
21. Increase to at least 75% the proportion of primary care providers who provide nutrition assessment and counseling and/or referral to qualified nutritionists or dietitians. (Baseline: Physicians provided diet counseling for an estimated 40% to 50% of patients in 1988.)

From USDH. 1990. *Healthy people 2000: National health promotion and disease prevention objectives.* Washington, DC: U.S. Department of Health and Human Services, Public Health Service.

for assessing adequate growth. The ability to evaluate dietary intake and interpret laboratory data and physical signs and symptoms reflecting nutritional status would be important in understanding some of the causes of diminished growth and in planning interventions to improve growth. Objective 5, reducing dietary fat intake to less than 30% of calories, requires a working knowledge of dietary survey methods to initially assess fat intake and to monitor long-term adherence to the objective.

In Hospitals

Hospitals continue to offer many opportunities for health professionals trained in nutritional assessment. **Protein-energy malnutrition (PEM)**, an excessive loss of lean body mass resulting from inadequate consumption of energy and/or protein, is commonly seen in residents of long-term care facilities and patients of acute-care hospitals.[15] Depending on the criteria used, the reported prevalence of PEM in long-term facilities ranges from 19% to 27%, while in acute-care hospitals the prevalence ranges from 33% to 58%.[15] One nutrition researcher characterized this situation by saying, "Malnutrition is the skeleton in the hospital's closet."[16]

Although the relationship between malnutrition and hospital outcome often is obscured by other factors that can affect the outcome of a patient's hospital stay (for example, the nature and severity of the disease process), several researchers have reported that patients with PEM tend to have a longer hospital stay, a higher incidence of complications, and a higher mortality rate.[17,19,20]

Identifying patients at nutritional risk is a major activity necessary for providing cost-effective medical treatment and helping to contain health care costs.[7] Good medical practice and economic considerations make it imperative that hospital patients be nutritionally assessed and that steps be taken, if necessary, to improve their nutritional status. Evaluation of a patient's weight, height, midarm muscle area, and triceps skinfold thickness and values from various laboratory tests can be valuable aids in assessing protein and energy nutriture.[9,16,18] Some researchers believe that rapid, nonpurposeful weight loss is the single best predictor of malnutrition currently available.[9] These and other assessment techniques for hospitalized patients will be discussed in detail in Chapter 8.

Diabetes Mellitus

Nutritional assessment has been an important component of managing diabetes in recent decades. However, nutritional assessment plays a major role in the American Diabetic Association's most recent nutrition recommendations and principles for people with diabetes.[20] Goals for the person with diabetes are based on dietary history, nutrient intake, and clinical data. A thorough knowledge of the patient gained through nutritional assessment will assist the dietitian—the primary provider of nutrition therapy—in guiding the patient to a successful treatment outcome. The role of nutritional assessment in managing diabetes is discussed further in Chapter 8.

Weight Management

The increasing number of Americans who are **overweight** or **obese** has focused attention on an important public health concern for which no efficacious, practical, and long-lasting preventive or therapeutic solution has yet been identified.[22] According to current estimates, 31.6% of males and 35.0% of females age 20 to 74 years are overweight (Figure 1-3).[23] Data from a national survey of Americans conducted between 1988 and 1991 show that the **prevalence** of overweight increased 8% compared with the prevalence during the late 1970s. During this time, average body weights of adult U.S. males and females increased 3.6 kg (7.9 lb).[22]

One of the Year 2000 Objectives is to reduce overweight among people age 20 through 74 years to a prevalence of no more than 20%.[14]

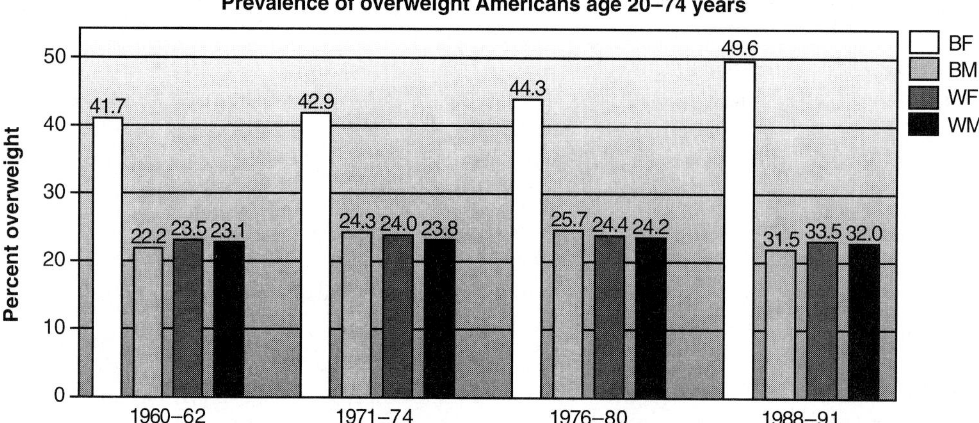

Figure 1-3 Close to one out of every three American adults is considered overweight, but the prevalence of overweight among black women is much higher. Adapted from the National Center for Health Statistics.

According to the 1990 National Health Interview Survey, 44 million Americans aged 25 years and older were trying to lose weight.[24] Recent surveys of the U.S. population estimate that about 40% of American women and 24% of American men are trying to lose weight at any given time.[25] Methods used include diets, exercise, behavior modification, and drugs. Participants who faithfully follow their weight loss program typically lose about 10% of their body weight. About one third to two thirds of this weight is regained within 1 year, and almost all is regained within 5 years. Unfortunately, many who are not overweight, particularly young women, are trying to lose weight, which may have adverse physical and psychological consequences.[25]

National surveys provide important nutritional assessment data such as prevalence of overweight and obesity in a particular population. Dietary methods can be valuable in initially assessing the quantity and quality of caloric intake and in monitoring dietary intake throughout treatment for obesity. Anthropometry is important in monitoring changes in percent body fat to help ensure that decrements in weight primarily come from body fat stores and that losses of lean body mass (mostly viscera and skeletal muscle) are minimized. Techniques for monitoring changes in percent body fat will be discussed in Chapter 6.

Heart Disease and Cancer

Heart disease and cancer are the first and second leading causes of death in the United States, respectively. Together they accounted for 56% of all deaths in 1993. Dietary factors playing a major role in heart disease are high intake of saturated fat, high intake of dietary cholesterol, and an imbalance between energy intake and energy expenditure leading to obesity.[26] Risk factors for coronary heart disease are shown in Box 1-2. Four of these factors (high blood pressure, elevated total blood cholesterol, diabetes, and obesity) are related to diet.

Despite a decline of more than 50% in the **age-adjusted death rate** from 1970 to 1990, heart disease remains the leading cause of death in the United States and accounts for 33% of all deaths. Because dietary therapy is the cornerstone of lowering blood cholesterol, nutritional assessment skills are vitally important in its management.[26] Proficiency in measuring diet, for example, would enable a dietitian to assess a client's consumption of saturated fat and cholesterol and suggest appropriate dietary changes. Chapter 3 includes a discussion of a recently developed questionnaire for assessing adherence to a cholesterol-lowering diet. Chapter 9 covers nutritional assessment in preventing heart disease.

BOX 1-2

Coronary Heart Disease Risk Factors

Major risk factors that cannot be changed
- heredity
- male sex
- increasing age

Major risk factors that can be changed
- cigarette smoking
- high blood pressure (≥140/90 mm Hg)
- elevated total blood cholesterol (≥200 mg/dl)
- physical inactivity

Other contributing factors
- diabetes
- obesity (more than 30% overweight)
- stress

From the American Heart Association.

BOX 1-3

Guidelines for Preventing Cancer Risk

- stop smoking
- avoid excessive sun exposure
- avoid excessive ionizing radiation exposure
- maintain desirable weight
- eat a varied diet
- include a variety of vegetables and fruits in the daily diet
- eat more high-fiber foods such as fruits, vegetables, and whole grain cereals, breads, and pasta
- cut down on total fat intake
- limit consumption of alcohol, if you drink at all
- limit consumption of salt-cured, smoked, and nitrite-cured foods

From the American Cancer Society. 1994. *Cancer facts & figures,* 1994. Atlanta: American Cancer Society.

Cancer accounted for 23% of all deaths among Americans in 1994 and resulted in more than 540,000 deaths.[27] Americans have an approximately 33% chance of dying of cancer. Cancers of 10 sites—lung, colon-rectum, breast, prostate, pancreas, leukemia, stomach, ovary, bladder, and liver and bile-conducting structures—account for about 72% of all cancer deaths in the United States and are variably associated with dietary factors.[28] The percentage of cancers attributable to diet is estimated to be 35% overall, with a range of 10% to 70%.[29]

The American Cancer Society's guidelines for preventing cancer are shown in Box 1-3.[30] Methods for assessing dietary levels of total fat, fiber, and alcohol, and intake of fruits, vegetables, and foods that are salt cured, salt pickled, or smoked will be necessary in applying these guidelines, as will anthropometric skills.

Nutrition Monitoring

Nutrition monitoring is defined as "those activities necessary to provide timely information about the contributions of food and nutrient consumption and nutritional status to the health of the U.S. population."[31] A recent milestone in nutrition monitoring in the United States was passage of the National Nutrition Monitoring and Related Research Act of 1990. Key provisions of the act are development of a 10-year comprehensive plan for coordinating the activities of 22 different federal agencies involved in nutrition monitoring and assurance of the collaboration and coordination of nutrition monitoring at federal, state, and local levels.[31] This includes all data collection and analysis activities associated with health and nutrition status measurements, food composition measurements, dietary knowledge, attitude assessment, and surveillance of the food supply.[4] Considerable nutrition assessment expertise is required for administering such surveys as the National Health and Nutrition Examination Survey and the Continuing Surveys of Food Intakes by Individuals. These will be discussed in Chapter 4.

Nutritional Epidemiology

Practically all nutrition research undertaken by universities, private industry, or government involves some aspect of nutritional assessment. An understanding of the theory behind assessment techniques, an awareness of the strengths and weaknesses of assessment methods, and proficiency in their use are essential skills for anyone currently involved in or contemplating a career in **nutritional epidemiology**.

For example, to arrive at valid conclusions about the relationships between the intake of antioxidant nutrients such as β-carotene and risk of cancer or heart disease, nutritional epidemiologists need to know which methods best assess β-carotene nutriture and how to appropriately use those methods. Failing to do so, they would likely arrive at erroneous conclusions and disseminate inaccurate information about diet-health relationships. Methods for measuring diet are discussed in Chapter 3, and measurement of vitamin A status is presented in Chapter 9.

Epidemiologists examining the prevention and treatment of **osteoporosis** must understand, among other things, the strengths and weaknesses of various techniques to assess changes in bone mineralization. Such techniques will be discussed in Chapter 8. Researchers investigating the influence of diet and/or exercise on weight loss and changes in percent body fat use a variety of dietary and anthropometric methods to monitor caloric intake and changes in weight and body composition.

Major limitations of research investigating the relationship between diet and disease are uncertainty in measuring diet and inadequate information on the quantity of certain nutrients and components in food.[32,33] Consequently, there is considerable need for improved methods of measuring diet, assessing the body's vitamin and mineral status, and for better data on the nutrient composition of foods.

SUMMARY

1. The relationship between nutrition and health has long been recognized. Scientific evidence confirming this relationship began accumulating as early as the mid-eighteenth century when James Lind showed that consumption of citrus fruits cured scurvy.
2. During the nineteenth and first half of the twentieth centuries, infectious disease was the leading cause of death throughout the world, and nutrition deficiency diseases were common. Because of sanitation measures, improved health care, vaccine development, mass immunization programs, and an improved food supply, infectious disease is no longer the leading cause of death in developed nations, and nutrient deficiency is relatively uncommon.
3. The current leading causes of death are chronic diseases such as coronary heart disease, cancer, and stroke. Although a number of factors are responsible, diet contributes in substantial ways to the development of these diseases and modification of diet can contribute to their prevention. Diet plays a prominent role in 5 of the 15 leading causes of death in America. Excessive alcohol consumption is a factor in at least another 4 of the 15.
4. The main conclusion of the 1988 *Surgeon General's Report on Nutrition and Health* is that "overconsumption of certain dietary components is now a major concern for Americans. While many food factors are involved, chief among them is the disproportionate consumption of foods high in fats, often at the expense of foods high in complex carbohydrates and fiber that may be more conducive to health."
5. The continuing presence of nutrition-related disease makes it important that health professionals be able to assess nutritional status to identify who might benefit from nutrition intervention and which interventions would be appropriate.

6. Nutritional screening allows persons who are at nutritional risk to be identified so that a more thorough evaluation of the individual's nutritional status can be performed. Nutritional assessment is an attempt to evaluate the nutritional status of individuals or populations through measurements of food and nutrient intake and nutrition-related health. Nutritional assessment techniques can be classified according to four types: anthropometric, biochemical or laboratory, clinical, and dietary. Use of the mnemonic "ABCD" can help in remembering these four types.
7. Our expanded ability to alter the nutritional state of a patient and our increased knowledge of the relationship between nutrition and health has made nutritional assessment an important tool in health care.
8. Objectives related to nutrition and health have a prominent place in the Year 2000 Health Objectives. Skill in applying nutritional assessment techniques will play a major part in the health professional's efforts to help achieve those objectives.
9. It is estimated that as many as one quarter of all patients in long-term care facilities and half of all patients in acute-care hospitals suffer from protein-energy malnutrition (PEM). Patients with PEM tend to have longer hospital stays and higher incidence of complications and mortality. Relatively simple techniques often can identify patients at nutritional risk.
10. Nutritional assessment is now a major component of the American Diabetes Association's nutrition recommendations and principles for people with diabetes.
11. Nutritional assessment also plays a significant role in identifying diet-related risk factors for heart disease and cancer and monitoring efforts to reduce risk.
12. Nutritional assessment is central to current government efforts to monitor and improve the nutritional status of its citizens. It is also a skill essential for nutritional epidemiologists and other nutrition researchers investigating links between diet and health.

REFERENCES

1. Todhunter EN. 1976. Chronology of some events in the development and application of the science of nutrition. *Nutrition Reviews* 34:353–365.
2. Todhunter EN. 1962. Development of knowledge in nutrition. *Journal of the American Dietetic Association* 41:335–340.
3. U.S. Department of Health and Human Services. 1988. *The Surgeon General's report on nutrition and health*. Washington, DC: U.S. Government Printing Office.
4. U.S. Department of Health and Human Services. 1989. *Nutrition monitoring in the United States—An update report on nutrition monitoring*. Washington, DC: U.S. Government Printing Office.
5. U.S. Department of Health and Human Services. 1994. *Healthy People 2000 Review 1993*. Washington, DC: U.S. Government Printing Office.
6. Sox HC. 1994. Preventive health services in adults. *Journal of the American Medical Association* 330:1589–1595.
7. Posthauer ME, Dorse B, Foiles RA, et al. 1994. ADA's definitions for nutrition screening and nutrition assessment. *Journal of the American Dietetic Association* 94:838–839.
8. Beghin I, Cap M, Dujardin B. 1988. *A guide to nutritional assessment.* Geneva: World Health Organization.
9. Starker PM. 1990. Nutritional assessment of the hospitalized patient. *Advances in Nutritional Research* 8:109–118.
10. National Academy of Sciences. 1991. *Nutrition during pregnancy*. Washington, DC: National Academy Press.
11. National Academy of Sciences. 1991. *Nutrition during lactation*. Washington, DC: National Academy Press.
12. Shils ME, Olson JA, Shike M. 1994. *Modern nutrition in health and disease,* 8th ed. Philadelphia: Lea & Febiger.
13. Buzzard IM. 1994. Rationale for an international conference series on dietary assessment methods. *American Journal of Clinical Nutrition* 59(suppl):143S–145S.

14. U.S. Department of Health and Human Services. 1990. *Healthy people 2000: National health promotion and disease prevention objectives.* Washington, DC: U.S. Department of Health and Human Services, Public Health Service.
15. Dwyer JT. 1991. *Screening older Americans' nutritional health: Current practices and future possibilities.* Washington, DC: Nutrition Screening Initiative.
16. Butterworth CE. 1974. The skeleton in the hospital closet. *Nutrition Today* 9:4–8.
17. Weinsier RL, Hunker EM, Krumdieck CL, Butterworth CE. 1979. A prospective evaluation of general medical patients during the course of hospitalization. *American Journal of Clinical Nutrition* 32:418–426.
18. Roubenoff R, Roubenoff RA, Preto J, Balke CW. 1987. Malnutrition among hospitalized patients: A problem of physician awareness. *Archives of Internal Medicine* 147:1462–1465.
19. Grant JP. 1986. Nutritional assessment in clinical practice. *Nutrition in Clinical Practice* 1:3–11.
20. Bistrian BR, Blackburn GL, Vitale J, Cochran D, Naylor J. 1976. Prevalence of malnutrition in general medical patients. *Journal of the American Medical Association* 235:1567–1570.
21. Tinker LF, Heins JM, Holler HJ. 1994. Commentary and translation: 1994 nutrition recommendations for diabetes. *Journal of the American Dietetic Association* 94:507–511.
22. Kuczmarski RJ, Flegal KM, Campbell SM, Johnson CL. 1994. Increasing prevalence of overweight among U.S. adults. *Journal of the American Medical Association* 272:205–211.
23. U.S. Department of Health and Human Services. 1994. *Health, United States, 1993.* Washington, DC: U.S. Government Printing Office.
24. Horn J, Anderson K. 1993. Who in America is trying to lose weight? *Annals of Internal Medicine* 119:672–676.
25. Technology Assessment Conference Panel. 1993. Methods for voluntary weight loss and control: Technology Assessment Conference statement. *Annals of Internal Medicine* 1993:764–770.
26. National Institutes of Health. 1993. *Second report of the expert panel on detection, evaluation, and treatment of high blood cholesterol in adults.* Washington, DC: National Institutes of Health, National Heart, Lung, and Blood Institute.
27. Centers for Disease Control and Prevention. 1995. *Monthly vital statistics report, volume 43, Number 12.* Washington, DC: U.S. Centers for Disease Control, National Center for Health Statistics.
28. Wingo PA, Tong T, Bolden S. 1995. Cancer statistics, 1995. *CA-A Cancer Journal for Clinicians* 45:8–30.
29. Doll R, Peto R. 1981. The causes of cancer: Quantitative estimates of avoidable risks of cancer in the United States today. *Journal of the National Cancer Institute* 66:1191–1308.
30. American Cancer Society. 1994. *Cancer facts and figures—1994.* Atlanta, GA: American Cancer Society.
31. Kuczmarski MF, Moshfegh A, Briefel R. 1994. Update on nutrition monitoring activities in the United States. *Journal of the American Dietetic Association* 94:753–760.
32. Mertz W, Tsui JC, Judd JT, Reiser S, Hallfrisch J, Morris ER, Steele PD, Lashley E. 1991. What are people really eating? The relation between energy intake derived from estimated diet records and intake determined to maintain body weight. *American Journal of Clinical Nutrition* 54:291–295.
33. National Research Council. 1989. *Diet and Health—Implications for Reducing Chronic Disease Risk.* Washington, DC: National Academy Press.

TWO

STANDARDS FOR NUTRIENT INTAKE

OUTLINE

- Introduction
- Early Dietary Standards and Recommendations
  - Observational Standards
  - Beginnings of Scientifically Based Dietary Standards
- Recommended Dietary Allowances
  - Defining Recommended Dietary Allowances
  - Estimating Dietary Allowances
    - Reviewing the Literature
    - Estimating Average Nutrient Requirements
    - Creating a Safety Margin
    - Publishing *Recommended Dietary Allowances*
  - Purpose and Use of the RDAs
  - Estimated Safe and Adequate Daily Dietary Intakes
  - Electrolytes
  - Recommended Dietary Allowances and Dietary Assessment
    - Fixed Cutoff Points
    - Probability Approach
  - Revising the Recommended Dietary Allowances
- Nutrient Density
  - Index of Nutritional Quality
  - Evaluating Nutrient Content
  - Weaknesses of the Index of Nutritional Quality
- Diet Quality Index
- Dietary Guidelines
  - Early Dietary Guidelines
  - U.S. Dietary Goals
  - *Dietary Guidelines for Americans*
  - *Toward Healthful Diets*
  - *The Surgeon General's Report on Nutrition and Health*
  - *Diet and Health*
  - Other Dietary Guidelines
  - *Healthy People 2000*
- Nutritional Labeling of Food
  - U.S. Recommended Daily Allowances
  - The Nutrition Labeling and Education Act
  - Daily Values
    - Daily Reference Values
    - Reference Daily Intakes
- Food Guides
  - Food Guide Pyramid
  - Alternative Food Guides
    - Mediterranean Pyramid
    - Vegetarian Pyramid
- Food Exchange System
  - Using the Food Exchange System
- Summary
- References
- Assessment Activity 2.1 Using Standards to Evaluate Nutrient Intake
- Assessment Activity 2.2 Index of Nutritional Quality (INQ)
- Assessment Activity 2.3 Food Exchange System

INTRODUCTION

This chapter discusses a variety of standards for evaluating the quality of nutrient intake of groups and individuals. Although most of these guidelines originally were designed to serve as standards for nutritional adequacy, to aid in diet planning, or to improve nutritional and health status, they are also useful as standards for evaluating levels and proportions of macronutrients, micronutrients, and various food components in diets.

Prominent among these standards is the Recommended Dietary Allowances. You will learn how the Recommended Dietary Allowances evolved from early dietary standards, what their intended purposes are, what some of the problems encountered with their application are, and what future plans are for their revision. We will discuss the Reference Daily Intakes and Daily Reference Values developed by the Food and Drug Administration (FDA) for food labeling purposes and briefly consider nutritional labeling of food. You will learn what nutrient density is, how it is calculated, and how it can be used to evaluate dietary intake. This chapter also will discuss how the food exchange system can be used to plan meals and quickly approximate energy and macronutrient intake. Another important standard discussed in this chapter is the report *Healthy People 2000,* which outlines the U.S. health objectives for the year 2000. This chapter's Assessment Activities will give you the opportunity to develop a greater working knowledge of recommended nutrient intake standards, the index of nutritional quality, and the food exchange system.

Recognition of diet's role in health and disease has led to numerous efforts in the last several decades to formulate dietary guidelines and goals to promote health and prevent disease. A clear consensus has developed among most dietary guidelines and goals: dietary patterns are important factors in several of the leading causes of death, and dietary modifications can, in a number of instances, reduce one's risk of premature disease and death. Nutritional assessment is pivotal to improving dietary intake, thus reducing disease risk and improving health.

EARLY DIETARY STANDARDS AND RECOMMENDATIONS

The earliest formal dietary standard was established in the British Merchant Seaman's Act of 1835. The act made the provision of "lime" or lemon juice compulsory in the rations of British merchant seamen. This action followed the 1753 treatise by British Naval Surgeon James Lind stating that citrus fruits cured scurvy and the introduction in 1796 of lemon juice (known as "lime juice") for the British Navy.[1] Throughout the remainder of the nineteenth century, dietary standards for protein, carbohydrates, and fat were proposed by scientists in Europe, the United Kingdom, and North America. These dietary standards had two things in common. First, the catalyst for their development was the occurrence of starvation and the diseases associated with it, resulting from economic dislocation and unemployment.[1,2] Second, they were, for the most part, **observational standards** because they were based on *observed* intakes rather than *measured* needs.[1]

Observational Standards

Carl Voit, a distinguished German physiologist of the late 1800s, made extensive observations of the amounts and kinds of foods eaten by German laborers and soldiers. He concluded that the nutritional needs of a 70-**kilogram (kg)** male of his day doing moderate work would be met by a diet containing 118 g of protein, 500 g of carbohydrate, and 56 g of fat—a total of approximately 3000 **kilocalories (kcal)**.[3] In 1895, W. O. Atwater, a notable American physiologist and nutrition researcher who studied in Germany under Voit, observed the dietary habits of Americans. He recommended that men weighing 70 kg consume 3400 kcal and 125 g of protein each day.[2,3] For men engaged in more strenuous occupations, Voit and Atwater recommended 145 g and 150 g of protein per day, respectively. Rather than representing the actual physiological needs of the body, these recommendations were based on observations of what people ate when guided by their appetites and financial resources.[3]

One notable exception to the observational nature of dietary standards of the nineteenth century was the work of Edward Smith, a British physician and scientist. Smith conducted a dietary survey of unemployed British workers to determine what kind of diet would maintain health at the lowest cost.[2] His suggested allowances for protein, carbohydrate, and fat were based on actual laboratory measurements of caloric need and nitrogen excretion as well as clinical observations that included absence of edema and anemia, "firmness of muscle, elasticity of spirits, capability for exertion."[1] Smith recommended approximately 3000 kcal of energy and 81 g of protein per day and believed that a diet adequate in calories and protein also would provide sufficient quantities of other necessary nutrients.[1,2]

Beginnings of Scientifically Based Dietary Standards

Advances in the early twentieth century in the ability to more accurately estimate actual energy and nutrient needs led to recommendations based on physiological requirements for protein, carbohydrate, and fat. At the same time, tremendous strides were made in understanding the role of vitamins and minerals in human nutrition.[4] This led to a reassessment and scaling down of protein recommendations in standards established during the 1920s and 1930s by the United Kingdom, America, and the League of Nations. There was also an effort to include recommendations for vitamins and minerals and make allowances for nutritional needs during pregnancy, lactation, and growth.[2]

Concern about limited resources worldwide and food shortages in European countries during World War I led the British Royal Society to appoint a committee to establish a standard for human energy needs. After reviewing the energy expenditure data of several scientists, the Royal Society Committee accepted the results of calorimetry research conducted by G. Lusk as applicable to the population of the United Kingdom. Lusk recommended 3000 kcal/day as an average energy requirement for adult males, with an appropriate adjustment for the needs of women and children. This standard also was used in estimating food requirements for the United Kingdom, France, and Italy as a basis for American food exports to these countries during World War I. In addition, the Royal Society Committee recommended that daily protein intake for adult males not fall below 70 g to 80 g, with no less than 25% of calories coming from fat. The committee made no specific recommendation for vitamins and minerals, but it recommended that "processed" foods should not be allowed to constitute a large proportion of the diet and that all diets should include a "certain proportion" of fresh fruits and green vegetables.[1]

The economic depression following the stock market crash in 1929 was the impetus for several dietary standards developed by the United Kingdom, the League of Nations, and the United States. Foremost among these was the standard proposed by Hazel Steibeling of the USDA in 1933. Hers was the first dietary standard to make deliberate recommendations for minerals and vitamins and maintenance of health rather than maintenance of work capacity.[2] In addition to energy and protein, the desirable amounts of calcium, phosphorus, iron, and vitamins A and C were stated. In 1939, these recommendations were expanded to include thiamin and riboflavin.[1]

Beginning in 1935, the League of Nations Technical Commission issued a series of dietary recommendations that were less concerned with defining requirements of food constituents than with outlining desirable allowances of the "protective" foods that had been lacking in so many diets.[1] Consumption of such foods as fruits, leafy vegetables, milk, eggs, fish, and meat was encouraged. These were among what the outstanding American biochemist E.V. McCollum termed "protective foods," because of his early observations that they tended to protect against nutritional deficiencies. The recommendations also raised questions about the use of sugar, milled grain, and other foods low in vitamins and minerals.[2]

In 1939 the Canadian Council on Nutrition established a Canadian Dietary Standard. Based in part on the recommendations of the League of Nations and on information gathered by the Royal Society Committee, it included recommendations for calories, protein, fat, calcium, iron, iodine, ascorbic acid, and vitamin D.

RECOMMENDED DIETARY ALLOWANCES

In 1940 the U.S. federal government established the Committee of Food and Nutrition under the National Research Council of the National Academy of Sciences in Washington, D.C. In 1941, this committee was established on a permanent basis and renamed the Food and Nutrition Board.[2] The role of the committee was to advise government agencies on problems relating to food and nutrition of the people and on nutrition problems in connection with national defense.[5,6] In 1941 the committee prepared the first Recommended Dietary Allowances (RDAs), as shown in Table 2-1, "to serve as a guide for planning adequate nutrition for the civilian population of the United States."[7] However, it was not until 1943 that the first officially published edition of RDAs appeared.[2] Since then, the RDAs have been revised approximately every 5 years to reflect advances in nutritional science.

The 10th edition of *Recommended Dietary Allowances,* released in 1989, included recommendations for 19 nutrients (Table 2-2), energy (Table 2-3), the estimated safe and adequate daily dietary intakes of seven additional vitamins and minerals (Table 2-4), and the estimated minimum requirements for three electrolytes (Table 2-5).[8]

From their inception, the RDAs have served as the premier nutrient standard, not only for the United States, but for many other countries throughout the developed and developing world.[9] Currently, more than 40 countries have their own national RDAs. A number of countries use the recommendations of the United States or those of the World Health Organization.[10]

Defining Recommended Dietary Allowances

The first edition of *Recommended Dietary Allowances* was published with the objective of "providing standards to serve as a goal for good nutrition" for the civilian population. Since 1974, the Food and Nutrition Board has defined the RDAs as "the levels of intake of essential nutrients that, on the basis of scientific knowledge, are judged by the Food and Nutrition Board to be adequate to meet the known nutrient needs of practically all healthy persons."[8] The RDAs are, in other words, a dietary standard for most known vitamins and minerals established by a highly respected group of nutrition scientists to be used in evaluating the adequacy of diets.

Various countries have their own definitions for their nutrient intake standards. The Recommended Nutrient Intakes (RNI) for Canadians is "the intake of nutrients, for example vitamin, mineral, protein, believed to be sufficiently high to meet the requirements, including reducing the risk of chronic diseases, of almost all individuals in a group with specified characteristics (age, size, physiological state). Because these Recommended Nutrient Intakes are designed to meet the needs of all normal individuals (almost all), they must exceed the needs of most."[11] The United Kingdom defines its Reference Nutrient Intakes (RNI) as the amount of protein, vitamin, or mineral "that is enough, or more than enough, for about 97% of people in a group. If average intake of a group is at RNI, then the risk of deficiency in the group is very small."[12] The United Kingdom Dietary Reference Values and Canadian Recommended Nutrient Intakes are shown in Appendixes A and B, respectively.

Estimating Dietary Allowances

Since their establishment in 1941 by the Food and Nutrition Board of the National Research Council, the RDAs have been revised approximately every 5 years. This laborious process usually begins soon after a new edition of *Recommended Dietary Allowances* has been published and is handled by a committee of nutrition experts appointed by the National Research Council on the recommendation of the Food and Nutrition Board.[9,13] The committee's task falls into four general areas: reviewing the scientific literature, estimating average nutrient requirements, creating a safety margin, and issuing the report.

Text continued on p. 24.

TABLE 2-1 The 1941 recommended dietary allowances

	Recommended daily allowances for specific nutrients*									
	Kilocalories	Protein	Calcium	Iron	Vitamin A†	Thiamin	Ascorbic acid	Riboflavin	Nicotinic acid	Vitamin D
		Grams	*Grams*	*Milligrams*	*IU‡*	*Milligrams*	*Milligrams*	*Milligrams*	*Milligrams*	*IU*
Man (70 kg):										
Moderately active	3000	70	0.8	12	5000	1.8	75	2.7	18	§
Very active	4500	70	0.8	12	5000	2.3	75	3.3	23	
Sedentary	2500	70	0.8	12	5000	1.5	75	2.2	15	
Woman (56 kg):										
Moderately active	2500	60	0.8	12	5000	1.5	70	2.2	15	§
Very active	3000	60	0.8	12	5000	1.8	70	2.7	18	
Sedentary	2100	60	0.8	12	5000	1.2	70	1.8	12	
Pregnancy (latter half)	2500	85	1.5	15	6000	1.8	100	2.5	18	400–800
Lactation	3000	100	2.0	15	8000	2.3	150	3.0	23	400–800
Children up to 12 years:										
Under 1 year‖	100 per kg	3–4 per kg	1.0	6	1500	0.4	30	0.6	4	400–800
1–3 years¶	1200	40	1.0	7	2000	0.6	35	0.9	6	§
4–6 years	1600	50	1.0	8	2500	0.8	50	1.2	8	
7–9 years	2000	60	1.0	10	3500	1.0	60	1.5	10	
10–12 years	2500	70	1.2	12	4500	1.2	75	1.8	12	
Children over 12 years:										
Girls: 14–15 years	2800	80	1.3	15	5000	1.4	80	2.0	14	§
6–20 years	2400	75	1.0	15	5000	1.2	80	1.8	12	
Boys: 13–15 years	3200	85	1.4	15	5000	1.6	90	2.4	16	§
16–20 years	3800	100	1.4	15	6000	2.0	100	3.0	20	

*These are tentative allowances toward which to aim in planning practical dietaries. These allowances can be met by a good diet of natural foods that will also provide other minerals and vitamins, the requirements for which are less well known.

†Requirements may be less than the amounts stated if provided as vitamin A and greater if the source is chiefly the pro-vitamin carotene.

‡IU = International Units.

§Vitamin D is undoubtedly necessary for older children and adults. When not available from sunshine, it should be provided probably up to the minimal amounts recommended for infants.

‖Needs of infants increase from month to month. The amounts given are for infants approximately 6 to 18 months of age. The amounts of protein and calcium needed are less if from breast milk.

¶Allowances are based on the middle year for each group (as 2, 5, 8, etc.) and for moderate activity.

TABLE 2-2 Food and Nutrition Board, National Academy of Sciences–National Research Council Recommended Dietary Allowances,* revised 1989

Category	Age (years) or condition	Weight† (kg)	Weight† (lb)	Height† (cm)	Height† (in)	Protein (g)	Fat-soluble vitamins: Vitamin A (μg RE)‡	Vitamin D (μg)§	Vitamin E (mg α-TE)‖	Vitamin K (μg)
Infants	0.0–0.5	6	13	60	24	13	375	7.5	3	5
	0.5–1.0	9	20	71	28	14	375	10	4	10
Children	1–3	13	29	90	35	16	400	10	6	15
	4–6	20	44	112	44	24	500	10	7	20
	7–10	28	62	132	52	28	700	10	7	30
Males	11–14	45	99	157	62	45	1000	10	10	45
	15–18	66	145	176	69	59	1000	10	10	65
	19–24	72	160	177	70	58	1000	10	10	70
	25–50	79	174	176	70	63	1000	5	10	80
	51+	77	170	173	68	63	1000	5	10	80
Females	11–14	46	101	157	62	46	800	10	8	45
	15–18	55	120	163	64	44	800	10	8	55
	19–24	58	128	164	65	46	800	10	8	60
	25–50	63	138	163	64	50	800	5	8	65
	51+	65	143	160	63	50	800	5	8	65
Pregnant						60	800	10	10	65
Lactating	1st 6 months					65	1300	10	12	65
	2nd 6 months					62	1200	10	11	65

From National Academy of Sciences. 1989. *Recommended Dietary Allowances,* 10th ed. Washington, DC: National Academy Press.

*Designed for the maintenance of good nutrition of practically all healthy people in the United States. The allowances, expressed as average daily intakes over time, are intended to provide for individual variations among most normal persons as they live in the United States under usual environmental stresses. Diets should be based on a variety of common foods to provide other nutrients for which human requirements have been less well defined.

†Weights and heights of reference adults are actual medians for the U.S. population of designated age, as reported by the second National Health and Nutrition Examination Survey. The median weights and heights of those under 19 years of age were taken from Hamill PVV, Drizd TA, Johnson CL, Reed RB, Roche AF, Moore WM. 1979. Physical growth: National Center for Health Statistics percentiles. *American Journal of Clinical Nutrition* 32:607–629. The use of these figures does not imply that the height-to-weight ratios are ideal.

TABLE 2-2 Food and Nutrition Board, National Academy of Sciences–National Research Council Recommended Dietary Allowances,* revised 1989—cont'd

		Water-soluble vitamins							Minerals						
Category	Age (years) or condition	Vitamin C (mg)	Thiamin (mg)	Riboflavin (mg)	Niacin (mg NE)¶	Vitamin B_6 (mg)	Folate (μg)	Vitamin B_{12} (μg)	Calcium (mg)	Phosphorus (mg)	Magnesium (mg)	Iron (mg)	Zinc (mg)	Iodine (μg)	Selenium (μg)
Infants	0.0–0.5	30	0.3	0.4	5	0.3	25	0.3	400	300	40	6	5	40	10
	0.5–1.0	35	0.4	0.5	6	0.6	35	0.5	600	500	60	10	5	50	15
Children	1–3	40	0.7	0.8	9	1.0	50	0.7	800	800	80	10	10	70	20
	4–6	45	0.9	1.1	12	1.1	75	1.0	800	800	120	10	10	90	20
	7–10	45	1.0	1.2	13	1.4	100	1.4	800	800	170	10	10	120	30
Males	11–14	50	1.3	1.5	17	1.7	150	2.0	1200	1200	270	12	15	150	40
	15–18	60	1.5	1.8	20	2.0	200	2.0	1200	1200	400	12	15	150	50
	19–24	60	1.5	1.7	19	2.0	200	2.0	1200	1200	350	10	15	150	70
	25–50	60	1.5	1.7	19	2.0	200	2.0	800	800	350	10	15	150	70
	51+	60	1.2	1.4	15	2.0	200	2.0	800	800	350	10	15	150	70
Females	11–14	50	1.1	1.3	15	1.4	150	2.0	1200	1200	280	15	12	150	45
	15–18	60	1.1	1.3	15	1.5	180	2.0	1200	1200	300	15	12	150	50
	19–24	60	1.1	1.3	15	1.6	180	2.0	1200	1200	280	15	12	150	55
	25–50	60	1.1	1.3	15	1.6	180	2.0	800	800	280	15	12	150	55
	51+	60	1.0	1.2	13	1.6	180	2.0	800	800	280	10	12	150	55
Pregnant		70	1.5	1.6	17	2.2	400	2.2	1200	1200	320	30	15	175	65
Lactating	1st 6 months	95	1.6	1.8	20	2.1	280	2.6	1200	1200	355	15	19	200	75
	2nd 6 months	90	1.6	1.7	20	2.1	260	2.6	1200	1200	340	15	16	200	75

‡Retinol equivalents. 1 retinol equivalent = 1μg retinol or 6 μg β-carotene. See *Recommended Dietary Allowances,* 10th ed. for calculation of vitamin A activity of diets as retinol equivalents.

§As cholecalciferol. 10 μg cholecalciferol = 400 IU of vitamin D.

‖α-Tocopherol equivalents. 1 mg d-α-tocopherol = 1 α-TE. See *Recommended Dietary Allowances,* 10th ed. for variation in allowances and calculation of vitamin E activity of the diet as α-tocopherol equivalents.

¶1 NE (niacin equivalent) is equal to 1 mg of niacin or 60 mg of dietary tryptophan.

TABLE 2-3 Recommended energy intake for infants, children, and adults based on their weight and height

Category	Age (years) or condition	Weight		Height		REE*	Average energy allowance (kcal)†		
		(kg)	(lb)	(cm)	(in)	(kcal/day)	Multiples of REE	Per kg	Per day‡
Infants	0.0–0.5	6	13	60	24	320		108	650
	0.5–1.0	9	20	71	28	500		98	850
Children	1–3	13	29	90	35	740		102	1300
	4–6	20	44	112	44	950		90	1800
	7–10	28	62	132	52	1130		70	2000
Males	11–14	45	99	157	62	1440	1.70	55	2500
	15–18	66	145	176	69	1760	1.67	45	3000
	19–24	72	160	177	70	1780	1.67	40	2900
	25–50	79	174	176	70	1800	1.60	37	2900
	51+	77	170	173	68	1530	1.50	30	2300
Females	11–14	46	101	157	62	1310	1.67	47	2200
	15–18	55	120	163	64	1370	1.60	40	2200
	19–24	58	128	164	65	1350	1.60	38	2200
	25–50	63	138	163	64	1380	1.55	36	2200
	51+	65	143	160	63	1280	1.50	30	1900
Pregnant	1st trimester								+0
	2nd trimester								+300
	3rd trimester								+300
Lactating	1st 6 months								+500
	2nd 6 months								+500

From National Academy of Sciences. 1989. *Recommended Dietary Allowances,* 10th ed. Washington, DC: National Academy Press.

*Calculation based on Food Agriculture Organization equations, then rounded.

†In the range of light to moderate activity, the coefficient of variation is ±20%.

‡Figure is rounded.

TABLE 2-4 Estimated safe and adequate daily dietary intakes of selected vitamins and minerals*

Category	Age (years)	Vitamins: Biotin (μg)	Vitamins: Pantothenic acid (mg)
Infants	0–0.5	10	2
	0.5–1	15	3
Children and adolescents	1–3	20	3
	4–6	25	3–4
	7–10	30	4–5
	11+	30–100	4–7
Adults		30–100	4–7

Category	Age (years)	Trace elements†: Copper (mg)	Manganese (mg)	Fluoride (mg)	Chromium (μg)	Molybdenum (μg)
Infants	0–0.5	0.4–0.6	0.3–0.6	0.1–0.5	10–40	15–30
	0.5–1	0.6–0.7	0.6–1.0	0.2–1.0	20–60	20–40
Children and adolescents	1–3	0.7–1.0	1.0–1.5	0.5–1.5	20–80	25–50
	4–6	1.0–1.5	1.5–2.0	1.0–2.5	30–120	30–75
	7–10	1.0–2.0	2.0–3.0	1.5–2.5	50–200	50–150
	11+	1.5–2.5	2.0–5.0	1.5–2.5	50–200	75–250
Adults		1.5–3.0	2.0–5.0	1.5–4.0	50–200	75–250

From National Academy of Sciences. 1989. *Recommended Dietary Allowances*, 10th ed. Washington, DC: National Academy Press.

*Because there is less information on which to base allowances, these figures are not given in the main table of *Recommended Dietary Allowances* and are provided here in the form of ranges of recommended intakes.

†Since the toxic levels for many trace elements may be only several times usual intakes, the upper levels for the trace elements given in this table should not be habitually exceeded.

TABLE 2-5 Estimated sodium, chloride, and potassium minimum requirements of healthy persons*

Age	Weight (kg)*	Sodium (mg)*†	Chloride (mg)*†	Potassium (mg)‡
Months				
0–5	4.5	120	180	500
6–11	8.9	200	300	700
Years				
1	11.0	225	350	1000
2–5	16.0	300	500	1400
6–9	25.0	400	600	1600
10–18	50.0	500	750	2000
>18§	70.0	500	750	2000

From National Academy of Sciences. 1989. *Recommended Dietary Allowances,* 10th ed. Washington, DC: National Academy Press.

*No allowance has been included for large, prolonged losses from the skin through sweat.

†There is no evidence that higher intakes confer any health benefit.

‡Desirable intakes of potassium may considerably exceed these values (approximately 3500 mg for adults—see *Recommended Dietary Allowances,* 10th ed.).

§No allowance included for growth. Values for those below 18 years of age assume a growth rate at the 50th percentile. Reported by the National Center for Health Statistics (Hamill PVV, Drizd TA, Johnson CL, Reed RB, Roche AF, Moore WM 1979. Physical growth: National Center for Health Statistics percentiles. *American Journal of Clinical Nutrition* 32:607–629) and averaged for males and females. See *Recommended Dietary Allowances,* 10th ed. for information on pregnancy and lactation.

Reviewing the Literature

First, committee members conduct an exhaustive review of nutritional data in the scientific literature—that published since the last revision of *Recommended Dietary Allowances* and, in some instances, earlier studies upon which previous editions were based. In addition, committee members may spend considerable time evaluating the philosophical base of the RDAs and their uses and limitations, and considering alternative approaches to their development.[13]

Estimating Average Nutrient Requirements

Using a variety of data including that derived from measurements of nutrient requirements for individuals, the committee estimates the *average* or *mean* physiological requirement for an *absorbed* nutrient for each of the numerous groups based on sex, age, and condition (for example, pregnancy or lactation). Several factors complicate this task. There is a lack of scientific data upon which to base many estimates of mean nutrient requirement.[14] The requirements for a specific nutrient vary widely among apparently similar people. Also, experts use different criteria and definitions of adequate and deficient nutrient intake. For example, in children nutrient requirement may be based on the amount that will maintain satisfactory growth and development. For adults it may be the amount that will maintain body weight, maintain certain nutrient levels within body tissues, prevent failure of a specific bodily function, or prevent development of specific deficiency signs.

Because of difficulty in estimating requirements for certain nutrients, some allowances are based on average intakes of the particular nutrient. The RDA for vitamin E for adults "is based primarily on customary intakes from U.S. food sources."[8] The committee refers to this as "an arbitrary but practical allowance."

Creating a Safety Margin

The estimated mean requirement for each nutrient then is *increased,* creating a *safety margin* to compensate for variations in individual nutrient requirements within groups. To illustrate the importance of this safety margin, consider a hypothetical nutrient X. If the requirements of nutrient X in a given group of people of the same sex and similar age and condition were plotted as shown in Figure 2-1, a **normal,** or **Gaussian, distribution** might result, creating a bell-shaped curve. In reality, however, nutrient requirements often are not normally distributed, and in many instances they are unknown.[14,15]

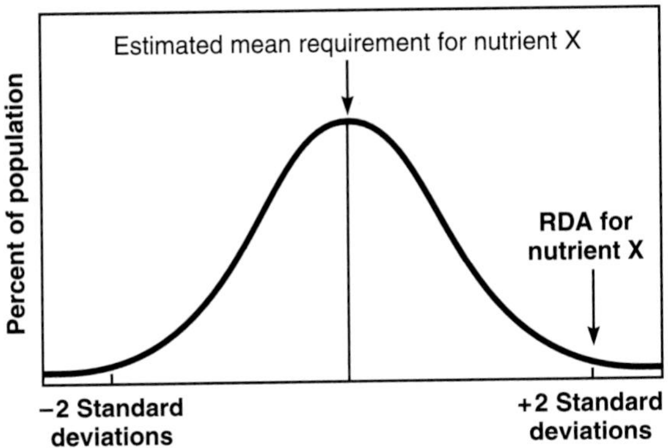

Figure 2-1 The distribution of the requirement for nutrient X for a group of people of the same age, sex, and condition. The estimated mean requirement for the group and the mean ±2 standard deviations are shown. The nutrient requirement level that is 2 standard deviations greater than the mean group requirement is the point often selected for the Recommended Dietary Allowance, except for energy. Adapted with permission from Beaton, GH. 1985. Uses and limits of the use of the Recommended Dietary Allowances for evaluating dietary intake. *American Journal of Clinical Nutrition* 41:155–164.

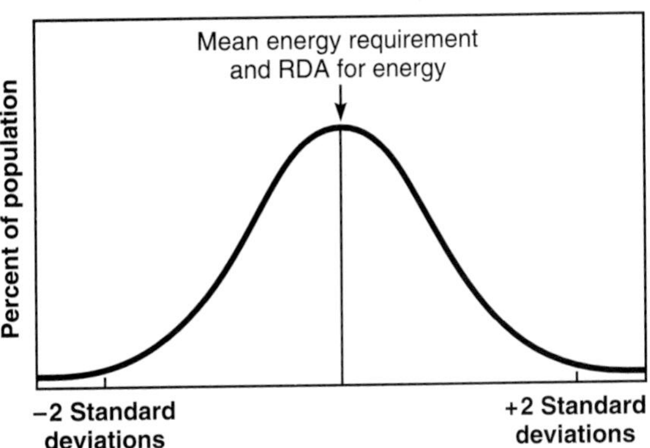

Figure 2-2 Distribution of the requirement for energy for a group of people of the same age, sex, and condition. The mean energy requirement is the point selected for the Recommended Dietary Allowance for energy. Adapted with permission from Beaton, GH. 1985. Uses and limits of the use of the Recommended Dietary Allowances for evaluating dietary intake. *American Journal of Clinical Nutrition* 41:155–164.

If the RDA of nutrient X were set at the *mean* requirement for a particular age/sex group, it would only meet the needs of half the group—those with an average or lower requirement for nutrient X. The need for X for the other half of the group—those with a greater-than-average requirement—would not be met. Thus to meet the needs of practically all persons in the group, the RDA is set at two **standard deviations (SD)** above the mean group requirement, as shown in Figure 2-1. The standard deviation indicates the degree of variation from the mean; in this case it indicates how similar or different the nutrient requirements of individual group members are from the group mean. At two standard deviations above the mean, the need for nutrient X would be met for nearly 98% of the group members.[15] This method or a similar one is followed in establishing the RDAs for all nutrients (except energy); they all have a built-in safety margin and are set sufficiently high to meet the needs of practically all healthy persons in the United States.[14,15]

A safety margin also is built into the RDA of a nutrient to compensate for its incomplete utilization by the body and to account for variations in the levels of the nutrient provided by various food sources. Adjustment also is made in some RDAs to account for the consumption of certain dietary components that are subsequently converted within the body to an essential nutrient. For example, the amino acid tryptophan can be converted to niacin within the body. Because the RDAs are sufficiently above mean physiological requirements, it cannot be automatically assumed that a nutrient deficiency exists whenever the recommendations are not completely met.[16] This presents a unique challenge that will be discussed in the section entitled "Recommended Dietary Allowances and Dietary Assessment" later in this chapter.

A somewhat different strategy is used to establish the RDAs for energy. The energy allowance is based on the estimated *mean population requirement with no added safety factor* for each age and sex group, as shown in Figure 2-2. One-half of persons are expected to have higher energy needs, and one-half are expected to have lower

TABLE 2-6 Uses of the Recommended Dietary Allowances

Category	Examples
Planning and procuring food supplies for groups	Schools, hospitals, health care facilities, the military, and the elderly
Evaluating dietary survey data and other scientific research	Reporting data of the Nationwide Food Consumption Surveys and the National Health and Nutrition Examination Surveys
Guides for food selection	Food Guide Pyramid
Food and nutrition information and education	Educational components of the Special Supplemental Food Program for Women, Infants, and Children and the Nutrition Education and Training Program
Food labeling	Daily Values
Food fortification	Standard fortification policies for milled grain products, milk, salt, etc.
Developing new or modified food products	Military combat rations, space rations
Clinical dietetics	Therapeutic diets when additional metabolic information is taken into account
Nutrient supplements and special dietary food	Infant formulas
Establishing the poverty level	Poverty level used to determine eligibility for Food Stamp program, free school lunches, and WIC program

energy needs. Although energy needs vary from person to person within each group, no additional amount is added to cover this variation as is done with specific nutrients. A safety factor to cover this variation would be inappropriate because, over the long term, it could lead to obesity in persons with less-than-average energy requirements and thus be detrimental to health.[8]

Publishing Recommended Dietary Allowances

Finally, individual committee members are given responsibility to draft various segments of the report, which are then scrutinized and discussed by the entire committee. Many of these segments are circulated to nutrition authorities outside the committee for their evaluation and input.[9,13] The draft report then is reviewed until approved by the Food and Nutrition Board and then by the National Research Council. Final approval for publication is given by the president of the National Academy of Sciences.[9]

Purpose and Use of the RDAs

The first edition of the *Recommended Dietary Allowances* was published with the objective of "providing standards to serve as a goal for good nutrition" and to serve as a guide for advising "on nutrition problems in connection with national defense."[8] Since then, the RDAs have been used for a variety of other purposes, as outlined in Table 2-6. They often are used for planning and procuring food supplies for population subgroups such as schools, hospitals, penal institutions, and the military. The RDAs are used in interpreting food consumption records in national surveys like the Nationwide Food Consumption Survey and the National Health and Nutrition Examination Survey, which are discussed in Chapter 4.

The RDAs have inadvertently become powerful tools in shaping public policy, and attempts by nutritional scientists to change the RDAs can have significant political and economic implications. For example, the federal government's definition of poverty—the poverty level—is set at three times the cost of the USDA's Thrifty Food Plan, which must meet 100% of the RDAs for eight nutrients—protein, vitamins A and C, thiamin, riboflavin, niacin, calcium, and iron. Changing or reducing the RDAs could affect the Thrifty Food Plan and thus the government's definition of poverty. Eligibility for the Food Stamp Program, the Special Supplemental Food Program for Women, Infants, and Children (WIC), or other food assistance programs administered by the federal government, or being able to receive free or reduced-cost lunches through the School Lunch Program, is based, at least in part, on whether a family falls within the poverty level. Thus changing the RDAs can affect eligibility for these important programs as well as the nutritional contribution they make to the diets of participants.[9]

The RDAs also are used in evaluating the adequacy of food supplies in meeting national nutritional needs, designing nutrition education programs, and developing new food products. The seventh edition of *Recommended Dietary Allowances,* published in 1968, became the basis of the U.S. RDAs, which, until recently, were used as the basis for nutritional labeling of foods.[8] The RDAs also act as a standard in formulating military combat rations, the meals of astronauts, nutrient supplements, and special dietary foods like infant formulas.[9]

The RDAs are intended to be met through a diet composed of a variety of foods from diverse food groups. Such diets probably will be adequate in all other nutrients for which RDAs cannot currently be established because of insufficient information. *The RDAs are not intended to be met by reliance on fortified foods or through the use of vitamin and/or mineral supplements* (Figure 2-3). However, food fortification and individual supplementation are appropriate in the few instances where deficiency is commonly observed (for example, iron deficiency in women).[8]

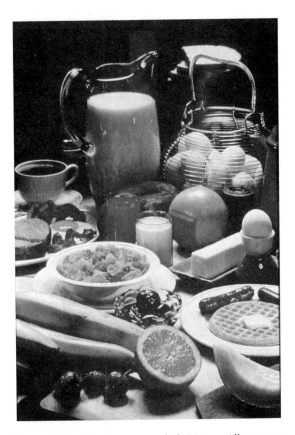

Figure 2-3 The Recommended Dietary Allowances are intended to be met through foods from diverse food groups, such as those shown in the above breakfast foods, not through the use of vitamin and/or mineral supplements.

Although the RDAs are expressed as recommended intakes of a nutrient *per day* or *daily,* these terms should actually be interpreted as *average intake over time.* The length of time over which averaging occurs depends on the nutrient, the body pool size, and the nutrient's turnover rate. The body's capacity to store most nutrients (for example, thiamin and vitamin C) is limited, and many nutrients are rapidly degraded. Total deprivation of such nutrients could lead to the development of symptoms within several days or weeks. If a nutrient requirement is not met on a particular day, tissue stores and a surplus consumed shortly thereafter will compensate for the lack. Thus, for most nutrients, the RDAs are intended to be average intakes over at least 3 days.

The body's capacity to store vitamins A, D, and B_{12}, on the other hand, is rather large, and these are slowly degraded. Several weeks or more of inadequate intake of these nutrients would not be problematic for someone with previously sufficient body stores and whose average intake over several months was adequate. Thus for a few nutrients, intakes can be averaged over several months.[8] Menus for congregate feeding, for example, should be so designed that the RDAs are met in a 5- to 10-day rotation.[8]

The RDAs are designed to apply to healthy persons. They do not cover the special nutritional needs associated with premature birth, metabolic disorders, injuries, chronic diseases, other medical conditions, and drug therapies.[8] Nutrition professionals can adapt the RDAs to meet the special needs of persons with special medical conditions.

The RDAs are not amounts of nutrients required by all individuals. Rather they are suggested levels of intake of nutrients (except for energy) sufficiently in excess of average nutritional requirements to meet the needs of nearly all healthy persons. Instead of being absolute nutritional standards, they are tentative and revisable "goals at which to aim in providing for the nutritional needs of groups of people."[5,17] They are based on the best knowledge available at the time of their formulation and are subject to change as more evidence becomes available.[15]

Estimated Safe and Adequate Daily Dietary Intakes

The category of **estimated safe and adequate daily dietary intakes (ESADDIs)** is for essential nutrients for which data are available to estimate a *range* of requirements but insufficient for developing a specific RDA. Included in this category are the vitamins biotin and pantothenic acid and the trace elements copper, manganese, fluoride, chromium, and molybdenum. These are shown in Table 2-4. The Food and Nutrition Board advises against habitually exceeding the upper limits for these trace elements because their toxic level may be only several times the usual intake.

Electrolytes

An electrolyte is a substance which, when in solution, becomes ionized and is capable of conducting an electrical current through the solution. Electrolytes commonly encountered in nutrition include sodium, chloride, and potassium. Table 2-5 shows the estimated minimum requirements of healthy persons for sodium, chloride, and potassium as established by the Food and Nutrition Board.

Recommended Dietary Allowances and Dietary Assessment

The RDAs are a useful standard for evaluating the adequacy of nutrient intake in groups and identifying individuals at relative risk of developing nutrient deficiency. Because the RDAs were not originally intended to be used in this way, the following points should be carefully noted.

Comparisons of dietary intake data with the RDAs alone cannot provide sufficient information to determine the nutritional status of individuals or population groups. *Such information only can be obtained when dietary intake data are combined with laboratory, anthropomorphic, and clinical measures.*[14]

In comparing the RDAs with estimates of individual or group dietary nutrient intake, such estimates should be representative of the individual's or group's *usual intake.* As will be discussed further in Chapter 3, observing a person's diet for only 1 or 2 days is rarely long enough to establish his or her usual intake.

Observations for several days over a 3- to 12-month period is better, but even then it may be inadequate.[15]

Nutrient requirements vary considerably among apparently similar individuals. Because of this and other factors, the RDAs include a safety margin and are set sufficiently high to meet the needs of practically all healthy persons in the United States. For many people this means that the RDA for a particular nutrient is set much higher than their own individual need and intake. Therefore, many people who receive less than the RDA for a specific nutrient will meet their own nutrient requirement; according to the RDA, they will be misclassified as having an inadequate intake when in reality it is adequate. These are called **false positives**—intakes misclassified as inadequate according to the RDA when in actuality they are adequate based on individual requirements. Failure to account for persons with nutrient requirements less than the RDA leads to *overestimation* of inadequate nutrient intakes.[14,18]

Fixed Cutoff Points

To prevent overestimation of inadequate nutrient intake, some nutrition professionals use a *fixed cutoff point,* such as two thirds or three fourths of the RDA, in determining inadequate nutrient intake for specific nutrients.[14] In other words, because the RDAs are set high enough to cover practically every person (except in the instance of energy), some nutritionists may not classify the intake of a particular nutrient as inadequate unless it is less than two thirds (or some other percentage) of the RDA. Thus using a fixed cutoff point results in fewer false positives.[14]

What about those persons whose high nutrient requirements caused the RDAs to be set much higher than the mean group requirement? If a cutoff point less than the actual RDA is used, some of these persons may be classified as having adequate intakes when actually they are inadequate. These are examples of **false negatives**—intakes misclassified as adequate when they are actually inadequate. Thus use of cutoff points has the advantage of reducing the number of false positives but the disadvantage of increasing the number of false negatives. Another problem is that RDAs for different nutrients have different margins of safety.[19] Further complicating cutoff points is the difficulty in determining which intakes are misclassified, when they are misclassified, and whether they are false positives or false negatives. Use of cutoff points has serious limitations. Thus an alternate method, called the probability approach, is recommended.[14,15]

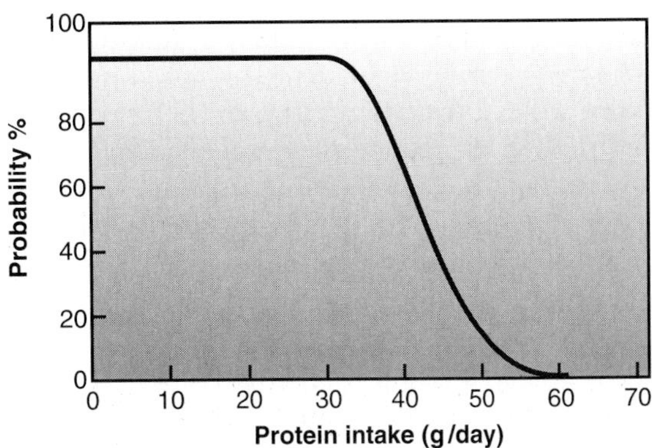

Figure 2-4 Distribution of protein requirements among adult men. The curve describes the probability, or risk, that an observed intake would be inadequate for a randomly selected male. From National Research Council. 1986. *Nutrient adequacy: Assessment using food consumption surveys.* Washington, DC: National Academy Press.

Probability Approach

The probability approach is based on the probability or likelihood that persons with a specific nutrient intake level will fail to meet their requirement for that nutrient. The approach does not identify specific individuals having inadequate intakes, only the prevalence or proportion of the population with inadequate intakes.[14]

Figure 2-4 shows the distribution of protein requirements among adult men. Protein intake in grams per day is shown along the horizontal axis, and the percent probability that an intake is inadequate to meet the protein requirement of this group is shown along the vertical axis. A very low intake (for example, 20 g/day) would be inadequate for everyone. Beyond about 30 g/day, the probability of inadequate protein intake decreases rapidly. At about 40 g to 45 g/day, the requirements of about 50% of group members are met. As protein intake exceeds about 60 g/day, the probability that protein intake is inadequate approaches zero.[14,15]

An example of the probability approach applied to protein intake is shown in Table 2-7. In the far left column, the distribution of protein intakes for adult males obtained from the 1977–78 Nationwide Food Consumption Survey (see Chapter 4) are shown arbitrarily divided into 11 groups or intervals based on level of protein intake. To the right of that column is the percentage of adult males having that level of protein intake. For example, only about 0.4% of group members have a protein intake of less than 24 g/day. The column labeled "Probability of inadequacy" shows the probability of each interval of intake being inadequate. With protein intakes less than 24 g/day, the probability of inadequacy is 1.0; thus everyone within that intake interval would be expected to have an inadequate protein intake. The probability of inadequacy eventually reaches zero when intakes are greater than 60 g/day. The percentage of the entire group of adult males expected to have inadequate intakes is estimated by multiplying the percentage of the total population in each intake interval by the probability of inadequate intake for that interval. This is shown in the far right column. When the percentages of inadequate intake at each intake interval are added together, the sum is 2.29%, the estimated prevalence of inadequate protein intake for that population of adult males.[14]

Using this approach, predictions of inadequate iron intakes among Canadian women were shown to be consistent with estimates of iron status based on laboratory data.[15] The probability approach is recommended by both the Food and Nutrition Board of the National Research Council and by the World Health Organization.[14]

Table 2-8 compares estimates of the prevalence of inadequate nutrient intakes derived by the probability approach with those based on the fixed cutoff approach. The table clearly demonstrates that the fixed cutoff approach may or may not give estimates of the prevalence of inadequate intakes similar to those generated with the probability approach. Because of this unpredictability, use of the probability approach is preferred over the fixed cutoff approach. However, some additional data are needed before the probability approach can be applied to all nutrients, including data on specific nutrient requirements and individual variation in requirements and more complete data on usual intakes of these nutrients. It is important to note that the probability approach cannot be applied to energy.[14,15]

The Food and Nutrition Board of the National Research Council has recommended that priority be assigned to the collection of the data necessary to apply the probability approach to more nutrients.[14]

Revising the Recommended Dietary Allowances

Although the RDAs serve an important role in nutritional science, they have limitations. The greatest area of concern regarding the RDAs is their failure to address the major nutrition-related problems of our time—chronic disease.[20,21] For example, there are no RDAs for carbohydrate, dietary fiber, fats, and cholesterol. This concern was at the heart of the National Research Council's decision to withhold release until 1989 of the 10th edition of *Recommended Dietary Allowances*. It originally had been scheduled for release in 1985. Committee members who prepared the report felt there were insufficient data on which to base nutrient recommendations for chronic disease prevention.[13] Those responsible for the report's release felt is should address diet and chronic disease-relationships and that the RDAs should be consistent with the recommended dietary guidelines for the maintenance of good health.[22]

TABLE 2-7 Predicted proportion of a population of adult males with protein intakes below their individual requirements: an application of the probability approach*

Protein intake interval (g/day)	Percentage of total population with observed protein intake in that interval	Probability of inadequacy	Estimated percentage of total population with inadequate intake†
<24	0.4	1.0	0.4
24–28	0.1	0.995	0.1
28–32	0.2	0.97	0.19
32–36	0.2	0.90	0.18
36–40	0.5	0.74	0.37
40–44	0.9	0.5	0.45
44–48	1.1	0.26	0.29
48–52	1.3	0.10	0.13
52–56	1.8	0.03	0.05
56–60	3.5	0.005	0.02
>60	91.0‡	0	0
			Total 2.29§

From National Research Council. 1986. *Nutrient adequacy: Assessment using food consumption surveys*. Washington, DC: National Academy Press.

*Based on 1977–78 *Nationwide Food Consumption Survey* data.

†Obtained by multiplying probability of inadequacy by the percentage of population in each intake interval.

‡Percentages do not add to 100 due to rounding.

§Prevalence of inadequate protein intake in this population of adult males, which is obtained by adding the percentage for each interval.

TABLE 2-8 Comparison of estimates of the prevalence of inadequate nutrient intakes for adults using the probability and fixed cutoff approaches*

Nutrient and sex group	Prevalence estimates (%) by approach method				
		Fixed cutoff approach			
	Probability approach	100% RDA†	80% RDA	70% RDA	60% RDA
Protein (males)	2.3	6.5	2.4	1.3	0.8
Vitamin C (males)	39.6	57.5	44.5	36.3	27.1
Iron (females)	23.0	98.2	91.2	81.6	62.5

From National Research Council. 1986. *Nutrient adequacy: Assessment using food consumption surveys*. Washington, DC: National Academy Press.

*Based on data from the 1977–78 *Nationwide Food Consumption Survey*.

†Recommended Dietary Allowance.

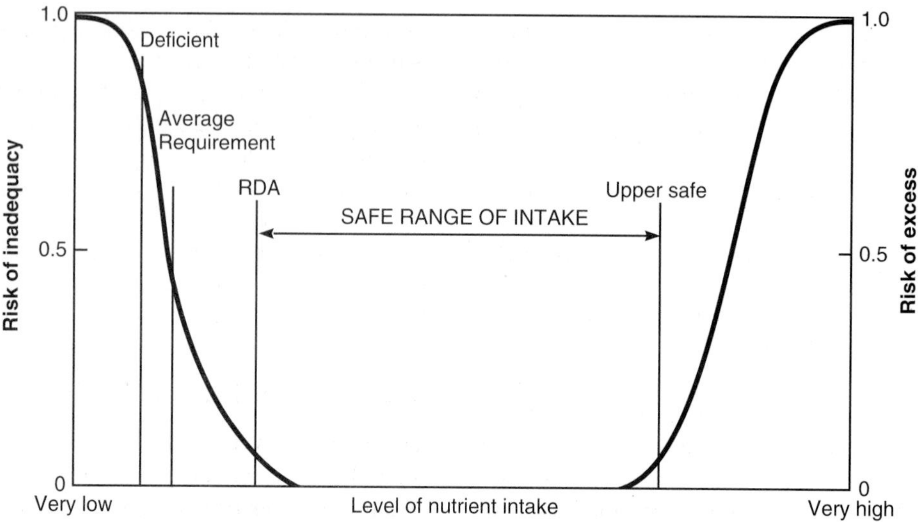

Figure 2-5 The risk of inadequate or excess intake varies according to the level of nutrient intake. When nutrient intake is very low, the probability of inadequate intake is high. When nutrient intake is very high, the probability of excessive intake is high. Between the RDA and an upper safe intake level is the safe range of intake that is associated with a very low probability of either inadequate or excessive nutrient intake. Adapted from Health and Welfare, Canada. 1983. *Recommended nutrient intakes for Canadians.* Ottawa: Canadian Publishing Centre.

Other concerns about the RDAs include the lack of specific nutrient recommendations for older persons, the tendency for people to use them for evaluating the diets of individuals (for which they were not intended), the need for more documentation explaining how specific nutrient recommendations are derived, whether recommendations should be expressed as single numbers or as a range, and whether recommended nutrient intake levels should be limited to amounts obtainable through diet alone.[21,23,24]

In response to these concerns, the Food and Nutrition Board has proposed sweeping changes in future editions of the RDAs.[23,24] The relationships between diet and chronic disease will be considered, as will pertinent interactions between nutrients. There will be recommendations for essential nutrients and important food components such as carbohydrate, dietary fiber, fats, specific fatty acids, dietary fiber, and β-carotene. Future reports will give more detail about how the recommendations were derived and provide more guidance in using the values for public policy and other uses. Through the use of various publications and symposia held at professional meetings, the Food and Nutrition Board will involve a greater number of nutritional scientists and professionals in developing the RDAs.

Rather than making a single nutrient intake recommendation for each age/sex group, as many as four levels of intake might be identified: deficient, average requirement, Recommended Dietary Allowance, and upper safe.[23,24] These are illustrated in Figure 2-5. This figure shows how the intake of nutrients is distributed in a population and how various levels of intake relate to risk of nutrient deficiency or excess. When intake of a nutrient or food component is very low, there is increased risk of deficiency. When intake is very high, there is increased risk of nutrient excess and probable toxicity. The vertical line labeled "deficient" is the nutrient intake level below which almost all healthy people could be expected, over time, to experience deficiency symptoms. The vertical line labeled "average requirement" is the amount of a nutrient or food component necessary to maintain desired biochemical and physiological function in 50% of people composing a certain age/sex group. The "RDA" is the amount necessary to meet the known nutritional needs of practically all healthy people in a particular age/sex group. "Upper safe" is the level of intake that is apparently safe for most healthy people in a particular group, but above which there is risk, over time, of experiencing toxic symptoms.

Another major departure from the past is the proposal that three separate reports related to the RDAs be published.[23,24] The first publication would discuss the essential nutrients and important food components relative to the above four proposed reference points. It would also address the role of nutrients and food components in reducing chronic disease risk as well as noteworthy interactions between nutrients. The second publication would describe the appropriate use of the RDAs for the various purposes they were intended. The third, targeted to the public, would explain the principles and scientific evidence underlying the RDAs and how they can be used in planning meals for persons of various sexes, ages, and ethnic dietary preferences.

NUTRIENT DENSITY

In the nutrient density approach, recommended nutrient intakes and nutritional composition of foods are expressed in terms of *nutrient quantity per 1000 kcal*. The basic concept of nutrient density is that if the quantity of nutrients per 1000 kcal is great enough, the nutrient needs of a person will be met when his or her energy needs are met.

In recent years there has been renewed interest in using the nutrient density concept as a criterion of the nutritional quality of diets.[25–28] Nutrient density addresses the issues of overconsumption and the relationships between diet and disease and allows the nutritional qualities of foods and diets to be evaluated and compared easily, quickly, and independently of serving size.

The nutritional value of foods also can be evaluated with respect to their caloric content. This is of particular importance to people consuming low-calorie diets. To achieve nutritional adequacy on a 1000-kcal to 1200-kcal reducing diet (which is roughly half the recommended calorie level for adults), most foods consumed should have a nutrient density approximately double the per 1000-kcal allowance. In other words, the foods selected should be both high in nutrients and low in calories to provide an adequate nutrient intake on a low-calorie diet. Nutrient density is a relatively simple approach to insuring nutritional adequacy for those on low-calorie diets.

Index of Nutritional Quality

The **index of nutritional quality (INQ)** is a concept related to nutrient density that allows the quantity of a nutrient per 1000 kcal in a food, meal, or diet to be compared with a nutrient standard. The first step in determining the INQ of a food or meal is to calculate a single-value nutrient recommendation for each nutrient from the RDAs or a similar recommended nutrient intake standard. Unlike the RDAs, which recommend nutrient intakes for *18 specific groups* of females and males of different ages and physiological conditions, the INQ generally uses only one recommendation for each nutrient for all people. The method used by scientists at Utah State University, who developed the INQ approach, is to divide the RDAs for each age/sex group by the average kilocalorie recommendation for the group and then multiply by 1000.[25,26] Table 2-9 shows nutrient recommendations per 1000 kcal for persons age 1 year and older derived from the 1989 revision of the RDAs. Several of the nutrient recommendations per 1000 kcal are constant or nearly so, and determining a single-value recommendation for these is simple. For nutrients whose per 1000-kcal values are not constant, the single-value recommendations approximate the recommendations for persons whose nutrient-to-calorie needs are the greatest. These are usually for persons having the lowest calorie needs (that is, persons in the 51+ year age group).[25] The bottom row of values in Table 2–9 gives the single-value recommendations selected by the authors using the method suggested by R.G. Hansen and others at Utah State University.[25,27]

TABLE 2-9 Nutrient allowances per 1000 kcal derived from the 1989 revision of the Recommended Dietary Allowances (Food and Nutrition Board)*†

Age and sex group	Energy (kcal)	Protein (g)	Fat-soluble vitamins				Water-soluble vitamins						
			Vitamin A (μg RE)	Vitamin D (μg)	Vitamin E (mg α-TE)	Vitamin K (μg)	Vitamin C (mg)	Thiamin (mg)	Riboflavin (mg)	Niacin (mg NE)	Vitamin B_6 (mg)	Folate (μg)	Vitamin B_{12} (μg)
Children													
1–3 yr	1300	12	307	8	5	12	31	0.5	0.6	7	0.8	38	0.5
4–6 yr	1800	13	278	8	4	11	25	0.5	0.6	7	0.6	42	0.6
7–10 yr	2000	14	350	5	4	15	24	0.5	0.6	7	0.7	50	0.7
Males													
11–14 yr	2500	18	400	4	4	18	20	0.5	0.6	7	0.7	60	0.8
15–18 yr	3000	20	333	3	3	22	20	0.5	0.6	7	0.7	67	0.7
19–24 yr	2900	20	345	3	3	24	21	0.5	0.6	7	0.7	69	0.7
25–50 yr	2900	22	345	2	3	28	21	0.5	0.6	7	0.7	69	0.7
51+ yr	2300	27	435	2	3	28	26	0.5	0.6	7	0.9	87	0.9
Females													
11–14 yr	2200	21	364	5	4	20	23	0.5	0.6	7	0.6	68	0.9
15–18 yr	2200	20	364	5	4	25	27	0.5	0.6	7	0.7	81	0.9
19–24 yr	2200	21	364	5	4	27	27	0.5	0.6	7	0.7	81	0.9
25–50 yr	2200	23	364	2	4	30	27	0.5	0.6	7	0.7	81	0.9
51+ yr	1900	26	421	3	4	34	32	0.5	0.6	7	0.8	95	1.1
Single value‡		27	430	5	4	30	30	0.5	0.6	7	0.8	90	1.0

*Nutrient values calculated by dividing the Recommended Dietary Allowances for each age/sex group by the average calorie allowance for the group and then multiplying by 1000.

†RE = retinol equivalents; α-TE = alpha-tocopherol equivalents; NE = niacin equivalents.

‡Single-value allowances are arrived at by either selecting those values that are constant (e.g., thiamin, riboflavin, and niacin) or approximating the allowances for persons having the greatest nutrient-to-calorie needs.

TABLE 2-9 Nutrient allowances per 1000 kcal derived from the 1989 revision of the Recommended Dietary Allowances (Food and Nutrition Board)*†—cont'd

	Minerals						
	Calcium (mg)	Phosphorus (mg)	Magnesium (mg)	Iron (mg)	Zinc (mg)	Iodine (µg)	Selenium (µg)
Children							
1–3 yr	615	615	62	8	8	54	15
4–6 yr	444	444	67	6	6	50	11
7–10 yr	400	400	85	5	5	60	15
Males							
11–14 yr	480	480	108	5	6	60	16
15–18 yr	400	400	133	4	5	50	17
19–24 yr	414	414	121	3	5	52	24
25–50 yr	276	276	121	3	5	52	24
51+ yr	348	348	152	4	7	65	30
Females							
11–14 yr	545	545	127	7	5	68	20
15–18 yr	545	545	136	7	5	68	23
19–24 yr	545	545	127	7	5	68	25
25–50 yr	364	364	127	7	5	68	25
51+ yr	421	421	147	5	6	79	29
Single value†	540	540	150	7	7	75	30

TABLE 2-10 Single-value nutrient density recommendations per 1000 kcal for Americans age 1 year and older*

Nutrient	Amount†
Vitamin A	430 μg RE
Vitamin D	5 μg
Vitamin E	4 mg α-TE
Vitamin K	30 μg
Vitamin C	30 mg
Thiamin	0.5 mg
Riboflavin	0.6 mg
Niacin	7 mg NE
Vitamin B_6	0.8 mg
Folate	90 μg
Vitamin B_{12}	1.0 μg
Calcium	540 mg
Phosphorus	540 mg
Magnesium	150 mg
Iron	7 mg
Zinc	7 mg
Iodine	75 μg
Selenium	30 μg
Protein	27 g
Carbohydrate (55% of kcal)	138 g
Total fat (30% of kcal)	33 g
Saturated fat (10% of kcal)	11 g
Polyunsaturated fat (10% of kcal)	11 g
Monounsaturated fat (10% of kcal)	11 g
Cholesterol (100 mg/1000 kcal)	100 mg
Dietary fiber	10 g
Sodium	1000 mg

*Recommendations were derived from the 1989 revision of the *Recommended Dietary Allowances* and "prudent diet" recommendations.

†RE = retinol equivalents; α-TE = alpha-tocopherol equivalents;
NE = niacin equivalents.

Table 2-10 shows these single values with the addition of several others (fat, cholesterol, and so on) that are not addressed by the RDAs.

The INQ of a food then is calculated using the following formula:[29]

$$\text{INQ} = \frac{\text{Amount of nutrient in 1000 kcal of food}}{\text{Allowance of nutrient per 1000 kcal of food}}$$

To calculate the INQ of nonfat or whole milk, for example, determine the amount of nutrients per 1000 kcal in milk from a food composition table or computerized nutritional software (see Chapter 5). Then divide the per 1000-kcal nutrient values by the single-value allowance for each nutrient.

Evaluating Nutrient Content

Figure 2-6 illustrates how the INQ simplifies the evaluation of the nutrient content of foods and allows easy comparison of two or more foods. It compares the INQ of whole milk with that of nonfat milk. When a horizontal bar extends to the right of the vertical line labeled "1," a 1000-kcal amount of the food supplies more than the single-value recommendation for that nutrient as given in Table 2-10. When the horizontal bar reaches the numbers "2" or "3," a 1000-kcal amount of the food supplies two or three times the single-value recommendation, respectively, for that nutrient. For most nutrients, this is desirable. However, in the case of fat (especially saturated fat), cholesterol, and sodium, a relatively low INQ is preferable. Because of the association between consumption of these food components and risk of certain diseases, it is best that they be eaten in relatively low amounts.

Irrespective of the quantity consumed, it is apparent from the figure that on an equal kilocalorie basis, nonfat milk provides significantly less cholesterol and fat and more protein and the vitamins and minerals shown than whole milk. The ease by which the INQ can convey the nutritional content of food is obvious.

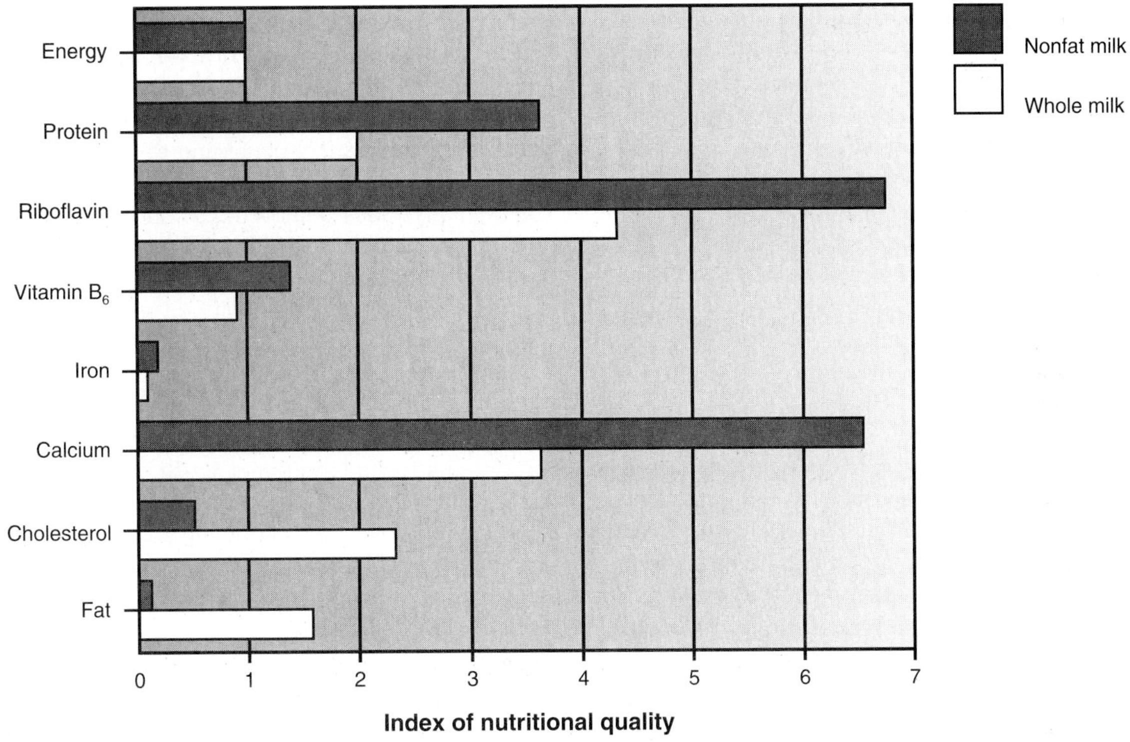

Figure 2-6 Index of nutritional quality of whole milk compared with that of nonfat milk.

A food with an overall INQ substantially greater than "1" is generally considered to be of good quality. It provides important nutrients in excess of calories. On the contrary, a food supplying calories in excess of nutrients would have an INQ less than "1," and a person would have to consume excessive calories to meet his or her recommended intake of nutrients. It is clear that nonfat milk, on a per 1000-kcal basis, is a much better source of nutrients than whole milk. This is mainly because fat (and other components such as sugar) *dilutes* the nutrient density of food.[27] On a *volume* basis, both foods contain approximately the same amount of calcium, riboflavin, and protein. The extra kilocalories from fat in whole milk, however, significantly reduce its contribution of calcium, riboflavin, and protein on a *per 1000-kcal* basis.

Weaknesses of the Index of Nutritional Quality

The INQ has its weaknesses. Defining the criterion for determining the single-value nutrient recommendation is a major issue of the approach. Dividing an average nutrient requirement plus two standard deviations (the RDA, which is sufficient for almost all group members) by an average energy requirement (sufficient for half of the group) is considered by some scientists as convenient but tenuous and lacking a good scientific basis.

Another criticism stems from the fact that nutrient requirements per 1000 kcal of energy expended will be higher in sedentary persons compared with physically active persons. Note that the recommendations for several nutrients in

Table 2-9 are highest for males and females in the 51+ year age group. This is because as people age, their energy requirements tend to decrease while their nutrient requirements, in most instances, remain about the same as younger adults. Some scientists object to arbitrarily setting single-value recommendations at an artificially high level to accommodate the needs of persons with a low energy requirement. "Why," they ask, "should the recommendations be so high when the nutrient requirements of more physically active persons can be met with a much lower nutrient quantity per 1000 kcal?"

Expecting a single-value nutrient recommendation to be appropriate for all persons age 1 year and older is an oversimplification. More than one single-value nutrient recommendation may be necessary—perhaps one for children, one for adolescents and adults, and yet another for pregnant and lactating females. When using nutrient density or INQ in meal planning or evaluating nutrient intake, individual activity levels and energy requirements also should be considered.

Despite its weaknesses, the INQ and nutrient density approach have definite advantages, making them useful tools for meal planning by nutrition professionals, as well as for nutrition education, evaluation of nutrient intake, and food labeling.

DIET QUALITY INDEX

The Diet Quality Index is an approach developed to measure overall diet quality and assess risk for chronic diseases related to overall dietary pattern.[30] It compares a person's or group's diet with selected dietary recommendations from the National Academy of Sciences publication *Diet and Health: Implications for Reducing Chronic Disease Risk* (see Box 2-6).[31] Table 2-11 shows the approach used by the Diet Quality Index for scoring diets. The diet is scored on the basis of the eight recommendations. A low score is preferred over a high score. If a person's diet derives ≤30% of energy from total fat, a score of 0 is assigned. If total fat supplies 31% to 40% or more than 40% of energy, that person's score is 1 or 2, respectively.

The first dietary recommendation shown on Box 2-6 (relating to intake of total fat, saturated fat, and cholesterol) was used to create the first three scoring criteria in Table 2-11. The recommendation in Box 2-6 pertaining to alcohol was not used in scoring because those developing the Diet Quality Index considered alcohol abuse and alcoholism as psychoactive substance abuse and not as dietary indiscretions. Fluoride and dietary supplement use were not included as scoring criteria because they "were not judged to be sufficiently important for the prevention of chronic disease to be included in the index."[30] Rather than basing judgments about diet on the intake of one or two individual nutrients or dietary components, the Diet Quality Index uses a number of nutrients and dietary components that have been identified as important factors in influencing risk of chronic disease.

DIETARY GUIDELINES

Dietary guidelines or goals can be defined as statements from authoritative scientific bodies translating nutritional recommendations into practical advice to consumers about their eating habits.[32] Rather than merely insuring adequate nutrient intake, *they are primarily intended to address the more common and pressing nutrition-related health problems such as heart disease, certain cancers, stroke, hypertension, and diabetes.* They often are expressed as nonquantitative changes from the present average national diet or from people's typical eating habits. Examples of guidelines are: "choose a diet low in fat, saturated fat, and cholesterol" and "choose a diet with plenty of vegetables, fruits, and grain products." Table 2-12 contrasts the RDAs and dietary guidelines.

Early Dietary Guidelines

Dietary guidelines have existed since time immemorial in the form of cultural practices, taboos, and religious teachings.[32] The first formal set of dietary guidelines of modern times, however, was published in Sweden in 1968.[33] There were a

TABLE 2-11 Diet Quality Index diet scoring guidelines

Recommendation	Intake	Score
Reduce total fat intake to 30% or less of energy	≤30%	0
	31%–40%	1
	>40%	2
Reduce saturated fatty acid intake to less than 10% of energy	<10%	0
	10%–13%	1
	>13%	2
Reduce cholesterol to less than 300 mg daily	<300 mg	0
	300–400 mg	1
	>400	2
Eat five or more servings daily of a combination of vegetables and fruits	5+ servings	0
	3–4 servings	1
	0–2 servings	2
Increase intake of starches and other complex carbohydrates by eating six or more servings daily of breads, cereals, and legumes	6+ servings	0
	4–5 servings	1
	0–3 servings	2
Maintain protein intake at moderate levels (levels lower than twice the Recommended Dietary Allowance [RDA])	≤100% RDA	0
	101%–150% RDA	1
	>150% RDA	2
Limit total daily intake of salt to 6 g (equivalent to 2400 mg of sodium)	≤2400 mg sodium	0
	2401–3400 mg sodium	1
	>3400 mg sodium	2
Maintain adequate calcium intake (approximately RDA levels)	≥100% RDA	0
	67%–99% RDA	1
	<67% RDA	2

Adapted from Patterson RE, Hainses PS, Popkin BM. 1994. Diet Quality Index: Capturing a multidimensional behavior. *Journal of the American Dietetic Association* 94:57–64 and Food and Nutrition Board, National Research Council. 1989. *Diet and health: Implications for reducing chronic disease risk.* Washington, DC: National Academy Press.

number of reasons for the guidelines.[10,33] Dietary surveys showed that the proportion of calories from fat in the Swedish diet had increased from an average of about 19% at the end of the nineteenth century to 42% by the mid-1960s. There was concern over the high intakes of saturated fat, calories, and refined sugars and low intakes of fruits, vegetables, cereal products, lean meats, and nonfat dairy products. Swedish health authorities were concerned about the association between such dietary practices and obesity, coronary heart disease, hypertension, stroke, and tooth decay.

The Swedish guidelines called for a reduced energy intake (when appropriate) to prevent overweight; decreased consumption of total fat, saturated fat, sugar, and sugar-containing products; increased consumption of vegetables, fruits, potatoes, nonfat milk, fish, lean meat, and cereal products; and regular physical activity, especially for those with sedentary occupations.[33]

These dietary trends were recognized in other Western nations such as Australia, New Zealand, the Netherlands, the United Kingdom, Germany, and Canada, which, in the early 1970s, issued dietary guidelines of their own.[10]

TABLE 2-12 The Recommended Dietary Allowances (RDAs) and dietary guidelines contrasted

The RDAs	Dietary guidelines
Developed earlier	Developed more recently
Expressed in quantitative terms as weight of nutrient per day	Often expressed as nonquantitative change from present average national diet
Intended to insure adequate nutrient intakes	Intended to help reduce risk of developing chronic degenerative disease
Needed now and every day	Can be target to aim for at some future time
More firmly established scientifically	More provisional, based more on indirect evidence
More concerned with micronutrients	Primarily deal with macronutrients
Specific for groups based on sex, age, and physiologic condition	Generally the same advice for everybody
Expressed in technical language	Expressed in less technical language and better understood by the public

From Truswell AS. 1987. Evolution of dietary recommendations, goals, and guidelines, *American Journal of Clinical Nutrition* 45:1060–1072.

During this time, a similar situation existed in the United States. Scientists were concerned about trends in the eating habits of Americans. Data from the USDA showed that the distribution of calories from carbohydrate and fat had changed significantly between 1909 and the 1970s. Based on the *disappearance* of food from the marketplace (see Chapter 4), the department concluded that the percentage of calories provided by fats had increased from 32% to about 43% while calories provided by carbohydrate had declined from 57% to 46%. The percent of calories from fats obtained from meat and dairy products had risen sharply while carbohydrate from fruits, vegetables, and grains had fallen precipitously.[30,33] At the same time, there was increasingly convincing evidence linking dietary habits to the major causes of death in America: heart disease, cancer, and stroke. Although scientists recognized that heredity, age, and numerous environmental factors besides diet were involved in the causation of these diseases, diet was one factor over which people had a certain amount of control. This led private agencies such as the American Medical Association, the American Heart Association, and the American Health Foundation to publish dietary guidelines.

U.S. Dietary Goals

In February 1977, the report ***Dietary Goals for the United States*** was issued by the U.S. Senate Select Committee on Nutrition and Human Needs.[34] This was the first of several government reports setting prudent dietary guidelines for Americans.

In its introduction, the Senate Select Committee made this statement:

> The overconsumption of foods high in fat, generally, and saturated fat in particular, as well as cholesterol, refined and processed sugars, salt and/or alcohol has been associated with the development of one or more of six to ten leading causes of death: heart disease, some cancers, stroke and hypertension, diabetes, arteriosclerosis and cirrhosis of the liver.[34]

The committee then submitted seven goals, listed in Box 2-1.

The Dietary Goals were to be accomplished through the changes in food selection and preparation listed in Box 2-2.

BOX 2-1

1977 Dietary Goals

1. To avoid overweight, consume only as much energy (calories) as is expended; if overweight, decrease energy intake and increase energy expenditure.
2. Increase the consumption of complex carbohydrates and "naturally occurring" sugars from about 28% of energy intake to about 48% of energy intake.
3. Reduce the consumption of refined and processed sugars by about 45% to account for about 10% of total energy intake.
4. Reduce overall fat consumption from approximately 40% to about 30% of energy intake.
5. Reduce saturated fat consumption to account for about 10% of total energy intake and balance that with polyunsaturated and monounsaturated fats, which should account for about 10% of energy intake each.
6. Reduce cholesterol consumption to about 300 milligrams per day.
7. Limit the intake of sodium by reducing the intake of salt to about 5 grams a day.

From Select Committee on Nutrition and Human Needs. 1977. *Dietary goals for the United States,* U.S. Senate.

BOX 2-2

Recommendations from Dietary Goals for the United States

1. Increase consumption of fruits, vegetables, and whole grains.
2. Decrease consumption of refined and other processed sugars and foods high in such sugars.
3. Decrease consumption of foods high in total fat and partially replace saturated fats, whether obtained from animal or vegetable sources, with polyunsaturated fats.
4. Decrease consumption of animal fat and choose meats, poultry, and fish, which will reduce saturated fat intake.
5. Except for young children, substitute low-fat and nonfat milk for whole milk, and low-fat dairy products for high-fat dairy products.
6. Decrease consumption of butterfat, eggs, and other high cholesterol sources. Some consideration should be given to easing the cholesterol goal for premenopausal women, young children, and the elderly to obtain the nutritional benefit of eggs in the diet.
7. Decrease consumption of salt and foods high in salt content.

From Select Committee on Nutrition and Human Needs. 1977. *Dietary goals for the United States,* U.S. Senate.

The reaction to *Dietary Goals for the United States* from U.S. nutrition scientists and professionals was swift, strong, and polarized.[10] *Nutrition Today* published opinions about the goals from some leading nutrition scientists and professionals.[35,36] Some felt the goals were "hastily conceived and based on fragmentary evidence," "premature . . . because the diet has not yet been tested," "blatant sensationalism," "speculation," and "a nutritional debacle." One professional declared that the "Senate Select Committee has perpetrated a hoax." Other scientists believed the goals were "long overdue," "a giant step forward in improving the health of our citizens," "a valid criticism of our current diet," "a significant achievement," and deserving "the broadest support from all who are concerned with the health and well-being of American citizens." Who was right? Time would tell.

It was immediately clear, however, that to meet the goals, Americans would need to change the way they ate. Figure 2-7 compares the 1977 U.S. Dietary Goals with the diet of that time and highlights the necessary changes.

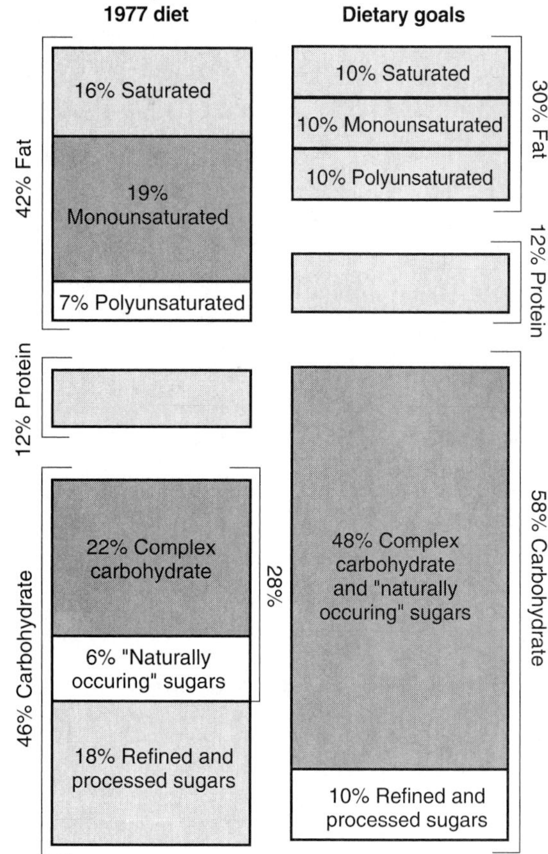

Figure 2-7 The 1977 U.S. Dietary Goals (right) compared with the American diet of that time.

Dietary Guidelines for Americans

In 1980 the U.S. Departments of Agriculture and Health and Human Services jointly issued *Nutrition and Your Health: Dietary Guidelines for Americans.*[37] The Dietary Guidelines appear to have been a modification and reissue of the earlier Dietary Goals. They contained all the essential elements of the earlier Dietary Goals—fewer animal products, more plant products, and less sugar, salt, and fat. They also were less forceful than the Dietary Goals, more brief, and nonquantitative.[10] For example, the three goals regarding overall fat consumption, saturated/polyunsaturated/monounsaturated fats, and cholesterol were combined into the guideline "avoid too much fat, saturated fat, and cholesterol," and a guideline regarding alcohol consumption was added. The Dietary Guidelines were revised in 1985 (guideline 2 was changed from "maintain ideal weight" to "maintain desirable weight") and again in 1990 and 1995.[38,39] The 1990 edition of *Dietary Guidelines for Americans* is shown in Figure 2-8, and the 1995 guidelines are listed in Box 2-3. The basic concepts of the second edition of the *Dietary Guidelines for Americans* were retained in the 1990 and 1995 editions but were presented in a more positive way. More extensive food selection guidance also was included.[40] Updates of the *Dietary Guidelines for Americans* are planned approximately every 5 years.

The Dietary Guidelines are for healthy Americans. According to the second edition of the report, "They do not apply to people who need special diets because of diseases or conditions that interfere with normal nutritional requirements. These people may need special instruction from registered dietitians, in consultation with their own physicians."[38]

Toward Healthful Diets

Toward Healthful Diets was a brief report released in 1980 by the Food and Nutrition Board of the National Research Council. It gave dietary recommendations that the Food and Nutrition Board believed would "improve general nutritional status, be beneficial in preventing or delaying the onset of some chronic degenerative diseases, and incur no appreciable risks."[41] The

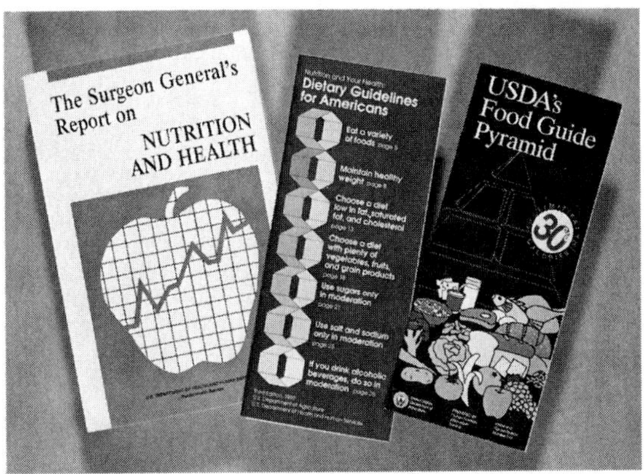

Figure 2-8 *The U.S. Surgeon General's Report on Nutrition and Health* serves as an authoritative source of information on which nutrition policy decisions have been based. The third edition of the *Dietary Guidelines for Americans* and the *USDA's Food Guide Pyramid* represent the U.S. federal government's official advice on how to achieve a healthy diet.

BOX 2-3

The 1995 Dietary Guidelines for Americans

- Eat a variety of foods.
- Balance the food you eat with physical activity; maintain or improve your weight.
- Choose a diet with plenty of grain products, vegetables, and fruits.
- Choose a diet low in fat, saturated fat, and cholesterol.
- Choose a diet moderate in sugars.
- Choose a diet moderate in salt and sodium.
- If you drink alcoholic beverages, do so in moderation.

From *Nutrition and your health: Dietary guidelines for Americans,* 4th ed., U.S. Department of Agriculture and U.S. Department of Health and Human Services, 1995.

recommendations were more conservative than either the Dietary Goals or Dietary Guidelines, except on the matter of salt.

The report appears to have been a response to concerns about the scientific soundness of the many, and sometimes confusing, dietary recommendations extant during the 1970s.[10,41] In the report's introduction, the Food and Nutrition Board stated its concern about

> the flood of dietary recommendations currently being made to the American public in the hope that a variety of chronic degenerative diseases may be prevented in some persons. These recommendations . . . often lack a sound scientific foundation, and some are contradictory to one another. In an effort to reduce the confusion in the mind of the public that has resulted from these many conflicting recommendations, the Board has prepared the following statement[41]

The report gave five recommendations (Box 2-4), which were targeted to adults.

The Surgeon General's Report on Nutrition and Health

In 1988, *The Surgeon General's Report on Nutrition and Health* (Figure 2-8) was issued.[42] This was a landmark publication summarizing the scientific evidence linking specific dietary factors to health maintenance and disease prevention and presenting recommendations for dietary change to improve the health of the American people.[43] The report recognized that what we eat can affect our risk for several of the leading causes of death and identified, as of primary importance, the need to reduce consumption of fat, especially saturated fat. It served as an authoritative source of information on which to base nutrition policy decisions and distinguished recommendations appropriate for the general public from those for special populations.[44] The report's recommendations are given in Box 2-5.

Diet and Health

In 1989, the book *Diet and Health: Implications for Reducing Chronic Disease Risk* was published by the Committee on Diet and Health of the National Research Council.[31] It represented the view that dietary recommendations should go beyond the prevention of nutrient deficiencies to the prevention of chronic disease. From their extensive

BOX 2-4

Recommendations of *Toward Healthful Diets*

1. Select a nutritionally adequate diet from the foods available by consuming appropriate daily servings of dairy products, meats or legumes, vegetables and fruits, and cereal and breads.
2. Select as wide a variety of foods in each of the major food groups as is practicable to ensure a high probability of consuming adequate quantities of all essential nutrients.
3. Adjust dietary energy intake and energy expenditure so as to maintain appropriate weight for height; if overweight, achieve appropriate weight reduction by decreasing total food and fat intake and by increasing physical activity.
4. If the requirement for energy is low (e.g., reducing diet), reduce consumption of foods such as alcohol, sugars, fats, and oils, which provide calories but few other essential nutrients.
5. Use salt in moderation; adequate but safe intakes are considered to range between 3 and 8 g of sodium chloride daily.

From Food and Nutrition Board, National Research Council. 1980. *Toward healthful diets*. Washington, DC: National Academy Press.

review of the scientific literature, the committee members concluded that in addition to genetic and environmental factors, "dietary patterns are important factors in the **etiology** of several major chronic diseases and that dietary modifications can reduce such risks." The influence of diet is "very strong" for coronary heart disease and hypertension and "highly suggestive" for certain cancers (esophagus, stomach, large bowel, breast, lung, and prostate). The committee stated that dietary habits also play a role in dental caries, chronic liver disease, and obesity, which increases the risk of **noninsulin-dependent diabetes mellitus (NIDDM)**. Of particular concern was the need for Americans to reduce consumption of fats, saturated fats, and cholesterol and increase intake of fruits, vegetables, legumes, and whole-grain cereals. The committee's dietary recommendations are summarized in Box 2-6.

In 1991 the Food and Nutrition Board published *Improving America's Diet and Health*, which proposes detailed strategies and options for the implementation of the dietary guidelines presented in *Diet and Health*.[45] In 1992 the Food and Nutrition Board published *Eat for Life*, a book intended to help translate the dietary guidelines in *Diet and Health* into practical guidelines for individuals and families.[46]

Other Dietary Guidelines

Since the U.S. Dietary Goals were issued in 1977, numerous scientific organizations and professional groups have studied the impact of American dietary practices on health and disease and have issued their own dietary guidelines. Only those considered most important have been discussed here. Some of the more important ones are summarized in Table 2-13.

There is a great deal of agreement among the various guidelines despite the 18-year transition from the release of the Dietary Goals in 1977 to publication of the revised Dietary Guidelines in 1995. Most of the dietary guidelines published since 1977 have supported the original Dietary Goals. This is true despite their differing emphases—some focusing on general improvement of dietary habits, others stressing prevention of heart disease or cancer or the nutritional management of diabetes. The different guidelines definitely agree on limiting total fat and saturated fat intake, increasing consumption of complex

BOX 2-5

Recommendations of *The Surgeon General's Report on Nutrition and Health*

Issues for most people

- *Fats and cholesterol:* Reduce consumption of fat (especially saturated fat) and cholesterol. Choose foods relatively low in these substances, such as vegetables, fruits, whole grain foods, fish, poultry, lean meats, and low-fat dairy products. Use food preparation methods that add little or no fat.
- *Energy and weight control:* Achieve and maintain a desirable body weight. To do so, choose a dietary pattern in which energy (caloric) intake is consistent with energy expenditure. To reduce energy intake, limit consumption of foods relatively high in calories, fats, and sugars, and minimize alcohol consumption. Increase energy expenditure through regular and sustained physical activity.
- *Complex carbohydrates and fiber:* Increase consumption of whole grain foods and cereal products, vegetables (including dried beans and peas), and fruits.
- *Sodium:* Reduce intake of sodium by choosing foods relatively low in sodium and limiting the amount of salt added in food preparation and at the table.
- *Alcohol:* To reduce the risk for chronic disease, take alcohol only in moderation (no more than two drinks a day), if at all. Avoid drinking any alcohol before or while driving, operating machinery, taking medications, or engaging in any other activity requiring judgment. Avoid drinking alcohol while pregnant.

Other issues for some people

- *Fluoride:* Community water systems should contain fluoride at optimal levels for prevention of tooth decay. If such water is not available, use other appropriate sources of fluoride.
- *Sugars:* Those who are particularly vulnerable to dental caries (cavities), especially children, should limit their consumption and frequency of use of foods high in sugars.
- *Calcium:* Adolescent girls and adult women should increase consumption of foods high in calcium, including low-fat dairy products.
- *Iron:* Children, adolescents, and women of childbearing age should be sure to consume foods that are good sources of iron, such as lean meats, fish, certain beans, and iron-enriched cereals and whole grain products. This issue is of special concern for low-income families.

From *The Surgeon General's report on nutrition and health,* U.S. Department of Health and Human Services, 1988.

carbohydrates, maintaining healthy body weight, and using alcoholic beverages in moderation, if at all. General agreement exists on limiting the intake of cholesterol and salt and increasing consumption of fiber-rich foods.

Healthy People 2000

In 1990 the U.S. Department of Health and Human Services (DHHS) released *Healthy People 2000: National Health Promotion and Disease Prevention Objectives.*[47] The report outlined objectives to be met by the year 2000 for improving the health of Americans. This was the second DHHS report setting objectives for improving health. The first, *Promoting Health/Preventing Disease: Objectives for the Nation* was published in 1980 and set health objectives for the year 1990.[48]

The 300 objectives in 22 priority areas included in *Healthy People 2000* were the result of nearly

BOX 2-6

Summary of Dietary Recommendations from *Diet and Health: Implications for Reducing Chronic Disease Risk*

1. Reduce total fat intake to 30% or less of calories. Reduce saturated fatty acid intake to less than 10% of calories and the intake of cholesterol to less than 300 mg daily. The intake of fat and cholesterol can be reduced by substituting fish, poultry without skin, lean meats, and low-fat or nonfat dairy products for fatty meats and whole-milk dairy products; by choosing more vegetables, fruits, cereals, and legumes; and by limiting oils, fats, egg yolks, and fried and other fatty foods.
2. Eat five or more servings every day of a combination of vegetables and fruits, especially green and yellow vegetables and citrus fruits. Also, increase intake of starches and other complex carbohydrates by eating six or more daily servings of a combination of breads, cereals, and legumes. (An average serving is equal to a half cup for most fresh or cooked vegetables, fruits, dry or cooked cereals and legumes, one medium piece of fresh fruit, one slice of bread, or one roll or muffin.)
3. Maintain protein intake at moderate levels.
4. Balance food intake and physical activity to maintain appropriate body weight.
5. The committee does not recommend alcohol consumption. For those who drink alcoholic beverages, the committee recommends limiting consumption to the equivalent of less than 1 oz of pure alcohol in a single day. This is the equivalent of two cans of beer, two small glasses of wine, or two average cocktails. Pregnant women should avoid alcoholic beverages.
6. Limit total daily intake of salt (sodium chloride) to 6 g or less. Limit the use of salt in cooking and avoid adding it to food at the table. Salty, highly processed salty, salt-preserved, and salt-pickled foods should be consumed sparingly.
7. Maintain adequate calcium intake.
8. Avoid taking dietary supplements in excess of the Recommended Dietary Allowance in any one day.
9. Maintain an optimal intake of fluoride, particularly during the years of primary and secondary tooth formation and growth.

From National Research Council: Food and Nutrition Board. 1989. *Diet and health: Implications for reducing chronic disease risk*. Washington, DC: National Academy Press.

3 years of work involving hundreds of organizations and experts, public hearings, and public comment. Twenty-one of the objectives specifically deal with nutrition. These are briefly discussed in Chapter 1 and shown in Box 1-1.

In addition to setting specific goals, the document set three overarching goals for the 1990s: increase the span of healthy life that Americans live, eliminate disparities in health and health care delivery among different population groups, and achieve access to preventive services for all people. According to the DHHS, the objectives reflect important recent changes in thinking about the protection and enhancement of personal health. Three such changes, especially, form the basis for the objectives: increased personal responsibility for healthy behavior, the need to extend the benefits of good health to every citizen, and the desire to reduce the cost of preventable illness.

Although public health experts have criticized the report for lacking an implementation plan, overemphasizing individual responsibility, and being diluted in some areas, it sets important and specific standards for improving personal nutrition and health and for gauging the nation's progress toward health for all.

TABLE 2-13 Summary of major dietary recommendations for Americans*

Recommendation	U.S. Dietary Goals, 1977	Surgeon General's Report on Nutrition and Health, 1988	Diet and Health NRC, 1989	Diet, Nutrition and Cancer, NRC, 1982	ACS Guidelines on Diet, Nutrition, and Cancer, 1991	Dietary Guidelines for Americans, USDA/DHHS, 1990	Dietary Guidelines for Healthy Adult Americans, AHA, 1988	American Diabetes Association, 1994
Limit or reduce total fat (% of kcal)	27%–33%	Yes	≤30%	~30%	<30%	Yes	<30%	≤30%
Reduce saturated fatty acids (% of kcal)	Yes	Yes	<10%	Yes	NC	Yes	<10%	<10%
Increase polyunsaturated fatty acids (% of kcal)	Yes	No	≤10%	No	NC	No	≤10%	No
Limit cholesterol (mg/day)	250–350	Yes	<300	NC	NS	Yes	<300	<300
Limit simple sugars	Yes	Yes	Yes	NC	NC	Yes	NS	Individualized based on meal plan
Increase complex carbohydrate (% of kcal)	Yes	Yes	≥55%	Through whole grains, fruits, vegetables	Through whole grains, fruits, vegetables	Yes	≥50%	Individualized based on meal plan
Increase fiber	Yes	Yes	Yes	NS	Yes	Yes	NS	20–35 g/day
Restrict sodium chloride (g/day)	8 g/day	Yes	≤6 g/day	Limit salt-cured, pickled, smoked foods	Limit salt-cured, pickled, smoked foods	Yes	≤3 g/day of sodium	≤2400 mg sodium for people with mild to moderate hypertension
Moderate alcohol	Yes	Yes	Yes	Yes	Yes	Yes	Yes	Yes
Maintain appropriate weight/exercise	Yes	Yes	Balance energy intake and expenditure	NC	Yes	Yes	Yes	Yes
Other	Reduce additives and processed foods	Foods rich in calcium and iron, fluoridated water for some people	Drink fluoridated water, eat wide variety of plant foods, avoid supplements	Emphasize fruits and vegetables, avoid high doses of supplements	Emphasize a variety of fruits and vegetables in the daily diet	Variety in diet	High-risk persons should especially restrict fat and cholesterol	Chromium and magnesium supplements recommended only when medically indicated

Adapted from National Cholesterol Education Program. 1990. *Report of the Expert Panel on Population Strategies for Blood Cholesterol Reduction*. Bethesda, Md: U.S. Department of Health and Human Services; Public Health Service, National Institutes of Health. Work Study Group on Diet, Nutrition, and Cancer. 1991. American Cancer Society guidelines on diet, nutrition, and cancer. *Ca-A Cancer Journal for Clinicians* 41(6):334–338. American Diabetes Association. 1994. Nutrition recommendations for people with diabetes. *Diabetes Care* 17:519–522.

*NRC = National Research Council; ACS = American Cancer Society; AHA = American Heart Association, USDA = U.S. Department of Agriculture; DHHS = Department of Health and Human Services.

NC = No comment; NS = Not specified

NUTRITIONAL LABELING OF FOOD

Nutritional labeling of food in the United States began in 1973 when the U.S. Food and Drug Administration (FDA) established labeling regulations. These included creation of the U.S. Recommended Daily Allowances and institution of specific guidelines for food labeling.

U.S. Recommended Daily Allowances

In 1973, the FDA issued regulations requiring the nutritional labeling of any food containing one or more added nutrients or whose label or advertising included claims about the food's nutritional properties or its usefulness in the daily diet. Nutrition labeling was voluntary for almost all other foods. The *U.S. Recommended Daily Allowances* (*U.S. RDAs*) were nutrient standards developed by the FDA at that time for use in regulating the nutritional labeling of food. They replaced the Minimum Daily Requirement, which had been in use since 1940 for labeling vitamin and mineral supplements, breakfast cereals, and some special foods.

The U.S. RDAs (shown in Appendix C) included 19 nutrients and recommendations for four categories of people. Three sets of nutrient standards (those for infants, children under 4 years of age, and pregnant and lactating females) were used for labeling specialty foods and supplements marketed specifically to infants, children, and pregnant or lactating women. The fourth and most familiar set was for males and nonpregnant, nonlactating females 4 or more years of age; this was the standard seen on most food labels in the United States. It was developed by selecting the highest value for each nutrient given in the 1968 RDA table for males and nonpregnant, nonlactating females 4 or more years of age, except for calcium and phosphorus, which were set at the midpoint of the RDA values for males and females.

The Nutrition Labeling and Education Act

Between 1973 and 1993 there was growing awareness that the major nutritional problem facing North Americans was overconsumption of foods rich in total fat, saturated fat, and cholesterol and low in complex carbohydrates. There were also major breakthroughs in our knowledge of essential nutrient requirements (for example, the RDAs were revised three times). Despite these advances, the U.S. RDAs were not updated, and food labeling regulations remained virtually unchanged. During the same period, the public and various professional and consumer interest groups called for food labels that were easily understood and truthful and that reflected awareness of the relationship between diet and health. In 1990, the FDA's **Nutrition Labeling and Education Act** (NLEA) was passed, mandating nutrition labeling for almost all processed foods regulated by the FDA and authorizing appropriate health claims on the labels of such products. It brought about the most extensive food labeling reform in U.S. history. The NLEA also called for activities to educate consumers about nutrition information on the label and the importance of using that information in maintaining healthful dietary practices. The NLEA's final regulations were published in the January 6, 1993 *Federal Register*. August 8, 1994 was the final deadline for manufacturers to comply. The USDA's Food Safety and Inspection Service, responsible for the inspection of meat and poultry, has issued parallel regulations that will govern the labeling of meat and poultry.

The NLEA requires about 90% of processed foods to carry nutrition information on the label (Figure 2-9). Foods exempted from the regulations include plain coffee and tea, some spices and flavorings, and other foods having insignificant nutritional value; ready-to-eat food prepared primarily on-site such as deli and bakery items; foods in very small packages; restaurant food;

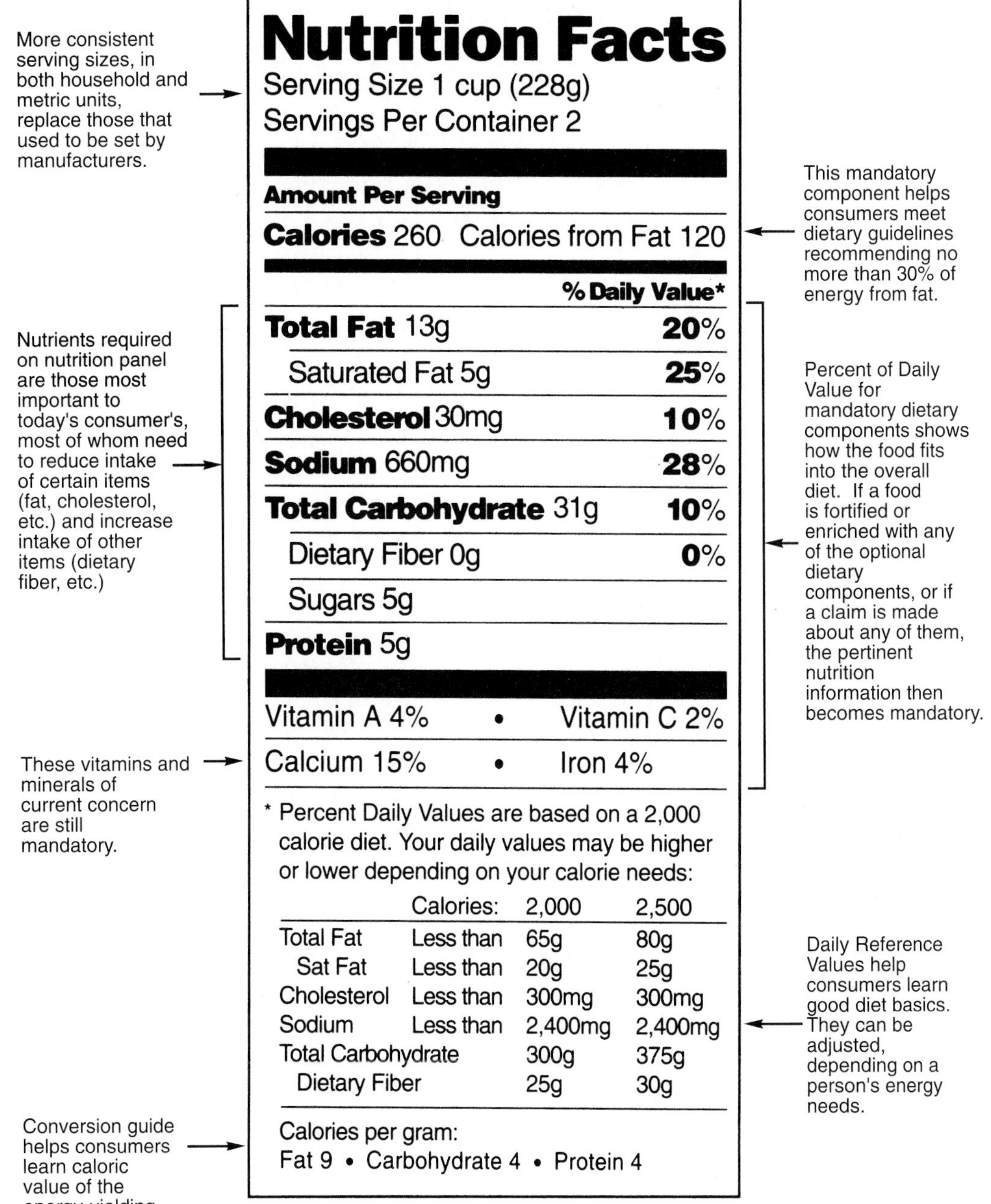

More consistent serving sizes, in both household and metric units, replace those that used to be set by manufacturers.
Nutrients required on nutrition panel are those most important to today's consumer's, most of whom need to reduce intake of certain items (fat, cholesterol, etc.) and increase intake of other items (dietary fiber, etc.)
These vitamins and minerals of current concern are still mandatory.
Conversion guide helps consumers learn caloric value of the energy-yielding nutrients.
This mandatory component helps consumers meet dietary guidelines recommending no more than 30% of energy from fat.
Percent of Daily Value for mandatory dietary components shows how the food fits into the overall diet. If a food is fortified or enriched with any of the optional dietary components, or if a claim is made about any of them, the pertinent nutrition information then becomes mandatory.
Daily Reference Values help consumers learn good diet basics. They can be adjusted, depending on a person's energy needs.
Nutrition Facts
Serving Size 1 cup (228g)
Servings Per Container 2
Amount Per Serving
Calories 260 Calories from Fat 120
% Daily Value*
Total Fat 13g 20%
Saturated Fat 5g 25%
Cholesterol 30mg 10%
Sodium 660mg 28%
Total Carbohydrate 31g 10%
Dietary Fiber 0g 0%
Sugars 5g
Protein 5g
Vitamin A 4% • Vitamin C 2%
Calcium 15% • Iron 4%
* Percent Daily Values are based on a 2,000 calorie diet. Your daily values may be higher or lower depending on your calorie needs:
Calories: 2,000 2,500
Total Fat Less than 65g 80g
Sat Fat Less than 20g 25g
Cholesterol Less than 300mg 300mg
Sodium Less than 2,400mg 2,400mg
Total Carbohydrate 300g 375g
Dietary Fiber 25g 30g
Calories per gram:
Fat 9 • Carbohydrate 4 • Protein 4

Figure 2-9 Key aspects of the Food and Drug Administration's Food Label Format.

BOX 2-7

Mandatory (in Italics) and Voluntary Nutrients and Dietary Components in the Order They Must Appear on Food Labels

- *total calories*
- *calories from fat*
- calories from saturated fat
- *total fat*
- *saturated fat*
- stearic acid (on meat and poultry products only)
- polyunsaturated fat
- monounsaturated fat
- *cholesterol*
- *sodium*
- potassium
- *total carbohydrate*
- *dietary fiber*
- soluble fiber
- insoluble fiber
- *sugars*
- sugar alcohols
- other carbohydrates
- *protein*
- *vitamin A*
- *vitamin C*
- *calcium*
- *iron*
- other essential vitamins and minerals

bulk food that is not resold; and foods produced by businesses with food sales of less than $50,000 per year or total sales less than $500,000 per year unless the food item contains a nutrition claim. Nutrition labeling is voluntary for most raw foods. The 20 most frequently eaten raw fruits, vegetables, and fish are included in the FDA's voluntary point-of-purchase nutrition information program. The 45 major cuts of meat and poultry are covered under the USDA's voluntary point-of-purchase program.

The nutrients and food components required on the label were selected because of their relationship to current health concerns, and the order in which they are listed reflects their public health significance. Box 2-7 shows the mandatory and voluntary nutrients and dietary components in the order they must appear on food labels. The mandatory nutrients and dietary components are required on all food labels. Listing of the voluntary ones is optional. If a food is fortified or enriched with any of the voluntary nutrients or dietary components, or if a health or nutrient content claim is made about any of them, the pertinent nutrition information then becomes mandatory. Total calories, total fat, total carbohydrate, protein, sodium, vitamins A and C, calcium, and iron were carryovers from the previous label. Saturated fat, cholesterol, sugars, dietary fiber, and calories from fat were added by the new regulations. Niacin, thiamin, and riboflavin are now voluntary nutrients.

Serving sizes listed on the label are specified by the FDA, are uniform across all product lines so consumers can more easily compare brands, and are closer to the amounts people actually eat. Using data from USDA food consumption surveys, the FDA determined the amounts of various foods that people customarily consume per eating occasion. These are called **reference amounts** and are expressed in metric units. The serving size listed on food labels is the amount in common household measures closest to the reference amount. It is important to note that serving sizes as defined by the FDA do not always agree with the serving sizes recommended in such dietary guidelines as the Food Guide Pyramid or the exchange system.

A list of all ingredients must appear on all processed and packaged foods. When appropriate, ingredient lists must include any FDA-certified color additives, the sources of any protein hydrolysates, a declaration that caseinate is a milk derivative when caseinate is found in foods claiming to be nondairy, and a declaration of the total percentage of juice in any beverage claiming to contain juice.

An important feature of the NLEA is that it regulates nutrient content claims and health claims on food labels or other labeling of food, such as advertisements. Nutrient content claims are those describing the amount of nutrients in foods, such as "cholesterol free," "low fat," "light," or "lean." Examples of these are shown in Table 2-14. Most nutrient claims are based on the reference amount of the food, not necessarily the serving size noted on the label. In addition to the nutrient claims shown in Table 2-14 are those using the words "reduced" or "less." A food making the claim "reduced or less sodium" would have to contain at least 25% less sodium per reference amount than an appropriate food used for comparison purposes. For example, potato chips labeled "low sodium" would have to contain at least 25% less sodium than comparable potato chips (the "reference food").

The FDA defines a health claim as any claim on the package label or other labeling of a food that characterizes the relationship of any nutrient or other substance in the food to a disease or health-related condition. According to FDA regulations, health claims are allowed only under certain circumstances and must be scientifically based and standardized. Allowable health claims are shown in Box 2-8. The NLEA stipulates that foods bearing health claims must not contain any nutrient or substance in an amount that increases the risk of a disease or a health condition. Foods bearing health claims must contain 20% or less of the Daily Value of fat, saturated fat, cholesterol, and sodium per serving. For example, whole milk (which is high in calcium) may not bear a calcium-osteoporosis claim because its fat content exceeds 20% of the Daily Value for fat. Skim and 1% fat milk easily qualify for the calcium-osteoporosis claim. According to FDA regulation, claims that a substance will prevent a disease are drug claims. Health claims on food labels are limited to saying that a food "may" or "might" reduce the risk of a disease or health condition.

Daily Values

The **Daily Values** are dietary reference values intended to help consumers use food label information to plan healthy diets. They serve as the basis for quantifying the amounts of various nutrients and food components on food labels. They are to be used for regulatory purposes only and are not intended to serve as recommended intakes. The basis for calculating the Daily Values are two separate sets of nutrient reference values: the **Daily Reference Values** (DRVs) and the **Reference Daily Intakes** (RDIs).

Daily Reference Values

The DRVs are reference values for nutrients and food components for which no set of standards (e.g., the RDAs or U.S. RDAs) previously existed. Table 2-15 shows the DRVs for 2000 kcal and 2500 kcal diets. For labeling purposes, 2000 kcal is the reference for calculating percent of Daily Values, although some labels may also include DRVs for a higher energy intake such as 2500 kcal. The DRVs include values for total fat, saturated fatty acids, cholesterol, total carbohydrate, dietary fiber, sodium, potassium, and protein. Some of the DRVs are based on recommendations to increase or maintain intake of the particular food component (carbohydrate, dietary fiber, and potassium), whereas other DRVs reflect levels that are limitations on intake (total fat, saturated fat, cholesterol, and sodium).

Four of the seven food components for which DRVs have been established require a specific energy intake to quantify reference values. Those for total fat, saturated fat, and carbohydrate are based on intake levels of approximately 30%, 10%, and 60% of total energy, respectively. The DRV for protein is based on 10% of energy from protein for adults and children 4 years of age and older. The reference value for dietary fiber is based on an intake of approximately 11.5 g per

TABLE 2-14 Examples and meanings of some allowable nutrient content claims

Example of nutrient content claim	Meaning of nutrient content claim
Sugar free	less than 0.5 g sugars per reference amount and per serving
Calorie free	fewer than 5 kcal per reference amount and per serving
Low calorie	40 kcal or less per reference amount (and per 50 g if reference amount is small)
Fat free	less than 0.5 g fat per reference amount and per serving
Saturated fat free	less than 0.5 g saturated fat and less than 0.5 g *trans* fatty acid per reference amount and per serving
Low fat	3 g or less per reference amount (and per 50 g if reference amount is small)
Low saturated fat	1 g or less per reference amount and 15% or less of calories from saturated fat
Cholesterol free	less than 2 mg of cholesterol and 2 g or less of saturated fat per reference amount and per serving
Low cholesterol	20 mg or less of cholesterol and 2 g or less of saturated fat per reference amount and per serving
Sodium free	less than 5 mg per reference amount and per serving
Low sodium	140 mg or less per reference amount (and per 50 g if reference amount is small)
Very low sodium	35 mg or less per reference amount (and per 50 mg if reference amount is small)
Lean meat or poultry	contains less than 10 g total fat, 4 g saturated fat, and 95 mg of cholesterol per reference amount and 100 g for individual foods
Extra lean meat or poultry	contains less than 5 g total fat, 2 g saturated fat, and 95 mg cholesterol per reference amount and 100 g for individual foods
High, rich in	contains 20% or more of Daily Value to describe protein, vitamins, minerals, dietary fiber, or potassium per reference amount
Good source of	10%–19% or more of the Daily Value per reference amount
More, added	10% or more of the Daily Value per reference amount
Light, lite	at least 50% less fat per reference amount or one third fewer calories if less than 50% of kcal come from fat

Adapted from Stehlin D. 1993. A little 'lite' reading. *FDA Consumer* 27(4):29–33; Wilkening VL. 1993. FDA's regulations to implement the NLEA. *Nutrition Today* 28(5):13–20; and Schor D, Edwards C. 1993. USDA's role: Nutrition labeling of meat and poultry products. *Nutrition Today* 28(5):21–23.

TABLE 2-15 The Food and Drug Administration's Daily Reference Values (DRVs) for 2000 kcal and 2500 kcal diets

Food Component	Daily Reference Value	
	2000 kcal	2500 kcal
Fat	<65 g	<80 g
Saturated fatty acids	<20 g	<25 g
Cholesterol	<300 mg	<300 mg
Total carbohydrate	300 g	375 g
Fiber	25 g	30 g
Sodium	<2400 mg	<2400 mg
Potassium	3500 mg	3500 mg
Protein*	50 g	63 g

*The DRV for protein applies only to children older than 4 years and adults. The RDIs for protein for infants, children 1 to 4 years, pregnant females, and nursing females are 14 g, 16 g, 60 g, and 65 g, respectively.

BOX 2-8

Health Claims Allowed on Food Labels

- Calcium and reduced risk of osteoporosis
- Sodium and increased risk of hypertension
- Dietary saturated fat and cholesterol and increased risk of coronary heart disease
- Dietary fat and increased risk of cancer
- Fiber-containing grain products, fruits, and vegetables and reduced risk of cancer
- Fruits, vegetables, and grain products that contain fiber, particularly soluble fiber, and reduced risk of coronary heart disease
- Fruits and vegetables and reduced risk of cancer
- Folic acid and reduced risk of neural tube defects

TABLE 2-16 The Food and Drug Administrations's Reference Daily Intakes (RDIs)*

Nutrient	Amount
Vitamin A	5000 IU†
Vitamin C	60 mg
Thiamin	1.5 mg
Riboflavin	1.7 mg
Niacin	20 mg
Calcium	1000 mg
Iron	18 mg
Vitamin D	400 IU
Vitamin E	30 IU
Vitamin B_6	2.0 mg
Folic acid	400 μg
Vitamin B_{12}	6 μg
Phosphorus	1000 mg
Iodine	150 μg
Magnesium	400 mg
Zinc	15 mg
Copper	2 mg
Biotin	300 μg
Pantothenic acid	10 mg

*Based on the National Academy of Sciences' 1986 Recommended Dietary Allowances
†IU international units

1000 kcal. The DRV for cholesterol is based on recommendations that individuals, regardless of energy intake, limit their consumption to less than 300 mg/day. The value for sodium resulted from recommendations that all persons limit their *salt* intake to less than 6 g/day, which is a sodium intake of less than 2.4 g/day. The DRV for potassium is 3500 mg, a level associated with decreased risk of hypertension.

Reference Daily Intakes

The RDIs serve as reference values for vitamins and minerals and are the familiar U.S. RDAs with a new name. The RDIs are shown in Table 2-16. In 1990, the FDA proposed updating the U.S.

RDAs but was temporarily prevented from doing so by Congress. Part of the rationale for changing the name of the U.S. RDAs to RDIs was to decrease confusion over the terms "RDA" and "U.S. RDA." The FDA plans to update the RDIs in the near future so they will be more representative of our contemporary understanding of nutrient requirements.

FOOD GUIDES

A food guide is a nutrition education tool translating scientific knowledge and dietary standards and recommendations into an understandable and practical form for use by those who have little or no training in nutrition.[33,49] Food guides are "problem oriented" and address specific nutritional problems identified within the targeted population. Typically, foods are classified into basic groups according to similarity of nutrient content or some other criteria. If a certain number of servings from each group is consumed, a balanced and adequate diet is thought likely to result.

The USDA has been at the forefront of food guide development in the United States. The major food guides developed by the USDA are outlined in Table 2-17. The USDA's first food guides are credited to Caroline Hunt, a nutrition specialist in USDA's Bureau of Home Economics.[50] In 1916 she developed *Food for Young Children,* followed in 1917 by *How to Select Foods.* In these, foods were categorized into five groups—milk and meat; cereals; vegetables and fruits; fats and fat foods; and sugars and sugary foods. These "buying guides" were designed to insure adequate energy intake from fat, carbohydrate, and protein while encouraging sufficient variety for minerals and some of the newly discovered body-regulating substances we now know as vitamins. The financial constraints imposed by the economic depression of the early 1930s led to the development of food guides providing advice to families for purchasing foods at various cost levels. Hazel Stiebeling, a food economist in USDA's Bureau of Home Economics, led in the development of these buying guides. She emphasized a balance between high-energy foods (e.g., fats and sweets) and "protective" or nutrient-dense foods supplying essential nutrients. Among the protective foods are milk, which supplies calcium, and fruits and vegetables, which supply vitamins A and C.[50]

Hunt and Stiebeling's buying guides gave way to food guides promoting "foundation diets." These food guides recommended a minimum number of servings from different food groups, which provided a foundation diet supplying a major portion of the RDAs. It was assumed that to meet their energy needs, most people would consume more food than the guide specified. This extra food would not only provide necessary energy, but additional nutrients as well. It was further assumed that such a diet would meet requirements for all essential nutrients, not just those included in the RDAs.[49,50] During the mid-1940s the USDA developed the "Basic Seven," which was widely used for many years. Its complexity and lack of specific serving sizes led to the development of the "Basic Four" in 1956.[49,50] The assumption underlying development of the Four Food Groups was that eating the specified numbers of servings from the different food groups would supply approximately 1200 kcal, approximately 100% of the RDAs for vitamins A and C and calcium, and at least 80% of the RDAs for the remaining five nutrients of the 1953 revision of the RDAs.[49] Vitamins A and C and calcium were given priority status because they were shown to be **shortfall nutrients** (nutrients whose intakes were below recommended levels among a significant part of the population).[49]

In 1979 the USDA issued the Hassle-Free Guide to a Better Diet. This was a revision of the Four Food Groups that gave more attention to micronutrients in food groups and included a fifth food group: fats, sweets, and alcohol. The purpose of including this fifth group was to help consumers recognize fats, sweets, and alcohol as empty

TABLE 2-17 Major USDA food guides (1916–1995) showing food groups and numbers of servings*

<table>
<tr><th rowspan="2">Food guide</th><th rowspan="2">Number of food groups</th><th colspan="2">Protein-rich foods</th><th rowspan="2">Breads</th><th rowspan="2">Vegetables</th><th rowspan="2">Fruits</th><th colspan="2">Other</th></tr>
<tr><th>Milk</th><th>Meat</th><th>Fats</th><th>Sugars</th></tr>
<tr><td>Caroline Hunt
Buying guides
(1916)</td><td>5</td><td colspan="2">Meats and other protein-rich foods
10% of energy from milk
10% of energy from other foods
1 c milk + 2–3 svgs of other foods
based on 3-oz svg</td><td>Cereals and other starchy foods
20% of energy
9 svgs
based on 1 oz or ¾ c dry cereal</td><td colspan="2">Vegetables and fruits
30% of energy
5 svgs
based on average 8-oz svg</td><td>Fatty foods
20% of energy
9 svgs
based on 1-Tbsp svg</td><td>Sugars
10% of energy
10 svgs
based on 1-Tbsp svg</td></tr>
<tr><td>H. K. Stiebeling
Buying guide
(1930s)</td><td>12</td><td>Milk
2c</td><td>Lean meat, poultry, fish
9–10 svgs/wk

Dry, mature beans, peas, nuts
1 svg/wk

Eggs
1</td><td>Flours, cereals
as desired</td><td>Leafy green, yellow
11–12 svgs per wk

Potato, sweet potato
1 svg

Other vegetables and fruit
3 svgs</td><td>Tomato and citrus
1 svg</td><td>Butter
—

Other fats
—</td><td>Sugars
—</td></tr>
<tr><td>Basic Seven
Foundation diet
(1940s)</td><td>7</td><td>Milk and milk products
2 or more svgs
svg = 1 c</td><td>Meat, poultry, fish, eggs, dried beans, peas, nuts
1–2 svgs</td><td>Breads, flour, and cereals
every day</td><td>Leafy green yellow
1 or more svgs

Potato and other fruits and vegetables
2 or more svgs</td><td>Citrus, tomato, cabbage, salad greens
1 or more svg</td><td colspan="2">Butter, fortified margarine
some daily</td></tr>
<tr><td>Basic Four
Foundation diet
(1956–70s)</td><td>4</td><td>Milk group
2 or more svgs</td><td>Meat group
2 or more svgs
2–3 oz svgs</td><td>Bread, cereal
4 or more svgs
1 oz dry, 1 slice
½–¾ c cooked</td><td colspan="2">Vegetable-fruit group
4 svgs
include dark green/yellow vegetables frequently, ½ c typical portion</td><td></td><td></td></tr>
<tr><td>Hassle-Free
Foundation diet
(1979)</td><td>5</td><td>Milk-cheese group
2 svgs
1 c, 1½ oz cheese</td><td>Meat, poultry, fish, and bean group
2 svgs
2–3 oz svg</td><td>Bread-cereal group
4 or more svgs
1 oz dry, 1 slice
½–¾ c cooked</td><td colspan="2">Vegetable-fruit group
4 svgs
include vitamin C source daily and dark-green/yellow vegetables frequently
½ c or typical portion</td><td colspan="2">Fats, sweets, alcohol group
use dependent on calorie needs</td></tr>
<tr><td>Food Guide
Pyramid
Total diet (1984)</td><td>6</td><td>Milk, yogurt, cheese
2–3 svgs
1 c, 1½ oz cheese</td><td>Meat, poultry, fish eggs, dry beans, nuts
2–3 svgs
5–7 oz total/day</td><td>Breads, cereals rice pasta
6–11 svgs
whole grain and enriched
1 slice, ½ c cooked</td><td>Vegetable
3–5 svgs
dark green
deep yellow
starchy/legumes
other
½ c raw,
½ c cooked</td><td>Fruit
2–4 svgs
citrus
other
½ c or average</td><td colspan="2">Fats, oils, sweets
total fat not to exceed 30% of energy
sweets vary according to energy need</td></tr>
</table>

From Human Nutrition Information Service. 1993. *USDA's food guide: Background and development*. Hyattsville, Md: USDA, Human Nutrition Information Service.

*Number of servings are daily unless noted otherwise; svg = serving

TABLE 2-18 A daily food guide

Food group	Suggested servings
Vegetables	3–5
Fruits	2–4
Breads, cereals, rice, and pasta	6–11
Milk, yogurt, and cheese	2–3
Meats, poultry, fish, dry beans and peas, eggs, and nuts	2–3

Eat a variety of foods daily, choosing different foods from each group. Most people should have at least the lower number of servings suggested from each food group. Some people may need more because of their body size and activity levels. Young children should have a variety of foods but may need small servings.
From USDA/USDHHS. 1990. *Nutrition and your health: Dietary guidelines for Americans,* 3rd ed. Washington, DC: U.S. Government Printing Office.

calories and to draw attention to the need for considering them in meal planning, since no servings from this group were recommended. The "Hassle-Free Guide" highlighted the need to use fat, sugars, and alcohol moderately and gave special attention to calories and dietary fiber.[50]

Publication of the *Dietary Goals for the United States* in 1977 (Figure 2-7, Box 2-1) was a turning point for dietary guidance and food guides. Following this landmark event, the USDA and USDHHS published the *Dietary Guidelines for Americans* in 1980, with revisions following every 5 years. In 1980, USDA began working on a new food guide to replace the "Basic Four." This led to development of the food guide shown in Table 2-18. Three key messages of this guide were variety (eating a selection of foods of various types that together meet nutritional needs); proportionality (eating appropriate amounts of various types of foods to meet nutritional needs); and moderation (avoiding too much of food components in the total diet that have been linked to diseases).[50]

Despite dissemination of the food guide in several publications developed by the USDA and other groups (including the 1990 edition of *Dietary Guidelines for Americans*), the perception remained among the public and professionals that the USDA was still using the "Basic Four" developed in the 1950s.[50,51] This led the USDA to develop a separate publication explaining the food guide and containing an appealing illustration conveying the key messages of the guide.

Food Guide Pyramid

In 1988 the USDA contracted with a private market research firm to develop and extensively test a publication and graphics to communicate the new food guide. Of the various graphic alternatives tested, a pyramid proved to be the most effective visual approach for communicating the messages of variety, proportionality, and moderation.[50,51] The Pyramid underwent extensive peer review by nutrition educators and was enthusiastically received by these groups. The Pyramid was the centerpiece of a colorful nutrition education brochure developed by the USDA and USDHHS that better reflected the current state of nutritional knowledge. On the day that printing of the brochure was to be completed, then Secretary of Agriculture Edward Madigan canceled the project. According to a former top USDA official, Secretary Madigan canceled the project ten days after meeting with members of the National Cattlemen's Association who were reportedly "incensed" over the pyramid graphic. The National Milk Producers Federation also voiced complaints about the graphic.[52,53] It was alleged that cancellation was to allow further testing of the pyramid graphic. However, the media widely reported that the project was killed because of meat and dairy industry objections to the Pyramid.[54–57] After a year of additional testing at a cost of $855,000, the USDA finally released the Food Guide Pyramid in 1992 (see Figure 2-10).

The Food Guide Pyramid graphically suggests the number of servings of foods from five major

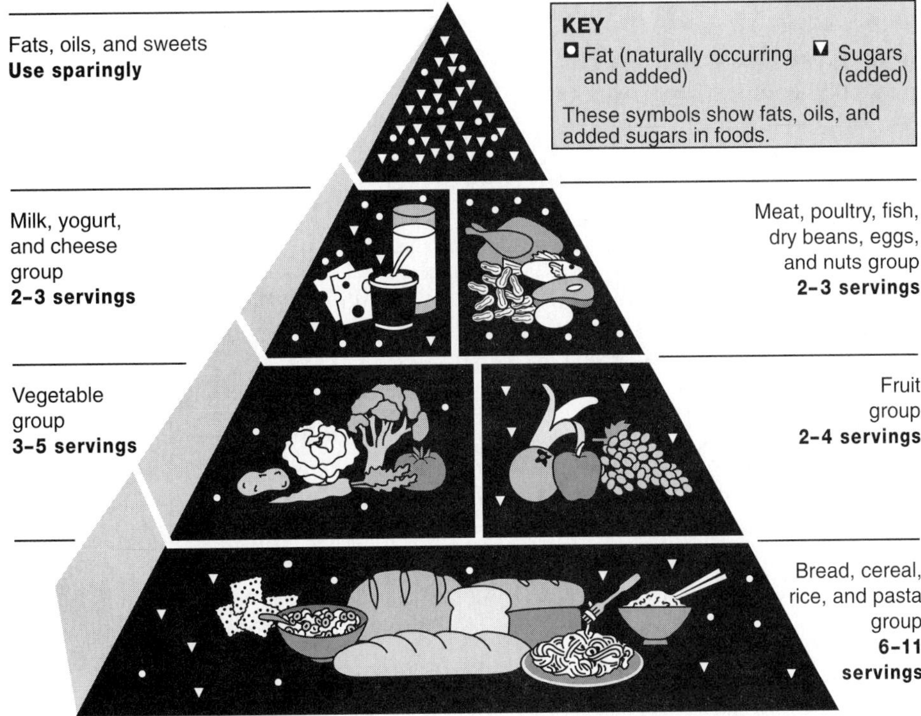

Figure 2-10 The U.S. Department of Agriculture's Food Guide Pyramid. USDA

groups in an easily understandable way. Recommendations are made for cereals/grains, vegetables, fruits, dairy products, and protein-rich foods. At the pyramid's bottom are the bread, cereal, rice, and pasta group; these should compose the largest portion of the diet, about 6 to 11 servings per day. At the very top of the pyramid are fats, oils, and sweets; placement there indicates caution to use these sparingly.

The Pyramid shows a range of food servings for each food group. The number of servings a person should eat depends on the number of kilocalories needed, which in turn depends on that person's age, sex, size, and physical activity. As shown in Table 2-19, the low number of servings from each group provides approximately 1600 kcal per day while the high number of servings from each group provides approximately 2800 kcal per day. Examples of serving sizes are shown in Table 2-20.

Alternative Food Guides

The Food Guide Pyramid has been criticized by some as representing "a mix of well-supported findings, educated guesses, and political compromises with powerful economic interests such as the dairy and meat industries."[58] Some feel that the recommended number of servings of meat (two to three per day) may be unhealthy and that

TABLE 2-19 Sample diets for a day at three energy levels

Food group	Lower, about 1600 kcal	Moderate, about 2200 kcal	Higher, about 2800 kcal
Bread group servings	6	9	11
Vegetable group servings	3	4	5
Fruit group servings	2	3	4
Milk group servings*	2–3	2–3	2–3
Meat group servings† (ounces)	5	6	7
Total fat (grams)	53	73	93
Total added sugars (teaspoons)	6	12	18

*Women who are pregnant or breastfeeding, teenagers, and young adults to age 24 years need 3 servings
†Meat group amounts are in total ounces

TABLE 2-20 Examples of serving sizes used in the Food Guide Pyramid

Bread, cereal, rice and pasta group	1 slice of bread
	1 oz ready-to eat cereal
	½ c cooked cereal, rice, or pasta
Vegetable group	1 c raw leafy vegetables
	½ c other vegetables, cooked, chopped, or raw
	¾ c vegetable juice
Fruit group	1 medium apple, banana, orange
	½ c chopped, cooked, canned fruit
	¾ c fruit juice
Milk, yogurt, and cheese group	1 c milk or yogurt
	1 ½ oz natural cheese
	2 oz processed cheese
Meat, poultry, fish, dry beans, eggs, and nut group	2–3 oz cooked lean meat, poultry, fish
	½ c cooked dry beans, 1 egg or 2 Tbsp peanut butter count as 1 oz of lean meat

the Food Guide Pyramid ignores important differences in types of fat, such as saturated and *trans* fatty acids as opposed to monounsaturated fatty acids.[58] Others object to the USDA's approach to grouping foods. For example, grouping nonfat dairy products (skim milk or nonfat yogurt, for example) with higher fat dairy products such as ice cream and many cheeses or grouping legumes with meat, many of which are high in fat. In response to these and other concerns, alternative "pyramids" have been developed. Among these are the Mediterranean Pyramid and the Vegetarian Pyramid.

Mediterranean Pyramid

The Mediterranean Pyramid (Figure 2-11) is based on the dietary patterns typically followed by persons living in Greece and Southern Italy in the 1960s. (Recently, however, diets in these countries have become more similar to those eaten in North America.) Persons in these countries had very low death rates from coronary heart disease and long life expectancies.[58] The Mediterranean Pyramid has several things in common with the USDA's Pyramid. Both emphasize making grain products the basis of the diet and liberal daily intake of fruits and vegetables. The Mediterranean

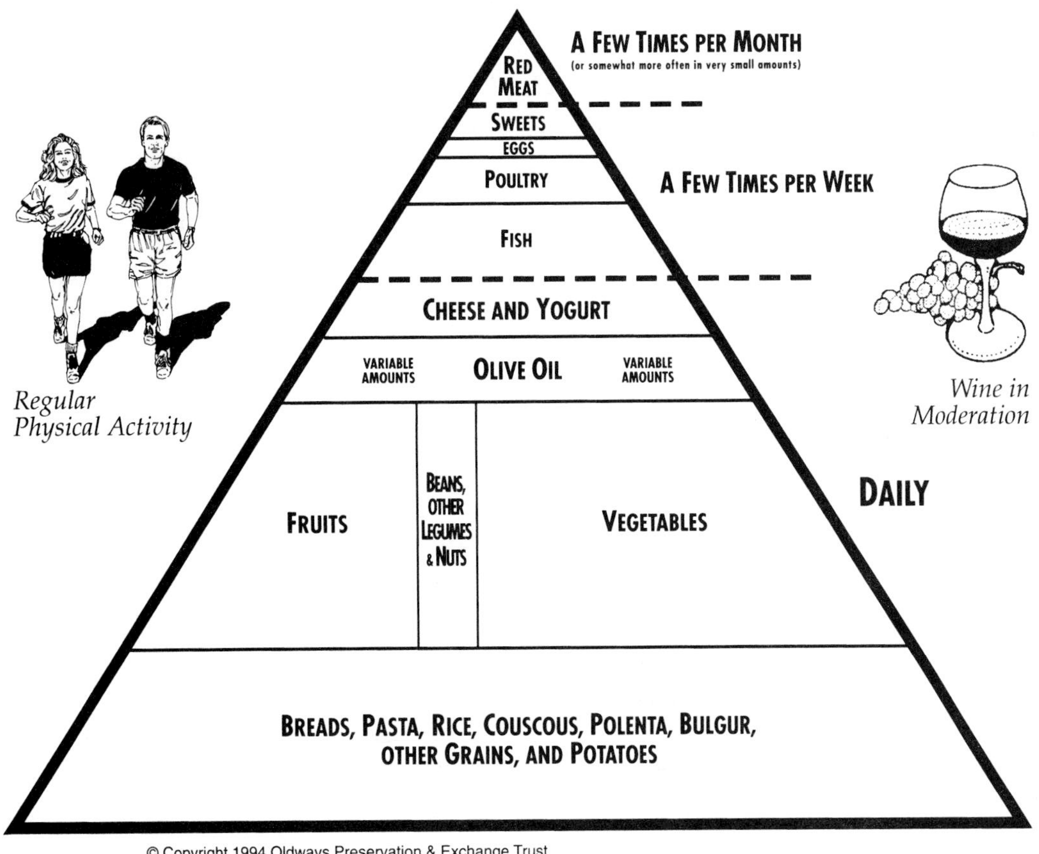

Figure 2-11 The Mediterranean Diet Pyramid.

Pyramid places greater emphasis on whole-grain foods than the USDA's Pyramid. The Mediterranean Pyramid recommends only small amounts of dairy products each day, eating poultry, sweets, and eggs only a few times a week, and eating lean red meats only a few times a month. It also identifies olive oil as the preferred type of fat. In addition to daily exercise, it suggests the controversial option of one glass of wine per day for women and up to two glasses per day for men, with the warning that drinking should be avoided when doing so might put the drinker or others at risk. Despite evidence suggesting that moderate alcohol consumption raises HDL-cholesterol, lowers risk of coronary heart disease, and lowers overall mortality, alcohol consumption is a major factor in motor vehicle accidents, homicide, suicide, and domestic violence. There is considerable evidence that even one or two drinks per day can increase risk of breast cancer in females.

Vegetarian Pyramid

The New York Medical College's Vegetarian Pyramid (Figure 2-12) was developed for use by nutritionists and dietitians in counseling their vegetarian clients. In many respects is it similar to the Food Guide Pyramid. There are some differences, however. Included with the bread, cereal, rice, and pasta group are starchy vegetables such as potatoes, green peas, and corn. Starchy vegetables are excluded from the vegetable group and no limit is set on vegetable consumption. The milk and milk substitute group includes fortified soy milk to provide vegans and ovo-vegetarians with nutrients they might otherwise be lacking. One cup of fortified soy milk contains 200 mg of calcium and 1000 IU vitamin D, roughly 20% of an adult's RDAs. This explains the upper limit of four servings from this group for those not consuming dairy products. The meat/fish substitutes group recommends such foods as beans, protein-rich seeds, peanut butter, and tofu. A cupful of cooked dry beans is considered a serving, and two or three servings per day are suggested. At the top of the pyramid is the "vegans must consume daily" group. This includes a tablespoon each per day of blackstrap molasses (supplies iron and calcium) and brewer's yeast (supplies riboflavin and B_{12}). The three to five teaspoons of vegetable oil serve as a source of added energy.

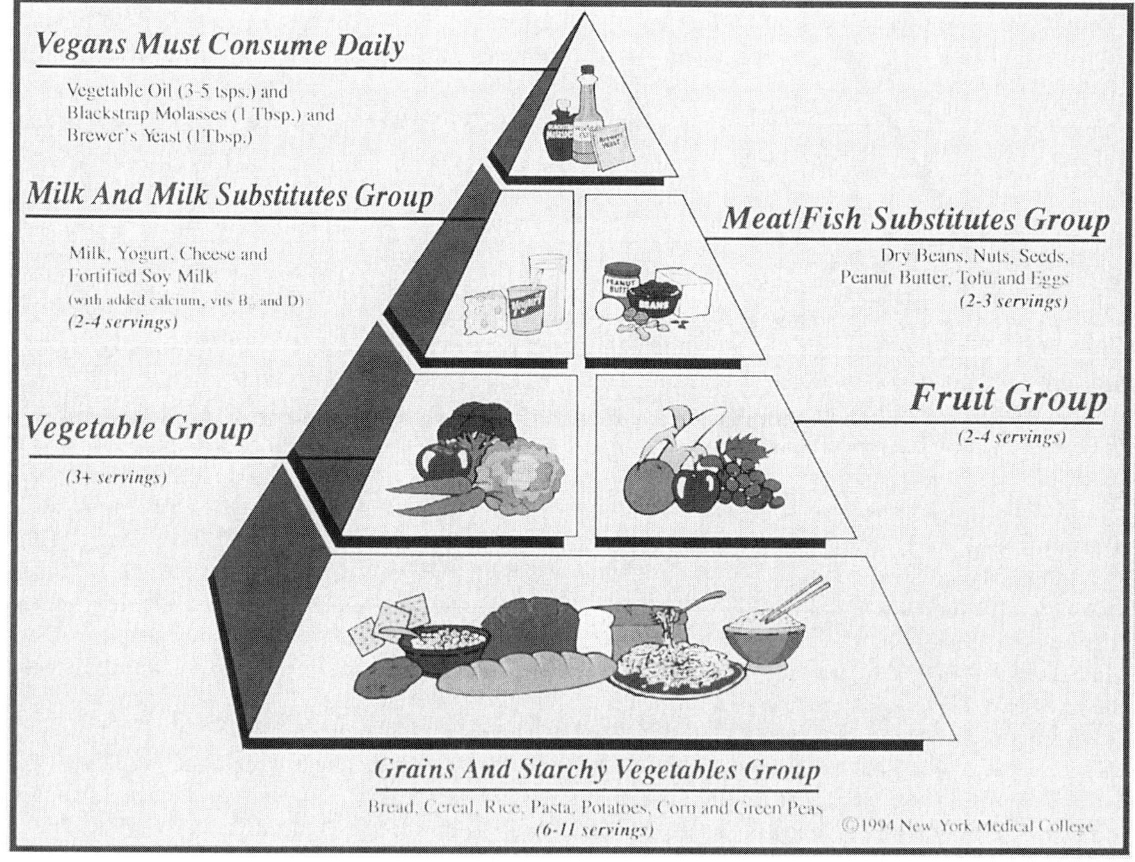

Figure 2-12 The New York Medical College Vegetarian Pyramid.

FOOD EXCHANGE SYSTEM

The **food exchange system** is a method of planning meals that simplifies controlling energy consumption (particularly from carbohydrate), helps ensure adequate nutrient intake, and allows considerable variety in food selection. Also, once a person becomes familiar with the system, he or she can use it to quickly approximate kilocalorie and macronutrient levels in individual foods or an entire meal.

The food exchange system and accompanying exchange lists originally were developed in 1950 by the American Dietetic Association and the American Diabetes Association in cooperation with the U.S. Public Health Service for use in planning diabetic diets.[59] Before then, no standardized method for planning diabetic diets existed, and many health professionals and people with diabetes complained that meal planning often was laborious and difficult to adapt to individual food preferences.

The system categorizes foods into three main groups—the carbohydrate group, the meat and meat substitute group, and the fat group. The carbohydrate group lists foods that supply most of their energy in the form of carbohydrate: starches, fruits, dairy products, vegetables, and other carbohydrates. The meat and meat substitute group includes foods that serve as good protein sources, supply variable amounts of fat, and generally provide little, if any, carbohydrate. Foods in this group are listed on the basis of the amount of fat they supply: very lean, lean, medium-fat, and high-fat. Foods in the fat group provide fat and little, if any, protein and carbohydrate. They are divided among three lists on the basis of the major fatty acid they supply: monounsaturated, polyunsaturated, and saturated. There is also a "free foods list" and a list of combination foods and fast foods.

These lists are referred to as "exchange lists" because foods on the same list provide, on average, a similar number of kilocalories and grams of carbohydrate, protein, and fat as shown in Table 2-21. When planning a meal, foods on the same list can be "exchanged" or traded for any other on the list without changing the approximate amount of carbohydrate, protein, fat, and energy supplied by the meal. At breakfast, for example, a person could exchange a slice of bread for ¾ cup of unsweetened, ready-to-eat cereal. Each of these foods equals one choice from the starch exchange list and, consequently, have about the same macronutrient and energy contents. A detailed listing of foods within the exchange lists and their serving sizes are given in Table 2-22. Unless otherwise indicated, portion sizes are for cooked foods. Note in Table 2-22 that serving sizes differ among the various foods within one exchange list. For example, ⅓ cup of grape juice and 1¼ cup of cubed watermelon are both considered a fruit exchange. Each provides approximately 15 g of carbohydrate and 60 kcal. However, because grape juice is a more concentrated source of energy compared with watermelon, its serving size is smaller.

Note that foods are not always where you might expect them to be. This is because foods are categorized primarily according to their carbohydrate, protein, and fat content. Olives and peanuts are considered monounsaturated fat exchanges. Corn is in the starchy vegetable exchange list because of its high carbohydrate content. The same is true of green peas, potatoes, and winter squash.

The American Dietetic Association and the American Diabetic Association have developed exchange lists for foods commonly eaten by a number of ethnic groups. Included among these ethnic groups are African Americans, Native Americans (Navajo), Chinese Americans, Hmong Americans, Indians, Eastern Europeans (Jewish), Mexican Americans, and Asian Americans. An exchange list for foods commonly eaten by vegetarians has also been developed. For information on these exchange lists contact the American Dietetic Association or the American Diabetic Association.

TABLE 2-21 Average kilocalorie and macronutrient contents of the exchange lists*

Group/List	Carbohydrate (g)	Protein (g)	Fat (g)	Calories
Carbohydrate group				
Starch	15	3	1 or less	80
Fruit	15	—	—	60
Milk				
Skim	12	8	0–3	90
Low-fat	12	8	5	120
Whole	12	8	8	150
Other carbohydrates	15	varies	varies	varies
Vegetables	5	2	—	25
Meat and meat substitute group				
Very lean	—	7	0–1	35
Lean	—	7	3	55
Medium-fat	—	7	5	75
High-fat	—	7	8	100
Fat group	—	—	5	45

From the American Diabetes Association, Inc. and the American Dietetic Association, 1995.

*The exchange lists are based on material in the Exchange Lists for Meal Planning prepared by committees of the American Diabetes Association, Inc. and the American Dietetic Association in cooperation with the National Institute of Arthritis, Metabolism, and Digestive Diseases and the National Heart, Lung, and Blood Institute, Public Health Service, U.S. Department of Health and Human Services.

Using the Food Exchange System

Sample meal plans using the exchange lists and providing 1500, 2000, and 2500 kcal/day are given in Table 2-23. A person following the 2000 kcal/day plan, for example, would eat eight servings from the starch/bread exchange list, seven from the meat list, three from the vegetable list, six from the fruit list, three from the milk list, and three from the fat list.

Ideally, when diabetes is diagnosed in a patient, a dietitian will work with the patient to design a meal plan individualized to the patient's dietary preferences, daily schedule, medications, body weight, serum lipid levels, and exercise habits. This meal plan can be expressed in terms of the number of foods from each of the six exchange lists. Many weight-management programs and meal plans for people with diabetes are based on the exchange system because it simplifies the task of counting calories. An outstanding feature of the exchange system is that rather than specifying a particular food, it gives a person an almost unlimited variety of foods from which to choose in planning meals. A person following one of the meal patterns in Table 2-23 could have selected a number of different foods from the starch list to get his or her exchanges from that list. The same is true for the protein, fruit, milk, or fat selections. The important thing is to select the specified *number* of exchanges and the correct *serving size* from each exchange list.

TABLE 2-22 The exchange lists for meal planning

Starch list

One starch exchange equals 15 g carbohydrate, 3 g protein, 0 to 1 g fat, and 80 calories.

Cereals, grains, pasta, breads, crackers, snacks, starchy vegetables, and cooked dried beans, peas, and lentils are starches. In general, one starch is:

- 1/2 cup of cereal, grain, pasta, or starchy vegetable.
- 1 ounce of a bread product such as 1 slice of bread.
- 3/4 to 1 ounce of most snack foods. (Some snack foods may also have added fat.)

Nutrition tips

1. Most starch choices are good sources of B vitamins.
2. Foods made from whole grains are good sources of fiber.
3. Dried beans and peas are a good source of protein and fiber.

Selection tips

1. Choose starches made with little fat as often as you can.
2. Starchy vegetables prepared with fat count as one starch and one fat.
3. Bagels or muffins can be 2, 3, or 4 ounces in size and can, therefore, count as 2, 3, or 4 starch choices. Check the size you eat.
4. Dried beans, peas, and lentils are also found on the meat and meat substitutes list.
5. Regular potato chips and tortilla chips are found on the other carbohydrates list.
6. Most of the serving sizes are measured after cooking.
7. Always check nutrition facts on the food label.

Bread	
Bagel	1/2 (1 oz)
Bread, reduced-calorie	2 slices (1 1/2 oz)
Bread, white, whole wheat, pumpernickel, rye	1 slice (1 oz)
Bread sticks, crisp, 4 in. long × 1/2 in.	2 (2/3 oz)
English muffin	1/2
Hot dog or hamburger bun	1/2 (1 oz)
Pita, 6 in. across	1/2
Roll, plain, small	1 (1 oz)
Raisin bread, unfrosted	1 slice (1 oz)
Tortilla, corn, 6 in. across	1
Tortilla, flour, 7–8 in. across	1
Waffle, 4 1/2 in. square, reduced fat	1
Cereals and grains	
Bran cereals	1/2 cup
Bulgur	1/2 cup
Cereals	1/2 cup
Cereals, unsweetened, ready-to-eat	3/4 cup
Cornmeal (dry)	3 Tbsp
Couscous	1/3 cup
Flour (dry)	3 Tbsp

Continued

TABLE 2-22 The exchange lists for meal planning—cont'd

Starch list—cont'd	
Cereals and grains—cont'd	
Granola, low-fat	1/4 cup
Grape-Nuts	1/4 cup
Grits	1/2 cup
Kasha	1/2 cup
Millet	1/4 cup
Muesli	1/4 cup
Oats	1/2 cup
Pasta	1/2 cup
Puffed cereal	1 1/2 cups
Rice milk	1/2 cup
Rice, white or brown	1/3 cup
Shredded wheat	1/2 cup
Sugar-frosted cereal	1/2 cup
Wheat germ	3 Tbsp
Starchy vegetables	
Baked beans	1/3 cup
Corn	1/2 cup
Corn on cob, medium	1 (5 oz)
Mixed vegetables with corn, peas, or pasta	1 cup
Peas, green	1/2 cup
Plantain	1/2 cup
Potato, baked or boiled	1 small (3 oz)
Potato, mashed	1/2 cup
Squash, winter (acorn, butternut)	1 cup
Yam, sweet potato, plain	1/2 cup
Crackers and snacks	
Animal crackers	8
Graham crackers, 2 1/2 in. square	3
Matzoh	3/4 oz
Melba toast	4 slices
Oyster crackers	24
Popcorn (popped, no fat added or low-fat microwave)	3 cups
Pretzels	3/4 oz
Rice cakes, 4 in. across	2
Saltine-type crackers	6
Snack chips, fat-free (tortilla, potato)	15–20 (3/4 oz)
Whole-wheat crackers, no fat added	2–5 (3/4 oz)
Dried beans, peas, lentils	
Count as 1 starch exchange plus 1 very lean meat exchange.	
Beans and peas (garbanzo, pinto, kidney, white, split, black-eyed)	1/2 cup
Lima beans	2/3 cup
Lentils	1/2 cup
Miso*	3 Tbsp

* = 400 mg or more of sodium per serving.

TABLE 2-22 The exchange lists for meal planning—cont'd

Starch list—cont'd

Starchy foods prepared with fat	
Count as 1 starch exchange, plus 1 fat exchange.	
Biscuit, 2 1/2 in. across	1
Chow mein noodles	1/2 cup
Corn bread, 2 in. cube	1 (2 oz)
Crackers, round butter type	6
Croutons	1 cup
French-fried potatoes	16–25 (3 oz)
Granola	1/4 cup
Muffin, small	1 (1 1/2 oz)
Pancake, 4 in. across	2
Popcorn, microwave	3 cups
Sandwich crackers, cheese or peanut butter filling	3
Stuffing, bread (prepared)	1/3 cup
Taco shell, 6 in. across	2
Waffle, 4 1/2 in. square	1
Whole-wheat crackers, fat added	4–6 (1 oz)

Some foods you buy uncooked will weigh less after you cook it. Starches often swell in cooking, so a small amount of uncooked starch will become a much larger amount of cooked food. The following table shows some of the changes.

Food (starch group)	Uncooked	Cooked
Oatmeal	3 Tbsp	1/2 cup
Cream of Wheat	2 Tbsp	1/2 cup
Grits	3 Tbsp	1/2 cup
Rice	2 Tbsp	1/3 cup
Spaghetti	1/4 cup	1/2 cup
Noodles	1/3 cup	1/2 cup
Macaroni	1/4 cup	1/2 cup
Dried beans	1/4 cup	1/2 cup
Dried peas	1/4 cup	1/2 cup
Lentils	3 Tbsp	1/2 cup

Fruit list

One fruit exchange equals 15 g carbohydrate and 60 calories. The weight includes skin, core, seeds, and rinds.

Fresh, frozen, canned, and dried fruits and fruit juices are on this list. In general, one fruit exchange is:

- 1 small to medium fresh fruit.
- 1/2 cup of canned or fresh fruit or fruit juice.
- 1/4 cup of dried fruit.

Continued

TABLE 2-22 The exchange lists for meal planning—cont'd

Fruit list—cont'd

Nutrition tips

1. Fresh, frozen, and dried fruits have about 2 g of fiber per choice. Fruit juices contain very little fiber.
2. Citrus fruits, berries, and melons are good sources of vitamin C.

Selection tips

1. Count 1/2 cup cranberries or rhubarb sweetened with sugar substitutes as free foods.
2. Read the nutrition facts on the food label. If one serving has more than 15 g of carbohydrate, you will need to adjust the size of the serving you eat or drink.
3. Portion sizes for canned fruits are for the fruit and a small amount of juice.
4. Whole fruit is more filling than fruit juice and may be a better choice.
5. Food labels for fruits may contain the words "no sugar added" or "unsweetened." This means that no sucrose (table sugar) has been added.
6. Generally, fruit canned in extra light syrup has the same amount of carbohydrate per serving as the "no sugar added" of the juice pack. All canned fruits on the fruit list are based on one of these three types of pack.

Fruit	
Apple, unpeeled, small	1 (4 oz)
Applesauce, unsweetened	1/2 cup
Apples, dried	4 rings
Apricots, fresh	4 whole (5 1/2 oz)
Apricots, dried	8 halves
Apricots, canned	1/2 cup
Banana, small	1 (4 oz)
Blackberries	3/4 cup
Blueberries	3/4 cup
Cantaloupe, small	1/3 melon (11 oz) or 1 cup cubes
Cherries, sweet, fresh	12 (3 oz)
Cherries, sweet, canned	1/2 cup
Dates	3
Figs, fresh	1 1/2 large or 2 medium (3 1/2 oz)
Figs, dried	1 1/2
Fruit cocktail	1/2 cup
Grapefruit, large	1/2 (11 oz)
Grapefruit sections, canned	3/4 cup
Grapes, small	17 (3 oz)
Honeydew melon	1 slice (10 oz) or 1 cup cubes
Kiwi	1 (3 1/2 oz)
Mandarin oranges, canned	3/4 cup
Mango, small	1/2 fruit (5 1/2 oz) or 1/2 cup
Nectarine, small	1 (5 oz)
Orange, small	1 (6 1/2 oz)
Papaya	1/2 fruit (8 oz) or 1 cup cubes
Peach, medium, fresh	1 (6 oz)

TABLE 2-22 The exchange lists for meal planning—cont'd

Fruit list—cont'd	
Fruit—cont'd	
Peaches, canned	1/2 cup
Pear, large, fresh	1/2 (4 oz)
Pears, canned	1/2 cup
Pineapple, fresh	3/4 cup
Pineapple, canned	1/2 cup
Plums, small	2 (5 oz)
Plums, canned	1/2 cup
Prunes, dried	3
Raisins	2 Tbsp
Raspberries	1 cup
Strawberries	1 1/4 cup whole berries
Tangerines, small	2 (8 oz)
Watermelon	1 slice (13 1/2 oz) or 1 1/4 cup cubes
Fruit juice	
Apple juice/cider	1/2 cup
Cranberry juice cocktail	1/3 cup
Cranberry juice cocktail, reduced-calorie	1 cup
Fruit juice blends, 100% juice	1/3 cup
Grape juice	1/3 cup
Grapefruit juice	1/2 cup
Orange juice	1/2 cup
Pineapple juice	1/2 cup
Prune juice	1/3 cup

Milk list

One milk exchange equals 12 g carbohydrate and 8 g protein.

Different types of milk and milk products are on this list. Cheeses are on the meat list and cream and other dairy fats are on the fat list. Based on the amount of fat they contain, milks are divided into skim/very low-fat milk, low-fat milk, and whole milk. One choice of these includes:

	Carbohydrate (g)	Protein (g)	Fat (g)	Calories
Skim/very low-fat	12	8	0–3	90
Low-fat	12	8	5	120
Whole	12	8	8	150

Nutrition tips

1. Milk and yogurt are good sources of calcium and protein. Check the food label.
2. The higher the fat content of milk and yogurt, the greater the amount of saturated fat and cholesterol. Choose lower-fat varieties.
3. For those who are lactose intolerant, look for lactose-reduced or lactose-free varieties of milk.

Continued

TABLE 2-22 The exchange lists for meal planning—cont'd

Milk list—cont'd	
Selection tips	
1. One cup equals 8 fluid ounces or 1/2 pint.	
2. Look for chocolate milk, frozen yogurt, and ice cream on the other carbohydrates list.	
3. Nondairy creamers are on the free foods list.	
4. Look for rice milk on the starch list.	
5. Look for soy milk on the medium-fat meat list.	
Skim and very low-fat milk (0-3 g fat per serving)	
Skim milk	1 cup
1/2% milk	1 cup
1% milk	1 cup
Nonfat or low-fat buttermilk	1 cup
Evaporated skim milk	1/2 cup
Nonfat dry milk	1/3 cup dry
Plain nonfat yogurt	3/4 cup
Nonfat or low-fat fruit flavored yogurt sweetened with aspartame or with a nonnutritive sweetener	1 cup
Low-fat (5 g fat per serving)	
2% milk	1 cup
Plain low-fat yogurt	3/4 cup
Sweet acidophilus milk	1 cup
Whole milk (8 g fat per serving)	
Whole milk	1 cup
Evaporated whole milk	1/2 cup
Goat's milk	1 cup
Kefir	1 cup

Other carbohydrates list

One exchange equals 15 g carbohydrate, or 1 starch, or 1 fruit, or 1 milk.

You can substitute food choices from this list for a starch, fruit, or milk choice on your meal plan. Some choices will also count as one or more fat choices.

Nutrition tips

1. These foods can be substituted in your meal plan, even though they contain added sugars or fat. However, they do not contain as many important vitamins and minerals as the choices on the starch, fruit, or milk lists.
2. When planning to include these foods in your meal, be sure to include foods from all the lists to eat a balanced meal.

Selection tips

1. Because many of these foods are concentrated sources of carbohydrate and fat, the portion sizes are often very small.
2. Always check nutrition facts on the food label. It will be your most accurate source of information.
3. Many fat-free or reduced-fat products made with fat replacers contain carbohydrate. When eaten in large amounts, they may need to be counted. Talk with your dietitian to determine how to count these in your meal plan.
4. Look for fat-free salad dressings in smaller amounts on the free foods list.

TABLE 2-22 The exchange lists for meal planning—cont'd

Food	Serving size	Exchanges per serving*
Angel food cake, unfrosted	1/12 cake	2 C
Brownie, small, unfrosted	2 in. square	1C, 1 F
Cake, unfrosted	2 in. square	1 C, 1 F
Cake, frosted	2 in. square	2 C, 1 F
Cookie, fat-free	2 small	1 C
Cookie or sandwich cookie with creme filling	2 small	1 C, 1 F
Cupcake, frosted	1 small	2 C, 1 F
Cranberry sauce, jellied	1/4 cup	2 C
Doughnut, plain cake	1 medium (1 1/2 oz)	1 1/2 C, 2 F
Doughnut, glazed	3 3/4 in. across (2 oz)	2 C, 2 F
Fruit juice bars, frozen, 100% juice	1 bar (3 oz)	1 C
Fruit snacks, chewy (pureed fruit concentrate)	1 roll (3/4 oz)	1 C
Fruit spreads, 100% fruit	1 Tbsp	1 C
Gelatin, regular	1/2 cup	1 C
Gingersnaps	3	1 C
Granola bar	1 bar	1 C, 1 F
Granola bar, fat-free	1 bar	2 C
Hummus	1/3 cup	1 C, 1 F
Ice cream	1/2 cup	1 C, 2 F
Ice cream, light	1/2 cup	1 C, 1 F
Ice cream, fat-free, no sugar added	1/2 cup	1 C
Jam or jelly, regular	1 Tbsp	1 C
Milk, chocolate, whole	1 cup	2 C, 1 F
Pie, fruit, 2 crusts	1/6 pie	3 C, 2 F
Pie, pumpkin or custard	1/8 pie	1 C, 2 F
Potato chips	12–18 (1 oz)	1 C, 2 F
Pudding, regular (made with low-fat milk)	1/2 cup	2 C
Pudding, sugar-free (made with low-fat milk)	1/2 cup	1 C
Salad dressing, fat-free†	1/4 cup	1 C
Sherbert, sorbet	1/2 cup	2 C
Spaghetti or pasta sauce, canned†	1/2 cup	1 C, 1 F
Sweet roll or Danish	1 (2 1/2 oz)	2 1/2 C, 2 F
Syrup, light	2 Tbsp	1 C
Syrup, regular	1 Tbsp	1 C
Syrup, regular	1/4 cup	4 C
Tortilla chips	6–12 (1 oz)	1 C, 2 F
Yogurt, frozen, low-fat, fat-free	1/3 cup	1 C, 0–1 F
Yogurt, frozen, fat-free, no sugar added	1/2 cup	1 C
Yogurt, low-fat with fruit	1 cup	3 C, 0–1 F
Vanilla wafers	5	1 C, 1 F

† = 400 mg or more of sodium per serving
* C = carbohydrate exchange; F = fat exchange

Continued

TABLE 2-22 The exchange lists for meal planning—cont'd

Vegetable list

One vegetable exchange equals 5 g carbohydrate, 2 g protein, 0 g fat, and 25 calories.

Vegetables that contain small amounts of carbohydrates and calories are on this list. Vegetables contain important nutrients. Try to eat at least 2 to 3 vegetable choices each day. In general, one vegetable exchange is:

- 1/2 cup of cooked vegetables or vegetable juice.
- 1 cup of raw vegetables.

If you eat 1 or 2 vegetable choices at a meal or snack, you do not have to count the calories or carbohydrates because they contain small amounts of these nutrients.

Nutrition tips

1. Fresh and frozen vegetables have less added salt than canned vegetables. Drain and rinse canned vegetables if you want to remove some salt.
2. Choose more dark green and dark yellow vegetables such as spinach, broccoli, romaine lettuce, carrots, chilies, and peppers.
3. Broccoli, brussels sprouts, cauliflower, greens, peppers, spinach, and tomatoes are good sources of vitamin C.
4. Vegetables contain 1 to 4 grams of fiber per serving.

Selection tips

1. A 1-cup portion of broccoli is a portion about the size of a light bulb.
2. Tomato sauce is different from spaghetti sauce, which is on the other carbohydrates list.
3. Canned vegetables and juices are available without added salt.
4. If you eat more than 4 cups of raw vegetables or 2 cups of cooked vegetables at one meal, count them as 1 carbohydrate choice.
5. Starchy vegetables such as corn, peas, winter squash, and potatoes that contain larger amounts of calories and carbohydrates are on the starch list.

Artichoke
Artichoke hearts
Asparagus
Beans (green, wax, Italian)
Bean sprouts
Beets
Broccoli
Brussels sprouts
Cabbage
Carrots
Cauliflower
Celery
Cucumber
Eggplant
Green onions or scallions
Greens (collard, kale, mustard, turnip)
Kohlrabi
Leeks
Mixed vegetables (without corn, peas, or pasta)
Mushrooms
Okra
Onions
Pea pods
Peppers (all varieties)
Radishes
Salad greens (endive, escarole, lettuce, romaine, spinach)

TABLE 2-22 The exchange lists for meal planning—cont'd

Vegetable list—cont'd

Selection tips—cont'd

Sauerkraut*
Spinach
Summer squash
Tomato
Tomatoes, canned
Tomato sauce*
Tomato/vegetable juice*
Turnips
Water chestnuts
Watercress
Zucchini

* = 400 mg or more sodium per exchange

Meat and meat substitutes list

Meat and meat substitutes that contain both protein and fat are on this list. In general, one meat exchange is:

- 1 oz of meat, fish, poultry, or cheese.
- 1/2 cup dried beans.

Based on the amount of fat they contain, meats are divided into very lean, lean, medium-fat, and high-fat lists. This is done so you can see which ones contain the least amount of fat. One ounce (one exchange) of each of these includes:

	Carbohydrate (g)	Protein (g)	Fat (g)	Calories
Very lean	0	7	0–1	35
Lean	0	7	3	55
Medium-fat	0	7	5	75
High-fat	0	7	8	100

Nutrition tips

1. Choose very lean and lean meat choices whenever possible. Items from the high-fat group are high in saturated fat, cholesterol, and calories and can raise blood cholesterol levels.
2. Meats do not have any fiber.
3. Dried beans, peas, and lentils are good sources of fiber.
4. Some processed meats, seafood, and soy products may contain carbohydrate when consumed in large amounts. Check the nutrition facts on the label to see if the amount is close to 15 g. If so, count it as a carbohydrate choice as well as a meat choice.

Selection tips

1. Weigh meat after cooking and removing bones and fat. Four ounces of raw meat is equal to 3 ounces of cooked meat. Some examples of meat portions are:
   - 1 ounce cheese = 1 meat choice and is about the size of a 1-inch cube
   - 2 ounces meat = 2 meat choices such as 1 small chicken leg or thigh, 1/2 cup cottage cheese or tuna
   - 3 ounces meat = 3 meat choices and is about the size of a deck of cards, such as 1 medium pork chop, 1 small hamburger, 1/2 of a whole chicken breast, 1 unbreaded fish fillet
2. Limit your choices from the high-fat group to three times per week or less.

Continued

TABLE 2-22 The exchange lists for meal planning—cont'd

Meat and meat substitutes list—cont'd

Selection tips—cont'd

3. Most grocery stores stock Select and Choice grades of meat. Select grades of meat are the leanest meats. Choice grades contain a moderate amount of fat, and Prime cuts of meat have the highest amount of fat. Restaurants usually serve Prime cuts of meat.
4. "Hamburger" may contain added seasoning and fat, but ground beef does not.
5. Read labels to find products that are low in fat and cholesterol (5 g or less of fat per serving).
6. Dried beans, peas, and lentils are also found on the starch list.
7. Peanut butter, in smaller amounts, is also found on the fats list.
8. Bacon, in smaller amounts, is also found on the fats list.

Meal planning tips

1. Bake, roast, broil, grill, poach, steam, or boil these foods rather than fry.
2. Place meat on a rack so that fat will drain off during cooking.
3. Use nonstick spray and a nonstick pan to brown or fry foods.
4. Trim off visible fat before or after cooking.
5. If you add flour, bread crumbs, coating mixes, fat, or marinades when cooking, ask your dietitian how to count it in your meal plan.

Very lean meat and substitutes list

One exchange equals 0 g carbohydrate, 7 g protein, 0–1 g fat, and 35 calories.
One very lean meat exchange is equal to any one of the following items:

Poultry:	Chicken or turkey (white meat, no skin), Cornish hen (no skin)	1 oz
Fish:	Fresh or frozen cod, flounder, haddock, halibut, trout; tuna fresh or canned in water	1 oz
Shellfish:	Clams, crab, lobster, scallops, shrimp, imitation shellfish	1 oz
Game:	Duck or pheasant (no skin), venison, buffalo, ostrich	1 oz
Cheese:	(1 g or less fat per ounce)	
	Nonfat or low-fat cottage cheese	1/4 cup
	Fat-free cheese	1 oz
Other:	Processed sandwich meats with 1 g or less fat per ounce such as deli thin, shaved meats, chipped beef,* turkey ham	1 oz
	Egg whites	2
	Egg substitutes, plain	1/4 cup
	Hot dogs with 1 g or less fat per ounce	1 oz
	Kidney (high in cholesterol)	1 oz
	Sausage with 1 g or less fat per ounce	1 oz
Count as one very lean meat and one starch exchange		
Dried beans, peas, lentils (cooked)		1/2 cup

* = 400 mg or more sodium per exchange

TABLE 2-22 The exchange lists for meal planning—cont'd

Meat and meat substitutes list—cont'd

Lean meat and substitutes list

One exchange equals 0 g carbohydrate, 7 g protein, 3 g fat, and 55 calories.
One lean meat exchange is equal to any one of the following items:

Beef:	USDA Select or Choice grades of lean beef trimmed of fat, such as round, sirloin, and flank steak; tenderloin; roast (rib, chuck, rump); steak (T-bone, porterhouse, cubed), ground round	1 oz
Pork:	Lean pork such as fresh ham; canned, cured, or boiled ham; Canadian bacon,* tenderloin, center loin chop	1 oz
Lamb:	Roast, chop, leg	1 oz
Veal:	Lean chop, roast	1 oz
Poultry:	Chicken, turkey (dark meat, no skin), chicken white meat (with skin), domestic duck or goose (well-drained of fat, no skin)	1 oz
Fish:	Herring (uncreamed or smoked)	1 oz
	Oysters	6 medium
	Salmon (fresh or canned), catfish	1 oz
	Sardines (canned)	2 medium
	Tuna (canned in oil, drained)	1 oz
Game:	Goose (no skin), rabbit	1 oz
Cheese:	4.5%-fat cottage cheese	1/4 cup
	Grated parmesan	2 Tbsp
	Cheeses with 3 g or less fat per ounce	1 oz
Other:	Hot dogs with 3 g or less fat per ounce*	1 1/2 oz
	Processed sandwich meat with 3 g or less fat per ounce such as turkey, pastrami, or kielbasa	1 oz
	Liver, heart (high in cholesterol)	1 oz

* = 400 mg or more sodium per exchange

Medium-fat meat and substitutes list

One exchange equals 0 g carbohydrate, 7 g protein, 5 g fat, and 75 calories.
One medium-fat meat exchange is equal to any one of the following items:

Beef:	Most beef products fall into this category (ground beef, meatloaf, corned beef, short ribs, Prime grades of meat trimmed of fat such as prime rib)	1 oz
Pork:	Top loin, chop, Boston butt, cutlet	1 oz
Lamb:	Rib roast, ground	1 oz
Veal:	Cutlet (ground or cubed, unbreaded)	1 oz
Poultry:	Chicken dark meat (with skin), ground turkey or ground chicken, fried chicken (with skin)	1 oz
Fish:	Any fried fish product	1 oz
Cheese:	(5 g or less fat per ounce)	
	Feta	1 oz
	Mozzarella	1 oz
	Ricotta	1/4 cup (2 oz)

Continued

TABLE 2-22 The exchange lists for meal planning—cont'd

Meat and meat substitutes list—cont'd

Medium-fat meat and substitutes list—cont'd

Other:	Egg (high in cholesterol, limit to 3 per week)	1
	Sausage with 5 g or less fat per ounce	1 oz
	Soy milk	1 cup
	Tempeh	1/4 cup
	Tofu	4 oz or 1/2 cup

High-fat meat and substitutes list

One exchange equals 0 g carbohydrate, 7 g protein, 8 g fat, and 100 calories.

Remember these items are high in saturated fat, cholesterol, and calories and may raise blood cholesterol level if eaten on a regular basis. One high-fat meat exchange is equal to any one of the following items:

Pork:	Spareribs, ground pork, pork sausage	1 oz
Cheese:	All regular cheeses such as American,* cheddar, Monterey Jack, Swiss	1 oz
Other:	Processed sandwich meats with 8 g or less fat per ounce such as bologna, pimento loaf, salami	1 oz
	Sausage such as bratwurst, Italian, knockwurst, Polish, smoked	1 oz
	Hot dog (turkey or chicken)	1 (10/lb)
	Bacon	3 slices (20 slices/lb)

Count as one high-fat meat plus one fat exchange.

Hot dog (beef, pork, or combination)*	1 (10/lb)
Peanut butter (contains unsaturated fat)	2 Tbsp

* = 400 mg or more sodium per exchange

Fat list

Fats are divided into three groups based on the main type of fatty acids they contain: monounsaturated, polyunsaturated, and saturated. Small amounts of monounsaturated and polyunsaturated fats in the foods we eat are linked with good health benefits. Saturated fats are linked with heart disease and cancer. In general, one fat exchange is:

- 1 teaspoon of regular margarine or vegetable oil.
- 1 tablespoon of regular salad dressings.

Nutrition tips

1. All fats are high in calories. Limit serving sizes for good nutrition and health.
2. Nuts and seeds contain small amounts of fiber, protein, and magnesium.
3. If blood pressure is a concern, choose fats in the unsalted form, such as unsalted peanuts, to help lower sodium intake.

TABLE 2-22 The exchange lists for meal planning—cont'd

Fat list—cont'd

Selection tips

1. Check the nutrition facts on food labels for serving sizes. One fat exchange is based on serving size containing 5 g of fat.
2. When selecting regular margarine, choose those with liquid vegetable oil as the first ingredient. Soft margarine are not as saturated as stick margarine. Soft margarines are healthier choices. Avoid those listing hydrogenated or partially hydrogenated fat as the first ingredient.
3. When selecting low-fat margarines, look for liquid vegetable oil as the second ingredient. Water is usually the first ingredient.
4. When used in smaller amounts, bacon and peanut butter are counted as fat choices. When used in larger amounts, they are counted as high-fat meat choices.
5. Fat-free salad dressings are on the other carbohydrates list and the free foods list.
6. See the free foods list for nondairy coffee creamers, whipped topping, and fat-free products, such as margarines, salad dressings, mayonnaise, sour cream, cream cheese, and nonstick cooking spray.

Monounsaturated fats list

One fat exchange equals 5 g fat and 45 calories.

Avocado, medium	1/8 (1 oz)
Oil (canola, olive, peanut)	1 tsp
Olives: ripe (black)	8 large
green, stuffed*	10 large
Nuts	
almonds, cashews	6 nuts
mixed (50% peanuts)	6 nuts
peanuts	10 nuts
pecans	4 halves
Peanut butter, smooth or crunchy	2 tsp
Sesame seeds	1 Tbsp
Tahini paste	2 tsp

* = 400 mg or more sodium per exchange

Polyunsaturated fats list

One fat exchange equals 5 g fat and 45 calories.

Margarine: stick, tub, or squeeze	1 tsp
lower-fat (30%–50% vegetable oil)	1 Tbsp
Mayonnaise: regular	1 tsp
reduced-fat	1 Tbsp
Nuts, walnuts, English	4 halves
Oil (corn, safflower, soybean)	1 tsp
Salad dressing: regular*	1 Tbsp
reduced-fat	2 Tbsp
Miracle Whip Salad Dressing®: regular	2 tsp
reduced-fat	1 Tbsp
Seeds (pumpkin, sunflower)	1 Tbsp

* = 400 mg or more sodium per exchange

Continued

TABLE 2-22 The exchange lists for meal planning—cont'd

Fat list—cont'd	
Saturated fats list*	
One fat exchange equals 5 g fat and 45 calories.	
Bacon, cooked	1 slice (20 slices/lb)
Bacon, grease	1 tsp
Butter: stick	1 tsp
whipped	2 tsp
reduced-fat	1 Tbsp
Chitterlings, boiled	2 Tbsp (1/2 oz)
Coconut, sweetened, shredded	2 Tbsp
Cream, half and half	2 Tbsp
Cream cheese: regular	1 Tbsp (1/2 oz)
reduced-fat	2 Tbsp (1 oz)
Fatback or salt pork†	
Shortening or lard	1 tsp
Sour cream: regular	2 Tbsp
reduced-fat	3 Tbsp

*Saturated fats can raise blood cholesterol levels.

†Use a piece 1 in. × 1 in. × 1/4 in. if you plan to eat the fatback cooked with vegetables. Use a piece 2 in. × 1 in. × 1/2 in. when eating only the vegetables with the fatback removed.

Free foods list

A *free food* is any food or drink that contains less than 20 calories or less than 5 g of carbohydrate per serving. Foods with a serving size listed should be limited to three servings per day. Be sure to spread them out throughout the day. If you eat all three servings at one time, it could affect your blood glucose level. Foods listed without a serving size can be eaten as often as you like.

Fat-free or reduced-fat foods	
Cream cheese, fat free	1 Tbsp
Creamers, nondairy, liquid	1 Tbsp
Creamers, nondairy, powdered	2 tsp
Mayonnaise, fat-free	1 Tbsp
Mayonnaise, reduce-fat	1 tsp
Margarine, fat-free	4 Tbsp
Margarine, reduced-fat	1 tsp
Miracle Whip®, nonfat	1 Tbsp
Miracle Whip®, reduced-fat	1 tsp
Nonstick cooking spray	
Salad dressing, fat-free	1 Tbsp
Salad dressing, fat-free, Italian	2 Tbsp
Salsa	1/4 cup
Sour cream, fat-free, reduced-fat	1 Tbsp
Whipped topping, regular or light	2 Tbsp

TABLE 2-22 The exchange lists for meal planning—cont'd

Free foods list—cont'd	
Sugar-free or low-sugar foods	
Candy, hard, sugar-free	1 candy
Gelatin dessert, sugar-free	
Gelatin, unflavored	
Gum, sugar-free	
Jam or jelly, low-sugar or light	2 tsp
Sugar substitutes*	
Syrup, sugar-free	2 Tbsp

*Sugar substitutes, alternatives, or replacements that are approved by the Food and Drug Administration are safe to use. Common brand names include:

- Equal® (aspartame)
- Sprinkle Sweet® (saccharin)
- Sweet One® (acesulfame K)
- Sweet-10® (saccharine)
- Sugar Twin® (saccharin)
- Sweet 'n Low® (saccharin)

Drinks	
Bouillon, broth, consomme*	
Bouillon or broth, low sodium	
Carbonated or mineral water	
Cocoa powder, unsweetened	1 Tbsp
Coffee	
Club soda	
Diet soft drinks, sugar-free	
Drink mixes, sugar-free	
Tea	
Tonic water, sugar-free	
Condiments	
Catsup	1 Tbsp
Horseradish	
Lemon juice	
Lime juice	
Mustard	
Pickles, dill*	1 1/2 large
Soy sauce, regular or light*	
Taco sauce	1 Tbsp
Vinegar	

Continued

TABLE 2-22 The exchange lists for meal planning—cont'd

Free foods list—cont'd

Seasonings

Be careful with seasonings that contain sodium or are salts, such as garlic or celery salt and lemon pepper.

Flavoring extracts
Garlic
Herbs, fresh or dried
Pimento
Spices
Tabasco® or hot pepper sauce
Wine, used in cooking
Worcestershire sauce

* = 400 mg or more of sodium per choice.

Combination foods list

Many of the foods we eat are mixed together in various combinations. These combination foods do not fit into any one exchange list. Often it is hard to tell what is in a casserole dish or prepared food item. This is a list of exchanges for some typical combination foods. This list will help you fit these foods into your meal plan. Ask you dietitian for information about any other combination foods you would like to eat.

Food	Serving size	Exchanges per serving*
Entrees		
Tuna noodle casserole, lasagna, spaghetti with meatballs, chili with beans, macaroni and cheese†	1 cup (8 oz)	2 C, 2 MFM
Chow mein (without noodles or rice)	2 cups (16 oz)	1 C, 2 LM
Pizza, cheese, thin crust†	1/4 of 10 in. (5 oz)	2 C, 2 MFM, 1 F
Pizza, meat topping, thin crust†	1/4 of 10 in. (5 oz)	2 C, 2 MFM, 2 F
Pot pie†	1 (7 oz)	2 C, 1 MFM, 4 F
Frozen entrees		
Salisbury steak with gravy, mashed potato	1 (11 oz)	2 C, 3 MFM, 3–4 F
Turkey with gravy, mashed potato, dressing	1 (11 0z)	2 C, 2 MFM, 2 F
Entree with less than 300 calories	1 (8 oz)	2 C, 3 LM

TABLE 2-22 The exchange lists for meal planning—cont'd

Combination Foods List—cont'd

Food	Serving size	Exchanges per serving*
Soups		
Bean†	1 cup	1 C, 1 VLM
Cream (made with water)†	1 cup (8 oz)	1 C, 1 F
Split pea (made with water)†	1/2 cup (4 oz)	1 C
Tomato (made with water)†	1 cup (8 oz)	1 C
Vegetable beef, chicken noodle, or other broth-type	1 cup (8 oz)	1 C

* C = carbohydrate exchange; VLM = very-lean meat exchange; LM = lean meat exchange; MFM = medium-fat meat exchange; F = fat exchange.

† = 400 mg or more sodium per exchange.

Fast foods*

Food	Serving size	Exchanges per serving†
Burritos with beef‡	2	4 C, 2 MFM, 2 F
Chicken nuggets‡	6	1 C, 2 MFM, 1 F
Chicken breast and wing, breaded and fried	1 each	1 C, 4 MFM, 2 F
Fish sandwich/tartar sauce‡	1	3 C, 1 MFM, 3 F
French fries, thin	20–25	2 C, 2 F
Hamburger, regular	1	2 C, 2 MFM
Hamburger, large‡	1	2 C, 3 MFM, 1 F
Hot dog with bun‡	1	1 C, 1 HFM, 1 F
Individual pan pizza‡	1	5 C, 3 MFM, 3 F
Soft-serve cone	1 medium	2 C, 1 F
Submarine sandwich‡	1 sub (6 inch)	3 C, 1 V, 2 MFM, 1 F
Taco, hard shell‡	1 (6 oz)	2 C, 2 MFM, 2 F
Taco, soft shell‡	1 (3 oz)	1 C, 1 MFM, 1 F

*Ask at your fast-food restaurant for nutrition information about your favorite fast foods.

† C = carbohydrate exchange; MFM = medium-fat meat exchange; HFM = high-fat meat exchange; F = fat exchange; V = vegetable exchange

‡ = 400 mg or more sodium per serving

The Exchange Lists are the basis of a meal planning system designed by a committee of the American Diabetes Association and the American Dietetic Association. While designed primarily for people with diabetes and others who must follow special diets, the Exchange Lists are based on principles of good nutrition that apply to everyone.

TABLE 2-23 Sample meal patterns using the exchange lists for meal planning

	1500 kilocalorie diet with two snacks				
	Breakfast	Lunch	Snack	Dinner	Snack
Starch	2	2	½	2	½
Meat, medium-fat	1	2	1	2	
Vegetable		1		1	
Fruit	1	1		1	
Milk, skim	½	½			½
Fat	1	1		1	
		Kcal	Carbohydrate	Protein	Fat
Total		1510	178 g	79 g	45 g
Percent of energy			50	22	28
	2000 kilocalorie diet with two snacks				
	Breakfast	Lunch	Snack	Dinner	Snack
Starch	2	2	½	3	½
Meat, medium-fat	1	2	1	2	1
Vegetable		1		2	
Fruit	2	2		2	
Milk, skim	1	1		1	
Fat	1	1		1	
		Kcal	Carbohydrate	Protein	Fat
Total		2005	261 g	103 g	50 g
Percent of energy			55	22	23
	2500 kilocalorie diet with two snacks				
	Breakfast	Lunch	Snack	Dinner	Snack
Starch	3	3	1	4	1
Meat, medium-fat	1	3	1	3	1
Vegetable		2		2	
Fruit	2	2		2	
Milk, skim	1	1		1	
Fat	1	1		1	
		Kcal	Carbohydrate	Protein	Fat
Total		2500	326 g	131 g	60 g
Percent of energy			55	22	23

SUMMARY

1. A number of tools and methods are available for nutrition professionals to use in evaluating dietary intakes of individuals and groups. Included among these are standards of recommended nutrient intake, measurements of nutrient density, dietary guidelines or goals, and food guides.
2. With a few exceptions, dietary standards up until the twentieth century were observational and lacked a firm scientific base. Advances in metabolic, vitamin, and mineral research during the early twentieth century led to the establishment of scientifically based estimates of human nutrient requirements by the League of Nations and several European countries, Canada, and the United States.
3. One of the earliest and most familiar of the dietary standards is the Recommended Dietary Allowance (RDA), developed in the United States by the Food and Nutrition Board of the National Research Council. RDAs provide specific nutrient intake recommendations for groups based on sex, age, pregnancy, and lactation. They are designed to be used primarily by nutrition professionals who are familiar with the complexities of their practical application.
4. The RDAs are revised approximately every 5 years by a group of distinguished nutrition scientists. Revision involves thoroughly reviewing the nutritional literature, estimating nutrient requirement, creating a safety margin to allow for individual variations in nutrient requirements, and drafting a report, which is scrupulously reviewed before being published.
5. The RDAs are not intended to be met by relying on fortified foods or supplements but on a diet composed of a variety of foods from diverse food groups. Such a diet probably will be adequate in all other nutrients for which RDAs cannot currently be established because of insufficient information.
6. Although the RDAs are a useful standard in evaluating the usual dietary intake of groups and individuals, they cannot provide sufficient information to determine the nutritional status of individuals or population groups. Such information can be obtained only when dietary intake data are combined with laboratory, anthropomorphic, and clinical measures.
7. To cover the needs of practically all healthy people, the RDAs exceed the requirements of most people (except for energy). To prevent nutrient intakes from being erroneously classified as deficient when in reality they are adequate (false positives), a fixed cutoff point of two thirds or three fourths of the RDA is used by some nutritionists as an acceptable standard. This method increases the chance that inadequate intakes are classified as adequate (false negatives) and is inferior to the probability approach.
8. The probability approach is based on the likelihood that persons with a specific nutrient intake level would fail to meet their requirement for that nutrient. It does not identify individuals having inadequate intakes, only the prevalence or proportion of the population with inadequate intakes.
9. A major weakness of the RDA is its failure to address the relationship between diet and chronic disease. In the future the National Research Council plans a major revision of the RDA, including nutrient and food component recommendations for the prevention of chronic disease.
10. In the nutrient density approach, recommended nutrient intakes and nutritional composition of foods are expressed in terms of nutrient quantity per 1000 kcal. It allows the nutritional qualities of foods and diets to be evaluated and compared easily, facilitates meal planning, addresses the issue of overconsumption, and allows the nutritive value of foods to be evaluated with respect to their caloric content.

11. The index of nutritional quality (INQ) of a food equals the amount of a nutrient in 1000 kcal of that food divided by the recommended allowance of that nutrient per 1000 kcal. A food with an overall INQ substantially greater than "1" has a high nutrient density and provides important nutrients in excess of calories.
12. Dietary guidelines or goals are dietary standards primarily intended to address the more common and pressing nutrition-related health problems of chronic disease. They often are expressed as nonquantitative change from the present average national diet or from people's typical eating habits.
13. Since the late 1960s, numerous dietary guidelines have been issued by Western governments and various health organizations. Overall, they have consistently called for maintenance of healthy body weight, decreased consumption of fat (especially saturated fat), increased consumption of complex carbohydrates, and use of alcoholic beverages in moderation, if at all.
14. U.S. health objectives for the year 2000 are outlined in the publication *Healthy People 2000*. The report contains 300 objectives, 21 of which specifically deal with nutrition. It sets important and specific standards for improving personal nutrition and health and for gauging the nation's progress toward health for all.
15. Nutrition labeling in the United States began in 1973 when the Food and Drug Administration established the U.S. Recommended Daily Allowances (U.S. RDAs). In 1990, Congress passed the Nutrition Labeling and Education Act, which made sweeping changes in nutrition labeling regulations, replaced the U.S. RDAs with the Reference Daily Intakes (RDIs), and established the Daily Reference Values (DRVs). The RDIs and DRVs are collectively referred to as the Daily Values.
16. Food guides are nutrition education tools that translate dietary standards and recommendations into understandable and practical forms for use by those who have little or no training in nutrition. Generally, foods are classified into groups according to similarity of nutrient content. If a certain number of servings from each group are consumed, a balanced and adequate diet is thought likely to result.
17. The food exchange system simplifies meal planning for persons limiting energy consumption and helps insure adequate nutrient intake. Originally developed to facilitate meal planning for persons with diabetes, it is easily adapted to personal food preferences and is useful for quickly approximating kilocalorie and macronutrient levels in foods. The specified serving sizes of foods within each exchange list are approximately equal in their contribution of energy and macronutrients.
18. With the help of a dietitian, people can develop an easily followed meal plan to control energy intake in which the number of servings to be selected from the various exchange lists for each meal is outlined. Meal planning simply involves selecting the correct number of servings from each list and observing the specified serving size.

REFERENCES

1. Leitch I. 1942. The evolution of dietary standards. *Nutrition Abstracts and Reviews* 11:509–521.
2. Harper AE. 1985. Origin of recommended dietary allowances—an historic overview. *American Journal of Clinical Nutrition* 41:140–148.
3. McCollum EV. 1957. *A History of Nutrition*. Boston: Houghton Mifflin.
4. Todhunter EN. 1976. Chronology of some events in the development and application of the science of nutrition. *Nutrition Reviews* 34:353–365.
5. Roberts LJ. 1958. Beginnings of the Recommended Dietary Allowances. *Journal of the American Dietetic Association* 34:903–908.
6. Miller DF, Voris L. 1969. Chronologic changes in the Recommended Dietary Allowances. *Journal of the American Dietetic Association* 54:109–117.

7. Committee on Food and Nutrition, National Research Council. 1941. Recommended allowances for the various dietary essentials. *Journal of the American Dietetic Association* 17:565–567.
8. Food and Nutrition Board, National Research Council. 1989. *Recommended Dietary Allowances,* 10th ed. Washington, DC: National Academy Press.
9. Smith J, Turner JS. 1986. A perspective on the history and use of the Recommended Dietary Allowances. *Currents* 2(1):4–11.
10. Truswell AS. 1987. Evolution of dietary recommendations, goals, and guidelines. *American Journal of Clinical Nutrition* 45:1060–1072.
11. Health and Welfare Canada. 1990. *Nutrition recommendations.* Ottawa: Canadian Government Publishing Centre.
12. Department of Health. 1991. *Dietary reference values for food energy and nutrients for the United Kingdom.* London: Her Majesty's Stationery Office.
13. Guthrie HA. 1985. The 1985 Recommended Dietary Allowance Committee: An overview. *Journal of the American Dietetic Association* 85:1646–1648.
14. National Research Council. 1986. *Nutrient adequacy: Assessment using food consumption surveys.* Washington, DC: National Academy Press.
15. Beaton GH. 1985. Uses and limits of the use of the Recommended Dietary Allowances for evaluating dietary intake data. *American Journal of Clinical Nutrition* 41:155–164.
16. Leverton RM. 1975. The RDAs are not for amateurs. *Journal of the American Dietetic Association* 66:9–11.
17. Harper AE. 1974. Recommended Dietary Allowances: Are they what we think they are? *Journal of the American Dietetic Association* 64:151–156.
18. Habicht JP. 1980. Some characteristics of indicators of nutritional status for use in screening and surveillance. *American Journal of Clinical Nutrition* 33:531–535.
19. U.S. Department of Health and Human Services. 1989. *Nutrition monitoring in the United States—An update report on nutrition monitoring.* Washington, DC: U.S. Government Printing Office.
20. Hegsted DM. 1993. Nutrition standards for today. *Nutrition Today* 28(2):34–36.
21. Lachance P, Langseth L. 1994. The RDA concept: Time for a change? *Nutrition Reviews* 52:266–270.
22. Press F. 1985. Postponement of the 10th edition of the RDAs. *Journal of the American Dietetic Association* 85:1644–1645.
23. Food and Nutrition Board. 1994. *How should the recommended dietary allowances be revised?* Washington, DC: National Academy Press.
24. Food and Nutrition Board. 1994. How should the Recommended Dietary Allowances be revised? A concept paper from the Food and Nutrition Board. *Nutrition Reviews* 52:216–219.
25. Hansen RG, Wyse BW. 1980. Expression of nutrient allowances per 1,000 kilocalories. *Journal of the American Dietetic Association* 76:223–227.
26. Hansen RG, Windham CT, Wyse BW. 1985. Nutrient density and food labeling. *Clinical Nutrition* 4:164–170.
27. Wyse BW, Windham CT, Hansen RG. 1985. Nutrition intervention: Panacea or Pandora's box? *Journal of the American Dietetic Association* 85:1084–1090.
28. Wretlind A. 1982. Standards for nutritional adequacy of the diet: European and WHO/FAO viewpoints. *American Journal of Clinical Nutrition* 36:366–375.
29. Windham CT, Wyse BW, Hansen RG. 1983. Nutrient density of diets in the USDA Nationwide Food Consumption Survey, 1977–1978. II. Adequacy of nutrient density consumption practices. *Journal of the American Dietetic Association* 82:34–43.
30. Patterson RE, Hainses PS, Popkin BM. 1994. Diet Quality Index: Capturing a multidimensional behavior. *Journal of the American Dietetic Association* 94:57–64.
31. Food and Nutrition Board, National Research Council. 1989. *Diet and health: Implications for reducing chronic disease risk.* Washington, DC: National Academy Press.
32. Berger S. 1987. The implementation of dietary guidelines—ways and difficulties. *American Journal of Clinical Nutrition* 45:1383–1389.
33. Truswell AS. 1994. Dietary goals and guidelines: National and international perspectives. In Shils ME, Olson JA, Shike M, eds. *Modern nutrition in health and disease,* 8th ed. Philadelphia: Lea & Febiger.

34. Select Committee on Nutrition and Human Needs, U.S. Senate. 1977. *Dietary Goals for the United States*. Washington, DC: U.S. Government Printing Office.
35. Twenty commentaries. 1977. *Nutrition Today* 12(6): 10–27.
36. Additional commentaries. 1978. *Nutrition Today* 13(1):30–32.
37. U.S. Department of Agriculture/U.S. Department of Health and Human Services. 1980. *Nutrition and your health: Dietary Guidelines for Americans*. Washington, DC: U.S. Government Printing Office.
38. U.S. Department of Agriculture/U.S. Department of Health and Human Services. 1985. *Nutrition and your health: Dietary Guidelines for Americans,* 2nd ed. Washington, DC: U.S. Government Printing Office.
39. U.S. Department of Agriculture/U.S. Department of Health and Human Services. 1990. *Nutrition and your health: Dietary Guidelines for Americans,* 3rd ed. Washington, DC: U.S. Government Printing Office.
40. Dietary Guidelines Advisory Committee. 1990. Report of the Dietary Guidelines Advisory Committee on the Dietary Guidelines for Americans, 1990. Hyattsville, Md: U.S. Department of Agriculture, Human Nutrition Information Service.
41. Food and Nutrition Board, National Research Council. 1980. *Toward healthful diets*. Washington, DC: National Academy Press.
42. U.S. Department of Health and Human Services. 1988. The Surgeon General's Report on Nutrition and Health. Washington, DC: U.S. Government Printing Office.
43. Nestle M. 1988. The Surgeon General's report on nutrition and health: New federal dietary guidance policy. *Journal of Nutrition Education* 20:252–254.
44. McGinnis JM, Nestle M. 1989. The Surgeon General's report on nutrition and health: Policy implications and implementation strategies. *American Journal of Clinical Nutrition* 49:23–28.
45. Food and Nutrition Board. 1991. *Improving America's diet and health: From recommendations to action*. Washington, DC: National Academy Press.
46. Food and Nutrition Board. 1992. *Eat for life: The food and nutrition board's guide to reducing your risk of chronic disease*. Washington, DC: National Academy Press.
47. U.S. Department of Health and Human Services. 1990. *Healthy People 2000: National Health Promotion and Disease Prevention Objectives*. Washington, DC: U.S. Government Printing Office.
48. U.S. Department of Health and Human Services. 1980. *Promoting health/preventing disease: Objectives for the nation*. Washington, DC: U.S. Government Printing Office.
49. Haughton B, Gussow JD, Dodds JM. 1987. An historical study of the underlying assumptions for United States Food Guides from 1971 through the Basic Four Food Group Guide. *Journal of Nutrition Education* 19:169–175.
50. Welsh SO, Davis C, Shaw A. 1993. USDA's Food Guide: Background and Development. Hyattsville, Md: U.S. Department of Agriculture, Human Nutrition Information Service.
51. Welsh S, Davis C, Shaw A. 1992. A brief history of food guides in the United States. *Nutrition Today* 27(6):6–11.
52. Combs GF. 1991. What's happening at USDA. *American Institute of Nutrition Notes* 27(3):6.
53. Anonymous. 1991. Official blows whistle on pyramid cancellation. *Community Nutrition Institute Nutrition Week* 21(46):6–7.
54. Nestle M. 1994. The politics of dietary guidance—a new opportunity. *American Journal of Public Health* 84: 713–715.
55. Nestle M. 1993. Food lobbies, the food pyramid, and U.S. nutrition policy. *International Journal of Health Services* 23:483–496.
56. Burros M. 1991. U.S. delays issuing nutrition chart. *New York Times,* April 27, p. A9.
57. Toufexis A. 1991. Playing politics with our food. *Time* 138(2):57–58.
58. Willett WC. 1994. Diet and health: what should we eat? *Science* 264:532–537.
59. Caso EK. 1950. Calculation of diabetic diets. *Journal of the American Dietetic Association* 26:575–583.

Assessment Activity 2-1

USING STANDARDS TO EVALUATE NUTRIENT INTAKE

Whether they are the recommended nutrient intakes (RNIs) from Canada, the reference nutrient intakes from the United Kingdom, or the recommended dietary allowances (RDAs) from America, nutrient standards are indispensable in establishing a benchmark from which to assess adequacy of nutrient intake. This activity will help you become familiar with the RNIs and the RDAs as you assess a defined diet and compare results from these various standards.

Table 2-24 shows mean intakes for five nutrients and energy by women age 20 to 49 years from the 1985–86 Continuing Survey of Food Intake by Individuals (see Chapter 4). The data were averaged from 24-hour dietary recalls conducted on 4 nonconsecutive days.

1. Locate the recommended intakes of the five nutrients and energy for females from the recommended nutrient intake tables for the United States (25–50 years old, Tables 2-2 and 2-3), Canada (25–49 years old, Appendix B), and the United Kingdom (19–50 years old, Appendix A). Record these in Table 2-24 in the appropriate "Standard" columns. (Note that values present in one table may not be found in another; enter "N/A" for any missing values.)
2. Calculate how intakes compare with each standard by using the following formula. Enter the percent of standard value in the appropriate "Percent of Standard" columns in Table 2-24.

$$\text{Percent of standard} = \frac{\text{Intake of certain nutrient}}{\text{Recommended level of intake for that nutrient}}$$

3. Which of the average nutrient intakes are greater than recommended? Which are lower than recommended?
4. Note that recommended nutrient levels vary among countries. The intake of calcium, for example, may exceed the recommended intake level of one country but not that of another.

TABLE 2-24 Mean intakes of selected nutrients and energy of U.S. females 20–49 years old and how they compare with Canadian, United Kingdom, and U.S. nutrient intake standards

		Canada		United Kingdom		United States	
Nutrient	Mean intake*	Standard	Percent of standard	Standard	Percent of standard	Standard	Percent of standard
Energy	1517 kcal	______	______	______	______	______	______
Protein	61 g	______	______	______	______	______	______
Vitamin C	78 mg	______	______	______	______	______	______
Folate	193 µg	______	______	______	______	______	______
Calcium	630 mg	______	______	______	______	______	______
Iron	10.1 mg	______	______	______	______	______	______

*From U.S. Department of Health and Human Services. 1989. *Nutrition monitoring in the United States—An update report on nutrition monitoring*. Washington, DC: U.S. Government Printing Office.

Assessment Activity 2-2

INDEX OF NUTRITIONAL QUALITY (INQ)

This activity will familiarize you with calculating the INQ and using it to compare different foods or meals. Table 2-25 provides values for energy and selected nutrients found in two meals as shown below.

Meal 1

1 cheeseburger with lettuce, tomato, pickle and mayonnaise
2 servings of French fries
24-ounce diet cola

Meal 2

1 broiled chicken breast sandwich with mayonnaise
1 baked potato topped with ¼ cup nonfat yogurt
1 small tossed salad
1 tablespoon of low-calorie dressing
8 fluid ounces of nonfat milk

Table 2-26 provides nutrient and energy values per 1000 kcal and INQs for the two meals. The energy levels per 1000 kcal for meals 1 and 2 already have been set at 1000 kcal, and nutrient values per 1000 kcal (rounded to the nearest whole number), and the INQs (rounded to the nearest tenth) for meal 1 already have been calculated. Your task is to calculate the nutrient values per 1000 kcal and the INQs for meal 2 and record them in the blank spaces of the table.

1. The first step in converting nutrient levels for meal 2 to a *per 1000-kcal* basis is to divide 1000 by the number of kilocalories provided by meal 2.

$$1000 \div 814 = 1.23$$

Store this number in your calculator's memory and multiply it by each of the nutrient values for meal 2 provided in Table 2-25. For example, the grams of protein *per 1000 kcal* provided by meal 2 is 52.

$$1.23 \times 42 \text{ g of protein} = 52 \text{ g of protein per 1000 kcal}$$

Perform the same calculations for each of the other nutrient values given for meal 2 and record these in Table 2-34 in the "Per 1000 kcal" column.

2. Use the following formula to calculate the INQs of meal 2. Nutrient allowances per 1000 kcal are given in Table 2-9.

$$\text{INQ} = \frac{\text{Amount of nutrients in 1000 kcal of food}}{\text{Allowance of nutrients per 1000 kcal}}$$

The INQ of protein in meal 2, for example, is 1.9. This value was reached by dividing the amount of protein per 1000 kcal in meal 2 (52 g) by the single-value protein recommendation per 1000 kcal (27 g) found in Table 2-9. Calculate the remaining INQs for meal 2 and record these in the "INQ" column.

3. Now compare the two meals on the basis of nutrient density (nutrients provided per 1000 kcal) and the INQ. Which of the two meals has an overall higher nutrient density? Which has an overall higher INQ?
4. What do you think is the primary difference between the two meals? Although they supply roughly the same number of kilocalories, the cheeseburger and French fries in meal 1 give it a significantly greater fat content. Fats and refined sugars are common *nutrient diluents* of the Western diet. Foods high in fat (like French fries or potato chips) will tend to have higher INQs for fat than low-fat foods (like baked or boiled potatoes with little or no added fat). Remember that although it is desirable to have a *high* INQ for most nutrients, it is preferable to have *low* INQs for fats (especially saturated fats), cholesterol, and sodium. Which of the meals has the lower INQs for total and saturated fats?

TABLE 2-25 Values for energy and selected nutrients found in two meals

Nutrient	Meal 1	Meal 2
Energy (kcal)	837	814
Protein (g)	24	42
Carbohydrate (g)	87	96
Total fat (g)	44	30
Saturated fat (g)	19	9
Calcium (mg)	230	523
Iron (mg)	5	7
Folate (μg)	72	139

TABLE 2-26 Nutrient and energy values per 1000 kcal and index of nutritional quality (INQ) for two meals

	Meal 1		Meal 2	
Nutrient	Per 1000 kcal	INQ	Per 1000 kcal	INQ
Energy (kcal)	1000	1	1000	1
Protein (g)	29	1.1	52	1.9
Carbohydrate (g)	104	0.8	—	—
Total fat (g)	53	1.6	—	—
Saturated fat (g)	23	2.1	—	—
Calcium (mg)	275	0.5	—	—
Iron (mg)	6	1.2	—	—
Folate (μg)	86	1.0	—	—

Assessment Activity 2-3

FOOD EXCHANGE SYSTEM

Using the food exchange system to plan meals and assess macronutrient intake is quite easy once you become accustomed to the technique and familiar with the exchange lists. Let's begin this activity by planning an evening meal and snack for two different days using the meal pattern in the far left column of Table 2-27. To manage energy intake and promote dental health, it is probably best for most people to limit eating to meal times and avoid snacking. However, persons taking insulin often need mid-afternoon and late-evening snacks to maintain adequate blood sugar levels.

1. In the spaces provided under "Meal plan 1" and "Meal plan 2," write foods from the exchange lists (see Table 2-22) and their serving sizes that would appropriately match the meal pattern. An example of three exchanges from the starch list would be a small baked potato, ½ cup of green peas, and a small, plain roll. One strength of the exchange system is that it allows almost unlimited variety and can be easily adapted to personal or cultural eating practices.
2. Once you become familiar with the exchange lists, you can use them to rapidly approximate energy and macronutrient levels in individual foods or entire meals. The far left column of Table 2-28 lists a typical American breakfast. Using Table 2-21 (which gives the average kilocalorie and macronutrient content of the six exchanges) and Table 2-22 (which details the food exchanges lists), enter in the appropriate columns the quantities of energy, carbohydrate, protein, and fat for each food and then total them.

TABLE 2-27 Planning meals and snacks using an exchange list meal pattern

Meal pattern	Meal plan 1	Meal plan 2
Evening meal		
Starch—3 exchanges	______	______
	______	______
	______	______
Lean meat and substitutes —2 exchanges	______	______
	______	______
Vegetables—2 exchanges	______	______
	______	______
Fruit—1 exchange	______	______
Fat—2 exchanges	______	______
	______	______
Evening snack		
Starch—1/2 exchange	______	______
Low-fat milk—1/2 exchange	______	______

TABLE 2-28 Estimating energy and macronutrient levels in foods using the exchange lists

Food	Energy (kcal)	Carbohydrate (g)	Protein (g)	Fat (g)
Bran Chex, 1 1/2 cup	______	______	______	______
Milk, 2% fat, 1 cup	______	______	______	______
Banana, 1/2	______	______	______	______
Orange, 1 medium	______	______	______	______
Bagel, 1/2	______	______	______	______
Cream cheese, 1 Tbsp	______	______	______	______
Totals	______	______	______	______

THREE

Measuring Diet

OUTLINE

INTRODUCTION

Measurement of nutrient intake is probably the most widely used indirect indicator of nutritional status. It is used routinely in national nutrition monitoring surveys, epidemiologic studies, nutrition studies of free-living participants (those living outside a controlled setting), and various federal and state health and nutrition program evaluations. To the uninitiated, measurement of nutrient intake may appear to be straightforward and fairly easy. However, estimating an individual's usual dietary and nutrient intake is difficult. The task is complicated by weaknesses of data-gathering techniques, human behavior, the natural tendency of an individual's nutrient intake to vary considerably from day to day, and the limitations of nutrient composition tables and databases. Despite these weaknesses, nutrient intake data are valuable in assessing nutritional status when used in conjunction with anthropometric, biochemical, and clinical data.

This chapter discusses the reasons for measuring diet and different ways of approaching the topic. Techniques for measuring diet are described along with their strengths and weaknesses. The issues of accuracy and validity are examined, and the number of days of individual dietary intake required to characterize the usual nutrient intake of groups and individuals is discussed.

In some instances, data on the kinds and amounts of food eaten by groups or individuals are important because they allow the estimation of nutrient intake. However, conversion of dietary intake data to nutrient intake data requires information on the nutrient content of foods. This is provided by food composition tables and nutrient databases, which are subject to certain limitations and potential sources of error.

REASONS FOR MEASURING DIET

Assessing dietary status includes considering the types and amounts of foods consumed and the intake of the nutrients and other components contained in foods. When food consumption data are combined with information on the nutrient composition of food, the intake of particular nutrients and other food components can be estimated.[1]

Why measure diet? The ultimate reason is to improve human health.[2–4] Nutritional problems are at the root of the leading causes of death, particularly in developed nations. Food and nutrient intake data are critical for investigating the relationships between diet and these diseases, identifying groups at risk of nutrient deficiency or excess, and formulating food and nutrition policies for disease reduction and health promotion.[5] In general, however, there are four major uses of dietary intake data: assessing and monitoring food and nutrient intake, formulating and evaluating government health and agricultural policy, conducting epidemiologic research, and uses for commercial purposes.[6] These are outlined in Box 3-1.

Planning national and international food and nutrition programs depends on estimates of per capita (per person) food, energy, and nutrient consumption. Although per capita consumption cannot easily be measured directly, estimates of food disappearance (or availability) (discussed in detail in Chapter 4) are frequently used indirect indicators of consumption. Food consumption data are used in formulating public and private agricultural policies for the production, distribution, and consumption of food.

Repeated surveys estimating food disappearance, such as those conducted by the U.S. Department of Agriculture (USDA), suggest important trends in overall patterns of food consumption over time. Among these are changes in the American diet since the early 1900s in sources of energy, composition of foods, consumption of specific food groups, and eating patterns such as snacking and eating away from home, all of which can have profound health, social, and economic implications. Dietary assessment is used in determining the extent of malnutrition in a population, developing nutrition intervention and consumer education programs, constructing food guides, devising low-cost food plans, and providing a basis for food and nutrition legislation. Comparisons of dietary practices and nutritional intake with the distribution of disease have demonstrated important links between diet and disease and have shown how dietary changes can modulate disease risk and enhance health.

APPROACHES TO MEASURING DIET

Various methods for collecting food consumption data are available. It is important to note, however, that no single best method exists, and diet measurement will always be accompanied by some degree of error.[7] Each method has its own advantages and disadvantages. Despite these disadvantages and the inevitability of error, properly collected and analyzed, dietary intake data have considerable value, as summarized in Box 3-1. Being informed about the strengths and weaknesses of the methods available will better enable you to scrutinize nutrition research and to draw your own conclusions about a study's results. It will also allow researchers to choose the approach best suited for the task and enable them to use the methods in ways that improve data quality. Selecting the appropriate measurement method, correctly applying it, and using proper

BOX 3-1

Reasons for Measuring Diet

Assessing and monitoring food and nutrient intake	
Ensuring adequacy of the food supply	Data from national surveys and food disappearance indicate the adequacy of food, energy, and nutrient supply.
Estimating the adequacy of dietary intakes of individuals and groups	Individual nutrient intake data combined with anthropometric, biochemical, and clinical measures allow assessment of nutritional status. The proportion of group members having adequate or inadequate intake of a particular nutrient can be determined when the average group intake and the distribution of that intake are known.
Monitoring trends in food and nutrient consumption	Trends in percent of energy from fat, carbohydrate, and protein per person can be derived from dietary surveys and food disappearance data.
Estimating exposure to food additives and contaminants	The FDA's Total Diet Study monitors average intakes of pesticides, toxins, industrial chemicals, and radioactive substances to determine whether they constitute a health risk.
Formulating and evaluating government health and agricultural policy	
Planning food production and distribution	Data indicating a marginal or inadequate supply of energy and/or nutrients can provide direction for planning food production, regulating food imports and exports, and setting priorities for food aid. Food consumption data allow certain groups or income levels to be targeted for food assistance programs such as WIC, food stamps, and the school lunch program.
Establishing food and nutrition regulations	National and individual consumption data allow identification of potential problems to be addressed by food regulations (e.g., labeling) and programs for food enrichment or fortification.

Continued

BOX 3-1

Cont'd

Establishing programs for nutrition education and disease risk reduction	The National Cholesterol Education Program is in part a response to dietary studies indicating that many Americans consume too much total fat, saturated fat, and cholesterol. National survey data showing increasing average body weights for Americans indicate the need for a national strategy for weight management.
Evaluating the success and cost-effectiveness of nutrition education and disease risk-reduction programs	The decline in the average serum total cholesterol of Americans suggests that cholesterol-lowering campaigns have been successful.
Conducting epidemiologic research	
Studying the relationships between diet and health	The purpose of many studies is to investigate the relationship between dietary and nutritional intake and health and disease, for example, the relationships between diet and coronary heart disease, cancer, hypertension, and anemia.
Identifying groups at risk of developing diseases because of their diet and/or nutrient intake	Nutrient consumption data show that women of childbearing age often have low folate intake, which increases the risk of their children being born with neural tube defects.
Commercial purposes	Data from national nutrition surveys are used by food manufacturers to develop advertising campaigns or new food products.

From Sabry JH. 1988. Purposes of food consumption surveys. In *Manual on methodology for food consumption studies*, Cameron ME, Van Staveren WA, eds. New York: Oxford University Press. (See also references 5 and 6).

data analysis techniques can make the difference between data showing a diet-disease relationship and data showing no relationship where one may actually exist. Choosing the appropriate method for measuring diet depends on such considerations as the research design, characteristics of the study participants, and available resources.

Research Design Considerations

Let's consider four types of research designs: correlational, survey or cross-sectional, case-control, and longitudinal or cohort. **Correlational studies** compare the level of some factor (e.g., saturated fat intake) with the level of another factor (e.g., coronary heart disease mortality) in the same population. They are considered most useful for generating hypotheses regarding the associations between suspected risk factors and disease risk. The data used in correlational studies often are only a rough estimate of dietary intake derived from food disappearance studies (discussed in Chapter 4) and are not based on actual dietary intake measurements obtained by methods discussed in this chapter. Much of these data are readily available from national and international agencies. Using such data, early researchers into the causes of coronary heart disease (CHD) showed that saturated fat consumption was positively correlated with risk of CHD. This association led to more definitive studies that demonstrated a cause-and-effect relationship between high saturated fat intake and increased risk of CHD.

Surveys or **cross-sectional studies** provide a "snapshot" of the health of a population at a specific point in time. Various health and dietary measurements are performed on a small segment of the population that has been selected using statistical sampling techniques. These data allow conclusions to be drawn about the health and dietary habits of the larger population from which the sample has been taken. Examples of surveys include the National Health and Nutrition Examination Survey, the Nationwide Food Consumption Survey, and the Continuing Survey of Food Intake of Individuals, all of which are discussed in Chapter 4. The goal is to collect information on the current diet or dietary habits in the immediate past. The 24-hour recall is the most common method used in surveys, although food records are sometimes used.[8]

Case-control studies compare levels of *past exposure* to some factor of interest (e.g., some nutrient or dietary component) in two groups of study participants (cases and controls) to determine how the past exposure relates to a currently existing disease. *Cases* are those people in whom the disease is already diagnosed (e.g., coronary heart disease, cancer, or osteoporosis). *Controls* do not have the disease but share certain similarities with the cases. The investigators then look *retrospectively* (or backward in time) to assess each group's level of exposure to the factor to determine if the disease was preceded by the exposure. Thus, case-control studies require methods that measure dietary intake in the recent past (e.g., the year before diagnosis) or in the distant past (e.g., 10 years ago or in childhood). Methods that focus on current behavior such as the 24-hour recall and food records are not suitable. The only good choices for case-control studies are food frequency questionnaires and diet history, which assess diet in the past.[8]

Case-control studies comparing intakes of total fat, different fatty acids, fiber, and fiber-rich foods in relation to different types of cancer have been carried out. Past intakes of these nutritional components among persons diagnosed with cancer (cases) have been compared with those of persons apparently free of cancer (controls). The results suggest that the risk of breast cancer and, to a possibly greater extent, of colon, prostate, and ovarian cancers, is associated with dietary fat.[9]

Longitudinal or **cohort studies** compare *future exposure* to various factors in a group or *cohort* of study participants in an attempt to determine how exposure to the factors relates to diseases that may develop. These are also known as *prospective* studies. Thus, longitudinal studies require methods that measure current diet or dietary habits in the immediate past, such as 24-hour recalls, food records, and food frequency questionnaires.[8, 10]

The Framingham Heart Study is an example of a longitudinal study. Initiated in 1949, the cohort consisted of more than 5000 30- to 62-year-old residents of Framingham, Massachusetts. Since joining the study, the participants have undergone regular examinations and dietary assessments in an attempt to identify factors contributing to the subsequent development of coronary heart disease and high blood pressure. Only 2% of the study participants have been lost to follow up, and approximately one half of the original participants are still alive. This and other prospective studies have shown that reducing fat intake, controlling body weight and blood pressure, avoiding smoking, and exercising regularly can reduce risk of coronary heart disease and stroke.

Sometimes the goal of dietary assessment is to quickly screen a group of people for probable dietary risk. In these instances, a brief questionnaire identifying people with a high intake of fat, cholesterol, or sodium or a low intake of dietary fiber, fruits, or vegetables can be administered. Two such instruments, the "fat screener" developed by researchers at the National Cancer Institute and the MEDFICTS questionnaire, are discussed later in this chapter. The food frequency questionnaire and the 24-hour recall are also suitable for this purpose.[10]

Time and budgetary constraints are major factors influencing the choice of a dietary measurement method. Analyzing the nutrient content of foods recorded in 24-hour recalls and food records can be labor intensive and costly. These methods also require research staff time in checking them over and reviewing them with study participants for completeness and accuracy (Figure 3-1).[5,6] Self-administered food frequency questionnaires, on the other hand, can save considerable time and expense. They can be mailed to study participants who can complete them on their own and then mail them back to the researchers for data entry and processing. Some food frequency questionnaires are designed to be optically scanned, thus resulting in further saving of staff time and expense.

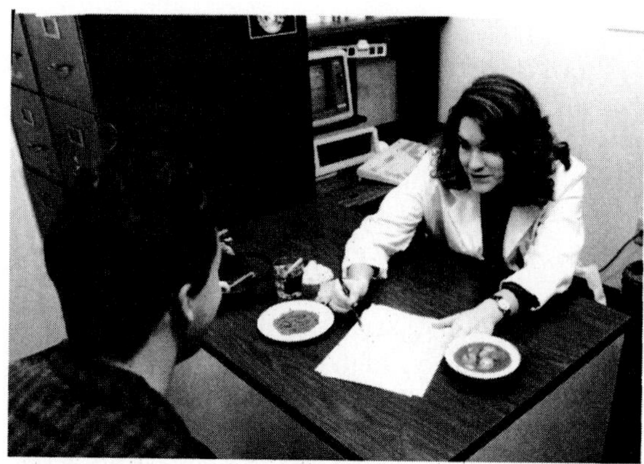

Figure 3-1 Studies of dietary practices and nutritional intake have shown the important role that diet plays in health and disease.

Characteristics of Study Participants

Factors influencing the selection of a dietary measurement technique include literacy, memory, commitment, age, ability to communicate, and culture. If some study participants are likely to be unable to read and/or write, the best methods would be the 24-hour recall or the food frequency questionnaire administered by a member of the research team. The food record or self-administered food frequency questionnaire would not be recommended. The 24-hour recall and food frequency questionnaire require the ability to remember past eating habits. Food records and self-administered food frequency questionnaires require the training and active participation of the study participants. The level of effort required can also lead participants to change their dietary patterns during the recording period. Consequently, there is concern about response rates, the comparability of recording skills among participants, and the quality of dietary intake results.[8]

The ability to communicate may be limited in study participants who are very young, elderly, developmentally disabled, victims of stroke or Alzheimer's disease, or deceased. In these instances, dietary intake data may have to be collected from another person familiar with the study participant such as a parent, spouse, child, or sibling. This other person is known as a **surrogate source**. Surrogate sources are discussed later in this chapter. A food inventory method can be useful for older persons living at home. Direct observation of eating habits of persons in institutional care facilities can also be done.[10] The eating habits of children has been assessed using the 24-hour recall, food records, and food frequency questionnaires. Assessing the diets of younger children may require information from surrogates or use of the "consensus recall method" in which the child and both parents give combined responses on a 24-hour recall. This approach has been shown to give more accurate information than a recall from either parent alone.[10]

Assessing the diets of ethnic populations requires modification of existing methods. If participants are interviewed, it is preferable that these be done by persons of the same ethnic or cultural background so that dietary information can be gathered more effectively. Nutrient analyses of ethnic foods and dishes will likely require changes in food composition data bases. Food frequency questionnaires will have to be modified to include food common to the ethnic group being studied.[10]

Available Resources

Some methods for measuring diet are more expensive and labor intensive to administer than others. Before a study begins, the budget must be carefully considered so that costs entailed will match the available resources. The 24-hour recall, for example, must be administered by a trained interviewer. If the food record is used, study participants should be trained to properly record their diets. Considerable labor is required to enter data from 24-hour recalls and food records into a computer for analysis. Food frequency questionnaires can be self-administered, and responses can be marked on a form that is then optically scanned. Data can then be downloaded into a computer for analysis, thus saving considerable time, effort, and expense. Food records and 24-hour recalls tend to be more feasible methods to use in research with smaller numbers of participants. Food frequency questionnaires, on the other hand, are often preferred by researchers studying large numbers of people.

TECHNIQUES IN MEASURING DIET

Measurement of dietary intake usually is conducted for one of three purposes: to compare average nutrient intakes of different groups, to rank individuals within a group, and to estimate an individual's usual intake. Dietary measurement techniques can be categorized as daily food consumption methods (food record and 24-hour recall) and recalled "usual" or average food consumption methods (diet history and food frequency questionnaire).[6] These techniques have also been categorized as meal-based (food record and 24-hour recall) and list-based (food frequency questionnaire).[5]

24-Hour Recall

In the dietary recall method, a trained interviewer asks the respondent to recall or remember in detail all the food and drink consumed during a period of time in the recent past. The interviewer then records this information for later coding and analysis. (In coding, a number is assigned to each kind of food, allowing it to be identified easily for purposes of computerized analysis.) In most instances, the time period is the previous 24 hours. Thus, the method is most commonly known as the **24-hour recall.**[11] Occasionally, however, the time period may be the previous 48 hours, the past 7 days, or, in rare instances, even the preceding month.[12] However, memories of intake may fade rather quickly beyond the most recent day or two, so that loss in accuracy may exceed gain in representativeness.[13,14]

In addition to recording responses, the interviewer helps the respondent remember all that was consumed during the period in question and assists the respondent in estimating portion sizes of foods consumed. (See Appendix D for an example of the 1987–88 Nationwide Food Consumption Survey 24-hour recall form.) A common technique of the 24-hour recall is to begin by asking what the respondent first ate or drank upon last awakening. The recall proceeds from the morning of the present day to the current moment. The interviewer then begins at the point exactly 24 hours in the past and works forward to the time of awakening. Some researchers ask respondents to recall their diet from midnight to midnight of the previous day. Asking the respondent about his or her activities during the day and inquiring how they might have been associated with eating or drinking can help in recalling food intake. An inquiry about the previous evening's activities, for example, will stimulate the respondent's memory and may help him or her recall the snack eaten while watching a favorite television program.

After the interview, the recall is checked for omissions and/or mistakes. If necessary, a respondent may have to be contacted later by telephone or mail to clarify an entry or to obtain information such as brand names, preparation methods, and serving sizes. The recall can then be analyzed using a computerized diet analysis program. Most programs allow research staff to enter the name of the food into the computer and then select the appropriate method of preparation, serving size, and number of servings from a list of choices displayed on the computer screen. In some instances, however, each individual food may have to be "coded" using a unique number or food code that identifies each particular food. For the food "green beans," there may be separate code numbers for cooked frozen green beans, canned green beans, cooked fresh green beans, and so on. This code then is entered into the analysis software (to identify the food) along with the serving size and number of servings to calculate the nutrients of that food.

Strengths and Limitations

The 24-hour recall has several strengths. It is inexpensive and quick to administer (20 minutes or less) and can provide detailed information on specific foods, especially if brand names can be recalled.[11,15] It requires only short-term memory. It is well accepted by respondents because they are not asked to keep records and their expenditure of time and effort is relatively low. Thus probability sampling within populations and individuals is possible. The method is considered by some to be more objective than the dietary history and food frequency questionnaire, and its administration does not alter the usual diet.[16,17] The 24-hour recall was selected as the primary instrument for measuring dietary intake in the third National Health and Nutrition Examination Survey (NHANES III).[6] Recalls were collected using an automated interview system known as the Dietary Data Collection System.[18] This system is discussed in greater detail in Chapter 4.

Recalls have several limitations. Respondents may withhold or alter information about what they ate because of poor memory or embarrassment or to please or impress the interviewer and researchers. Respondents tend to underreport binge eating, consumption of alcoholic beverages, and eating foods perceived as of unhealthful. Respondents also tend to overreport consumption of name-brand foods, expensive cuts of meat, and foods considered healthful.[15] Foods eaten but not reported are known as **missing foods**, while foods not eaten but reported are known as **phantom foods**.[19] Several researchers report that when their actual food consumption is low, respondents have a tendency to overestimate the amount recalled, and when their actual consumption is high, they underestimate the amount recalled. Some researchers call this phenomena the "flat-slope syndrome."[20–22] Energy intake often is underestimated if drinks, sauces, and dressings are not reported.

The primary limitation of the method is that data on a *single-day's diet,* no matter how accurate, are a very poor descriptor of an individual's *usual* nutrient intake because of day-to-day or **intraindividual variability**.[15,23] Even if several 24-hour recalls are collected from one person, it may be impossible to measure intake of infrequently eaten foods such as liver.[8] However, a sufficiently large number of 24-hour recalls may provide a reasonable estimate of the mean nutrient intake of a group.[11,12,15] Depending on the purpose for which data are used, multiple 24-hour recalls performed on an individual and spaced over various seasons may provide a reasonable estimate of that person's usual nutrient intake.[1,11,24] For example, approximately 3500 participants in NHANES III who were 50 years of age or older completed two additional and unscheduled 24-hour recalls that were collected by telephone interviews approximately 8 and 16 months after their initial 24-hour recall.[18] This was part of the Supplemental Nutrition Survey of Older Americans, a special study collecting data on the diets of older Americans.

The necessary number of days of data collection depends on several factors: whether estimates of usual intake are for individuals or groups, the nutrients of interest, sample size, and degree of intraindividual and interindividual variability.[1,25,26] Twenty-four-hour recalls can provide

BOX 3-2

Strengths and Limitations of the 24-Hour Recall

Strengths	Limitations
Requires less than 20 minutes to administer	One recall is seldom representative of a person's usual intake
Inexpensive	Underreporting/overreporting occurs
Easy to administer	Relies on memory
Can provide detailed information on types of food consumed	Omissions of dressings, sauces, and beverages can lead to low estimates of energy intake
Low respondent burden	May be a tendency to overreport intake at low levels and overreport intake at high levels of consumption
Probability sampling possible	Data entry can be very labor intensive
Can be used to estimate nutrient intake of groups	
Multiple recalls can be used to estimate nutrient intake of individuals	
More objective than dietary history	
Does not alter usual diet	
Useful in clinical settings	

reasonably accurate data about the preceding day's dietary intake, but reports of diet for the preceding week or month do not accurately characterize dietary intake during those periods.[27] Box 3-2 summarizes the strengths and limitations of the 24-hour recall method.

Food Record or Diary

In this method, the respondent records, at the time of consumption, the identity and amounts of all foods and beverages consumed for a period of time usually ranging from 1 to 7 days. An example of a food record form is given in Appendix E. Food and beverage consumption can be quantified by estimating portion sizes, using household measures, or weighing the food or beverage on scales. In many instances, household measures such as cups, tablespoons, and teaspoons or measurements made with a ruler are used to quantify portion size. Certain items such as eggs, apples, or 12-oz cans of soft drinks may be thought of as units and simply counted. This method is sometimes referred to as the **estimated food record** because portion sizes are estimated (that is, in terms of coffee cups, dippers, bowls, glasses, and so on) or household measures are used. When food is weighed, the record may be referred to as a **weighed food record**. Box 3-3 compares these two methods. The use of food scales is preferred by European nutrition researchers who consider it more accurate than using household measures, as is typically done by North American researchers. The degree of accuracy from household measures appears acceptable for most research purposes, especially when considering whether respondents will adhere to the program if they must weigh everything that they eat.

Strengths and Limitations

The food record does not depend on memory because the respondent ideally records food and beverage consumption (including snacks) at the time of eating. In addition, it can provide detailed food intake data and important information about eating habits (for example, when, where, and with whom meals are eaten and the respondent's mood when choosing certain foods). Data from a

BOX 3-3

Comparison of the Estimated Food Record and the Weighed Food Record

Estimated food record

Amounts of food and leftovers are measured in household measures (cups, tablespoons, teaspoons) or estimated using such measures as coffee cups, bowls, glasses, and dippers. The researchers then quantify these measures by volume and weight

Considered less accurate than the weighed food record

Considered an acceptable method for collecting group intake data

Puts less burden on the respondent than the weighed food record and thus cooperation rates are likely to be higher, especially over long recording periods

As effective in ranking subjects into thirds and fifths as weighed records

Weighed food record

Food and leftovers are weighed using scales or computerized techniques supplied by researchers

Considered more accurate than the estimated food record

Preferred by some researchers for gathering data on individuals

Requires a greater degree of subject cooperation than the estimated food record and thus is likely to have a greater impact on eating habits than the estimated food record

Cost of scales may be prohibitive in some instances

From Bingham SA, Nelson M, Paul AA, et al. 1988. Methods for data collection at an individual level. In Cameron ME and Van Staveren WA (eds) *Manual on methodology for food consumption studies*. New York: Oxford University Press.

multiple-day food record also would be more representative of usual intake than single-day data from either a 24-hour recall or a 1-day food record. However, multiple food records from nonconsecutive, random days (including weekends) covering different seasons are necessary to arrive at useful estimates of usual intake.[11,28,29]

Food records have several limitations. They require a literate and cooperative respondent who is able and willing to expend the time and effort necessary to record dietary intake. Individuals having the time, interest, and ability to complete several days of food records without assistance may not be representative of the general population.[21,30] The act of recording food intake after several days may cause the respondent to change his or her usual diet. It appears that after keeping detailed food records for 5 or 6 days, participants tend to simplify their eating and drinking to streamline the recording process.[11,15,21,23,31] Box 3-4 summarizes the strengths and weaknesses of the food record.

Food Frequency Questionnaire

The **food frequency questionnaire** or checklist assesses energy and/or nutrient intake by determining how frequently a person consumes a limited number of foods that are major sources of nutrients or of a particular dietary component in question. The questionnaire consists of a list of approximately 100 or fewer individual foods or food groups that are important contributors to the population's intake of energy and nutrients. Respondents indicate how many times a day, week, month, or year that they usually consume the foods.[11,15,23,24] In some food frequency question-

BOX 3-4

Strengths and Limitations of the Food Record

Strengths	Limitations
Does not depend on memory	Requires high degree of cooperation
Can provide detailed intake data	Response burden can result in low response rates when used in large national surveys
Can provide data about eating habits	Subject must be literate
Multiple-day data more representative of usual intake	Takes more time to obtain data
Reasonably valid up to 5 days	Act of recording may alter diet
	Analysis is labor intensive and expensive

naires, a choice of portion size is not given. These generally use "standard" portion sizes (the amounts customarily eaten per serving for various age/sex groups) drawn from large-population data.[11,12,23,24] An example of this format is given in Figure 3-2a. It simply asks how many times a year, month, week, or day a person eats string beans or green beans. This is sometimes referred to as a **simple** or **nonquantitative food frequency questionnaire** format. The **semiquantitative food frequency questionnaire** shown in Figure 3-2b gives respondents an idea of portion size. It asks how many times a year, month, week, or day a person eats a ½ cup serving of string beans or green beans. In addition to asking the frequency of consumption, the **quantitative food frequency questionnaire** shown in Figure 3-2c asks the respondent to describe the size of his or her usual serving as small, medium, or large relative to a standard serving.[15] The portion numbers and sizes then are entered into a computer database, which multiplies these by the nutrients contained in each food or food group and arrives at an estimated nutrient intake.[23,24,32] An alternative to this is for respondents to mark their answers on an answer sheet that can then be optically scanned so that their responses can be directly downloaded into a computer for analysis, thus saving the researchers considerable time and money. This feature makes food frequency questionnaires a cost-effective approach for measuring diet in large epidemiologic studies.

Some questionnaires have been designed to assess intake of individual nutrients or food components such as vitamin A, fat, or calcium for studies investigating the relationships between diet and such conditions as cancer and cardiovascular disease.[12,33–37] Others have been developed to assess a wide spectrum of macronutrients and micronutrients.[23] Figure 3-3 shows several questions from a nonquantitative food frequency questionnaire used in NHANES III. NHANES and other national surveys are discussed in detail in Chapter 4. The entire diet portion of the NHANES III questionnaire for respondents age 17 years and older is shown in Appendix F.

Figure 3-4 shows a 13-item questionnaire developed by researchers at the U.S. National Cancer Institute for identifying groups whose mean percent fat intake is high (or low).[33] The database and age- and sex-specific portion sizes for food items necessary to score the questionnaire are given in Appendix G. The screening tool, which can be administered either by the respondent or an interviewer, is intended to identify those who might be further studied for the health consequences of their high- (or low-) fat diet, who may need further dietary assessment, or who might benefit from dietary intervention. It takes about 4 minutes to administer and does essentially as well as three 4-day food records in ranking respondents in terms of their intake in grams of total fat and saturated, oleic, and linoleic fatty acids.[33]

A)

Food Item	Average Use During Past Year					
	< 1 month	1–3 month	1–4 week	5–7 week	2–4 day	5+ day
coffee						
dark bread						
ice cream						

B)

Food Item	Average Use During Past Year								
	< 1 month	1–3 month	1 week	2–4 week	5–6 week	1 day	2–3 day	4–5 day	6+ day
coffee (1 cup)									
dark bread (1 slice)									
ice cream (1/2 cup)									

C)

Food Item	Medium Serving	Your Serving Size			How Often?				
		S	M	L	Day	Week	Month	Year	Never
coffee	(1 cup)								
dark bread	(1 slice)								
ice cream	(1/2 cup)								

Figure 3-2 Examples of three different food frequency questionnaire formats: **(A)** the simple or nonquantitative format; **(B)** the semiquantitative format; **(C)** the quantitative format. Adapted from Bingham SA, Cummings JH. 1985. Urine nitrogen as an independent validatory measure of dietary intake: A study of nitrogen balance in individuals consuming their normal diet. *American Journal of Clinical Nutrition* 42:1276–1289.

A questionnaire developed to quickly estimate how frequently foods high in total fat, saturated fatty acids, and cholesterol are eaten is shown in Appendix H. It is called the MEDFICTS Dietary Assessment Questionnaire (Meats, Eggs, Dairy, Fried foods, In baked goods, Convenience foods, Table fats, Snacks) and is recommended by the National Cholesterol Education Program as a simple approach to assess a person's adherence to the Step-One and Step-Two diets.[38] These two diets are the foundation of the National Cholesterol Education Program's recommendations for the dietary control of elevated blood cholesterol levels and are discussed in Chapter 8.

MEDFICTS focuses on foods that are major contributors of total fat, saturated fat, and cholesterol commonly eaten by North Americans. Within each of the questionnaire's eight categories, foods are placed into either a high-fat, high-cholesterol group (Group 1) or a low-fat, low-cholesterol group (Group 2). Group 1 foods are major contributors of dietary fat and cholesterol, and to the right of these groups are a series of shaded boxes with numbers representing points under each box. Group 2 foods are minor contributors of fat and cholesterol, and to the right of these are unshaded boxes with no points assigned to these boxes. In completing the questionnaire, the respondent simply checks the shaded boxes representing his or her frequency of weekly consumption and typical serving size for each food group. The points for weekly consumption

N3. Fruit and Fruit Juices	
Next are fruit juices and fruit. Include all forms — fresh, frozen canned and dried.	
a. How often did you have orange juice, grapefruit juice, and tangerine juice?	____ per 1☐D 2☐W 3☐M or 4☐N 9☐DK
b. Other fruit juices such as grape juice, apple juice, cranberry juice, and fruit nectars	____ per 1☐D 2☐W 3☐M or 4☐N 9☐DK
c. Citrus fruits including oranges, grapefruits, and tangerines	____ per 1☐D 2☐W 3☐M or 4☐N 9☐DK
d. Melons including cantaloupe, honeydew, and watermelon	____ per 1☐D 2☐W 3☐M or 4☐N 9☐DK
e. Peaches, nectarines, apricots, guava, mango, and papaya	____ per 1☐D 2☐W 3☐M or 4☐N 9☐DK
f. How often did you have any other fruits such as apples, bananas, pears, berries, cherries, grapes, plums, and strawberries? (include plantains.)	____ per 1☐D 2☐W 3☐M or 4☐N 9☐DK

Figure 3-3 Several questions from a food frequency questionnaire used in the third National Health and Nutrition Examination Survey. Note that portion size is not assessed. From National Center for Health Statistics

	Medium Serving	Your Serving Size			How Often?					Office Use
		S	M	L	Day	Week	Month	Year	Rarely/Never	
EXAMPLE: Hamburgers, cheeseburgers, meat loaf	**1 medium**									
Hamburger, cheeseburgers, meat loaf	1 medium									11 _ _ _ _
Beef steaks, roasts	4 oz.									15 _ _ _ _
Pork, including chops, roast	2 chops or 4 oz.									19 _ _ _ _
Hot dogs	2 dogs									23 _ _ _ _
Ham, lunch meats	2 slices									27 _ _ _ _
Whole milk not incl. on cereal	8 oz. glass									31 _ _ _ _
Cheese, excluding cottage	2 slices or 2 oz.									35 _ _ _ _
Doughnuts, cookies, cake, pastries	1 pc. or 3 cookies									39 _ _ _ _
Eggs	1 egg = small, 2 eggs = medium									43 _ _ _ _
White bread, rolls, bagels, etc., incl. on sandwiches	2 slices, 3 crackers									47 _ _ _ _
Margarine or butter	2 pats									51 _ _ _ _
Salad dressing or mayonnaise (incl. on sandwiches)	2 Tblsp.									55 _ _ _ _
French fries, fried potatoes	3/4 cup									59 _ _ _ _
Do you eat the following foods every day?										
Breakfast cereal ☐ Yes ☐ No										63 _
Dark bread such as whole wheat, rye, or pumpernickel? ☐ Yes ☐ No										64 _

Figure 3-4 A thirteen-item screening questionnaire for fat intake. See Appendix G for information on coding and scoring. Courtesy of Dr. Gladys Block.

(shown below each shaded box) are multiplied by the points for serving size and totaled in the score column. The points from each side of the questionnaire are totaled and compared with the key. A total score of 40 to 70 points suggests that a person is following the recommendations of the Step-One diet for intake of total fat, saturated fat, and cholesterol. A score less than 40 points suggests that a person is adhering to the somewhat more stringent recommendations of the Step-Two diet. Thus, a lower score should correspond to a lower intake of total fat, saturated fat, and cholesterol. Studies suggest that the MEDFICTS does a good job of estimating intake of total fat, saturated fat, and cholesterol, compared to intake estimates based on three-day and seven-day food records.[39,40]

The two most extensively tested semiquantitative food frequency questionnaires that are in widespread use are those developed by Willett and coworkers at Harvard University and Block and coworkers at the National Cancer Institute.

The Willett Questionnaire

Beginning in 1979, a team of Harvard University nutritionists and epidemiologists headed by Walter C. Willett developed a series of self-administered semiquantitative food frequency questionnaires to conduct epidemiologic research on the relationships between nutrient and food intake and risk of chronic disease. Over the years their original 61-item questionnaire was modified several times.[15,41–43] A more recently developed 131-item questionnaire (shown in Appendix I) was designed to classify individuals according to levels of average daily intake of nutrients and certain foods and food components during the past year.[44] Its format is similar to that shown in Figure 3-2b. It is self-administered and machine-readable, thus making it convenient for use in large epidemiologic studies. Foods included in the questionnaire are those that are major sources of the nutrients, foods, and food components of interest to the researchers. Open-ended questions are also included to identify specific brands of margarine, ready-to-eat cereals, cooking oils, vitamin/mineral supplements, and other foods eaten at least once per week.[44] For each item on the questionnaire, respondents are given nine choices ranging from less than once per month to six or more times per day. Nutrient values are calculated by multiplying nutrient content of each item by frequency of use.

The questionnaires have been designed to be self-administered by nurses and other health professionals in such epidemiologic studies as the Nurses' Health Study and the Health Professionals Follow-up Study with populations of more than 80,000 female nurses and nearly 40,000 male health professionals, respectively.[45,46] However, the questionnaire has been used successfully in a group of socioeconomically diverse group of older women living in Iowa.[47] Among the diet-disease relationships reported in studies using these questionnaires are the following: significant reductions in coronary heart disease risk in males and females using vitamin E supplements; a lack of association between dietary fat intake and breast cancer; increased risk of colon cancer in females consuming diets high in animal fat; increased risk of coronary heart disease in men consuming alcoholic beverages; and an association between intake of vitamin A, niacin, and zinc and progression of human immunodeficiency virus (HIV) infection to acquired immunodeficiency syndrome (AIDS) in HIV-positive homosexual and bisexual males.[45,46,48–51]

Researchers at Harvard University Medical School and Brigham and Women's Hospital in Boston have developed a food frequency questionnaire for assessing the diets of children and adolescents ages 9 to 18 years old. Known as the Youth/Adolescent Questionnaire (YAQ), it is self-administered and includes a list of 151 foods. According to reproducibility studies it has a reasonable ability to assess the eating habits of children and adolescents. It is shown in Appendix J.

The Block Questionnaire

The food frequency questionnaire shown in Appendix K (Health Habits and History Questionnaire) was developed by Gladys Block and coworkers at the National Cancer Institute to collect data on diet and well-established risk factors for cancer and total mortality. Although the questionnaire originally was designed to supplement data from more specific questionnaires collecting data on the relationships between disease and potential causative factors, it has proven useful in assessing total dietary intake.[23,32] The questionnaire was developed using data from the 24-hour recalls of a statistically representative sample of nearly 12,000 American adults who participated in the second National Health and Nutrition Examination Survey (NHANES II) conducted from 1976 to 1980.[23] The 2244 different food codes recorded in these 24-hour recalls were grouped into 147 conceptually similar food items based on several criteria, including similarity in nutrient content per usual serving (for example, 11 different codes for green beans were consolidated into one food item labeled "string beans, green beans"). The decision of whether an item should be included on the food list was based on its energy and nutrient content, the frequency of its consumption by the population, and the typical serving size. Foods that were important contributors of energy and nutrients in the NHANES II database were included in the questionnaire. Items included in the food list represent 94% of all food items reported in the NHANES II data, 93% of the nation's total caloric intake, and more than 90% of each of 17 additional nutrients. Table 3-1 details how comprehensively the questionnaire assesses energy and nutrient intake in the American diet.

TABLE 3-1 Percent of total U.S. population intake for energy and 17 nutrients represented by the food list of the Health Habits and History Questionnaire

Energy or nutrient	Percent of total population intake
Energy (kcal)	92.9
Protein	95.0
Total fat	94.7
Carbohydrate	92.1
Calcium	96.5
Phosphorus	95.3
Iron	92.4
Sodium	92.2
Potassium	94.3
Vitamin A	96.4
Thiamin	93.6
Riboflavin	95.2
Niacin	94.6
Vitamin C	95.7
Saturated fat	95.0
Oleic acid	91.9
Linoleic acid	90.0
Cholesterol	96.9

From GS Block, AM Hartman, CM Dresser, MD Carroll et al. 1986. A data-based approach to diet questionnaire design and testing. *American Journal of Epidemiology* 124:453–469.

Portion sizes for items on the food list also were developed using data from NHANES II rather than convenient but arbitrary household measures. Portion sizes were determined in NHANES II using three-dimensional models during collection of the 24-hour recalls, and the large database of NHANES II allowed developers to identify age- and sex-specific portion sizes on the list. Thus, portion sizes can be adjusted during analysis of the questionnaire and computation of nutrient intake to reflect the age and sex of the respondent.

Population data from NHANES II also were used in developing the nutrient database of the questionnaire. Many of the items on the food list consist of several foods grouped together. For instance, an item on the list is labeled "other potatoes, including boiled, baked, potato salad." Even the item labeled "string beans, green beans" is a composite of 11 different types of green beans or ways of preparing them.[23] Using the NHANES II data, researchers determined how frequently the various types of green beans were consumed by the nearly 12,000 persons interviewed. Thus, nutrient composition values for each item on the food list reflect the frequency of consumption of the different varieties included within that item. As discussed in Assessment Activity 3-3, software is available from the National Cancer Institute for analyzing data collected by the questionnaire.

Strengths and Limitations

Food frequency questionnaires have several strengths. They place a modest demand on the time and energy of respondents and generate estimates of food and nutrient intake that may be more representative of usual intake than a few days of diet records. They are relatively quick to administer. Approximately 30 minutes are required to complete the diet section of the Health Habits and History Questionnaire in Appendix K, and another 12 to 15 minutes are needed for the nondiet section.[32] They can be self-administered and machine readable and thus are relatively economical to use in large-scale studies.[11,43,52,53] However, data quality may be better when the questionnaire is administered by a trained interviewer.[54] Estimates of nutrient and food intake from repeat administrations of food frequency questionnaires generally compare favorably, showing reasonable reproducibility (see the section on reproducibility later in this chapter).[15,41–44,53]

There are questions about how well food frequency questionnaires estimate the actual average nutrient intakes of individuals and groups—what is called validity. Studies comparing nutrient or food intake estimates obtained from food frequency questionnaires with estimates obtained from "criterion methods" such as multiple food records or 24-hour recalls suggest that food frequency questionnaires are appropriate for estimating mean intakes of energy and some nutrients for groups and for ranking persons as having a low, average, or high consumption of energy and certain nutrients.[41,42,44,47,54,55] Some investigators, however, challenge these conclusions.[56,57] Food frequency questionnaires do not appear appropriate for estimating the nutrient intake of groups (see the section on validity later in this chapter).

Food frequency questionnaires have definite limitations. Because the food list is limited to approximately 100 to 150 foods and food groups, these must be representative of the most common foods consumed by respondents in the sample. Short questionnaires are faster and easier to administer but lack comprehensiveness. Long questionnaires may do a better job of assessing nutrient intake but also require respondents to make an almost overwhelming number of decisions. Longer food frequency questionnaires have the disadvantage of being tedious to complete. Individual foods listed on the questionnaire are more likely to be remembered than foods grouped under such headings as "any other fruit" or "any other vegetable" unless a trained interviewer carefully probes the respondent.[52] Grouping foods under broad categories precludes the ability to collect information about specific food items.[56] For example, the Block questionnaire groups doughnuts, cookies, cakes, and pastry within a single group. Portion sizes allow limited choices as well, and they must be the most typical of what is usually eaten. Questionnaires lacking portion size selections or having poorly chosen ones may only identify individuals at the extremes of the nutrient-intake distribution. However, the usefulness of such portion size information is questioned by research suggesting that defined portion sizes may not be meaningful to some respondents.[27] However, frequency is a more important determinant of nutrient intake than portion size.[58] Another limitation is reliance on the ability of the respondent to describe his or her diet.[13,52,59]

It is important that food frequency questionnaires be culturally sensitive. The Block questionnaire, for example, is best suited for white, middle-class people, who composed the majority of the NHANES II population. Failure to include foods commonly eaten by various groups may result in underestimates of nutrient intake, particularly if the foods are major sources of certain nutrients or food components. The Block and Willett questionnaires address this shortcoming by providing space for respondents to write in foods that they at least occasionally eat but that are not included in the food list. Food lists also must be periodically updated to keep pace with the thousands of new food products entering the marketplace each year.

BOX 3-5

Strengths and Limitations of Food Frequency Questionnaires

Strengths	Limitations
Can be self-administered	May not represent usual foods or portion sizes chosen by respondents
Machine readable	Intake data can be compromised when multiple foods are grouped within single listings
Modest demand on respondents	Depends on ability of subject to describe diet
Relatively inexpensive for large sample sizes	Not appropriate for determining absolute nutrient intake in large surveys like NHANES III
May be more representative of usual intake than a few days of diet records	
Design can be based on large population data	
Considered by some as the method of choice for research on diet-disease relationships	

Despite these limitations, the food frequency questionnaire was used in NHANES III to collect information on water and alcohol consumption, the intake of selected foods and food groups, food sources of calcium and vitamins A and C, and milk intake, although the 24-hour recall was the primary approach for measuring diet.[6] The food frequency questionnaire is considered by some as the method of choice for research on diet-disease relationships on both the macronutrient and micronutrient levels.[11,58]

Box 3-5 summarizes the strengths and weaknesses of food frequency questionnaires.

Diet History

Diet history is used to assess an individual's usual dietary intake over an extended period of time such as the past month or year.[11,60,61] Traditionally, the diet history approach has been associated with the method of assessing usual diet developed by B. S. Burke during the 1940s.[62]

Burke's original method involved four steps: (1) collect general information about the respondent's health habits, (2) question the respondent about his or her usual eating pattern, (3) perform a cross-check on the data given in step two, and (4) have the respondent complete a 3-day food record.[62]

A trained nutritionist begins the interview by asking questions about the number of meals eaten per day, appetite, food dislikes, the presence or absence of nausea and vomiting, use of nutritional supplements, cigarette smoking, habits related to sleep, rest, work, and exercise, and so on. This allows the interviewer to become acquainted with the respondent in ways that may be helpful in obtaining further information. This is followed by a 24-hour recall in which the interviewer also inquires about the respondent's usual pattern of eating during and between meals, beginning with the first food or drink of the day. The interviewer records the respondent's description of his or her usual food intake, including types of food eaten, serving sizes, frequency and timing, and significant seasonal variations.

With the respondent's stated usual dietary practices recorded, the interviewer then cross-checks the data by asking specific questions about the respondent's dietary preferences and habits. For example, the respondent may have said that he or she drinks an 8-oz glass of milk every morning. The interviewer then should inquire about the participant's milk drinking habits to clarify and verify the information given about the respondent's milk intake. Finally, the participant is asked to complete a 3-day food record, which serves as an additional means of checking the usual intake.

BOX 3-6

Strengths and Limitations of the Diet History Method

Strengths	Limitations
Assesses usual nutrient intake	Lengthy interview process
Can detect seasonal changes	Requires highly trained interviewers
Data on all nutrients can be obtained	Difficult and expensive to code
Can correlate well with biochemical measures	May tend to overestimate nutrient intake
	Requires cooperative respondent with ability to recall usual diet

Burke admits that this is the least helpful part of the method, and it generally is omitted by the few researchers who currently use this method.

Strengths and Limitations

Strengths of the diet history approach are that it assesses the respondent's usual nutrient intake, including seasonal changes, and data on all nutrients can be obtained.[11] The method is one of the preferred methods for obtaining estimates of usual nutrient intake.[11,60] Estimates of protein intake by the method correlate well with measures of nitrogen excretion. If what is needed for research purposes is a list of items that is typical of an individual's diet rather than a specific list of items eaten during a certain period of time, the diet history appears adequate to determine the typical diet. Most people are able to report what they typically eat, even if they cannot report exactly what they ate during some specific period of time.[27]

Among the method's limitations are that 1 to 2 hours are required to conduct the interview, highly trained interviewers are needed, coding is difficult and expensive, and nutrient intake tends to be overestimated.[11,61,62] The method also requires a cooperative respondent with the ability to recall usual diet.

Box 3-6 summarizes the strengths and limitations of the diet history method.

Duplicate Food Collections

Collection of food consumption data generally is not an end in itself but rather a means of eventually arriving at an estimate of nutrient intake. Limitations of using food consumption data to arrive at nutrient intake are the incompleteness of food composition tables, mistakes in coding and entering data, and nutrient losses during food storage and preparation that may not be accounted for in food composition tables.[4] A more direct method of calculating nutrient intake that avoids these particular problems is **duplicate food collections.**

When performing duplicate food collections, participants place in collection containers an identical portion of all foods and beverages consumed during a specified period.[63] This then is chemically analyzed at a laboratory for nutrient content. To prevent bacterial decomposition of the duplicate samples, they should be kept refrigerated and delivered to the laboratory daily.

Strengths and Limitations

The method has the strength of potentially providing a more accurate determination of actual nutrient intake compared with calculations based on food composition data. Values in composition tables may not be representative of nutrient levels in the particular foods that respondents consume because of seasonal or regional differences,

BOX 3-7

Strengths and Limitations of the Duplicate Food Collection Method

Strengths	Limitations
Can provide more accurate measurements of actual nutrient intake than calculations based on food composition tables	Expense and effort of preparing more food Effort and time to collect duplicate samples May underestimate usual intake

agricultural practices, and losses during marketing and preparation. A participant may have eaten a food that was introduced recently into the marketplace that is not listed in a food composition table or database. Among the method's limitations are the necessity of preparing the additional amount of food to be collected and the work involved in measuring or weighing exact duplicate portions of food and beverage. In the Beltsville 1-year dietary intake study, respondents kept daily food records throughout the 1-year period and provided duplicate food collections for 1 week during each of the four seasons of the year.[63,64] The participants' mean calculated nutrient intake was 12.9% less during the 4 weeks when duplicate food collections were done. Reductions were greatest for foods rich in fat and protein—often the most expensive foods. The respondents may have felt guilty about "wasting" food that went into the collection jar or were concerned about the food's expense, despite receiving payment for their participation in the study. Thus intakes during food collection periods may not be representative of habitual nutrient intake.

Box 3-7 summarizes the strengths and limitations of the duplicate food collection method.

Food Accounts

Food accounts are used to measure dietary intake within households and institutions where congregate feeding is practiced, such as penal institutions, nursing homes, military bases, and boarding schools.[65] The method accounts for all food on hand in the home or institution at the beginning of the survey period, all that is purchased or grown throughout the period, and all that remains by the end of the survey. Inventories establish amounts of food on hand at the beginning and ending of the survey period, and invoices or other accounting methods provide records of food purchased or obtained from farm or garden. Trained personnel make site visits at the beginning and ending of the survey period and as necessary throughout the period to assist in record keeping.

The daily mean consumption per person is calculated for each food item from the total amount of food consumed during the survey period and the number of people in the household or institution.[65] This method was used in the Finnish Mental Hospital Study, which showed that when soft margarine and skim milk with added soy oil replaced butter and whole milk in the diets of institutionalized persons, serum cholesterol levels and heart disease mortality dropped in contrast to a similar institution where no such dietary changes were made.[66,67]

When used to measure household food consumption, the usual survey period is 2 to 4 weeks. To capture seasonal variations, some researchers may record consumption over different seasons for shorter periods. In addition to the amounts of different foods consumed by family members, it is necessary to account for the number of people present at each meal, the number of meals eaten away from home, and the number served to visitors.[65]

BOX 3-8

Strengths and Limitations of the Food Account Method

Strengths	Limitations
Suitable for use with large sample sizes	Does not account for food losses
Can be used over relatively long periods	Respondent literacy and cooperation necessary
Gives data on dietary patterns and habits of families and other groups	Not appropriate for measuring individual food consumption
Less likely to lead to alterations in diet than some other methods	
Relatively economical	

Strengths and Limitations

The strengths of the method are that the survey can include a large sample size, food consumption can be monitored for a relatively long period of time, and data on the annual mean consumption and general food patterns and habits of the population can be obtained. The likelihood that the method will alter the diet is less than with the food record method. The method is also relatively economical because personnel need only make periodic visits for supervising and controlling the recording.[65]

Included among the limitations of the method are its inability to account for food that is given to animals, thrown away due to spoilage, or discarded as plate waste or for other reasons. Because respondent literacy and cooperation are necessary, families or institutions willing to keep food accounts may not be representative of the population of interest. Accuracy may suffer from forgetfulness or lack of faithfulness in maintaining food accounts. The method only provides information on the mean daily consumption of the whole family; it does not indicate how food is distributed among the various family members. Thus, it is only appropriate for measuring food consumption of groups.[65]

Box 3-8 summarizes the strengths and limitations of the food account method.

Food Balance Sheets

The **food balance sheet** is a method of indirectly estimating the amounts of food consumed by a country's population at a certain time. It provides data on food *disappearance* (sometimes referred to as *food availability*) rather than actual food consumption. It is calculated using beginning and ending inventories, figures on food production, imports and exports, and adjustments for nonhuman food consumption (for example, cattle feed, pet food, seed, and industrial use). Food disappearance can be thought of as the amount of food that "disappears" from the food distribution system. Much of this is purchased by consumers at supermarkets; however, a considerable amount is lost due to spoilage.

Mean per capita annual amounts are calculated by dividing total disappearance of food by the country's population.[65] This method has been valuable for detecting trends in the amount of food that disappears from the food distribution system within a country over time and thus has been used to roughly indicate likely trends in consumption as well. It is useful for promoting agricultural production in various parts of the world and encouraging a more even distribution of food among different countries.[65] Because these data are collected in a roughly similar manner in countries around the world, they are useful in epidemio-

BOX 3-9

Strengths and Limitations of the Food Balance Sheet

Strengths	Limitations
Can give a total view of a country's food supplies	Accuracy of data may be questionable
Indicates food habits and dietary trends	Only represents food available for consumption
Used to plan international nutrition policies and food programs	Does not represent food actually consumed
May be the only data available on a country's food consumption practices	Does not indicate how food was distributed
	Does not account for wasted food

logic research across countries.[9] We will discuss food disappearance data in greater detail in Chapter 4 in connection with national surveys.

Strengths and Limitations

Strengths of the method are that it can give a total view of the food supplies of a country, can be used in drawing conclusions about general food habits and dietary trends within a country, and is valuable in planning international nutrition policy and formulating food programs.[65] In some instances, information on food disappearance may be the only accessible data representing a country's food consumption practices.

The method has a number of limitations. The accuracy of data depends on available statistics, the quality of which can vary greatly depending on a country's level of development. The data only represent the total amount of food that reportedly leaves the food distribution system, apparently for consumption. Note that it is not an estimate of what was actually consumed. It also does not show how food was distributed among individuals or groups within a particular country. The method also does not account for food that is wasted or fed to animals (for example, pets).[65]

Box 3-9 summarizes the strengths and limitations of the food balance sheet.

Telephone Interviews

Telephone interviewing has, in recent years, become an accepted and widely used method for collecting dietary intake data. Investigators have used the technique to administer 24-hour recalls and food frequency questionnaires, particularly to follow-up face-to-face interviews. This approach was used in NHANES III as part of a study of the eating habits of Americans age 50 years and older. After a face-to-face 24-hour recall, a series of two additional 24-hour recalls were collected by telephone from a subset of older respondents.[6,10,18] Telephone interviewing was also used in the Continuing Survey of Food Intakes by Individuals conducted by the USDA in 1985 and 1986.[10] Preadolescent children were shown to be able to provide 24-hour recall data during telephone interviews that compared favorably to written records of their intake unobtrusively collected by parents.[68] Recalls obtained by telephone interview showed good agreement with the observed intake of both college students and elderly participants.[69,70] Telephone reporting has been shown to be an acceptable method of collecting food record data whether the data are reported directly to an individual or left on a recording device such as a telephone answering machine.[69,71]

BOX 3-10

Strengths and Limitations of Telephone Interviewing

Strengths	Limitations
One quarter to one half the cost of a comparable personal interview	Subject to many of the same disadvantages of collecting 24-hour recall and food record data
Fewer time, logistical, and personnel constraints	Estimating portion sizes in recalls may be difficult unless steps are taken to address the problem
Lower respondent burden	
Gives respondent more personal security	

Strengths and Limitations

Telephone interviewing has several strengths. Cost of the method has been reported to be approximately one fourth to one half that of comparable personal interviews.[71–74] It also has the potential of easing time, logistical, and personnel constraints associated with nutrition surveys.[75] Telephone surveys have higher response rates than mail surveys.[10] The respondent burden may be somewhat lower with this method compared with personal interviews. In an era of pervasive suspicion of strangers resulting from rising crime rates, some respondents may find this method more conducive to personal safety than interviews within their home.[76]

Twenty-four-hour recall or food frequency data collected over the telephone will be subject to the same limitations as that collected in personal interviews. One additional problem is estimation of portion sizes. Investigators have addressed this shortcoming by providing respondents with measuring cups and a ruler[43] or with two-dimensional food models for estimating portion sizes.[68,75] Although 97% of the U.S. population has a telephone, there is lower telephone coverage among blacks, Hispanics (except for Cuban-Americans), unemployed persons, and the poor. Households in the South are twice as likely to be without telephones than those in other areas of the United States.[74]

Box 3-10 summarizes the strengths and limitations of telephone interviewing.

Visual Records

Several investigators have developed photographic and video methods to record dietary intake in an attempt to reduce respondent burden and increase validity of dietary intake data.[77–80] In one approach, respondents were provided with an easily operated camera with a built-in electronic flash.[77] Participants photographed all their food before eating it (on plates, in bowls, and so on) and what was left over after eating. In a manual, they recorded descriptions of their food and preparation methods, especially those that would not be apparent in the photographs. The exposed slide film was returned to the investigators for development and evaluation. The slides were projected on a screen, and estimates were made of each food. Using a second projector, slides of known food portions could be projected beside the respondent's slide to help in estimating portion sizes.

When compared with results of weighed food records, the photographic method was reported to provide very similar results with no significant difference in nutrient calculations between the two methods.[78] In another validation study conducted in a cafeteria setting, on-site observers recorded the identity of foods selected by participants. This record compared favorably with the identification of foods from slides.[79]

More recently, the validity and reproducibility of video recordings to assess dietary intake were tested.[80] Video recordings of test trays containing foods of known volume or weight were evaluated independently by two trained observers. Food amounts estimated from the videos were closely correlated with measured amounts, indicating that this method has good validity. Results obtained independently by the two observers who identified food items on the same set of videotaped meals then were compared. These were shown to agree favorably, indicating that the method has good reproducibility.

Strengths and Limitations

The validity of the photographic and video methods appears to be good, as does the reproducibility of video records.[78–80] The actual time to record food intake using the methods is less than that for 24-hour recalls, food records, or weighed-food records. Respondent burden also is considerably less with the two methods, and the practice of photographing food within the home was acceptable to participants. These advantages may lead to fewer of the alterations in diet that inevitably result from the recording process. The methods appear useful for evaluation of food selection in institutional settings such as retirement facilities, nursing homes, or cafeterias. They may be especially well suited for assessing intake of groups with cognitive, visual, or verbal impairment.[80]

Considerable initial expense is involved in both methods. Aside from the cost of video equipment or cameras, a greater amount of labor and expense is required in developing comparison photographs or slides of standard foods of known portion size. However, these costs may be offset by the greater efficiency and reduced long-term costs of the methods. Considerable skill is needed to interpret the slide or video records, and the coding procedure and time needed for clerical work remains the same as for traditional methods.[53] The methods are not suited to distinguishing between visually similar foods (for example, skim milk versus whole milk or premium ice cream versus ice milk). Some form of written or verbal records will continue to be necessary to document preparation methods and identify visually similar foods.[78,79] The likelihood of technical problems spoiling the data will increase as the sophistication of recording devices increases.

Box 3-11 summarizes the strengths and limitations of the photographic and video methods.

Computerized Techniques

To reduce respondent burden and increase validity of dietary intake data and the cost-effectiveness of collecting such data, computerized techniques to record dietary intake have been developed. Researchers at the USDA's Western Human Nutrition Research Center have developed what they call a Nutrition Evaluation Scale System.[81–84] A team from the United Kingdom has developed what they call a Food Recording Electronic Device.[86,87]

Nutrition Evaluation Scale System

The Nutrition Evaluation Scale System (NESSy) (Figure 3-5) is an electronic scale interfaced to a laptop computer with a built-in modem.[81–84] The user enters the identity of foods into the system by typing a brief description of the food into the computer prior to eating. The user then matches this description with the appropriate food item within the laptop's database. The computer then directs the user through the weighing of foods, containers, and leftovers. Users do not need to know how to operate the scale or computer, only how to respond to visual and audio instructions from the computer. The software is user-friendly, using icons, sounds, and on-screen prompts to guide users through the process of entering data. The identity and weights of foods consumed are saved in the computer's memory. These data then can be transferred via modem or disk to another

BOX 3-11

Strengths and Limitations of Photographic and Video Methods

Strengths

- Photographic method has good validity
- Video method has good validity and reproducibility
- Recording food intake takes less time than 24-hour recalls or food records
- Respondent burden is less
- Methods appear to be acceptable to subjects
- Eating habits may be less affected by recording
- Well suited for institutional settings and for disabled persons

Limitations

- Large initial expense involved, but this may be offset by lower long-term costs
- Periodic revalidations are recommended
- Unable to distinguish visually similar foods or document preparation methods
- Subject to technical problems caused by sophisticated equipment

computer for review by a dietitian and eventual analysis using a food composition database.

In a validation study, nine participants used the NESSy to record their food intake during a 16-day period. These data were compared with those obtained from weighed food records kept at the same time by research staff. There were no significant differences in group means between the two methods for energy or any nutrient.[84] When the two methods were compared on the basis of time required to weigh and record food, the NESSy provided savings in time and labor of about 80%.[82] Research has shown the instrument to be a reliable and valid method of measuring dietary intake by persons of both sexes and by free-living teenagers, adults, and older persons having no more than about 12 years of formal education.[83,85] The NESSy shows considerable promise as a method of providing precise quantitative data of an individual's dietary intake while significantly reducing the labor, time, and costs associated with collecting such data. The instrument was commercially available for purchase in 1995.

Food Recording Electronic Device

The Food Recording Electronic Device (FRED) is an electronic scale interfaced to a microprocessor and keyboard with over one hundred food record and control keys.[86] Because the number of keys is far smaller than the number of individual foods a user is likely to eat during the survey period, the food record keys represent *food groups* rather than *individual foods*. The food groups included in the FRED are determined by a questionnaire that each user initially completes. The instrument has 90 keys labeled with different foods or food groups, plus 5 keys that can be customized to suit a user's individual eating habits. Data are collected by setting an empty plate on the scale and, after each food item is added to the plate, depressing the key representing the food or food group to which the food item belongs. After eating, leftovers are weighed and accounted for in a similar manner. The instrument stores in its memory the weight and identity of each item until the data are downloaded to a larger computer for calculation of nutrient levels.[86]

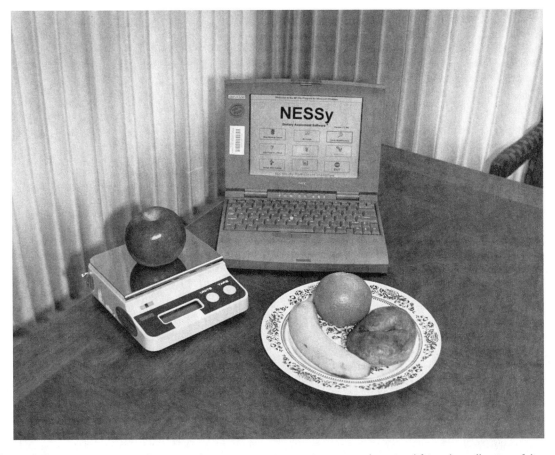

Figure 3-5 The Nutrition Evaluation Scale System is an innovative approach to simplifying the collection of dietary intake data. Photo courtesy of Dr. MJ Kretsch, USDA, ARS, San Francisco.

To test the validity of the FRED, consumption of energy, protein, and fat was measured for 7 days with the device. These results were compared with those of a conventional weighed-food record kept at the same time.[87] It was reported that the literate and motivated participants had little difficulty using the device and that use of food groups was not a source of error. However, technical problems with the device resulted in significant underestimations of energy, protein, and fat intake. Although the investigators expressed confidence that future improvements would lead to elimination of these problems, the instrument has not undergone any further development or testing in recent years.

Surrogate Sources

There are times when a respondent may not be able to provide the dietary intake data that investigators desire. In some instances, a respondent may have a problem with hearing, speech, or memory due to disease, trauma, or advanced age. This is especially a problem with elderly respondents participating in case-control studies. In such instances, obtaining information from **surrogate sources** may improve information quality and provide data otherwise unavailable from deceased or incompetent participants. Potential surrogate respondents include the respondent's spouse or partner, children, other close relatives, and friends.[10,88]

Several investigators have studied the use of surrogate sources of dietary intake. A review of these studies demonstrates that "surrogate respondents can provide dietary information, but that incomplete responses must be anticipated."[88] In some cases, surrogate respondents may provide more valid data than the respondents themselves. Surrogate sources often can provide good information on specific foods or nutrients. The availability of data from surrogate respondents varies with the relationship of the surrogate to the participant, the sex of the surrogate (e.g., females provide more accurate data about the eating habits of males than males do about the eating habits of females), and the number of shared meals. There may be considerable difference in the quality of surrogate data between spouses or partners of deceased participants and spouses or partners of living participants.[10]

Surrogate sources are good in studies where there is rapid mortality of study participants, concern about biased recall from participants, or where participants have problems with memory impairment or difficulty communicating because of such causes as stroke or Alzheimer's disease. In some instances, data from surrogates may be good enough for ranking persons in quintiles (one of five levels) in terms of their nutrient intake (i.e., as having an intake that is very low, low, average, high, or very high). In any event, surrogate sources must be carefully selected and data closely scrutinized because misclassification of dietary intake can occur easily when relying on surrogate sources alone.[10,88]

CONSIDERATIONS FOR CERTAIN GROUPS

Special adaptations in dietary measurement can be made for certain groups such as young persons, the reading impaired, individuals having problems recalling their diet, persons who are visually or hearing impaired, and the obese. These considerations, summarized in Box 3-12, facilitate ccollection of intake data from persons who otherwise might have difficulty participating in surveys.

ISSUES IN DIETARY MEASUREMENT

Validity

Validity is the ability of an instrument to actually measure what it is intended to measure.[31,97,98] In most instances, investigators are interested in knowing what a respondent's *usual intake* is or has been. Thus, validating an instrument involves comparing estimates of intake obtained by that instrument with a respondent's usual intake. Because it is difficult if not impossible to know a person's true usual intake, investigators must turn to *relative* or *criterion validity*. Relative or criterion validity is defined as the comparison of a new instrument with another instrument (a so-called "gold standard") that has a greater degree of *demonstrated* or *face validity*.[31,98] However, if the two instruments fail to compare favorably, the question must be asked, "Which instrument (if any) gave the best estimate of usual intake?" The failure of one instrument to compare favorably with another may not lie in the instrument being validated; it actually may have given the best estimate of usual intake. The fault may lie in the criterion instrument.

The validity of food frequency questionnaires has been examined by comparing estimates of food and nutrient intake obtained from food frequency questionnaires with estimates obtained from multiple food records or 24-hour recalls, which are thought to give a more detailed and quantitative estimate of dietary intake over an extended period.[41,42,98–100] Researchers at Harvard University, for example, collected four 1-week weighed-diet records over the course of a year from 173 participants.[41] These served as an estimate of usual intake during the 1-year period and the criterion against which intake data from the food frequency questionnaire were compared. Results of the study showed that a simple self-administered food frequency questionnaire could provide useful information about individual

BOX 3-12

Considerations when Measuring Diet in Certain Groups

Group	Considerations
Young persons	Dietary intake data on children under 8 years of age are best obtained from the person responsible for meals. For information on food eaten away from home, interview the child in the presence of parent or guardian. Data on meals eaten at school, kindergarten, or day care center can be obtained from those responsible for their meals. Reliable data on intake in the previous 24 hours can be obtained from children 8 years of age and older.
Persons with recall problems	There appears to be no firm evidence that memory of past diet is impaired during aging despite popular belief to the contrary. The ability to recall past diet may be more a function of how much attention is paid to what is eaten.[30] Diet recall can be helped through the use of checklists and visual aids such as food models and photographs.[30] Information obtained from surrogates (spouse, sibling, or caregiver) can improve quality of data.[88] Reproducibility of recall of diet many years in the past by older persons has been shown to be good but is reduced by older age, cognitive impairment, and male sex.[89]
Persons with impaired vision or hearing	Intake measurement instructions can be communicated to the visually impaired through large print materials, tape recordings, radio, telephone, personal interview, and Braille. Some visually impaired persons have video equipment that will enlarge print to a readable size. Data can be collected through personal interview, by telephone or tape recorder, or specially equipped computer systems. Communication of instructions to and collection of data from hearing-impaired persons is easily done with self-explanatory and well-prepared printed materials. Use of an interpreter of sign language and visual aids such as food models or photographs can be helpful. Verbal responses to an interviewer can facilitate collection of data.

Continued

BOX 3-12

Cont'd

Persons who cannot read well	Personal interviews, tape recorders, and telephone contacts can all be used in collecting dietary intake data from the reading impaired. Persons with limited reading ability may be able to use printed materials having an appropriate vocabulary. Food models and photographs are especially helpful. Printed forms relying heavily on pictures may be appropriate for collecting data.
The obese	Several studies have questioned the validity of reported energy intake in obese persons, indicating a tendency to underreport energy intake using the dietary history[90] and food records.[90–94] Other studies indicate this is a problem seen in both obese and normal-weight populations.[95,96]

From Cameron ME, Van Staveren WA. 1988. *Manual on methodology for food consumption studies*. New York: Oxford University Press, and other indicated sources.

nutrient intakes over a 1-year period. To study the questionnaire's ability to assess diet in the recent past, the researchers administered it to the same group of participants 3 to 4 years after the weighed-food records were collected and concluded that the questionnaire was useful in estimating nutrient intake 4 years in the past.[42] A number of other validation studies have been done as well.[44,47,54,55] Nutrient estimates derived from food frequency questionnaires compared favorably with those derived from criterion methods, suggesting that food frequency questionnaires can be appropriate to use in epidemiologic research. Overall, these studies support the use of food frequency questionnaires for estimating a group's average intake for energy and some nutrients. They also suggest that the method is appropriate for ranking individuals in terms of nutrient intake (e.g., categorizing individuals as having a low, average, or high intake of some nutrient).[41,99] Other investigators, however, question the use of food frequency questionnaires in epidemiologic research.[56,57]

The validity of a food frequency questionnaire depends in large part on items included in the food list and assumptions about portion size and nutrient content of the various groups.[24] Another important consideration in validation studies is the appropriateness of the criterion instrument. Given the weaknesses of food records and 24-hour recalls in characterizing usual intake, how appropriate are they to use as a "truth" measure against which to judge another instrument such as the food frequency questionnaire? If, in a validation study, data from food frequency questionnaires compare unfavorably to data from a criterion method, is it necessarily the fault of the food frequency questionnaire? A proposal for circumventing this dilemma is to include a biological marker as a *third* criterion method in the validation process.[58] Biological markers are discussed in the next section.

Some investigators have compared estimates of dietary intake using various methods with respondents' *actual* intake, which the investigators observed surreptitiously.[20–22,52] Usually the respondents ate all or at least most of their meals in a cafeteria or residential metabolic research facility where their food intake could be observed. Different assessment methods then could be used to measure respondents' intake during the period when their diet was observed. Among these were the 24-hour recall,[21,22,69,101,102] food records,[21,52] and food frequency questionnaires.[52] However, such comparisons over relatively short periods of time in monitored or controlled situations fail to adequately validate a method intended to assess the usual, self-selected diets of free-living persons.[98] Validation studies of the various diet measurement techniques are summarized in Box 3-13.

Use of Biologic Markers

Another approach to validating dietary measurement methods is to compare intake data with certain biologic markers associated with dietary intake.[10,58,110–113] Biologic markers offer the advantage of being easily accessible (urine, feces, blood, tissue samples) and providing a validity check of dietary intake independent of respondents' accuracy and truthfulness. A major problem, however, is that many factors other than dietary intake can affect nutrient concentrations in tissues, even in well-fed persons.[10] Although many biologic markers have potential for use, only a limited number have been investigated. Among these are nitrogen and sodium in urine, fatty acids in adipose tissue, and assessment of energy expenditure and body weight.[58,110–115]

Analysis of nitrogen in multiple 24-hour urine samples, the most well-known biologic marker, has been used to verify protein intake in dietary surveys.[110,112,115] If acceptable agreement exists between urinary nitrogen excretion and estimated protein intake, it can be assumed that intake of other nutrients is fairly well represented. Use of this method depends on several assumptions: that respondents are in nitrogen balance (there is no accumulation of protein for growth or repair or unusual losses due to starvation or injury); that estimates of extrarenal nitrogen excretion sufficiently cover losses through the feces, hair, skin, and other routes; and that all urine has been collected over the course of the collection period.[110,112] Researchers have attempted to use urinary levels of 3-methylhistidine, an amino acid released during muscle catabolism and excreted unchanged in the urine, in assessing meat consumption. Unfortunately, correlations between meat intake and 3-methylhistidine excretion have been low, apparently because of wide variability in 24-hour baseline excretion among individuals even when not consuming meat.[110] The presence of creatinine in meat makes 24-hour urine creatinine measurements ill suited for validating dietary estimates.[112]

Urinary sodium is a useful measure of dietary sodium intake, especially because amounts used at the table and in cooking are difficult to assess. Fecal sodium losses are minimal, and in temperate climates it is assumed that amounts in sweat are negligible. Differences in urinary sodium and estimated dietary intakes have been shown to be as low as 5%.[110] Because fecal losses of potassium are greater and more variable than with sodium, urinary potassium has not proven as suitable for validating dietary potassium intake.

A potential problem with measurements of nitrogen and sodium in 24-hour urine samples is the necessity of obtaining a *complete* 24-hour urine sample—a requirement some participants will have difficulty adhering to. One approach to checking on the completeness of 24-hour urine samples is use of the para-amino-benzoic acid (PABA) marker. Participants take one PABA tablet three times a day with their meals. The PABA is excreted in the urine. A 24-hour urine collection containing less than 85% of the PABA marker is considered unsatisfactory, either because the participant did not take all the PABA tablets or one or more urine specimens was omitted from the collection.[112]

Measurement of the urine osmolality (the number of dissolved particles per kilogram of urine) has been suggested as a method of assessing accuracy of reported dietary intake.[111] Urine osmolality is determined largely by nitrogen-containing substances and sodium and potassium salts in urine. It is measured using a 24-hour urine sample. It also can be predicted from dietary intake data obtained from food records and 24-hour dietary recalls. A measured osmolality significantly less than the predicted value indicates a lower food intake than that reported by

BOX 3-13

Summary of Studies Validating Diet Measurement Techniques

Measurement technique	Results of validation studies
24-hour recall	Can be validated directly by comparing with actual intake observed surreptitiously as in a cafeteria,[69] congregate meal site,[21,22] summer camp,[101] school lunch program,[102] or hospital. Comparisons with 7-day food record[27] or diet history[73] may not be appropriate since these methods measure diet over a different time frame than 24-hour recall. For most groups validity of the 24-hour recall is good for average group intakes of energy and certain nutrients.[103,104] Some researchers report overestimates of average group intakes in children[101] and the elderly.[22,105] Other researchers report the validity of 24-hour recalls for estimating group means when used in conjunction with food records.[106]
Food record or diary	In a direct validation study (actual weighed intake of noon meals over 7 days was compared with records of those meals) food records underestimated actual intake of energy and thiamin while no significant differences were seen for other nutrients studied.[21] Attempts to validate food records with periodic duplicate food collections have proved unsuccessful because of a decrease in energy and nutrient intake when duplicate food portions are collected.[97,98] Over a 7-day period, diet records for first 2 days were more valid than those for last 3 days. Education and motivation of respondents will affect validity of the last several days of diet records kept over a 7-day period.[21]
Food frequency questionnaire (FFQ)	This method has been compared against actual intake observed over 28 days in a cafeteria[59] and during 2 weeks in a metabolic unit.[52] The former study showed that a large percentage of college students could accurately estimate their intake with the FFQ while others had difficulty. In the latter study, the FFQ underestimated energy and nutrient intake. In comparison against food records, people report frequency of food consumption with reasonable accuracy.[27]

BOX 3-13

Cont'd

Food frequency questionnaire (FFQ)—*Cont'd*	Intake data from a semiquantitative FFQ compared favorably with that obtained from four 1-week weighed food records collected over a 12-month period.[41] A follow-up study using the FFQ to assess diet 3 to 4 years in the past showed the FFQ to be useful in assessing past diet.[42] In a similar study, correlations between a FFQ and diet records were lowest for selenium and vitamin A and highest for dietary fiber and polyunsaturated fats.[99] Comparisons with the diet history method show good correlations in terms of group averages but not for individuals.[61] When compared with reference methods, correlations tend to be low for highly variable nutrients such as vitamin A. However, the fault may not lie entirely with FFQs, as the reference data may not reflect usual intake.[98]
Diet history	In the few validation studies done, diet histories tend to overestimate group mean intakes compared with the reference method, which is generally 7-day estimated or weighed records.[61] As noted with FFQs, when compared with reference methods, correlations tend to be low for highly variable nutrients such as vitamin A. Again, the fault may not lie entirely with the diet history method since reference data may not be representative of usual intake.[98] Researchers attempting to measure past dietary intake using the diet history have noted that current diet can influence perceptions of past diet.[107–108]

From Gibson RS. 1990. *Principles of nutritional assessment*. New York: Oxford University Press, and other indicated sources.

the participant. A measured osmolality significantly greater than predicted indicates a greater food intake than that reported by the participant. As with urine nitrogen and sodium, the usefulness of this method depends on participants' obtaining complete 24-hour urine specimens.

Linoleic acid in adipose tissue can be used as an index of dietary intake of linoleic acid over the past 2 to 3 years, whereas the linoleic acid content of erythrocytes (red blood cells) can be an index of dietary linoleic acid during the past 6 to 8 weeks.[116] A small piece of adipose tissue can be easily removed from beneath the skin and measured for linoleic acid. This can be an independent way of estimating dietary fat intake. Such measurements have been shown to compare favorably with estimates of usual intake based on 2 weeks of weighed-food records and a food frequency questionnaire.[113] Another study showed that concentrations of monounsaturated and polyunsaturated fatty acids in adipose tissue compared closely with the type of fatty acids consumed by groups as assessed by 2-day food records.[110]

Energy Expenditure and Weight Maintenance

Another approach to validating dietary measurement methods is to compare reported energy intake with body weight and energy expenditure calculated from an equation or estimated using the doubly labeled water method. Self-reported energy intake has been compared with energy expenditure determined through use of the doubly labeled water method (discussed in greater detail in Chapter 8). Briefly, participants drink a known amount of water labeled with deuterium (^2H) and oxygen-18 ($^2H_2{}^{18}O$).[117] They provide periodic urine and blood samples over the next 2 weeks or so, which allow monitoring of the body's elimination of deuterium and oxygen-18. Knowledge of the rates at which these isotopes are eliminated allows researchers to calculate energy expenditure in free-living participants with considerable accuracy and precision, despite certain limitations discussed in Chapter 8. These studies show a consistent underreporting of energy intake by participants, especially among obese individuals.[117-119]

Researchers at the USDA Beltsville Human Nutrition Research Center compared self-reported energy intakes with the amount of energy the participants actually required to maintain their body weight to within ± 0.9 kg. The data, collected from 266 research participants over a 14-year period, showed that only 11% of self-reported energy intakes were accurate to within ± 100 kcal and that 81% of participants underreported their energy intake by 700 kcal ± 379 kcal (mean ± standard deviation).[120] Although some well-motivated and trained participants can reliably record their habitual food intake, it appears that most Americans underreport their habitual intake, resulting in an average discrepancy between reported and actual intake of about 18%.[120] During a 10-day field exercise in the Canadian Arctic, the self-reported energy intake of 20 infantrymen was 39% less than their actual energy expenditure measured by doubly labelled water.[121] A recent literature review reports that the energy expenditure of persons in energy balance (neither losing or gaining appreciable amounts of weight) averages about 18% less than reported energy intake. Underreporting of energy intake may be as high as 27% and 36% in obese and previously obese women, respectively.[94] Other investigators have reported a tendency for some obese persons to underreport food intake and overreport energy expenditure.[93] However, obesity may not be a universal predictor of the tendency to underreport.[112]

The findings of the Beltsville researchers led them to the hypothesis of the "uncertainty principle of food-intake measurements: the degree of deviation of reported from real intake is proportional to the degree of attention focused on the intake."[120] Although the task of maintaining food records resulted in an 18% underestimate of energy intake, collection of duplicate food portions resulted in a decline of an additional 13%.[63,120] Thus, although the collection of dietary data is critical to our understanding of nutrition, *dietary intake data must be interpreted with considerable caution,* whether self-reported or obtained by observers of whose presence respondents are aware.[117,120] These findings led another research team to recommend that "ideally, all dietary studies should include independent measures of validity."[94]

A simple check for underreporting of usual intake is to compare **resting energy expenditure** (REE) calculated from the equations in Table 3-2 with reported energy intake. If a participant's reported usual energy intake is < 1.2 times his or her calculated REE, underreporting of energy, and therefore nutrient, intake is highly likely.[94,122]

TABLE 3-2 Equations for calculating resting energy expenditure*

World Health Organization		
Females	3–9 years old	22.5 W + 499
	10–17 years old	12.2 W + 746
	18–29 years old	14.7 W + 496
	30–60 years old	8.7 W + 829
	>60 years old	10.5 W + 596
Males	3–9 years old	22.7 W + 495
	10–17 years old	17.5 W + 651
	18–29 years old	15.3 W + 679
	30–60 years old	11.6 W + 879
	>60 years old	13.5 W + 487
Harris-Benedict (values rounded for simplicity)		
Females	REE = 655 + 9.6W + 1.9S – 4.7A	
Males	REE = 66 + 13.8W + 5S – 6.8A	

*REE = resting energy expenditure; W = body weight in kg; S = stature in cm; A = age in years

Factors Affecting Validity

Several factors can affect the validity of an instrument. Among these are differences between usual diet and that measured in the study, inherent limitations or weaknesses of assessment methods, respondent characteristics, and observer characteristics. Examples of these are shown in Box 3-14. Sources of error in the different methods of measuring food intake are summarized in Table 3-3.

Reproducibility

Reproducibility or **reliability** can be defined as the ability of a method to produce the same estimate on two or more different occasions, assuming that nothing has changed in the interim.[98] Reproducibility is only concerned with whether a method is capable of providing the *same or similar answer* two or more times and does not necessarily indicate whether the answer is *correct*. Reproducibility studies can partially answer the validity question; a method cannot give a correct answer every time unless it gives approximately the same answer each time.[98] Problems in instrument design, respondent instructions, or quality control also can be uncovered by reproducibility studies.

How Many Days?

In studies comparing dietary and nutrient intakes with measures of health and disease, it is important to know how long dietary intake must be measured before a sufficiently reliable estimate of *usual intake* is obtained.[10,25,26,123] A few days of dietary observations, whether it be by 24-hour recall or food records, are not sufficient to adequately estimate an individual's usual intake. Because eating patterns vary between weekdays and weekends and across seasons, it is important to capture eating behavior in all parts of the week and in all seasons of the year.[10]

Investigators have tested approaches for calculating the number of days that dietary intake data must be collected.[25,26,123] Although a detailed discussion of these calculations is beyond the scope of this text, it should be noted that the number of days that data must be collected before usual intake can be estimated is related to an

BOX 3-14

Sources of Variation Between Actual Dietary Intake and that Measured by Various Methods

Causes of variation	Examples
Differences between usual diet and that measured in the study	Study group is unrepresentative of the general population.
	Individual's diet is unrepresentative of usual diet because sampling method fails to capture the type of variability that is present (e.g., weekday versus weekends, season to season, spells of illness, periodic episodes of weight-reduction diets, binges among bulimics, eating at home versus at business, travel, alternating day and night shifts).
	Number of observations made is inadequate.
Assessment method	Retrospective methods involve forgetting, which may be selective or nonuniform from food to food and may be influenced by frequency of consumption (seldom-eaten items remembered poorly), "telescoping," or including two weekends in one week.
	Prospective methods may lead to unconscious alteration of usual diets during reporting periods, especially in the first few days.
	Errors are present in food composition tables or nutrient database.
Respondent	Underreporting common among: Those who are nonadherent to therapeutic diets; Obese persons (especially early in reporting period for snacks, sweets, desserts); Heavy drinkers and alcoholics (for alcohol).

individual's day-to-day variation in nutrient intake (intraindividual variation) and the degree to which various individuals differ from one another in their nutrient intake (interindividual variation).[124,125] Estimation of usual dietary intake is facilitated when intraindividual variation is small in relation to interindividual variation. When the opposite condition exists (intraindividual variation is large relative to interindividual variation), characterization of usual intake requires a greater number of days.[124,125]

Other factors affecting the number of days of data collection include the purpose of the study, the sex and age of the group surveyed, and the nutrient(s) of interest. For most nutrients, fewer days are required to characterize the usual intake of persons 4 years old or younger (who typically consume a less varied diet) than for older children, adolescents, and adults (who generally consume a more varied diet).[26] The largest number of days is required for such nutrients as copper, vitamin A, vitamin B_{12}, and polyunsaturated fats.[25,26]

BOX 3-14

Cont'd

Respondent—*cont'd*	Overreporting common among: Recipients of food or meal program benefits; Anorectics and parents of infants with nonorganic failure to thrive; Those embarrassed about meager intakes. Alterations of a selective type: Respondents report their preconceived notions of ideal or desirable intakes; Respondents report what they think interviewers wish them to eat, especially respondents who have high needs for social approval or who fear loss of benefits or chastisement from those in power.
Observer	It is difficult to collect data about: Very old, very young persons (infants and children); Ill, retarded, or confused persons (mentally ill, alcoholics, drug addicts); Non–English-speaking persons or persons who cannot read; Subjects who lack interest or motivation; Subjects who desire to conceal true intake; Subjects who have chaotic and/or unstructured food intakes.

Table by Dwyer JT, used with permission from Stallones RA, 1982. Comments on the assessment of nutritional status in epidemiological studies and surveys of populations. *American Journal of Clinical Nutrition* 35:1290–1291.

Table 3-4 illustrates the problem of trying to estimate usual intake with a single 24-hour recall.[98] The precision of a single 24-hour recall in estimating kilocalorie intake for a typical male would be ± 51%. In other words, if a 24-hour recall estimated energy intake at 2300 kcal, the true long-term intake could be 51% greater or less than that estimate and thus could range from 1150 to 3450 kcal. Estimates for vitamin A have a precision of only ± 293% for males and ± 224% for females.

Data from the Beltsville 1-year dietary intake study have been used to calculate the number of days of food records needed to estimate an individual's true usual intake.[123,126] In the Beltsville study, 29 individuals kept food records for 365 consecutive days while consuming their customary diets. The ranges and averages for males and females, shown in Table 3-5, indicate the number of days of food records required for estimates of nutrient intake to be within ± 10% of true usual intake 95% of the time (that is, to have a *confidence index [CI] of 95%*).

It is apparent from Table 3–5 that the number of days needed to estimate usual intake of individuals varies among different participants and for

TABLE 3-3 Sources of error in methods estimating food consumption*

Sources of error	Duplicate portion	Weighed record	Estimated record	24-hour recall	Dietary history
Response errors					
Omitting foods	−	±	±	+	+
Adding foods	−	−	−	+	+
Estimating weight of foods	−	−	+	+	+
Estimating frequency of consumption of foods	−	−	−	−	+
Day-to-day variation	+	+	+	+	−
Changes in diet	+	+	±	−	−
Coding errors	−	+	+	+	+
Errors in conversion of nutrients					
Food composition tables	−	+	+	+	+
Sampling errors	+	−	−	−	−
Direct analysis	+	−	−	−	−

From Bingham SA, Nelson M, Paul AA, Haraldsdottir J, Loken EB, Van Staveren WA. 1988. Methods for data collection at an individual level. In Cameron ME, Van Staveren WA (eds.) *Manual on methodology for food consumption studies.* New York: Oxford University Press. Reprinted by permission of Oxford University Press.

*− indicates error is unlikely; + indicates error is likely.

different nutrients. Energy requires the least number of records whereas vitamin A requires the greatest number. A minimum of 14 days of records was required for capturing usual intake of energy of the 29 participants, but one male required 84 days of records and one female required 60 days.[123] These differences among different individuals, sexes, and nutrients reflect intraindividual variability in nutrient intake. Nutrient intake over several days tends to vary less in some persons than in others. Among all persons, day-to-day fluctuations in energy intake are much less than for nutrients such as vitamin C or vitamin A.

In contrast with estimating the usual intake of individuals, fewer days of data collection are necessary if the study's purpose is to estimate usual intake of groups or to rank the nutrient intake of individuals.[123,125] Data from the Beltsville study (Table 3-6) indicate the number of days of food records needed to estimate true average intake for groups of individuals with a precision of ± 10% and a CI of 95%.[123]

ESTIMATING PORTION SIZE

A variety of approaches can be used to help participants estimate portion sizes. Among the simplest and least costly are "food models" composed of various geometric shapes cut out of poster board, as shown in Figure 3-6. Circles of various diameters can be used to help estimate the diameter of round foods such as apples, oranges, tomato slices, hamburger patties, hamburger buns, and cookies. Square and rectangular pieces are useful in estimating the length and width of bread, cake, some cuts of meat, and cheese. Pie-shaped pieces of various radii can be used in estimating portion sizes of pie, round cake, watermelon, and pizza. Two-dimensional

TABLE 3-4 Precision of estimates from one 24-hour recall*

Nutrient	Males (%)	Females (%)
Kilocalories	± 51	± 63
Protein	± 71	± 62
Carbohydrate	± 59	± 72
Total fat	± 62	± 79
Polyunsaturated fat	± 100	± 150
Cholesterol	± 105	± 109
Vitamin C	± 134	± 130
Vitamin A	± 293	± 224

From Block GS and Hartman AM. 1989. Issues in reproducibility and validity of dietary studies. *American Journal of Clinical Nutrition* 50:1133–1138.

*Data from Beaton GH, Milner J, McGuire V, Feather TE, Little JA. 1983. Source of variance in 24-hour dietary recall data: implications for nutrition study design and interpretation. Carbohydrate sources, vitamins, and minerals. *American Journal of Clinical Nutrition* 37:986–995; and Beaton GH, Milner J, McGuire V, Feather TE, Little JA. 1979. Sources of variance in 24-hour dietary recall data: Implications for nutrition study design and interpretation. *American Journal of Clinical Nutrition* 32:2456–2459.

food models have been shown to be as effective as three-dimensional models for estimating portion size in nutritional research.[127]

Pieces of polyurethane foam 3 to 4 inches square and of varying thicknesses can be used to help respondents estimate the thickness of foods. Individual pieces can be used, or several can be stacked to achieve the desired thickness. An alternate approach is to have a number of pieces of cardboard cut 3 to 4 inches square, which can then be stacked to aid in estimating the thickness of food. Polystyrene balls of various diameters are useful in estimating sizes of round food objects. Bowls, plates, measuring cups and spoons, and drinking cups of various sizes also can be used to help respondents estimate serving sizes of soup, breakfast cereal, salad, beverages, sugar, and margarine.

Some investigators have used photographs to facilitate portion size estimation.[128] The photographs, similar to the one shown in Figure 3-7, illustrated each food in the three most frequent serving sizes. The plate used in the photograph was available to provide a sense of scale.

When, during an interview, identification of particular brand names of foods consumed is important, a notebook containing photographs of various foods, pictures cut from magazine advertisements, or actual food labels can be used. A photograph of a supermarket dairy case, for example, can help respondents identify the brand of margarine used at home. During the course of a 24-hour recall, for example, a child is likely to remember the brand of potato or corn chips he or she ate but perhaps not the particular bag size. Including in the notebook an assortment of snack food wrappers (for candy, chips, and chewing gum of various brands and sizes) can be helpful in collecting accurate intake data. Lifelike food models such as those shown in Figure 3-8 also can be used to help respondents estimate food portion sizes. Recent research suggests that memory of food portion sizes is not long lasting and that food models are only useful for collecting very crude portion size information.

FOOD COMPOSITION TABLES

A primary function of dietary measurement data is estimating the intake of particular nutrients and other food components consumed by groups and/or individuals. This is done by combining data on food consumption with information on the nutrient composition of food obtained from food composition tables and databases.[1]

Early Tables

Food composition tables, like the science of nutrition, are a relatively recent development. The earliest known data on nutrient composition was reported in 1795 by the English scientist

TABLE 3-5 Ranges and averages of number of days required to estimate true average intake for an individual with given statistical confidence*

	Range and average number of days required					
	Males (n = 13)			Females (n = 16)		
Component	Minimum	Average	Maximum	Minimum	Average	Maximum
Food energy	14	27	84	14	35	60
Iron	18	68	130	28	66	142
Vitamin A	115	390	1724	152	474	1372
Protein	23	36	72	23	48	70
Fat	34	57	131	32	71	114
Saturated fat	30	71	156	42	87	149
Oleic acid	35	68	163	31	85	145
Linoleic acid	77	145	225	82	166	237
Cholesterol	85	139	195	104	200	443
Carbohydrate	10	37	177	16	41	77
Crude fiber	43	82	146	51	86	138
Calcium	30	74	140	35	88	168
Phosphorus	18	32	62	19	41	62
Potassium	17	34	67	25	48	83
Sodium	27	58	140	36	73	116
Thiamin	46	138	405	41	198	728
Riboflavin	13	57	135	31	90	231
Niacin	27	53	89	48	78	126
Vitamin C	90	249	900	83	222	328

From Basiotis PP, Welsh SO, Cronin FJ, Kelsay JL, Mertz W. Number of days of food intake records required to estimate individual and group nutrient intakes with defined confidence. *Journal of Nutrition* 117:1638–1641.

*Estimated using intake data from 1-year dietary intake study by the U.S. Department of Agriculture's Beltsville Human Nutrition Research Center.

Pearson, who analyzed the composition of potatoes. Development of a simplified system of food analysis by German scientists in the mid-1800s allowed a large number of chemists from several countries to begin the systematic analysis of foods, and the early food composition tables were developed.[129–132]

The first comprehensive table for American foods was published by W. O. Atwater and C. D. Woods in 1896 as USDA Bulletin No. 28, *The Chemical Composition of American Food Materials*.[133,134] Values were expressed as percent available of refuse, water, protein, fat, carbohydrate, and ash, with energy stated as kilocalories per pound. By 1945, tables began to include values for several vitamins and minerals.[132] Improved analytical techniques, an increasing number of nutrients recognized as essential, interest in relationships between diet and health, and development of new food products have made the revision of existing tables and the creation of new tables an ongoing process.

Current Tables and Databases

Of any organization in the world, the USDA maintains the most comprehensive system for collecting food composition data. The Human

TABLE 3-6 Number of days required to estimate true average intake for groups of individuals with given statistical confidence*

Component	Estimated number of days required for each group	
	Males ($n = 13$)	Females ($n = 16$)
Food energy	3	3
Iron	7	6
Vitamin A	39	44
Protein	4	4
Fat	6	6
Saturated fat	8	7
Oleic acid	6	7
Linoleic acid	13	12
Cholesterol	13	15
Carbohydrate	5	4
Crude fiber	9	9
Calcium	10	7
Phosphorus	4	5
Potassium	4	5
Sodium	6	6
Thiamin	13	16
Riboflavin	7	7
Niacin	5	6
Vitamin C	33	19

From Basiotis PP, Welsh SO, Cronin FJ, Kelsay JL, Mertz W. 1987. Number of days of food intake records required to estimate individual and group nutrient intakes with defined confidence. *Journal of Nutrition* 117:1638–1641.

*Estimated using intake data from 1-year dietary intake study by the U.S. Department of Agriculture's Beltsville Human Nutrition Research Center.

Nutrition Information Service (HNIS) of the USDA maintains the National Nutrient Data Bank (NNDB), the ultimate source from which data are drawn for a variety of published and machine-readable databases, including the nutrient databases for assessing diets reported in national food consumption surveys.[135] The HNIS obtains some food composition data through its contracts with universities and food-testing laboratories. However, 85% of the data in the NNDB comes from either the food industry or scientific literature.[135] The rapid expansion of food composition data, both in the number of food items analyzed and different nutrients reported, has necessitated a computerized data management system. The NNDB provides several computerized databases for estimating nutrient intake from dietary intake data. These are provided through the National Technical Information Service and will be further discussed in Chapter 5. These food composition data are available to the general public in two major sources: the HNIS's National Nutrient Data Bank Electronic Bulletin Board (see Chapter 5 for details on accessing the bulletin board and downloading files) and Handbooks 8 and 456 and Home and Garden Bulletin No. 72.

The USDA's Handbook No. 8, *Composition of Foods, Raw, Processed, Prepared* is the most extensive food composition table in the world and serves as the published standard reference for food composition in the United States.[135] Since first published as a single volume in 1950, it has grown into a 21-volume work, with each volume covering nutrient values for a major food group. The 1950 edition included values for 15 food components and nutrients for 751 foods. The 1963 edition provided values for 20 food components and nutrients for nearly 2500 foods. The current edition provides values for water, protein, lipids, carbohydrate, ash, nine minerals (calcium, iron, magnesium, phosphorus, potassium, sodium, zinc, copper, and manganese), nine vitamins (ascorbic acid, thiamin, riboflavin, niacin, pantothenic acid, vitamin B_6, folate, vitamin B_{12}, and vitamin A), individual fatty acids, cholesterol, total phytosterols, 18 amino acids, and dietary fiber.

To facilitate continual and rapid updating, the handbook is published in loose-leaf form, and each page contains the nutrient profile of a single food item. The USDA publishes an annual supplement to update selected items and to add data for new items. The supplements contain loose-leaf pages for insertion into the existing handbook sections. Individual sections of the handbook and annual supplements can be obtained through the U.S. Government Printing Office. Data used in revising Handbook No. 8 are

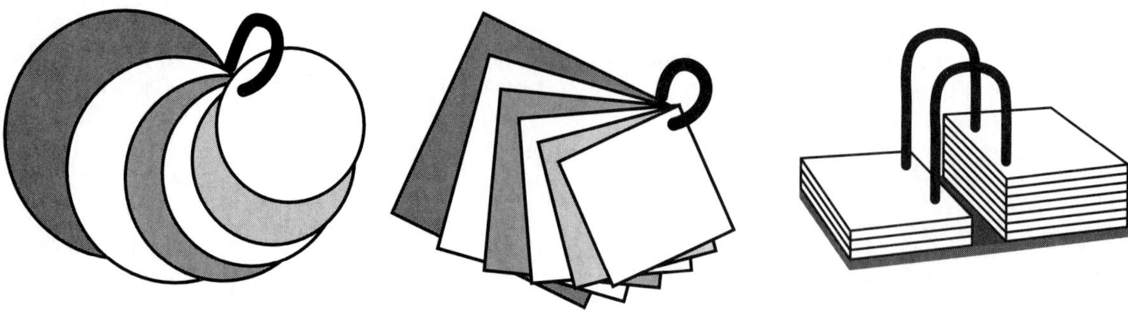

Figure 3-6 Simple, geometric shapes representing foods are sometimes used to help survey participants estimate food portion size. Each piece has a known dimension (surface area of thickness) and is made from poster board or other materials.

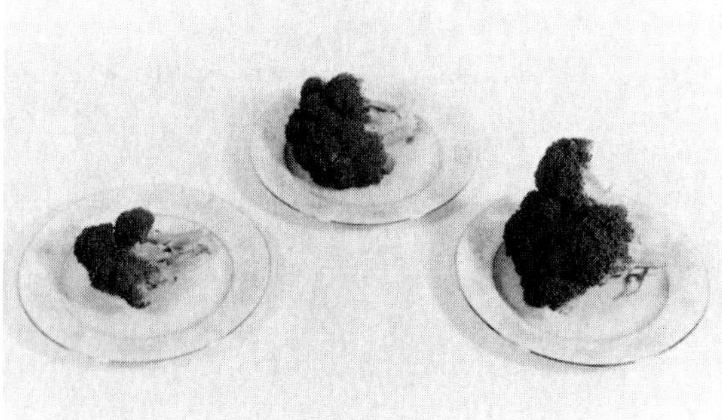

Figure 3-7 Some investigators use photographs to help respondents more accurately estimate food portion size.

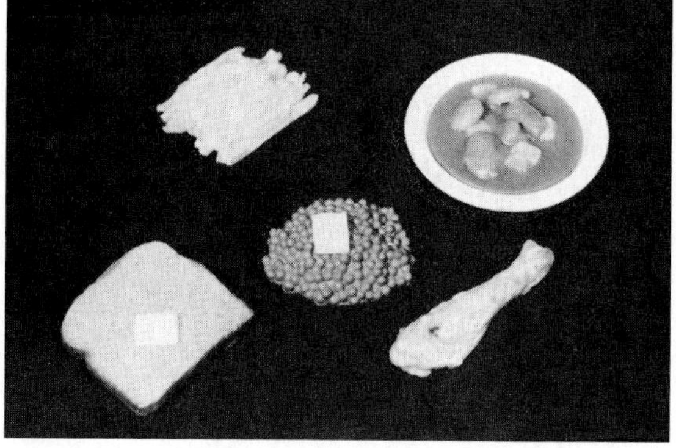

Figure 3-8 Lifelike food models can be used to improve accuracy in estimating food portion sizes.

supplied through the cooperation of private industry, government agencies, academic institutions, and contract research. The data are compiled by using the USDA's computerized NNDB. Table 3-7 outlines the current food groups covered by the different sections of Handbook No. 8.

Agriculture Handbook No. 456, *Nutritive Value of American Foods in Common Units,* was published in 1975. It contains nutrient data on 1500 foods using common household measures and market units. Values are given for water, energy, protein, carbohydrate, five minerals (calcium, phosphorus, iron, sodium, and potassium) and five vitamins (vitamin A, thiamin, riboflavin, niacin, and ascorbic acid), total fat, and fatty acids (total saturated, oleic, and linoleic). Foods are identified by the same numbering system used in Handbook No. 8. It is still available from the U.S. Government Printing Office.

USDA Home and Garden Bulletin No. 72, *Nutritive Value of Foods,* was first published in 1960 and was revised in 1991. It provides values for 15 food components and nutrients for 730 different foods based on average serving sizes or common household measures. It is based on data from Handbook No. 8.

Bowes and Church's Food Values of Portions Commonly Used has remained a popular source of nutrient data since it was first published in 1937. From its inception, its purpose has been "to supply

TABLE 3-7 Status of Handbook No. 8 sections

Section number*	Food group	Year of revision
AH-8–1	Dairy and egg products	1976
AH-8–2	Spices and herbs	1977
AH-8–3	Baby foods	1978
AH-8–4	Fats and oils	1979
AH-8–5	Poultry products	1979
AH-8–6	Soups, sauces, and gravies	1980
AH-8–7	Sausages and luncheon meats	1980
AH-8–8	Breakfast cereals	1982
AH-8–9	Fruits and fruit juices	1982
AH-8–10	Pork products	1983
AH-8–11	Vegetables and vegetable products	1984
AH-8–12	Nut and seed products	1984
AH-8–13	Beef products	1990
AH-8–14	Beverages	1986
AH-8–15	Finfish and shellfish products	1987
AH-8–16	Legumes and legume products	1986
AH-8–17	Lamb, veal, and game products	1989
AH-8–18	Baked products	1992
AH-8–19	Snacks and sweets	1991
AH-8–20	Cereal, grains, and pasta	1989
AH-8–21	Fast foods	1988

*AH-8–1 = Agriculture Handbook No. 8, section No. 1, etc.

authoritative data on the nutritional values of foods in a form for quick and easy reference."[136] Based largely on USDA data, it also includes values from the food industry and scientific literature. Features distinguishing it from Handbook No. 8 include its listing of foods by groups, use of household measures and gram weights, and identification of some foods by brand name.

Sources of Error in Food Composition Data

Errors can be introduced into food composition data from three major sources: values in a table that differ from the nutrient content of a food because of the way the food was grown, stored, or processed; biases due to incorrect identification of food items, use of inappropriate analytical methods, and use of imputed values; and differences in the bioavailability of individual nutrients.[137]

The nutrient content of foods can vary depending on plant variety, animal breed, geographic location, season of production, growing conditions, maturity, and transport and storage conditions.[1,9] The ascorbic acid content of oranges has been shown to vary from 20 to 80 mg per 100 g, depending on such factors as variety, production site, season of production, and maturity. Potatoes stored for 3 months can lose as much as half of their original ascorbic acid content.[138] Because of this, values in food composition tables are average values and apply to food as it is usually produced and marketed for year-round and countrywide use by consumers. The actual amount of a nutrient in any food may vary substantially from the average value given in food composition tables. It is thought, however, that use of representative or average values does not contribute greatly to the variability in the estimate of usual nutrient intake.[1]

Items listed in food composition tables must be clearly identified to avoid confusion with other items having different nutritive values. When the nutrient content of a diet is estimated, foods consumed should be carefully matched with those in food composition tables.[132]

The use of inappropriate analytical techniques can result in erroneous nutrient data. Some methods may not measure all the biologically active forms of a nutrient or may be inhibited by certain food components and thus result in underreporting of nutrient content. Certain assays may react to forms of the nutrient that are not biologically active or to food components other than the nutrient in question and thus overstate its presence.[137] A recent report from the U.S. General Accounting Office (GAO) was critical of the Human Nutrition Information Service for incorporating into the National Nutrient Data Base food composition data with "little or no supporting information on the testing and quality assurance procedures used to develop the data."[135] According to the GAO, some of the data in Handbook No. 8 on fast-food came primarily from brochures produced by fast-food chains. The brochures generally did not explain how the nutrient values were determined. The GAO recommended that the Human Nutrition Information Service develop specific quality control criteria for evaluating food composition data obtained from other sources and improved procedures to better direct the generation of food composition data under HNIS's contracts.

When certain nutrient data are unavailable, compilers of food composition tables may substitute missing data with **imputed data**, which are obtained from similar foods or ingredients for which data are more complete. Nutrient data on prepared dishes, for example, often are derived from data on ingredients rather than from direct analysis of the prepared foods themselves. Inaccuracies in imputed data can be a potential source of error in using nutrient data.[132,137]

Providing data on all nutrients in all types of food consumed is an overwhelming task. The most accurate and complete food composition data in the NNDB are for those foods most commonly consumed within the United States and for those nutrients for which a requirement or disease relationship has long been recognized. Nutrient content data are lacking for some nutrients because accurate, precise, and affordable analytical methodologies currently are not available.[1] However, the amount of data for the nutrient content of food has increased markedly in recent years. Table 3-8 shows changes in the percentage of analytical data for certain nutrients in the USDA's Primary Data Set from 1987 to 1991.[139] Progress was most noteworthy for copper, folate, dietary fiber, and alpha-tocopherol. Efforts are underway by the Nutrient Data Research Branch of the Human Nutrition Information Service to increase the percentage of analytical data for alpha-tocopherol and dietary fiber.[139]

Every year, an increasing variety and number of commercially prepared foods are introduced into the marketplace. Data on these foods supplied by the food industry are limited to nutrients required by labeling regulations and are compiled solely on the basis of the "as purchased" state. There is a great need for nutrient information on foods as they are consumed, which takes into account processing and preparation either at home or at retail establishments or institutions.[140] Also needed are more complete data on highly processed or manufactured foods such as snack foods, baked products, convenience foods, restaurant meals, fast foods, and frozen dinners.[9] The USDA's Nutrient Composition Laboratory recently has undertaken a program of nationwide sampling of foods and analysis for important nutrients. Foods to be analyzed have been prioritized based on the frequency of their consumption.[140]

The bioavailability of certain nutrients can be influenced by a number of factors. The absorption of iron, for example, is affected by its chemical

TABLE 3-8 Changes in the percentage of analytical data for a given nutrient in the U.S. Department of Agriculture's Primary Data Set from 1987 to 1991

Nutrient	Percentage in 1987*	Percentage in 1991
Vitamin C	92	95
Vitamin B_{12}	70	95
Carotene	88	93
Vitamin A (RE)†	73	92
Vitamin B_6	72	92
Zinc	79	91
Magnesium	72	90
Copper	71	88
Folate	69	87
Dietary fiber	40	82
α-tocopherol	39	47

From Matthews RH (ed). 1991. *16th National Nutrient Databank Conference Proceedings*. Ithaca, N.Y.: The CBORD Group, Inc.

*Data from Hepburn FN. 1987. Food Consumption/Food Composition Interrelationships. Human Nutrition Information Service, HNIS Report No. Adm-382. Hyattsville, Md: USDA.

†Retinol equivalents.

form in the diet, certain dietary components and nutrients that promote or inhibit its absorption, and physiologic requirements. Food composition tables do not account for factors influencing iron bioavailability. Consequently, although estimates of iron intake based solely on tables may indicate consumption, they may not represent what is actually biologically available.[137]

SUMMARY

1. The ultimate reason for measuring diet is to improve human health. Other reasons include assessing and monitoring food and nutrient intake, formulating and evaluating government health and agricultural policy, conducting epidemiologic research, and uses for commercial purposes.
2. No single best method exists for measuring dietary intake. Each method possesses certain advantages and disadvantages. The method used depends on research design considerations, characteristics of the study participants, available resources, and whether the intent is to estimate average group intake, rank individuals within a group, or estimate an individual's usual intake.
3. In the 24-hour recall method, a trained interviewer asks the respondent to remember all foods and beverages consumed during the past 24 hours. The 24-hour recall is quickly administered, has a low respondent burden, but does not give data representative of an individual's usual intake.
4. When keeping a food record or diary, the respondent records, at the time of consumption, the identity and amounts of all foods and beverages consumed during a 1- to 7-day period. Foods either can be quantified using household measures or weighed, in which case the method is called weighed-food record. This method does not rely on memory, can provide detailed intake data, requires a high degree of respondent cooperation, and may result in alterations of diet.
5. A food frequency questionnaire assesses nutrient intake by determining the frequency of consumption of a limited number of foods known to be major sources of the dietary components of interest. Respondents indicate how many times a day, week, month, or year the foods usually are consumed. Relatively high-quality data can be gathered on large groups of respondents; data may be more representative of usual intake than a few days of diet records; respondents must be able to describe their diets; and foods and portion sizes included in questionnaires must be carefully chosen.
6. Collection of duplicate food portions is a more direct method of assessing nutrient intake that avoids some of the problems

associated with coding and entering data and the limitations of food composition tables such as nutrient losses during food storage and preparation. Respondents collect identical portions of all foods and beverages consumed during a specified period, which are then analyzed at a laboratory for nutrient content. Respondent concern about the expense of duplicate portions can alter eating habits, resulting in underestimates of nutrient intake.

7. Food accounts estimate dietary intake within households and institutions where congregate feeding is practiced. The food inventory at the end of the survey period is subtracted from the sum of the beginning inventory and food obtained during the study period. Daily mean consumption per person is calculated by dividing total food consumed by number of meals served. This is a relatively economical method of assessing dietary intake of large groups. It does not account for food losses or meals eaten outside the group and cannot provide estimates of individual food intake.
8. The food balance sheet provides data on food disappearance (or availability) rather than actual food consumption. Mean per capita annual amounts are calculated by dividing total food disappearance by the country's population. It detects trends in food availability within a country over time and generates data that are useful in epidemiologic research across countries. The data only represent food that disappeared from the food distribution system and may be of questionable accuracy.
9. The high cost of research has led to innovations in the collection of dietary intake data. Included among these are telephone interviewing, photographic and video records, and computers interfaced with electronic scales for recording the identities and weights of foods consumed. Some of these methods have the potential of reducing respondent burden and increasing the validity of dietary intake data and the cost-effectiveness of collecting such data.
10. Surrogate sources are necessary when intake data are needed from persons unwilling or unable to provide them. Potential surrogate respondents include the spouse, partner, children, other close relatives, and friends of the respondent.
11. Validity is the ability of an instrument to measure what it is intended to measure. Validating a method involves comparing measurements of intake obtained by that method with estimates obtained using another method that is thought to have a greater degree of demonstrated or face validity. Some biologic markers can provide a validity check of dietary intake independent of respondents' accuracy and truthfulness.
12. Reproducibility or reliability is the ability of a method to produce the same estimate on two or more different occasions, assuming that nothing has changed in the interim. Reproducibility studies are important in partially answering the validity question; a method cannot give a correct answer every time unless it gives approximately the same answer each time.
13. To estimate usual nutrient intake, diet must be measured for multiple days, different days of the week (weekdays vs. weekends), and throughout the seasons of the year. The number of days required largely depends on the nutrient of interest, whether individuals or groups are studied, the degree of interindividual variation in nutrient intake, and the desired degree of precision.
14. Estimates of portion sizes can be sources of error in measuring dietary intake. A number of tools have been developed to assist respondents in accurately reporting amounts of foods consumed. These include photographs of food, geometric shapes of various sizes, measuring devices, and lifelike plastic food models.

15. Food composition tables allow nutrient intake to be estimated from data on food consumption. The USDA maintains the most comprehensive system for collecting food composition data in the world, including several published tables and computerized databases.
16. Errors can be introduced into food composition data from three major sources: values in a table that differ from the nutrient content of a food because of the way the food was grown, stored, or processed; biases due to incorrect identification of food items, use of inappropriate analytical methods, and use of imputed values; and differences in the bioavailability of individual nutrients.

REFERENCES

1. U.S. Department of Health and Human Services. 1989. *Nutrition monitoring in the United States—An update report on nutrition monitoring.* Washington, DC: U.S. Government Printing Office.
2. Begin I, Cap M, Dujardin B. 1988. *A guide to nutritional assessment.* Geneva: World Health Organization.
3. Stamler J. 1994. Assessing diets to improve world health: Nutritional research on disease causation in populations. *American Journal of Clinical Nutrition* 59(suppl):146S–156S.
4. Sabry JH. 1988. Purposes of food consumption surveys. In Cameron ME, Van Staveren WA, eds. *Manual on methodology for food consumption studies.* New York: Oxford University Press.
5. Buzzard IM. 1994. Rationale for an international conference series on dietary assessment methods. *American Journal of Clinical Nutrition* 59 (suppl):143S–145S.
6. Sempos CT, Briefel RR, Johnson C, Woteki CE. 1992. Process and rationale for selecting dietary methods for NHANES III. In National Center for Health Statistics. *Dietary methodology workshop for the Third National Health and Nutrition Examination Survey.* Hyattsville, Md: U.S. Department of Health and Human Services, Public Health Service, Centers for Disease Control.
7. Beaton GH. 1994. Approaches to analysis of dietary data: Relationship between planned analyses and choice of methodology. *American Journal of Clinical Nutrition* 59(suppl):253S–261S.
8. Liu K. 1992. Statistical issues related to the design of dietary survey methodology for NHANES III. In National Center for Health Statistics. *Dietary methodology workshop for the Third National Health and Nutrition Examination Survey.* Hyattsville, Md: U.S. Department of Health and Human Services, Public Health Service, Centers for Disease Control.
9. Food and Nutrition Board, National Research Council. 1989. *Diet and health: Implications for reducing chronic disease risk.* Washington, DC: National Academy Press.
10. Thompson FE, Byers T. 1994. Dietary assessment resource manual. *Journal of Nutrition* 124(suppl):2245S–2317S.
11. Block G. 1989. Human dietary assessment: Methods and issues. *Preventive Medicine* 18:653–660.
12. Lee Han H, McGuire V, Boyd NF. 1989. A review of the methods used by studies of dietary measurement. *Journal of Clinical Epidemiology* 42:269–279.
13. Block G. 1982. A review of validations of dietary assessment methods. *American Journal of Epidemiology* 115:492–505.
14. Dwyer JT, Krall EA, Coleman KA. 1987. The problem of memory in nutritional epidemiology research. *Journal of the American Dietetic Association* 87:1509–1512.
15. Feskanich D, Willett WC. 1993. The use and validity of food frequency questionnaires in epidemiologic research and clinical practice. *Medicine, Exercise, Nutrition, and Health* 2:143–154.
16. Briefel RR. 1994. Assessment of the U.S. diet in national nutrition surveys: National collaborative efforts and NHANES. *American Journal of Clinical Nutrition* 59(suppl):164S–167S.
17. Guenther PM. 1994. Research needs for dietary assessment and monitoring in the United States. *American Journal of Clinical Nutrition* 59 (suppl):168S–170S.

18. National Center for Health Statistics. 1994. *Plan and operation of the Third National Health and Examination Survey, 1988–94*. Hyattsville, Md: U.S. Department of Health and Human Services, Public Health Service, Centers for Disease Control.
19. Crawford PB, Obarzanek E, Morrison J, Sabry ZI. 1994. Comparative advantage of 3-day food records over 24-hour recall and 5-day food frequency validated by observation of 9- and 10-year-old girls. *Journal of the American Dietetic Association* 94:626–630.
20. Karvetti RL, Knuts LR. 1985. Validity of the 24-hour dietary recall. *Journal of the American Dietetic Association* 85:1437–1442.
21. Gersovitz M, Madden JP, Smiciklas-Wright H. 1978. Validity of the 24-hour dietary recall and seven-day record for group comparisons. *Journal of the American Dietetic Association* 73:48–55.
22. Madden JP, Goodman SJ, Guthrie HA. 1976. Validity of the 24-hour recall. Analysis of data obtained from elderly subjects. *Journal of the American Dietetic Association* 68:143–147.
23. Block G, Hartman AM, Dresser CM, Carroll MD, Gannon J, Gardner L. 1986. A data-based approach to diet questionnaire design and testing. *American Journal of Epidemiology* 124:453–469.
24. Block G. 1992. Dietary assessment issues related to cancer for NHANES III. In National Center for Health Statistics. *Dietary methodology workshop for the Third National Health and Nutrition Examination Survey*. Hyattsville, Md: U.S. Department of Health and Human Services, Public Health Service, Centers for Disease Control.
25. Beaton GH, Milner J, McGuire V, Feather TE, Little JA. 1983. Source of variance in 24-hour dietary recall data: Implications for nutrition study design and interpretation. Carbohydrate sources, vitamins, and minerals. *American Journal of Clinical Nutrition* 37:986–995.
26. Nelson M, Black AE, Morris JA, Cole TJ. 1989. Between- and within-subject variation in nutrient intake from infancy to old age: Estimating the number of days required to rank dietary intakes with desired precision. *American Journal of Clinical Nutrition* 50:155–167.
27. Smith AF. 1991. Cognitive processes in long-term dietary recall. *Vital and Health Statistics* 6(4). Hyattsville, Md: National Center for Health Statistics.
28. Tarasuk V, Beaton GH. 1992. Statistical examination of dietary parameters: Implications of patterns in within-subject variation—a case of sampling strategies. *American Journal of Clinical Nutrition* 55:22–27.
29. Larkin FA, Metzner HL, Guire KE. 1991. Comparison of three consecutive-day and three random-day records of dietary intake. *Journal of the American Dietetic Association* 91:1538–1542.
30. Hankin JH. 1989. Development of a diet history questionnaire for studies of older persons. *American Journal of Clinical Nutrition* 50:1121–1127.
31. Dwyer JT. 1994. Dietary Assessment. In Shils ME, Olson JA, Shike M, eds. *Modern nutrition in health and disease,* 8th ed. Philadelphia: Lea & Febiger.
32. Smucker R, Block G, Coyle L, Harvin R, Kessler L. 1989. A dietary and risk factor questionnaire and analysis system for personal computers. *American Journal of Epidemiology* 129:445–449.
33. Block G, Clifford C, Naughton MD, Henderson M, McAdams M. 1989. A brief dietary screen for high fat intake. *Journal of Nutrition Education* 21:199–207.
34. Cummings SR, Block G, McHenry K, Baron RB. 1987. Evaluation of two food frequency methods of measuring dietary calcium intake. *American Journal of Epidemiology* 126:796–802.
35. Samet JM, Humble CG, Skipper BE. 1984. Alternatives in the collection and analysis of food frequency interview data. *American Journal of Epidemiology* 120:572–581.
36. Hankin JH, Nomura AMY, Lee J, Hirohata T, Kolonel LN. 1983. Reproducibility of a diet history questionnaire in a case-control study of breast cancer. *The American Journal of Clinical Nutrition* 37:981–985.
37. Brown JL, Griebler R. 1993. Reliability of a short and long version of the Block food frequency form for assessing changes in calcium intake. *Journal of the American Dietetic Association* 93:784–789.
38. National Institutes of Health. 1993. *Second Report of the Expert Panel on Detection, Evaluation, and Treatment of High Blood Cholesterol in Adults*. Washington, DC: National Institutes of Health, National Heart, Lung, and Blood Institute.

39. Srinath U, Shacklock F, Shannon BM, Mitchell DC, Kris-Etherton PM, Scott L, Jaax S, Pearson TA. 1993. MEDFICTS—a dietary assessment instrument for evaluating fat, saturated fat, and cholesterol intake. *Circulation* 88(no. 4, part 2):I-634.
40. Srinath U, Shacklock F, Scott LW, Jaax S, Kris-Etherton PM. 1993. Development of MEDFICTS—a dietary assessment instrument for evaluating fat, saturated fat, and cholesterol intake. *Journal of the American Dietetic Association* 93:A-105.
41. Willett WC, Sampson L, Stampfer MJ, Rosner B, Bain C, Witschi J, Hennekens CH, Speizer FE. 1985. Reproducibility and validity of a semi-quantitative food frequency questionnaire. *American Journal of Epidemiology* 122:51–65.
42. Willett WC, Sampson L, Browne ML, Stampfer MJ, Rosner B, Hennekens CH, Speizer FE. 1988. The use of a self-administered questionnaire to assess diet four years in the past. *American Journal of Epidemiology* 127:188–189.
43. Feskanich D, Rimm EB, Giovannucci EL, Colditz GA, Stampfer MJ, Litin LB, Willett WC. 1993. Reproducibility and validity of food intake measurements from a semiquantitative food frequency questionnaire. *Journal of the American Dietetic Association* 93:790–796.
44. Rimm EB, Giovannucci EL, Stampfer MJ, Colditz GA, Litin LB, Willett WC. 1992. Reproducibility and validity of an expanded self-administered semiquantitative food frequency questionnaire among male health professionals. *American Journal of Epidemiology* 135:1114–1126.
45. Stampfer MJ, Hennekens CH, Manson J, Colditz GA, Rosner B, Willett WC. 1993. Vitamin E consumption and the risk of coronary heart disease in women. *New England Journal of Medicine* 328:1444–1449.
46. Rimm EB, Stampfer MJ, Asker A, Giovannucci E, Colditz GA, Willett WC. 1993. Vitamin E consumption and the risk of coronary heart disease in men. *New England Journal of Medicine* 328:1450–1456.
47. Munger RG, Folsom AR, Kushi LH, Kaye SA, Sellers TA. 1992. Dietary assessment of older Iowa women with a food frequency questionnaire: Nutrient intake, reproducibility, and comparison with 24-hour dietary recall interviews. *American Journal of Epidemiology* 136:192–200.
48. Willett WC, Hunter DJ, Stampfer MJ, et al. 1992. Dietary fat and fiber in relation to risk of breast cancer: An 8-year follow-up. *Journal of the American Medical Association* 268:2037–2044.
49. Willett WC, Stampfer MJ, Colditz GA, Rosner BA, Speizer FE. 1990. Relation of meat, fat, and fiber intake to the risk of colon cancer in a prospective study among women. *New England Journal of Medicine* 323:1664–1672.
50. Rimm EB, Giovannucci EL, Willett WC, Colditz GA, Asker A, Rosner B, Stampfer MJ. 1991. Prospective study on alcohol consumption and risk of coronary heart disease in men. *Lancet* 338:464–468.
51. Tang AM, Graham NMH, Kirby AJ, McCall D, Willett WC, Saah AJ. 1993. Dietary micronutrient intake and risk of progression to acquired immunodeficiency syndrome (AIDS) in human immunodeficiency virus type 1 (HIV-1)-infected homosexual men. *American Journal of Epidemiology* 138:937–951.
52. Krall EA, Dwyer JT. 1987. Validity of a food frequency questionnaire and a food diary in a short-term recall situation. *Journal of the American Dietetic Association* 87:1374–1377.
53. Zulkifli SN, Yu SM. 1992. The food frequency method for dietary assessment. *Journal of the American Dietetic Association* 92:681–685.
54. Sobell J, Block G, Koslowe P, Tobin J, Andres R. 1989. Validation of a retrospective questionnaire assessing diet 10–15 years ago. *American Journal of Epidemiology* 130:173–187.
55. Block G, Woods M, Potosky, Clifford C. 1990. Validation of a self-administered diet history questionnaire using multiple diet records. *Journal of Clinical Epidemiology* 43:1327–1335.
56. Briefel RR, Flegal KM, Winn DM, Loria CM, Johnson CL, Sempos CT. 1992. Assessing the nation's diet: Limitations of the food frequency questionnaire. *Journal of the American Dietetic Association* 92:959–962.
57. Liu K. 1994. Statistical issues related to semiquantitative food-frequency questionnaires. *American Journal of Clinical Nutrition* 59 (suppl):262S–265S.
58. Willett WC. 1994. Future directions in the development of food-frequency questionnaires. *American Journal of Clinical Nutrition* 59 (suppl):171S–174S.

59. Mullen BJ, Krantzler NJ, Grivetti LE, Schutz HG, Meiselman HL. 1984. Validity of a food frequency questionnaire for the determination of individual food intake. *American Journal of Clinical Nutrition* 39:136–143.
60. Van Staveren WA, de Boer JO, Burema J. 1985. Validity and reproducibility of a dietary history method estimating the usual food intake during one month. *American Journal of Clinical Nutrition* 42:554–559.
61. Jain M. 1989. Diet history: Questionnaire and interview techniques used in some retrospective studies of cancer. *Journal of the American Dietetic Association* 89:1647–1652.
62. Burke BS. 1947. The dietary history as a tool in research. *Journal of the American Dietetic Association* 23:1041–1046.
63. Kim WW, Mertz W, Judd JT, Marshall MW, Kelsay JL, Prather ES. 1984. Effect of making duplicate food collections on nutrient intakes calculated from diet records. *American Journal of Clinical Nutrition* 40:1333–1337.
64. Mertz W. 1992. Food intake measurements: Is there a "gold standard"? *Journal of the American Dietetic Association* 82:1463–1465.
65. Pekkarinen M. 1970. Methodology in the collection of food consumption data. *World Review of Nutrition and Dietetics* 12:145–171.
66. Turpeinen O, Karvonen MJ, Pekkarinen M, Miettinen M, Elosuo R, Paavilainen E. 1979. Dietary prevention of coronary heart disease: The Finish Mental Hospital Study. *International Journal of Epidemiology* 8:99–118.
67. Turpeinen O, Miettinen M, Karvonen MJ, Roine P, Pekkarinen M, Lehtosuo EJ, Alivirta P. 1968. Dietary prevention of coronary heart disease: Long-term experiment. *American Journal of Clinical Nutrition* 21:255–276.
68. Van Horn LV, Gernhofer N, Moag-Stahlberg A, Ferris R, Hartmuller G, Lasser VI, Stumbo P, Craddick S, Ballew C. 1990. Dietary assessment in children using electronic methods: Telephones and tape recorders. *Journal of the American Dietetic Association* 90:412–416.
69. Krantzler NJ, Mullen BJ, Schutz HG, Grivetti LE, Holden CA, Meiselman HL. 1982. Validity of telephoned diet recalls and records for assessment of individual food intake. *American Journal of Clinical Nutrition* 36:1234–1242.
70. Dubois S, Boivin JF. 1990. Accuracy of telephone dietary recalls in elderly subjects. *Journal of the American Dietetic Association* 90:1680–1687.
71. Schucker RE. 1982. Alternative approaches to classic food consumption measurement methods: Telephone interviewing and market data bases. *American Journal of Clinical Nutrition* 35:1306–1309.
72. Weeks MF, Kulka RA, Lessler JT, Whitmore RW. 1983. Personal versus telephone surveys for collecting household health data at the local level. *American Journal of Public Health* 73:1389–1394.
73. Morgan KJ, Johnson SR, Rizek RL, Reese R, Stampley GL. 1987. Collection of food intake data: An evaluation of methods. *Journal of the American Dietetic Association* 87:888–896.
74. Fox TA, Heimendinger J, Block G. 1992. Telephone surveys as a method for obtaining dietary information: A review. *Journal of the American Dietetic Association* 92:729–732.
75. Posner BM, Borman CL, Morgan JL, Borden WS, Ohls JC. 1982. The validity of a telephone-administered 24-hour dietary recall methodology. *American Journal of Clinical Nutrition* 36:546–553.
76. Medlin C, Skinner JD. 1988. Individual dietary intake methodology: A 50-year review of progress. *Journal of the American Dietetic Association* 88:1250–1257.
77. Elwood PC, Bird G. 1983. A photographic method of diet evaluation. *Human Nutrition: Applied Nutrition* 37A:474–477.
78. Bird G, Elwood PC. 1983. The dietary intakes of subjects estimated from photographs compared with a weighed record. *Human Nutrition: Applied Nutrition* 37A:470–473.
79. Weiss EH, Kien CL, Clark G. 1988. Validation of a photographic method for recording the selection of foods by individuals. *Journal of the American Dietetic Association* 88:599–600.
80. Brown J, Tharp TM, Dahlberg-Luby EM, Snowdon DA, Ostwald SK, Buzzard IM, Rysavy DM, Wieser MA. 1990. Videotape dietary assessment: Validity, reliability, and comparison of results with 24-hour dietary recalls from elderly women in a retirement home. *Journal of the American Dietetic Association* 90:1675–1679.

81. Kretsch MJ. 1989. New computerized techniques for assessing food intake. In Livingston GE, ed. *Nutritional Status Assessment of the Individual.* Trumbull, Conn: Food & Nutrition Press.
82. Fong AKH, Kretsch MJ. 1990. Nutrition evaluation scale system reduces time and labor in recording quantitative dietary intake. *Journal of the American Dietetic Association* 90:664–670.
83. Kretsch MJ, Fong AKH. 1993. Validity and reproducibility of a new computerized dietary assessment method. Effects of gender and educational level. *Nutrition Research* 13:133–146.
84. Kretsch MJ, Fong AKH. 1990. Validation of a new computerized technique for quantitating individual dietary intake: The Nutrition Evaluation Scale System (NESSy) vs the weighed food record. *American Journal of Clinical Nutrition* 51:477–484.
85. Kretsch MJ. Personal communication, 23 November 1994.
86. Stockley L, Chapman RI, Holley ML, Jones FA, Prescott EHA, Broadhurst AJ. 1986. Description of a food recording electronic device for use in dietary surveys. *Human Nutrition: Applied Nutrition* 40A:13–18.
87. Stockley L, Hurren CA, Chapman RI, Broadhurst AJ, Jones FA. 1986. Energy, protein and fat intake estimated using a food recording electronic device compared with a weighed diary. *Human Nutrition: Applied Nutrition* 40A:19–23.
88. Samet JM. 1989. Surrogate measures of dietary intake. *American Journal of Clinical Nutrition* 50:1139–1144.
89. Cumming RG, Klineberg RJ. 1994. A study of the reproducibility of long-term recall in the elderly. *Epidemiology* 5:116–119.
90. Andersson I, Rössner S. 1989. Energy intake of obese women. *International Journal of Obesity* 13:247–253.
91. Bandini LG, Schoeller DA, Cyr HN, Dietz WH. 1990. Validity of reported energy intake in obese and nonobese adolescents. *American Journal of Clinical Nutrition* 52:421–425.
92. Lansky D, Brownell KD. 1982. Estimates of food quantity and calories: Errors in self-report among obese patients. *American Journal of Clinical Nutrition* 35:727–732.
93. Lichtman SW, Pisarska K, Berman ER, Pestone M, Dowling H, Offenbacher E, Weisel H, Heshka S, Matthews DE, Heymsfield SB. 1992. Discrepancy between self-reported and actual caloric intake and exercise in obese subjects. *New England Journal of Medicine* 327:1893–1898.
94. Black AE, Prentice AM, Goldberg GR, Jebb SA, Bingham SA, Livingstone MBE, Coward WA. 1993. Measurements of total energy expenditure provide insights into the validity of dietary measurements of energy intake. *Journal of the American Dietetic Association* 93:572–579.
95. Blake AJ, Guthrie HA, Smiciklas-Wright H. 1989. Accuracy of food portion estimation by overweight and normal-weight subjects. *Journal of the American Dietetic Association* 89:962–964.
96. Myers RJ, Klesges RC, Eck LH, Hanson CL, Klem ML. 1988. Accuracy of self-reports of food intake in obese and normal-weight individuals: Effects of obesity on self-reports of dietary intake in adult females. *American Journal of Clinical Nutrition* 48:1248–1251.
97. Cameron ME, Van Staveren WA. 1988. *Manual on methodology for food consumption studies.* New York: Oxford University Press.
98. Block G, Hartman AM. 1989. Issues in reproducibility and validity of dietary studies. *American Journal of Clinical Nutrition* 50:1133–1138.
99. Pietinen P, Hartman AM, Haapa E, Räsänen L, Haapakoski J, Palmgren J, Albanes D, Virtamo J, Huttunen JK. 1988. Reproducibility and validity of dietary assessment instruments. I. A self-administered food use questionnaire with a portion size picture booklet. *American Journal of Epidemiology* 128:655–666.
100. Pietinen P, Hartman AM, Haapa E, Räsänen L, Haapakoski J, Palmgren J, Albanes D, Virtamo J, Huttunen JK. 1988. Reproducibility and validity of dietary assessment instruments. II. A qualitative food frequency questionnaire. *American Journal of Epidemiology* 128:667–676.
101. Carter RL, Sharbaugh CO, Stapell CA. 1981. Reliability and validity of the 24-hour recall. *Journal of the American Dietetic Association* 79:542–547.
102. Emmons L, Hayes M. 1973. Accuracy of 24-hour recalls of young children. *Journal of the American Dietetic Association* 62:409–415.

103. Stunkard AJ, Waxman M. 1981. Accuracy of self-reports of food intake. *Journal of the American Dietetic Association* 79:547–551.
104. Greger JL, Entyre GM. 1978. Validity of 24-hour recalls by adolescent females. *American Journal of Public Health* 68:70–72.
105. Campbell VA, Dodds ML. 1967. Collecting dietary information from groups of older people. *Journal of the American Dietetic Association* 51:29–33.
106. Lytle LA, Nichaman MZ, Obarzanek E, Glovsky E, Montgomery D, Nicklas T, Zive M, Feldman H. 1993. Validation of 24-hour recalls assisted by food records in third-grade children. *Journal of the American Dietetic Association* 93:1431–1436.
107. Van Staveren WA, West CE, Hoffmans MDAF, Bos P, Kardinaal AFM, Poppel GAFG, Schipper HJA, Hautvast JGJA, Hayes RB. 1986. Comparison of contemporaneous and retrospective estimates of food consumption made by a dietary history method. *American Journal of Epidemiology* 123:884–893.
108. Jain MG, Howe GR, Johnson KC, Miller AB. 1980. Evaluation of a diet history questionnaire for epidemiologic studies. *American Journal of Epidemiology* 111:212–219.
109. Herbert JR, Miller DR. 1988. Methodologic considerations for investigating the diet-cancer link. *American Journal of Clinical Nutrition* 47:1068–1077.
110. Bingham SA. 1987. The dietary assessment of individuals: Methods, accuracy, new techniques and recommendations. *Nutrition Abstracts and Reviews* 57:705–743.
111. Roberts SB, Ferland S, Young VR, Morrow F, Heyman MB, Melanson KJ, Gullans SR, Dallal GE. 1991. Objective verification of dietary intake by measurement of urine osmolality. *American Journal of Clinical Nutrition* 54:774–782.
112. Bingham SA. 1994. The use of 24-h urine samples and energy expenditure to validate dietary assessments. *American Journal of Clinical Nutrition* 59(suppl):227S–231S.
113. Hunter DJ, Rimm EB, Sacks FM, Stampfer MJ, Colditz GA, Litin LB, Willett WC. 1992. Comparison of measures of fatty acid intake by subcutaneous fat aspirate, food frequency questionnaire, and diet records in a free-living population of U.S. men. *American Journal of Epidemiology* 135:418–427.
114. Roberts SB, Morrow FD, Evans WJ, Shepard DC, Dallal GE, Meredith CN, Young VR. 1990. Use of *p*-aminobenzoic acid to monitor compliance with prescribed dietary regimens during metabolic balance studies in man. *American Journal of Clinical Nutrition* 51:485–488.
115. Bingham SA, Cummings JH. 1985. Urine nitrogen as an independent validatory measure of dietary intake: A study of nitrogen balance in individuals consuming their normal diet. *American Journal of Clinical Nutrition* 42:1276–1289.
116. Feunekes GIJ, Van Staveren WA, De Vries JHM, Burema J, Hautvast JGAJ. 1993. Relative and biomarker-based validity of a food-frequency questionnaire estimating intake of fats and cholesterol. *American Journal of Clinical Nutrition* 58:489–496.
117. Schoeller DA. 1990. How accurate is self-reported dietary energy intake? *Nutrition Reviews* 48:373–379.
118. Prentice AM, Black AE, Coward WA, Davies HL, Goldberg GR, Murgatroyd PR, Ashford J, Sawyer M, Whitehead RG. 1986. High levels of energy expenditure in obese women. *British Medical Journal* 292:983–987.
119. Lisner L, Habicht JP, Strupp BJ, Levitsky DA, Haas JD, Roe DA. 1989. Body composition and energy intake: Do overweight women overeat and underreport? *American Journal of Clinical Nutrition* 49:320–325.
120. Mertz W, Tsui JC, Judd JT, Reiser S, Hallfirsch J, Morris ER, Steele PD, Lashley E. 1991. What are people really eating? The relation between energy intake derived from estimated diet records and intake determined to maintain body weight. *American Journal of Clinical Nutrition* 54:291–295.
121. Jones PJH, Jacobs I, Morris A, Duchmarme MB. 1993. Adequacy of food rations in soldiers during an arctic exercise measured by doubly labeled water. *Journal of Applied Physiology* 75:1790–1797.
122. Goldberg GR, Black AE, Jebb SA, Cole TJ, Murgatroyd PR, Coward WA, Prentice AM. 1991. Critical evaluation of energy intake data using fundamental principles of energy physiology I. Derivation of cut-off limits to identify under-recording. *European Journal of Clinical Nutrition* 45:569–581.

123. Basiotis PP, Welsh SO, Cronin J, Kelsay JL, Mertz W. 1987. Number of days of food intake records required to estimate individual and group nutrient intakes with defined confidence. *Journal of Nutrition* 117:1638–1641.
124. Beaton GH, Milner J, McGuire V, Feather TE, Little JA. 1979. Sources of variance in 24-hour dietary recall data: Implications for nutrition study design and interpretation. *American Journal of Clinical Nutrition* 32:2456–2459.
125. Liu K, Stamler J, Dyer A, McKeever J, McKeever P. 1978. Statistical methods to assess and minimize the role of intra-individual variability in obscuring the relationship between dietary lipids and serum cholesterol. *Journal of Chronic Diseases* 31:399–418.
126. Mertz W, Kelsay JL. 1984. Rationale of the Beltsville one-year dietary intake study. *The American Journal of Clinical Nutrition* 40:1323–1326.
127. Posner BM, Smigelski C, Duggal A, Morgan JL, Cobb J, Cupples A. 1992. Validation of two-dimensional models for estimating portion size in nutrition research. *Journal of the American Dietetic Association* 92:738–741.
128. Hankin JH. 1986. 23rd Lenna Frances Cooper Memorial Lecture: A diet history method for research, clinical, and community use. *Journal of the American Dietetic Association* 86:868–875.
129. Todhunter EN. 1969. Food composition tables in the U.S.A. *Journal of the American Dietetic Association* 37:209–214.
130. Watt BK. 1962. Concepts in developing a food composition table. *Journal of the American Dietetic Association* 40:297–300.
131. McMasters V. 1963. History of food composition tables of the world. *Journal of the American Dietetic Association* 43:442–450.
132. Hertzler AA, Hoover LW. 1977. Development of food tables and use with computers. *Journal of the American Dietetic Association* 70:20–31.
133. Atwater WO, Woods CD. 1986. *The chemical composition of American food materials.* USDA Bulletin No. 28. Washington, DC: U.S. Department of Agriculture.
134. Smith JL. 1994. Atwater to the present: What have we learned about our food supply? *Journal of Nutrition* 124:1780S–1782S.
135. U.S. General Accounting Office. 1993. *Better guidance needed to improve reliability of USDA's food composition data.* Washington, DC: General Accounting Office, Publication No. GAO/RCED-94–30.
136. Pennington JAT. 1994. *Bowes and Church's food values of portions commonly used,* 16th ed. Philadelphia: Lippincott.
137. National Research Council. 1986. *Nutrient adequacy: Assessment using food consumption surveys.* Washington, DC: National Academy Press.
138. Watt BK. 1962. Concepts in developing food composition tables. *Journal of the American Dietetic Association* 40:297–300.
139. Matthews RH. 1991. Current HNIS nutrient data research. In Murphy SP, ed. *16th national nutrient databank conference proceedings.* Ithaca, N.Y.: The CBORD Group, Inc.
140. Hepburn FN. 1982. The USDA national nutrient data bank. *American Journal of Clinical Nutrition* 35:1297–1301.
141. Block G, Coyle LM, Hartman AM, Scoppa SM. 1994. Revision of dietary analysis software for the Health Habits and History Questionnaire. *American Journal of Epidemiology* 139:1190–1196.

Assessment Activity 3-1

COLLECTING A 24-HOUR RECALL

The 24-hour recall is probably the most commonly used technique for measuring diet. Consequently, it is important that health professionals involved in nutritional assessment understand, practice, and master this technique. In this Assessment Activity, you will collect a 24-hour recall from a classmate and calculate that person's intake of kilocalories, protein, carbohydrate, total fat, calcium, and iron from a food composition table. Be sure to have a classmate collect a 24-hour recall from you, too. This will provide you with additional experience with recalls. You also will need your own 24-hour recall for an Assessment Activity in Chapter 5.

This Assessment Activity also will help you become more familiar with using food composition tables. Experience in using food composition tables is valuable. Sometimes it is faster and easier to refer to a food composition table for a nutrient value than to use a computer. Familiarity with food composition tables will also make that task easier.

1. For this Assessment Activity, we suggest you use a photocopy of the form provided on page 145. It not only provides space for recording the names and quantities of foods and beverages consumed, it also allows you to easily record values for energy and nutrients for reported foods.
2. Familiarize yourself with the form *before* beginning your interview. Enter the name of the person being interviewed and the day and date.
3. After completing the recall form, manually calculate the intakes of kilocalories, protein, carbohydrate, total fat, calcium, and iron using the food composition table in Appendix L. If you cannot find a particular food or beverage in the food composition table, use a similar food or beverage or refer to another food composition table.
4. As you do this assignment, think about the following questions:
   How representative of your respondent's usual dietary intake is this one day of intake data?
   Did you have any difficulty finding any foods in the food composition table?
   If you had to substitute one food for another, how do you think that substitution affected the total nutrient values?

24-hour recording form for Assessment Activity 3.1

Name of person interviewed ________________ **Date** ________ **Day of week** ________

Food/Drink	Type/How prepared	Quantity	Kilocalories	Protein	Carbohydrate	Total fat	Calcium	Iron
Total								

Assessment Activity 3-2

COMPLETING A 3-DAY FOOD RECORD

Obtaining dietary intake data that is representative of the usual intake of *individuals* requires data from multiple days. According to the research reported in Table 3-5, estimating usual intake of energy (kilocalories) required an average of approximately 30 days of intake data. Vitamin A required approximately 400 days of data. Fewer days of data are required when characterizing the average intake of groups, as shown in Table 3-6.

Although this Assessment Activity will not even come close to giving you the data necessary to estimate your usual nutrient intake, it will give you an idea of what is involved in collecting multiple-day intake data. In this assignment, you will complete a 3-day food record on yourself using the food diary recording form in Appendix E or one provided by your professor. In Assessment Activity 5-1 you may analyze your food record using the diet analysis software available from the publisher or at your school's computer lab.

1. Familiarize yourself with the form in Appendix E and accompanying instructions *before* beginning your diary.
2. Record your food and beverage intake for two weekdays (Monday through Friday) and one weekend day (Saturday or Sunday). Because most people eat differently on weekend days than during weekdays, this will make your record more representative of your usual intake throughout the entire week.
3. Do not alter your normal diet during the recording period. Provide responses that are as accurate as possible. Record your food and beverage intake as soon after eating as possible.
4. You may save your completed food record for later analysis using a diet analysis software program.

Assessment Activity 3-3

HEALTH HABITS AND HISTORY QUESTIONNAIRE

Compared with other techniques for measuring diet, the food frequency questionnaire is a recent development. There is considerable interest in the food frequency questionnaire as a relatively simple and inexpensive approach to characterizing the usual dietary and nutrient intake of individuals. A food frequency questionnaire commonly used in nutrition research is the Health Habits and History Questionnaire reprinted in Appendix K. Take a close look at it. Note that its questions go beyond nutrition and deal with areas such as smoking, body weight, and medical history. Review its instructions, questions, and flow. Researchers and public health agencies can obtain the necessary software for analyzing the Health Habits and History Questionnaire from the National Cancer Institute.[141] The software, designed for IBM-compatible computers, is menu-driven and user-friendly. It requires only 2 megabytes of available hard disk space and 640 kilobytes of random-access memory. It is capable of analyzing several versions of the questionnaire, including a 98-item, a 60-item, and a machine-readable version, as well as questionnaires developed by the user. The software produces estimates of 33 nutrients and food components and has space for 17 more that can be added by the user or in future revisions based on NHANES III data. A computer-assisted interview program is also included for use with either the 98-item or the 60-item questionnaires.

For information on obtaining the software and accompanying documentation contact:

Applied Research Branch
Division of Cancer Prevention and Control
National Cancer Institute
Executive Plaza North, Room 313
9000 Rockville Pike
Bethesda, Maryland 20892

FOUR

NATIONAL DIETARY AND NUTRITION SURVEYS

OUTLINE

INTRODUCTION

Nutritional monitoring is an important activity for any government serious about promoting its citizens' health. The principle goal of nutritional monitoring is to accurately measure the dietary and nutritional status of a population and the quality, quantity, and safety of the food it consumes.[1] Data on the nutritional and health status of a population that are generated by nutritional monitoring are used for many purposes. They can identify nutritional problems of the country as a whole (e.g., excessive fat and cholesterol consumption) and groups at nutritional risk (e.g., low calcium intake by adolescent females). These data are used to justify changes in government policy and the spending of billions of dollars for planning and implementing programs related to food, nutrition, and health promotion, such as the Special Supplemental Food Program for Women, Infants, and Children (WIC) and the National Cholesterol Education Program. They are important in evaluating the cost effectiveness of such programs, particularly when voters and legislators express concern about reducing budget deficits and controlling the high cost of government. These data are also critical to research into the relationships between nutrition and health. This chapter discusses nutrition monitoring in the United States and the most important surveys comprising the federal government's nutrition and health surveillance activities. It also discusses the major findings of these surveys.

IMPORTANCE OF NATIONAL DIETARY AND NUTRITION SURVEYS

National dietary and nutrition surveys have a number of important functions and can provide much valuable information. They can show how food supplies are distributed according to such demographic factors as region, income, sex, race, and ethnicity. Survey data are important in monitoring nutritional status of a country's population. By observing trends in the health and dietary practices of a population, relationships between diet and health can be elucidated. They identify groups that are at nutritional risk and that may benefit from food assistance programs. They are important for developing the Thrifty Food Plan, which forms the basis for determining benefit levels for participants of the Food Stamp Program. They are also used for evaluating the effectiveness of various USDA food assistance programs. For example, a before-and-after comparison of food consumption practices by Food Stamp Program participants revealed that the program allowed families to purchase more nutritious foods and increased the market for surplus agricultural products. After analyzing nutritional and health survey data, the U.S. General Accounting Office (GAO) reported that women participating in the WIC program had a 25% reduction in low birth weight births (under 2500 g or 5.5 lb) and a 44% reduction in very-low birth weight births (under 1500 g or 3.3 lb) compared with similar women not participating in the WIC program.[2] The GAO estimated that for each tax dollar invested in WIC benefits, nearly $3.00 were saved within the first year by federal, state, and local governments and private insurance companies in reduced health-care costs and special education. These and other uses of data from nutrition and health surveys are summarized in Box 4-1.

Data from dietary surveys can be used to track food consumption trends over time, examine current dietary practices of specific groups of people, and monitor average intakes of pesticides, toxic substances, radioactive substances, and industrial chemicals. Studies of nutritional status allow monitoring of the general health of a population through health and medical histories, dietary interviews, physical examinations, and laboratory measurements.[3]

Dietary and nutrition surveys are important to government agencies that supervise their country's agriculture and food industries. Data from surveys provide a sound basis for development of policies and programs related to agricultural production, marketing of agricultural products, projecting supply and demand, and determining the adequacy of the available food supply.[4] These data provide early warning of impending food shortages and can indicate how such crises may be prevented or alleviated.[5] They have been used to develop the *Dietary Guidelines for Americans* and the nutrition and related health objectives included in *Healthy People 2000.*

Using food balance sheets (see Chapter 3), a government can estimate the "disappearance" of food from its food distribution system and thus arrive at an indirect and rough estimate of food consumption by its citizens. As discussed later in this chapter, data on food disappearance or "availability" do not measure actual food consumption, only what enters and leaves the food distribution system. However, these data allow comparisons among different countries and creation of a world food picture. These comparisons, in turn, can serve as the basis for the formulation of international policies designed to improve the world food and nutrition situation and prevent imbalances in dietary standards among countries.[6]

BOX 4-1

Uses of Data from Nutrition and Health Surveys

Public policy

Monitoring surveillance:

- Identify high-risk groups and geographic areas with nutrition-related problems to facilitate implementation of public health intervention programs and food assistance programs
- Evaluate changes in agricultural policy that may affect the nutritional quality and healthfulness of the U.S. food supply
- Assess progress toward achieving the nutrition objectives in *Healthy People 2000*
- Evaluate the effectiveness of nutritional initiatives of military feeding systems
- Report health and nutrition data from state-based programs to comply with federal administrative program requirements
- Monitor food production and marketing

Nutrition-related programs:

- Nutrition education and dietary guidance (*Dietary Guidelines for Americans*)
- Food assistance programs
- Nutrition intervention programs
- Public health programs

Regulatory:

- Food labeling
- Food fortification
- Food safety

Scientific research

- Nutrient requirements (*Recommended Dietary Allowances*)
- Diet-health relationships
- Knowledge and attitudes and their relationship to dietary and health behavior
- Nutrition monitoring research—national and international
- Food composition analysis
- Economic aspects of food consumption
- Nutrition education research

From various surveys conducted by the U.S. Department of Health and Human Services and the U.S. Department of Agriculture.

NUTRITIONAL MONITORING IN THE UNITED STATES

Nutritional monitoring can be defined as "the assessment of dietary or nutritional status at intermittent times with the aim of detecting changes in the dietary or nutritional status of a population."[7] It involves data collection and data analysis in five general areas:[1]

- nutritional and health status measurements
- food consumption measurements
- food composition measurement and nutrient data banks
- dietary knowledge, behavior, and attitude assessments
- food supply and demand determinations

Since about the middle of the twentieth century, the U.S. government has sought to obtain objective data on which to base decisions regarding nutrition-related public policies. This was done by the U.S. Department of Agriculture (USDA), which collected food disappearance data and began conducting national household food consumption surveys.

More recently, the federal government has evaluated the food intake of individual Americans through the USDA's Nationwide Food Consumption Survey and Continuing Survey of Food Intakes by Individuals and assessed the nutritional and health status of the public through the U.S. Department of Health and Human Service's (DHHS) National Health and Nutrition

Examination Survey.[8] These three nationwide surveys constitute the heart of the federal government's nutritional monitoring activities.

NATIONAL NUTRITION MONITORING AND RELATED RESEARCH PROGRAM

In the past several decades, Congress, the nutrition community, various private groups, and expert panels have expressed concern about problems with the federal government's nutrition monitoring program and the lack of coordination between USDA and DHHS. Issues have been raised about the frequency and costs of data collected by the two agencies, delays in reporting data, the low response rates seen in some surveys, and, in certain instances, the poor quality of data.[1,8–10] Problems in the two agencies' nutrition monitoring activities have been addressed by a number of reports by the National Research Council, the Federation of American Societies for Experimental Biology, and the General Accounting Office (a research arm of Congress that audits government programs and highlights areas of waste and fraud). These reports have called for the agencies to develop better methods for collecting dietary intake data, to use standardized data collection techniques that allow data to be compared across the different surveys, and to improve coverage of groups at nutritional risk such as pregnant and lactating women, infants, preschool children, adolescents, and older persons.[1]

Since the late 1970s, the USDA and DHHS have developed three separate plans to better integrate their activities and address weaknesses in their surveys. Despite some gains by the agencies, growing recognition of the need to improve nutrition monitoring led to passage of the National Nutrition Monitoring and Related Research Act of 1990 (PL 101–445). This legislation requires the Secretaries of the USDA and DHHS to prepare and implement a comprehensive 10-year plan for integrating the nutrition monitoring activities of the two agencies. This 10-year coordinated effort is called the National Nutrition Monitoring and Related Research Program (NNMRRP).[1,11] The legislation also calls for the creation of an Interagency Board for Nutrition Monitoring and Related Research and a National Nutrition Monitoring Advisory Council.

The NNMRRP is intended to coordinate the nutrition monitoring activities of 22 federal agencies under the joint direction of the USDA and DHHS. The program encompasses a group of over 50 surveys and surveillance activities assessing the health and nutritional status of the U.S. population.[12] The program's goal is to "establish a comprehensive nutrition monitoring and related research program for the federal government by collecting quality data that are continuous, coordinated, timely, and reliable; using comparable methods for data collection and reporting of results; and efficiently and effectively disseminating and exchanging information with data users."[11] Critical to the success of reaching this goal are three overall national objectives and three objectives addressing state and local nutrition monitoring efforts. The three national objectives are (1) to achieve continuous and coordinated data collection, (2) to improve the comparability and quality of data collected by the USDA and DHHS, and (3) to improve the research base for nutrition monitoring. The three state and local objectives are (1) to develop and strengthen state and local capacities for continuous and coordinated data collection, (2) to improve methodologies to enhance comparability of NNMRRP data across federal, state, and local levels, and (3) to improve the quality of state and local nutrition monitoring data.[1,11] The NNMRRP also addresses the need for better nutrition monitoring information about selected population subgroups, more efficient and effective data dissemination to users, and better ways to meet the needs of data users.

The National Nutrition Monitoring and Related Research Act of 1990 places responsibility for coordinating the NNMRRP with the USDA and DHHS. The Interagency Board for Nutrition Monitoring and Related Research assists in implementing the NNMRRP. The Board's members come from approximately 20 other federal agencies (e.g., the Departments of Labor, Commerce, Defense, Veterans Affairs, and the Environmental Protection Agency) and are responsible for representing their agencies in all areas of nutrition monitoring. The Board's activities include preparing an annual budget report on nutrition monitoring, preparing biennial reports on the progress of the coordinated program, and preparing periodic scientific reports on the nutritional and related health status of the population.[11]

The act also requires the establishment of the National Nutrition Monitoring Advisory Council. The Council is composed of the Secretaries of the USDA and DHHS and nine voting members with expertise in the areas of public health, nutrition monitoring research, and food production and distribution. Five of these voting members are appointed by the President and the other four by Congress. The Council provides scientific and technical input to the Board, evaluates the scientific and technical quality of the comprehensive plan and the effectiveness of the coordinated program, and recommends areas for improvement.[11] The organizational structure of the NNMRRP and members of the Interagency Board are shown in Figure 4-1.

To facilitate data dissemination, the National Nutrition Monitoring and Related Research Act of 1990 requires the publishing of a scientific report on the dietary, nutritional, and health-related status of the U.S. population every 2 to 5 years by a nonfederal scientific body. Intermediate to the publishing of these scientific reports, the National Center for Health Statistics is required to publish a *Nutrition Monitoring Chartbook.* The Chartbook highlights and updates nutrition monitoring data, information, and research in a user-friendly format, using graphics and brief narratives. To improve communication among data users, a *Directory of Federal Nutrition Monitoring Activities* is published every 3 years. The Directory contains information about federal and state nutrition monitoring activities, the sponsoring agency, contact persons, and the survey's purpose, date, target population, and design.[13] Depending on the survey, data are available in such forms as journal articles, government publications, magnetic tapes, CD-ROM, and computer diskettes. These are summarized in the *Catalog of Publications,* which is published annually by the National Center for Health Statistics. Food composition data are published by the USDA's Human Nutrition Information Service in *Composition of Foods—Raw, Processed, Prepared: Agriculture Handbook No. 8, Nutritive Value of American Foods in Common Units: Agriculture Handbook No. 456,* and in Home and Garden Bulletin No. 72, *Nutritive Value of Foods.*

ROLE OF THE U.S. DEPARTMENT OF AGRICULTURE

The earliest efforts at nutritional monitoring in the United States were carried out by the USDA. The USDA's primary contributions to nutrition monitoring involve collecting data on food disappearance, individual food consumption (through the Continuing Survey of Food Intakes by Individuals) and household food consumption (through the Household Food Consumption Survey).[1,4,14] Recent, current, and planned nutrition monitoring activities of the USDA and DHHS are described in Table 4-1.

Food Disappearance

Since about the middle of the twentieth century, the USDA has developed annual estimates of the amount of food that has "disappeared" from the U.S. food distribution system. Known as *food disappearance,* these estimates are also referred to as food available for consumption by the public or *per capita food availability.*[15,16] These are not direct measures of actual food consumption but estimates of food that has left the wholesale and retail food distribution system. These estimates, also known as the U.S. Food Supply Series, were the outgrowth of several factors: the need to track food surpluses during World War I, legislation in the early 1930s to ensure an adequate food supply for domestic consumption, and concerns about potential food shortages during the droughts of

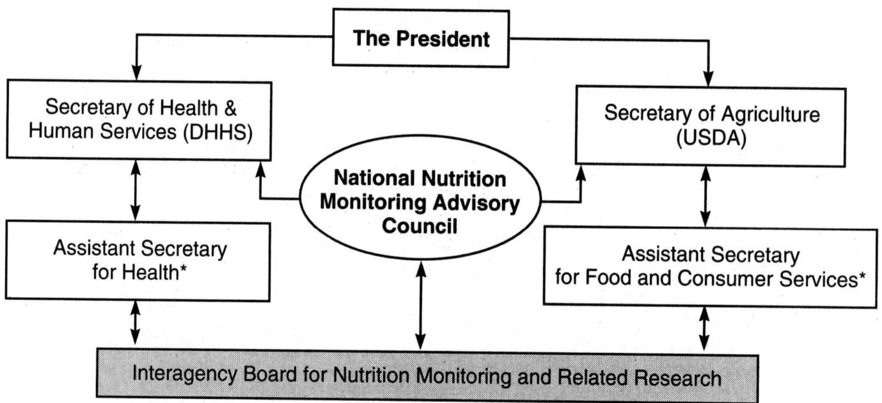

Members:

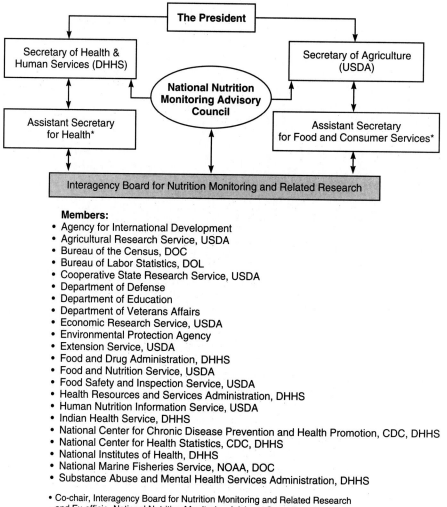

- Agency for International Development
- Agricultural Research Service, USDA
- Bureau of the Census, DOC
- Bureau of Labor Statistics, DOL
- Cooperative State Research Service, USDA
- Department of Defense
- Department of Education
- Department of Veterans Affairs
- Economic Research Service, USDA
- Environmental Protection Agency
- Extension Service, USDA
- Food and Drug Administration, DHHS
- Food and Nutrition Service, USDA
- Food Safety and Inspection Service, USDA
- Health Resources and Services Administration, DHHS
- Human Nutrition Information Service, USDA
- Indian Health Service, DHHS
- National Center for Chronic Disease Prevention and Health Promotion, CDC, DHHS
- National Center for Health Statistics, CDC, DHHS
- National Institutes of Health, DHHS
- National Marine Fisheries Service, NOAA, DOC
- Substance Abuse and Mental Health Services Administration, DHHS

* Co-chair, Interagency Board for Nutrition Monitoring and Related Research and Ex-officio, National Nutrition Monitoring Advisory Council

Figure 4-1 Organizational structure of the National Nutrition Monitoring and Related Research Program and members of the Interagency Board Data from the U.S. Department of Health and Human Services, U.S. Department of Agriculture. 1994. Ten-year comprehensive plan for the National Nutrition Monitoring and Related Research Program; notice. *Federal Register* 58(111): 32751–32806.

1934 and 1936. Estimates of food disappearance for approximately 300 foods were first summarized by the USDA in 1941 to assess food requirements and supplies during World War II. In 1949, food disappearance data from as far back as 1909—the first year for which reliable data were available—were compiled and published.[4]

Food disappearance data are derived using the **balance sheet approach.** Annual data on food exports, food not meant for human consumption (for example, livestock feed, seed, and food used for industrial purposes), military procurements, and year-end inventories are subtracted from data on beginning-year inventories, total food

TABLE 4-1 Recent, current, and planned nutrition monitoring activities of the USDA and DHHS

Date	Dept.	Agency	Survey	Target U.S. population
Nutrition and related health measurements				
Annual	DHHS	CDC/NCHS	National Health Interview Survey (NHIS)	Civilian, noninstitutionalized individuals
Annual	DHHS	CDC/NCHS	National Hospital Discharge Survey	Discharges from non-Federal general and short-stay specialty hospitals
Continuous	DHHS	CDC/NCHS	Vital Statistics Program	Total U.S. population
Continuous	DHHS	CDC/ NCCDPHP	Pregnancy Nutrition Surveillance System	Low-income, high-risk pregnant women
Continuous	DHHS	CDC/ NCCDPHP	Pediatric Nutrition Surveillance System	Low-income, high-risk children, age birth–17 years
Annual	DHHS	CDC/NCHS	National Ambulatory Medical Care Survey	Office visits to non-Federal, office-based physicians
1992—continuous	DHHS	CDC/NCHS	NHANES II Mortality Follow-up Survey	Individuals examined in NHANES II, age 35–75 years at baseline
1992—continuous	DHHS	CDC/NCHS	Hispanic HANES (HHANES) Mortality Follow-up Survey	Individuals interviewed in HHANES, age 20–74 years of baseline
1992—annual	DHHS	CDC/NCHS	National Hospital Ambulatory Medical Care Survey	Visits to hospital emergency and outpatients departments of non-Federal, short-stay, general and specialty hospitals
1992—continuous	DHHS	CDC/NCHS	NHANES III Longitudinal Follow-up Survey	Individuals interviewed and examined in NHANES III, age 20+ years at baseline
1992—continuous	DHHS	CDC/NCHS	Research on statistical methods: Model-based estimates of NHIS items for states	NA
1994—continuous	DHHS	CDC/ NCCDPHP	Adult Nutrition Surveillance System	Adults, age 18+ years participating in local public health programs
(1997 +)	DHHS	CDC/NCHS	National Health and Nutrition Examination Survey (NHANES '97+)	U.S. noninstitutionalized population
Continuous	USDA	ARS	Determination of Nutrient Requirements	U.S. population
Continuous	USDA	ARS	Methods of Assessing Nutritional Status	NA

Continued

TABLE 4-1 Recent, current, and planned nutrition monitoring activities of the USDA and DHHS—cont'd

Date	Dept.	Agency	Survey	Target U.S. population
Nutrition and related health measurements—cont'd				
Continuous	DHHS	CDC/NCEH	Methods of Assessing Nutritional Status	NA or varies
Continuous	USDA	CSRS	Nutrition Research in Support of Nutrition Monitoring	NA or varies
Continuous	DHHS	NIH	Nutrition Research in Support of Nutrition Monitoring	NA or varies
Periodic	DHHS, USDA	TBA	User conferences	NA
Food and nutrient consumption				
1994–96—annual	USDA	HNIS	Continuing Survey of Food Intakes by Individuals (CSFII)	Individuals of all ages residing in eligible households nationwide; oversampling of individuals in low-income households
1996	USDA	HNIS	Household Food Consumption Survey	Civilian households, oversampling of low-income households
(1997+)	DHHS	CDC/NCHS	NHANES '97+	See NHANES listing above
Annual	DHHS	FDA	Total Diet Study	Representative diets of specific age-sex groups
Continuous	DOD	USARIEM	Nutritional Evaluation of Military Feeding Systems and Military Populations	Enlisted personnel of the Army, Navy, Marine Corps, and Air Force
Continuous	DOL	BLS	Consumer Expenditure Survey	Civilian, noninstitutionalized population and a portion of the institutionalized population in the U.S.
Continuous	DOC	Census	Survey of Income and Program Participation	Civilian, noninstitutionalized population of the U.S.
Continuous	USDA	ERS	Research Program on Food Demand	NA
Periodic	DHHS, USDA	TBA	User conferences	NA
Knowledge, attitudes, and behavior assessments				
Biennial	DHHS	CDC/ NCCDPHP	Youth Risk Behavior Survey	Civilian, noninstitutionalized adolescents, age 12–18 years
1994–96	USDA	HNIS	Diet and Health Knowledge Survey	Selected adults, age 20+ years in households and noninstitutionalized group quarters participating in the CSFII

TABLE 4-1 Recent, current, and planned nutrition monitoring activities of the USDA and DHHS—cont'd

Date	Dept.	Agency	Survey	Target U.S. population
Knowledge, attitudes, and behavior assessments—cont'd				
Continuous	DHHS	CDC/NCCDPHP	Behavioral Risk Factor Surveillance System	Individuals, age 18+ years, residing in participating states in households with telephones
Biennial	DHHS	FDA	Health and Diet Survey	Civilian, noninstitutionalized individuals in households w/telephones, age 18+ years
Periodic	DHHS, USDA	TBA	User conference	NA
Food composition and nutrient data bases				
Annual	DHHS	FDA	Total Diet Study	See listing above
Biennial	DHHS	FDA	Food Label and Package Survey	NA
Continuous	USDA	HNIS	National Nutrient Data Bank	NA
Continuous	USDA	HNIS	Survey Nutrient Data Base	NA
Continuous	USDA	ARS	Nutrient Composition Laboratory	NA
Continuous	DHHS	NIH	Measurement of Nutrients in Foods	NA
Periodic	USDA	TBA	User conferences	NA
Food supply determinations				
Annual	DOC	NOAA/NMFS	Fisheries of the United States	NA
Annual	USDA	ERS	U.S. Food and Nutrition Supply Series	NA
	USDA	HNIS	Estimate of Food Available	
			Estimate of Nutrients	
Periodic	USDA	TBA	User conferences	NA

Data from the U.S. Department of Health and Human Services and the U.S. Department of Agriculture.

ARS = Agricultural Research Service (USDA); CDC = Centers for Disease Control and Prevention (DHHS); CSRS = Cooperative State Research Service (USDA); (Date) = tentative date; DHHS = U.S. Department of Health and Human Service; DOC = Department of Commerce; DOD = Department of Defense; DOL = Department of Labor; FDA = Food and Drug Administration (DHHS); HHANES = Hispanic Health and Nutrition Examination Survey; HNIS = Human Nutrition Information Service (USDA); NA = not applicable; NCCDPHP = National Center for Chronic Disease Prevention and Health Promotion (DHHS); NCEH = National Center for Environmental Health (DHHS); NCHS = National Center for Health Statistics (DHHS); NHANES = National Health and Nutrition Examination Survey; NIH = National Institutes of Health (DHHS); NMFS = National Marine Fisheries Service (DOC/NOAA); NOAA = National Oceanic and Atmospheric Administration; TBA = to be announced; USARIEM = United States Army Research Institute of Environmental Medicine (DOD); USDA = U.S. Department of Agriculture production, and imports to arrive at an estimate of food available for domestic consumption.[3,4] This estimate then is divided by the U.S. population count to derive per person disappearance (or per capita availability) of food. Per capita availability of energy and a number of nutrients are then calculated using food composition tables.[3,4]

This approach has several drawbacks. It depends almost entirely on data collected for other purposes. The data can vary considerably in adequacy, accuracy, and accessibility. These estimates fail to account for food fed to pets and food losses due to spoilage, disposal of inedible parts, and trimming by the consumer. It does not provide information relating to food consumption on a regional, household, or individual basis. Consequently, these data must be interpreted with care.[4]

Despite these weaknesses, however, the data reflect changes in overall patterns of food disappearance over time and have been the only source of information on food and nutrient trends since the beginning of the century.[3,7,14] When used in conjunction with similar data developed in other countries, epidemiologists have been able to study the relationships between diet and disease. For example, scientists have investigated how different levels of dietary fat and cholesterol intake across countries relate to coronary heart disease death rates in those countries.[3] Food disappearance data also serve as a rough check on the reasonableness of results from household food consumption surveys.[4] Trends in the per capita availability of energy and nutrients in the U.S. food supply are summarized later in this chapter.

Individual Food Consumption

The USDA has estimated individual food and nutrient consumption using two surveys, the Nationwide Food Consumption Survey (NFCS) and the more recently initiated Continuing Survey of Food Intakes by Individuals (CSFII). The USDA recently decided to discontinue conducting the NFCS because the collection of two types of data (individual and household) in one survey contributed to a heavy respondent burden and low response rates. The NFCS has been replaced by the CSFII, which collects individual intake data, and the Household Food Consumption Survey, which collects household food intake data.[1,11]

Continuing Survey of Food Intakes by Individuals

In 1985 the Human Nutrition Information Service of the USDA began a national survey of individual dietary intake known as the *Continuing Survey of Food Intakes by Individuals (CSFII)*. The CSFII was initially designed to be conducted annually except for those years when data were being collected for the NFCS.[7,14] However, it has only been conducted during 1985–86, 1989–91, and 1994–96. The CSFII has replaced the NFCS as the USDA's primary survey for estimating individual food and nutrient intake.[1] The CSFII provides timely information on U.S. diets; allows further study of the dietary habits of certain population groups thought to be at nutritional risk (e.g., low-income people); provides data on "usual" diets by measuring several days of data collected over the course of a year; and demonstrates how diets vary over time for individuals and groups of people.

The 1985–86 CSFII targeted females 19 to 50 years old and their children ages 1 to 5 years who were in one of two household types: households of any income level and low-income households (having income ≤130% of the poverty guidelines).[1,17,18] It also targeted males 19 to 50 years of age.[4,7]

In the 1985–86 CSFII, dietary intake data were collected using 24-hour recalls. In the surveys of women and children, basic household information was obtained and six 24-hour recalls were collected at approximately 2-month intervals. This not only provided data somewhat more representative of usual dietary intake, but diminished seasonal influence on dietary intake because data were collected throughout the year.

All information was collected by trained interviewers employed by a private contracting agency. Basic household information and the first of the six 24-hour recalls on all age-eligible participants were obtained from the female head of the household or the main meal planner/preparer.[7] An attempt was made to obtain subsequent 24-hour recalls by telephone interview. In the 1985 CSFII, about 90% of subsequent 24-hour recalls were obtained by telephone. In households not having a telephone or where the respondent requested to be interviewed in person, succeeding 24-hour recalls were collected by personal interview.[4,7]

The 1994–96 CSFII collected two nonconsecutive days of food intake using two in-person 24-hour recalls. Unlike previous CSFIIs, which were limited to the 48 contiguous states, it included persons in all 50 states. It sampled a disproportionately larger number of low-income people, young children, and older persons to better ascertain their dietary practices. This is known as "oversampling." Respondents were also asked questions on attitudes and knowledge about diet and health, as part of the Diet and Health Knowledge Survey. These questions were designed to examine the relationships between an individual's attitudes and knowledge about food and nutrition and the same individual's food choices and nutrient intake.

Nationwide Food Consumption Survey

The Nationwide Food Consumption Surveys were conducted in 1977–78 and again in 1987–88. Populations targeted by the two surveys included private households in the 48 contiguous states and persons residing in those households. The surveys included two samples: a basic sample of all households and a low-income sample of households with incomes at or below 130% of the poverty level—a level consistent with eligibility for the Food Stamp Program. As mentioned earlier, the USDA no longer conducts the NFCS, using instead the CSFII and the Household Food Consumption Survey.

Statistical sampling techniques were used to select households that would yield a sample representative of the U.S. population.[7,14] To control for seasonal variations in food intake, the 1987–88 NFCS conducted interviews during all four seasons. After collecting household food intake data, the interviewer obtained a 24-hour recall from the food manager who also was asked to recall all the food and beverages consumed at home and away from home by all children up to 10 years of age in the household. The food manager then was given instructions on keeping a 2-day food record for himself or herself and for all children in the household up to 10 years of age. Teens and adults provided interviewers with their own 24-hour recalls and kept their own food records.[14] Although interviews required from 80 minutes to 5½ hours to conduct, each family was given only $2.00 for participating in the survey.[19]

Once the data were collected, each food reported by the individual was given a unique food code, and the quantity consumed was converted to grams of the edible portion of food. The nutrient contribution of each of the 3 days was calculated and compared with the appropriate Recommended Dietary Allowance.[4,14]

The 1987–88 NFCS found no mean nutrient intake that was less than 70% of the 1989 Recommended Dietary Allowances.[20] However, because of the low response rate, data from the 1987–88 NFCS may not have accurately reflected true population mean intakes and therefore should be interpreted with caution, as discussed below.

Problems with the 1987–88 NFCS

A potential problem with any survey of this nature is bias resulting from a low rate of response from subjects. The goal of the 1987–88 NFCS was to obtain 3 days of dietary intake data from approximately 25,000 individuals.[14,21] The response rates were considered very low—approximately 38% at the household level with only 31% of individuals providing 1 day of intake data and only 25% of individuals providing 3 days of intake data.[19,22] If the diets of those who did not respond (nonrespondents) were significantly different from those who responded (respondents), then the survey results could be *biased* and not representative of the target population.

Concerns about this low rate of response prompted the USDA to direct the Life Sciences Research Office of the Federation of American Societies for Experimental Biology to appoint a panel of scientists to examine the data. The panel concluded that "it is not possible, with absolute certainty, to demonstrate either the presence or absence of nonresponse bias in the 1987–88 NFCS data. . . . The Expert Panel does not recommend use of the data from the 1987–88 NFCS. However, if the HNIS chooses to publish estimates of mean consumption of foods, food groups, or nutrients, the greatest caution must be employed."[22]

Among the expert panel's recommendations to improve response rate was to increase remuneration to respondents from $2.00 to $20.00, payable by check to the primary household respondent *before* the interview is conducted. This would help establish a bond of trust and goodwill with the respondent. Research indicates that promises to pay *after* an interview of this nature are not as effective in eliciting respondent cooperation as a cash payment in advance. The report suggested that individual members asked to complete 24-hour recalls and food records be paid $5.00. These amounts would be a fraction of the more than $1000.00 per household cost of the 1987–88 NFCS (according to the report, the survey cost $7.5 million).

The report stated that it "appeared that insufficient training and monitoring of interviewers, possible high rates of turnover of interviewers, and/or interviewers' failure to follow prescribed schedules may have contributed to the low response occurring in the survey. The need for improved management of personnel is an important consideration for improvement of response rate." The report also stated that the respondent burden was "very great" and that "modification of the survey design and instruments to lighten respondent burden may also improve response in future surveys."[22]

Household Food Consumption Survey

The USDA has conducted household food consumption surveys for about 100 years.[4,23] The earliest surveys, limited in the number of people and groups surveyed, gave way to the Household Food Consumption Surveys (HFCS) conducted in 1936–37, 1942, 1948, and 1955, which attempted to assess household food intake on the national level.[1,4,8] In these surveys persons responsible for food preparation in their households recalled the amounts and costs of foods used by their households during a 7-day period. Beginning with the 1965–66 HFCS, measurement of food intake at the individual level was added, and the survey was subsequently known as the Nationwide Food Consumption Survey (NFCS).[8] With the elimination of the NFCS, the USDA is estimating individual food consumption using the CSFII and household food consumption using the HFCS. Because the HFCS may duplicate data available from other sources or provide data that could be available from other surveys, the USDA will delay conducting the HFCS until the cost of the survey can be justified.[1]

The earliest surveys used the **food inventory record**, in which total household food use was calculated by subtracting food on hand at the end of the survey period (ending inventory) from the sum of food on hand at the start of the survey period (beginning inventory) and food brought into the household during the survey. In the 1930s, this cumbersome method was replaced by the simpler **food list-recall approach**, which is still in use.[4]

Food list recall involves an interview with the respondent, who recalls the amount of food used by the household during the preceding week and the amount paid for any purchased items. The interviewer uses a detailed listing of foods and enters responses manually on the food list. The approach results in a higher subject response rate, a factor important in obtaining data that are representative of the entire population from which subjects are selected.[4]

As the number of foods available to consumers increased, so did the complexity of the food list–recall approach. In 1948, the food list contained about 200 items. By 1978 it had grown to nearly 3000 items. Beginning with the 1987–88 survey, the list was replaced by a laptop computer.

Questions appeared on the computer's display, and the interviewer entered responses directly into the computer.[4,14] This process is known as computer-aided personal interviewing. The interviewer asked the food manager (the person most knowledgeable about meal planning and preparation within the household) to recall, with the aid of the computerized food list and any memory aids (store receipts, menus, shopping lists, etc.) the kinds and amounts of food used during the previous 7 days. This included all food that was prepared, eaten, discarded as waste, or fed to pets. The food manager also was asked to provide the price of each food used and to give information about several household characteristics.[14]

Data from household consumption surveys indicate the kinds, quantities, money value, and nutrient content of food used at home by the nation's households.[4,23] They provide data for determining the effects of income, household size, and other factors on total food and food group consumption. They show how diets on the household level conform to nutritional, budgeting, and other criteria. The 1936–37 survey, for example, showed that one third of the nation's families consumed diets rated poor by nutritional standards. Data from the survey helped fuel efforts to initiate school lunch programs, improve nutrition education, and enrich refined flour with iron, niacin, riboflavin, and thiamin.[23] Household surveys also supply basic information for developing the USDA family food plans at different cost levels; an example is the Thrifty Food Plan, which is the legal standard for benefits in the Food Stamp Program administered by the USDA.[4,23] One drawback to these data is that they do not provide data on how food is divided among individuals within the household or on the kinds and amounts of food consumed away from home.[4]

Other USDA Nutrition Monitoring Activities

Among the many other important roles of the USDA in nutrition monitoring are development of food composition and nutrient data bases, reporting of food and nutrient disappearance data, and oversight of the Diet and Health Knowledge Survey. The USDA compiles, reviews, evaluates, and makes available data on the nutrient composition of foods through development and maintenance of the National Nutrient Data Bank (NNDB) (see Chapters 3 and 5). Data from the NNDB are used to estimate nutrient levels in the U.S. food supply and for the major national nutrition surveys, including the CSFII and NHANES. As discussed later in this chapter, the USDA reports data on the disappearance of foods and nutrients from the U.S. food distribution system. The USDA has compiled food and nutrient disappearance data as far back as 1909, making it the only source of information on trends in the levels of foods and nutrients in the American diet since the beginning of the twentieth century.

The USDA's Diet and Health Knowledge Survey (DHKS) is a survey studying how attitudes and knowledge about healthy eating affect actual dietary practices. The DHKS provides data on knowledge and attitudes about dietary guidance, food preparation practices, use of nutrition information on food labels, and food safety concerns. The survey assesses respondents' accuracy of perceptions about how their diet rates relative to current dietary guidance, attitudes toward the importance of dietary guidance, and potential barriers to following the types of dietary guidance supported by federal nutrition policy. Data from the DHKS, shown in Figure 4-2, indicated that among female meal planners and preparers there was greater awareness of health problems related to the amount of salt or sodium in the diet and less awareness of health problems related to the amount of fiber. The DHKS is linked with the CSFII and is conducted annually during the years when the CSFII is conducted. In each of the households surveyed in the CSFII, one member is identified as the main meal planner or preparer. About 6 weeks following the CSFII, this person is contacted in a telephone follow-up, and the DHKS interview is conducted.[11]

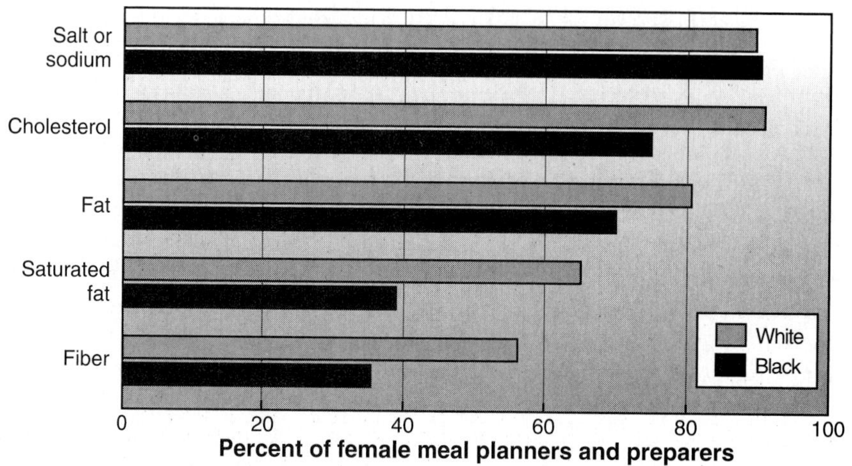

Figure 4-2 Awareness of health problems related to dietary components by race, 1989. This is an example of data collected by the Diet and Health Knowledge Survey. Data from the USDA Human Nutrition Information Service, Diet and Health Knowledge Survey.

ROLE OF THE U.S. DEPARTMENT OF HEALTH AND HUMAN SERVICES

The primary nutrition monitoring activity of the DHHS is the National Health and Nutrition Examination Survey (NHANES). The DHHS has been involved in nutrition and health-related monitoring since the 1960s, at which time it was known as the Department of Health, Education and Welfare or DHEW. Its current name was adopted in 1979. During the 1960s it conducted three National Health and Examination Surveys. These were followed by the landmark Ten-State Nutrition Survey and then the National Health and Nutrition Examination Surveys, including the Hispanic Health and Nutrition Examination Survey and the Navajo Health and Nutrition Survey. In addition to these, the DHHS is responsible for a number of other surveys related to diet and nutrition, health, knowledge and attitudes, and food labeling. Included among these are the Adult Nutrition Surveillance System, the National Health Interview Survey, the Pediatric Nutrition Surveillance System, the Total Diet Study, the Health and Diet Study, the Behavioral Risk Factor Surveillance System, and the Food Label and Package Survey. These and other surveys related to nutrition monitoring are outlined in Box 4-2.

BOX 4-2

The Five Primary Goals of NHANES III

1. Estimate the national prevalence of selected diseases and risk factors
2. Estimate national population reference distributions of selected health parameters
3. Document and investigate reasons for secular trends in selected diseases and risk factors
4. Contribute to an understanding of disease etiology
5. Investigate the natural history of selected diseases

National Health Examination Surveys

The National Health Examination Surveys (NHES) were a series of three health surveys conducted by the National Center for Health Statistics of the DHHS. NHES I was conducted from 1960 to 1962 and examined the prevalence of selected chronic diseases and health conditions in nearly 7000 Americans 18 to 79 years of age.[24] Using a variety of physical and physiologic measurements, such as blood pressure, serum cholesterol, skinfold measurements, height and weight, and electrocardiography, NHES I was able to focus on such conditions as coronary heart disease, arthritis, rheumatism, and diabetes.[24]

NHES II was conducted from 1963 to 1965 and sampled more than 7000 children 6 to 11 years old. From 1966 to 1970, NHES III studied nearly 7000 persons 12 to 17 years old. A primary task of NHES I and NHES II was to measure growth and development in American children and adolescents. This provided much of the data used by the National Center for Health Statistics in formulating its growth charts (described in Chapter 6 and shown in Appendix M). Because these two surveys sampled some of the same children, multiple measurements over time (known as *longitudinal measurements*) could be made on 2271 children, allowing their growth and development to be followed.[24]

Ten-State Nutrition Survey

The Ten-State Nutrition Survey was the nation's first comprehensive survey to assess the nutritional status of a large segment of the U.S. population.[8] During the 1960s, concerns about hunger and malnutrition in America escalated, leading legislators, health professionals, and private citizens to investigate the problem. Their reports revealed "chronic hunger and malnutrition in every part of the United States"[25] and described the situation as "shocking" and having reached "emergency proportions."[8] Congress responded by mandating the Department of Health, Education and Welfare to conduct a "comprehensive survey of the incidence and location of serious hunger and malnutrition and health problems incident thereto in the United States."[8]

The Ten-State Nutrition Survey targeted geographic areas having high proportions of low-income persons, inner-city residents, and migrant workers. Between 1968 and 1970, data were collected in the following ten states: California, Kentucky, Louisiana, Massachusetts, Michigan, New York (including New York City), South Carolina, Texas, Washington, and West Virginia.[8]

Although the survey helped reveal the extent and severity of hunger and malnutrition in America, groups surveyed were not representative of the general U.S. population, and consequently its findings could not be extrapolated to the overall population. The survey also demonstrated the difficulty and complexity of assessing nutritional status and recognized the need for additional data on the nutritional status of the U.S. population and the need for a continuing program of national nutritional surveillance. This led to the addition of a nutritional assessment component to the National Health Examination Survey and the beginning of the National Health and Nutrition Examination Survey.[8,26]

National Health and Nutrition Examination Survey

The **National Health and Nutrition Examination Survey (NHANES)** is conducted by the National Center for Health Statistics (NCHS), an agency of the DHHS. Its purpose is to monitor the overall nutritional status of the U.S. population through detailed interviews and comprehensive examinations. Interviews include dietary, demographic, socioeconomic, and health-related questions. Examinations consist of a medical and dental examination, physiological measurements, and laboratory tests.[12,26,27]

First National Health and Nutrition Examination Survey

NHANES I, conducted from 1971 to 1975, was designed to assess general health status, with particular emphasis on nutritional status and health of the teeth, skin, and eyes. Its target population was a representative sample of approximately 29,000 noninstitutionalized civilian Americans age 1 to 74 years. The nutrition component of NHANES I consisted of four major parts: dietary intake based on a 24-hour recall and food frequency questionnaire; biochemical levels of various nutrients based on assays of whole blood, serum, and urine samples; clinical signs of nutritional deficiency disease; and anthropometric measurements.[28] Although NHANES I originally was designed to provide data on the population's health and nutritional status at the time of the survey (in other words, a **cross-sectional survey**), the NHANES I Epidemiologic Follow-up Study, conducted in 1982–84, allowed subjects to be reexamined to assess the influence of nutritional status on development of disease and death.

Second National Health and Nutrition Examination Survey (NHANES II)

NHANES II was conducted from 1976 to 1980. It targeted nearly 28,000 noninstitutionalized civilian Americans 6 months to 74 years of age, of which more than 25,000 (91%) were interviewed and more than 20,000 (73%) were examined. Examination components included dietary interviews, anthropometric measurements, a variety of biochemical assays on whole blood, serum, and urine, glucose tolerance tests, blood pressure measurement, electrocardiography, and radiography of the chest and cervical and lumbar spine.[7]

Hispanic Health and Nutrition Examination Survey (HHANES)

HHANES was the largest and most comprehensive Hispanic health survey ever conducted in the United States. Planning for the survey began in 1979, and the actual data were collected from 1982 to 1984 under the direction of the NCHS.[29] The survey collected health and nutritional data on the three largest subgroups of Hispanics living in the 48 contiguous states: nearly 9500 Mexican-Americans residing in five Southwestern states (Arizona, California, Colorado, New Mexico, and Texas); more than 2000 Cuban-Americans living in Dade County, Florida; and more than 3500 Puerto Ricans residing in the New York City metropolitan area (selected counties in New York, New Jersey, and Connecticut).[29,30] Response rates ranged from 79% to 89% for interviews and from 61% to 75% for physical examinations. Because HHANES was not designed as a national Hispanic survey, its results do not necessarily apply to all Hispanics living in the United States. However, the sampled population included about 76% of the Hispanic-origin population of the United States as of 1980.[29]

Rather than providing a comprehensive picture of the health status or total health care needs of Hispanics, HHANES was designed to obtain basic data on certain chronic conditions and baseline health and nutritional information. As in NHANES, HHANES used five data-collecting techniques: interviews, physical examinations, diagnostic testing, anthropometrics, and laboratory tests.[29,31,32] Interviews were conducted at the homes of survey participants, followed by examinations at a mobile examination center, which consisted of three connected semitrailers that were specially designed and equipped for testing.[31] The nutritional component included an evaluation of iron status and anemia, serum vitamin A levels, and food consumption as related to diabetes, digestive diseases, overweight, dental health, and alcohol consumption.[29]

Third National Health and Nutrition Examination Survey (NHANES III)

Data collection for NHANES III began October 1988 and ended October 1994.[12,27,33] The survey was conducted in two phases of equal length and sample size. A total of approximately 40,000 noninstitutionalized Americans aged 2 months and older were asked to complete an extensive examination and interview. The response rates for the interview and examination were 86% and 78%, respectively.[12] Four population groups were specially targeted for examination: children aged 2 months to 5 years, persons 60 years of age and older, black Americans, and Mexican-Americans.[27] A disproportionately large number of persons in these four groups were examined to appropriately assess their nutritional and health status.[27] The five primary goals of NHANES III are shown in Box 4-2.

In planning for the survey in 1985, the NCHS intended it to provide several types of data: prevalence estimates of compromised nutritional status and trends in nutrition-related risk factors; data on the relationships among diet, nutritional status, and health; prevalence estimates of overweight and obesity in the U.S. population; and anthropometric data on children and adolescents, allowing revision of the NCHS growth charts (see Chapter 6 and Appendix M), which currently are based on data collected before 1976.[34] Four areas received special emphasis: child health, health of older Americans, occupational health, and environmental health.

The Food and Drug Administration (FDA) is using data from NHANES III to evaluate the need to change fortification regulations for the nation's food supply. NHANES III data have been used in evaluating public education efforts such as the National Cholesterol Education Program. Thirty-three of the health objectives for year 2000, including six in the nutrition priority area, rely on data from NHANES III. The National Institute of Occupational Safety and Health is comparing certain data (for example, pulmonary and central nervous system functioning) with those obtained in smaller studies of worker's health in various occupational settings.[26]

Examination and interviews were conducted in specially equipped and designed mobile examination centers (MEC) that travelled to survey locations throughout the country. Each MEC consisted of four trailers, approximately 48 feet long by 8 feet wide, providing about 1570 square feet of space. Several days before a survey was to begin at a particular location, the trailers were transported to the survey site, aligned, and leveled (as shown in Figure 4-3), and all connections of the passageways, electricity, water, and sewer were made. Each MEC contained a laboratory, examination rooms for physical, dental, and x-ray examinations, a computer room, and other rooms for conducting interviews and collecting specimens.[27] The floor plan of the MEC is shown in Figure 4-4. There were three MECs and two separate examination teams. Therefore a set of trailers could always be moved from one survey site to another, parked, set-up, and be ready by the time an examination team arrived.

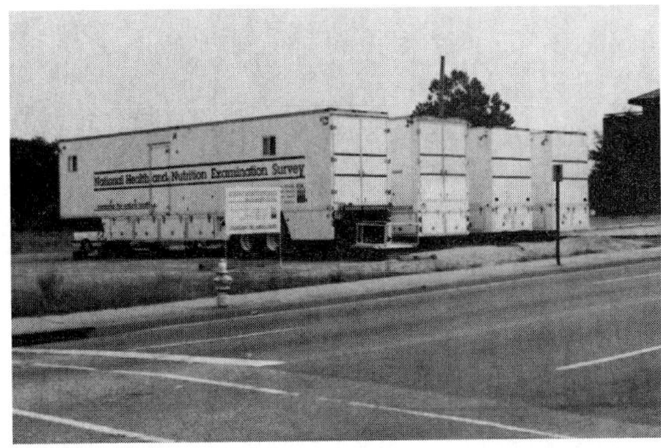

Figure 4-3 The Mobile Examination Center used in the third National Health and Nutrition Examination Survey.

In NHANES III, the 24-hour recall served as the primary dietary assessment method. Recalls were collected in the MEC (unless participants were unable to leave home). Most of the food frequency questionnaires were completed at home at the same time a detailed health questionnaire was completed by each participant. Recalls were completed using an automated, interactive, microcomputer-based interview procedure called the NHANES III Dietary Data Collection (DDC) system. The DDC was developed by the University of Minnesota's Nutrition Coordinating Center and includes a standardized interview format and automated probes to obtain detailed information about foods, including brand names, food preparation methods, and ingredients used in food preparation, particularly ingredients that contribute fat and sodium.[35] Information recorded in

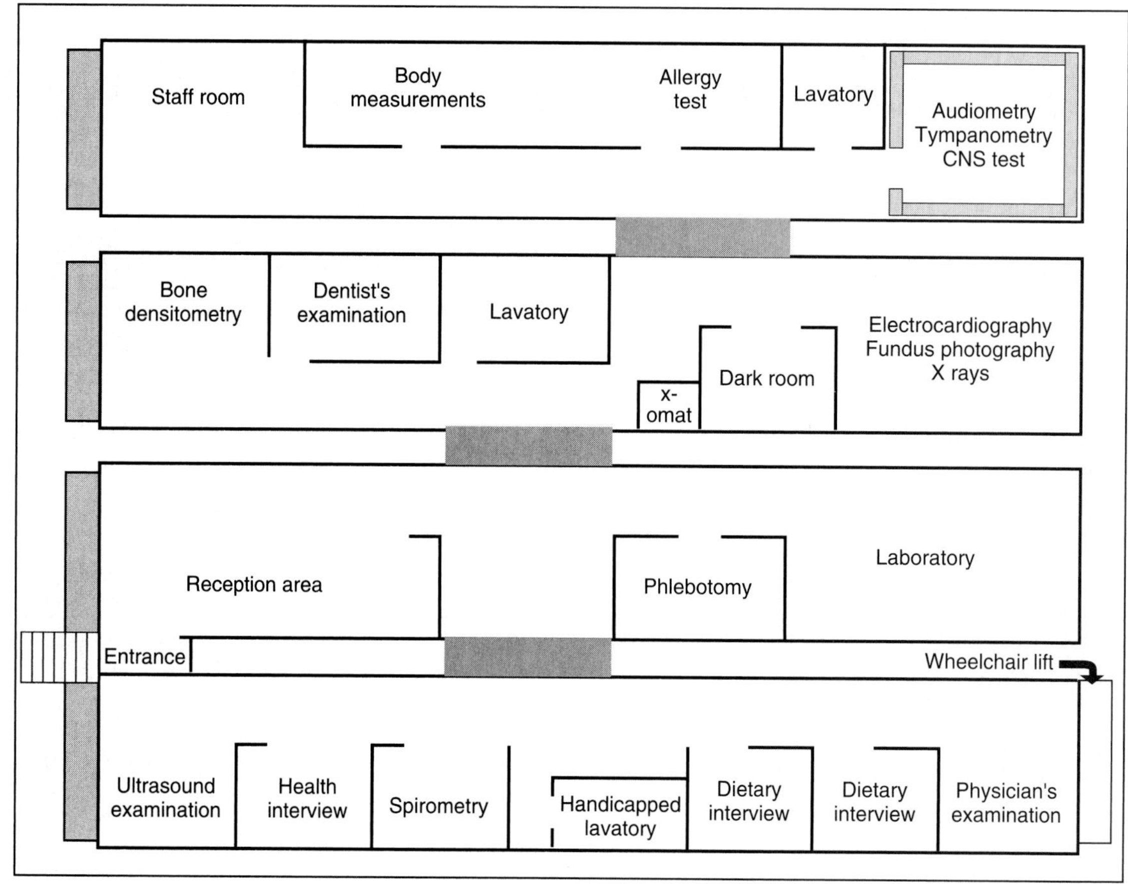

Figure 4-4 The floor plan of the Mobile Examination Centers used in the third National Health and Nutrition Examination Survey. Adapted from the National Center for Health Statistics. 1994. *Plan and operation of the Third National Health and Examination Survey, 1988–1994*. Hyattsville, Md: U.S. Department of Health and Human Services, Public Health Service; Centers for Disease Control and Prevention.

the 24-hour recalls included the time foods were consumed, food names, type of meal or snack, and where the foods were consumed.

Approximately 3500 participants in NHANES III who were 50 years of age or older completed two additional and unscheduled 24-hour recalls that were collected by telephone interviews approximately 8 and 16 months after the initial 24-hour recall.[27] This was part of the Supplemental Nutrition Survey of Older Americans, a special study collecting data on the diets of older Americans.

NHANES III also used a food frequency questionnaire to provide supplemental information on food and food group consumption, intake of alcohol, calcium, caffeine, and vitamin and mineral supplement use. The questionnaire was designed to provide qualitative data for ranking respondents by intake of specific foods and food groups. It was not intended to collect quantitative data on the actual amounts of nutrients consumed. It used a 1-month reference period and did not collect information on portion sizes. Researchers were

TABLE 4-2 Nutrition-related information collected in NHANES III by respondent age and information type.

Information	Age
24-hour dietary recall	2 months and over
Food security*	2 months and over
Food program participation*	2 months and over
Drinking water source* and quantity	2 months and over
Vitamin and mineral supplement usage	2 months and over
Salt use frequency and type	2 months and over
Instant food frequency	2–11 months
Breakfast practices	1 year and over
Dietary changes for health reasons	1 year and over
Infant feeding practices, including breast feeding	2 months–5 years
Food frequency	12 years and over
Alcohol use	12 years and over
Antacids use	17 years and over
Lifetime milk frequency	20 years and over
Self- (or proxy-) reported height and weight	2 months and over
Self- (or proxy-) assessed weight status	2 months and over
Birth weight	2 months–11 years
Weight loss practices and reasons	1 year and over
Desired weight	12 years and over
Weight history	25 years and over

From National Center for Health Statistics. 1994. *Plan and operation of the Third National Health and Examination Survey, 1988–1994*. Hyattsville, Md: U.S. Department of Health and Human Services, Public Health Services, Centers for Disease Control and Prevention.

*Also collected at the household (family) level.

particularly interested in foods containing nutrients related to risk of cancer, cardiovascular disease, and osteoporosis. As part of data collected to study osteoporosis, adults were asked to report their milk consumption during five age periods: 5–12 years, 13–17 years, 18–35 years, 36–65 years, and 65 years of age and older. Responses were recorded as "more than once per day," "once per day," "less than once per day, but more than once per week," "once per week," "less than once per week," or "never." Additional questions were asked about water intake, use of vitamin and mineral supplements, meal and snack patterns, infant feeding practices, and alcohol intake.

NHANES III also studied the impact of food insecurity on dietary intake, nutritional status, and health. At the family level, questions were asked about the number of days per month on which there was no food or money to buy food and the reasons for the problem. Individuals were asked the frequency of and reasons for skipping meals and going without food. Table 4-2 summarizes the nutrition-related information collected in NHANES III by respondent age and information type.

Each of the two examination teams consisted of a group of 16 persons who worked and traveled together. They included two dietary interviewers, a physician, a dentist, an ultrasonographer, four x-ray technicians, a phlebotomist, three medical technologists, a health interviewer, a home examiner, and a coordinator. Two locally hired staff supplemented the team at each site. Most of the staff, especially the interviewers, were fluent in both Spanish and English. Although the interviewing staff were not required to have academic credentials, most were experienced interviewers who represented a cross-section of society. A large staff of interviewers conducted the household interviews. In each location, local health and government officials were notified of the upcoming survey. Households in the survey received an advance letter and booklet to introduce the survey.

Participants were provided with transportation to and from the MEC. Participants received $30.00 cash for completing the 4-hour examination and an additional $20.00 if they arrived at the MEC on time and, if requested, were fasting. As shown in Table 4-3, all participants received a physical examination, various anthropometric measures, hearing tests, and a dietary interview. Depending on the participant's age, additional examination components were performed. In general, the older the participant, the more extensive the examination. Those unable to come to the MEC were given a less extensive examination in their homes.

NHANES III included several diagnostic procedures not used in previous NHANES studies, including bioelectrical impedance (see Chapter 6) and bone densitometry measurements using dual-energy x-ray absorptiometry (see Chapter 9). A variety of measures were used to assess nutritional status in NHANES III (see Figure 4-5). In addition to numerous biochemical tests, a variety of anthropometric measures were performed on participants as shown in Table 4-4.

The next NHANES (1997 NHANES) will begin in 1997 and will be conducted over a period of 2 to 3 years. The 1997 NHANES will provide national population estimates for non-Hispanic whites, non-Hispanic blacks, Mexican-Americans, and all Hispanics. Major objectives for the 1997 NHANES are:

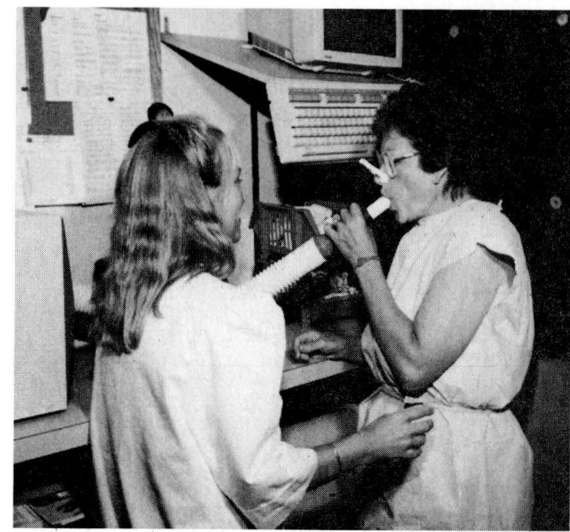

Figure 4-5 An example of the many types of diagnostic procedures performed as part of the Third National Health and Nutrition Examination Survey.

- to estimate the number and percentage of persons in the U.S. population and designated subgroups with selected diseases and risk factors
- to monitor trends in the prevalence, awareness, treatment, and control of selected diseases
- to monitor trends in risk behaviors and environmental exposures
- to analyze risk factors for selected diseases
- to study the relationships between diet, nutrition, and health
- to explore emerging public health issues

Other DHHS Surveys

Other surveys providing important food and nutrient intake data include the Total Diet Study, the Navajo Health and Nutrition Survey, the Pediatric Nutrition Surveillance System, the Pregnancy Nutrition Surveillance System, and the Health and Diet Survey.

TABLE 4-3 Examination components of NHANES III by age group

2 months–5 years	6–19 years	20–39 years	40–59 years	60–74 years	75 years and over
Physician's examination	Physician's examination	Physician's examination	Physician's examination	Physician's examination	Physician's examination
Dental examination*	Dental examination	Dental examination	Dental examination	Dental examination	Dental examination
Body measurements†	Body measurements	Body measurements†	Body measurements†	Body measurements†	Body measurements†
Venipuncture*	Venipuncture	Venipuncture†	Venipuncture†	Venipuncture†	Venipuncture†
Dietary interview	Dietary interview	Dietary interview	Dietary interview	Dietary interview	Dietary interview
Health interview	Health interview	Health interview	Health interview	Health interview	Health interview
	Urine collection	Urine collection	Urine collection	Urine collection	Urine collection
	Spirometry‡	Spirometry†	Spirometry†	Spirometry†	Spirometry†
	Bioelectric impedance§	Bioelectric impedance	Bioelectric impedance	Bioelectric impedance	Bioelectric impedance
	Allergy test	Allergy test‖	Allergy test‖	...	...
	Audiometry	...	...	...	...
	Tympanometry	...	...	...	...
	Cognitive test¶	...	...	Cognitive test†	Cognitive test†
		Bone density examination	Bone density examination	Bone density examination	Bone density examination
		Ultrasound examination	Ultrasound examination	Ultrasound examination	...
		CNS test‖	CNS test‖	...	...
			Fundus photography	Fundus photography	Fundus photography
			Electrocardiography	Electrocardiography	Electrocardiography
				Performance test†	Performance test†
				Hand/knee x-rays	Hand/knee x-rays

From National Center for Health Statistics. 1994. *Plan and operation of the Third National Health and Examination Survey, 1988–1994*. Hyattsville, Md: U.S. Department of Health and Human Services, Public Health Service, Centers for Disease Control and Prevention.

* 1 year of age and over.
† Also included in the home examination.
‡ 8 years of age and over.
§ 12 years of age and over.
‖ Half-sample only.
¶ 6–16 years of age.
NOTE: CNS is central nervous system.

TABLE 4-4 Anthropometric measures performed in NHANES III by age group*

	2–23 months	24–47 months	4–7 years	8–19 years	20–59 years	60+ years
Standing height		X	X	X	X	X
Recumbent length	X	X				
Sitting height		X	X	X	X	X
Knee height						X
Upper-leg length		X	X	X	X	X
Upper-arm length	X	X	X	X	X	X
Head circumference	X	X	X			
Midthigh circumference		X	X	X	X	
Calf circumference		X	X	X	X	X
Waist circumference		X	X	X	X	X
Buttocks circumference		X	X	X	X	X
Midupper-arm circumference	X	X	X	X	X	X
Subscapular skinfold	X	X	X	X	X	X
Suprailiac skinfold		X	X	X	X	X
Midthigh skinfold		X	X	X	X	
Triceps skinfold	X	X	X	X	X	X
Biiliac breadth		X	X	X	X	X
Elbow breadth		X	X	X	X	X
Wrist breadth		X	X	X	X	X
Biacromial breadth		(36–47 months)†	X	X	X	X
Weight	X	X	X	X	X	X
Bioelectrical impedance				(12+ years)	X	X

From Woteki CE, Briefel RR, Kuczmarski R. 1988. Contributions of the National Center for Health Statistics. *American Journal of Clinical Nutrition* 47:320–328.

*NHANES III = Third National Health and Examination Survey.

†Numbers in parentheses indicate ages of participants who received certain examinations. For example, (36–47 months) indicates that a particular test within the age group only was conducted on participants age 36 to 47 months.

The Total Diet Study is conducted annually by the Food and Drug Administration. It provides national estimates of average dietary intakes for 11 nutritional elements, four toxic metals, and various pesticide residues, industrial chemicals, additives, and radionuclides for 14 age-sex groups. Four or more times a year, the FDA purchases foods in grocery stores in selected cities in four geographic areas of the United States. These foods are among a group of approximately 265 "core" foods in the U.S. diet (i.e., foods that are among the most commonly eaten by Americans). These foods are then analyzed for nutrients, toxic metals, and pesticides, among other things. Data from these analyses are then combined with food consumption data from the CSFII and NHANES to arrive at estimates of daily intakes of these substances. The Total Diet Study allows the FDA to monitor the exposure of Americans to these substances, some of which are harmful if consumed in excess. If necessary, the FDA can take action to limit the use of pesticides, additives, and industrial chemicals in agriculture and food processing to maintain the public's exposure to these substances within desirable ranges.[11]

The Navajo Health and Nutrition Survey was planned by the Indian Health Service to establish prevalence data on nutrition-related chronic diseases and to generate a valid description of nutritional status and dietary behaviors of the Navajo people in general and for selected subgroups within that population. The sample size goal was 1700, and data collection took place over a 5-month period during 1991–92. Information was collected on dietary intake, food frequency, anthropometric measurements, lipid profiles, blood pressure, and full blood chemistries, including glucose tolerance tests.[11]

The Pregnancy Nutrition Surveillance System, conducted by the Centers for Disease Control and Prevention (CDC), is designed to monitor the prevalence of nutrition-related problems and behavioral risk factors that are related to infant mortality and low birth weight among high-risk prenatal populations. These include overweight, underweight, smoking, and alcohol consumption. The system also is studying the relationship of nutritional status to weight gain during pregnancy and birth outcome. Data are collected from health, nutrition, and food assistance programs for pregnant women such as WIC and prenatal clinics funded by Maternal and Child Health Block Grant and state monies.[11]

The Pediatric Nutrition Surveillance System, conducted by the CDC, is designed to continuously monitor the prevalence of major nutritional problems among high-risk, low-income infants and children from birth to 17 years of age. The system is based on information routinely collected by health, nutrition, and food assistance programs such as WIC; Early and Periodic Screening, Diagnosis, and Treatment (EPSDT); Head Start; and child health clinics operating under the Maternal and Child Health Block Grant. The Pediatric Nutrition Surveillance System was designed to improve the management of state child health programs and to allow states to develop and monitor state-based nutrition objectives. Program managers use this information to target high-risk subgroups of the population for interventions and to evaluate the effectiveness of interventions designed to reduce nutrition problems in infants and children.[11] An example of data collected by the Pediatric Nutrition Surveillance System is shown in Figure 4-6. This figure shows that between 1980 and 1991, the prevalence of short stature for low-income Asian children 2 to 5 years of age (represented by a height-for-age less than the 5th percentile) declined. This indicates that the nutritional status of this group (predominantly Southeast Asian refugees) improved markedly. During the same time growth status remained stable for the other groups represented in the figure.[36]

The Health and Diet Survey is a telephone survey of a nationally representative sample of American households conducted biennially (every two years) by the FDA. Participants are asked a core set of questions relating to health and nutrition that are included in each survey and additional questions that provide timely information on current health and diet issues or special topics. Topics covered by the survey include knowledge and perceptions about sodium, cholesterol, fats, and food labels; self-reported health-related behaviors such as dieting, sodium avoidance, efforts to lower blood pressure and blood cholesterol levels; and beliefs about the relationships between diet and cancer, high blood pressure, and heart disease. Survey data have been used to evaluate the effectiveness of public education initiatives of various federal agencies such as the National Cholesterol Education Program.[11]

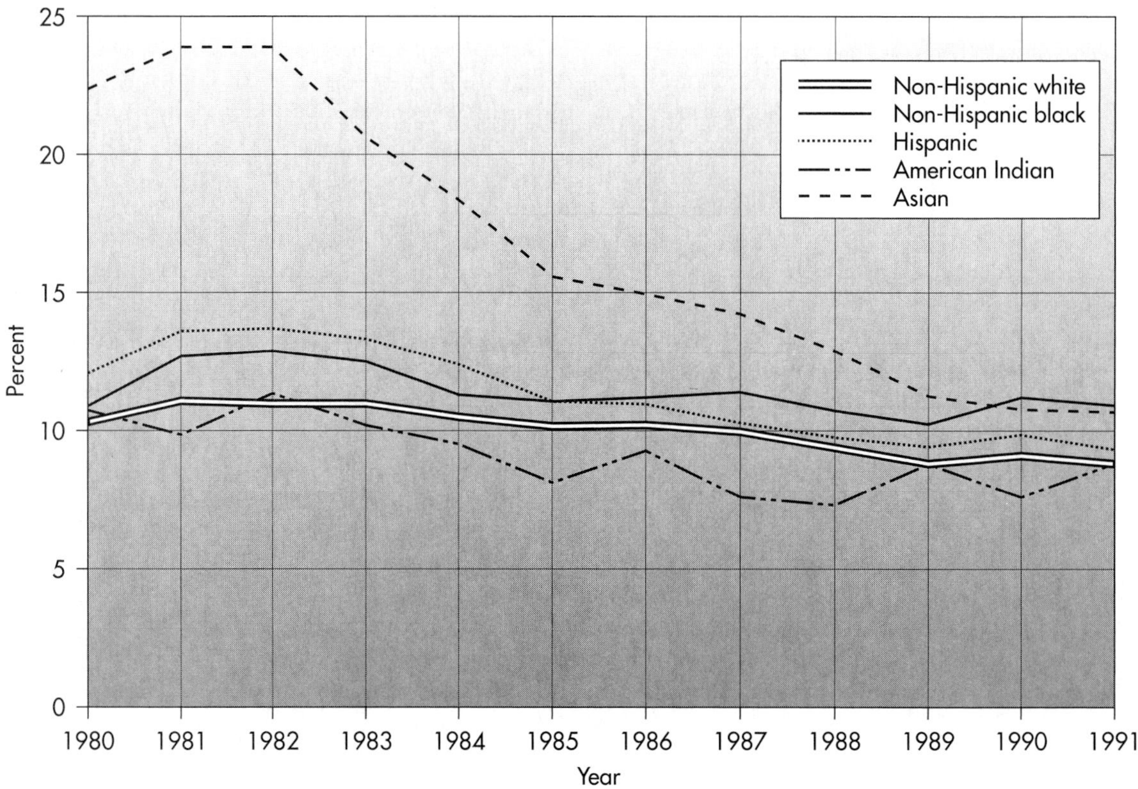

Figure 4-6 Percent of children 2 to 5 years of age with height-for-age less than the 5th percentile, by race and ethnicity, 1980–1991. This is an example of data collected by the Pediatric Nutrition Surveillance System. Data from the Centers for Disease Control and Prevention, National Center for Chronic Disease Prevention and Health Promotion, Division of Nutrition, Pediatric Nutrition Surveillance System.

DIETARY TRENDS

Data on food disappearance and consumption at the household and individual levels have revealed a number of significant changes in the American diet.[3] These include changes in the sources of food energy, average amounts of energy consumed by Americans, use of specific food groups including alcoholic and nonalcoholic beverages, and changes in eating patterns such as snacking and eating away from home. In the following material, some of the data presented is based on food disappearance (or availability), whereas other data are derived from surveys that measured actual food consumption (or at least attempted to). As discussed earlier in this chapter, food disappearance data fail to consider food lost from spoilage, cooking, removing inedible parts of food, or food fed to animals.

Sources of Food Energy

The distribution of food energy from carbohydrate, fat, and protein has changed since the USDA's Economic Research Service first began compiling food disappearance data. This is shown in Figure 4-7. From 1909 to 1990, energy available from protein remained essentially unchanged at 11% to 12% of total kilocalories. Percentage of kilocalories available from carbohydrate declined from 57% in 1909 to 46% in the 1970s and then increased modestly to about

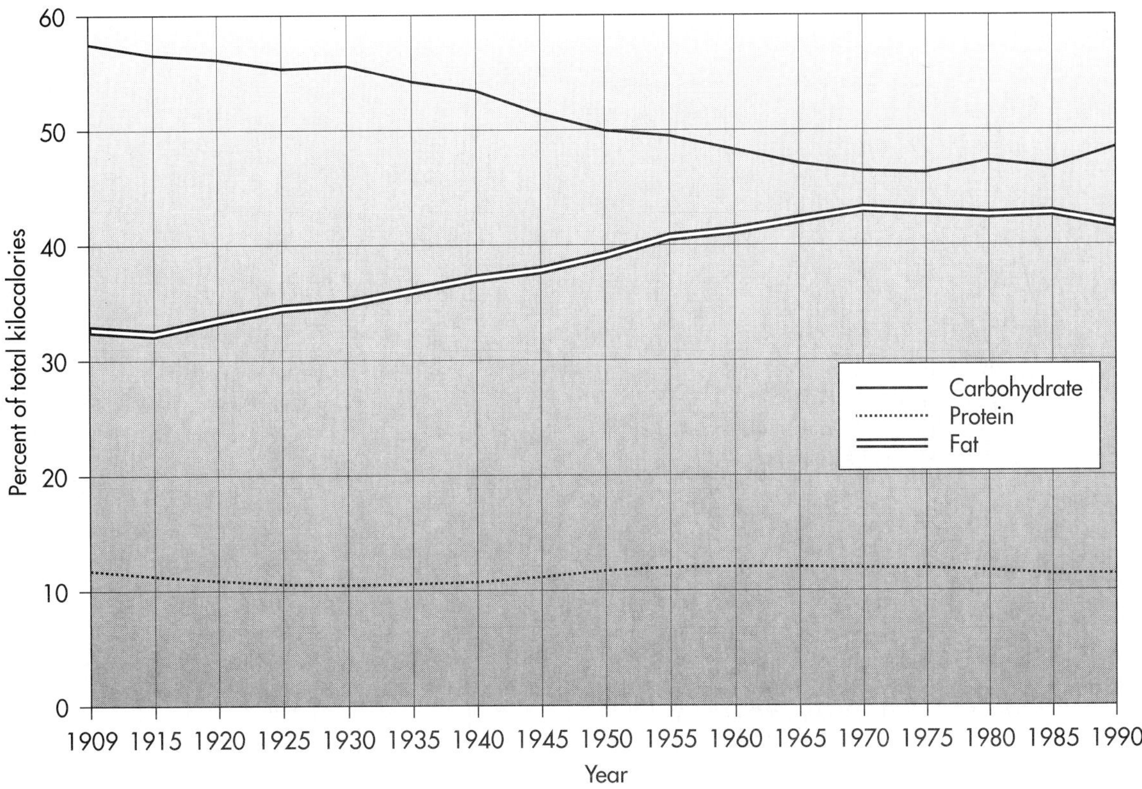

Figure 4-7 Percent of food energy (percent of total kilocalories) contributed by carbohydrate, protein, and fat from 1909 to 1990 based on U.S. Department of Agriculture. Data from Gerrior SA, Zizza C. 1994. *Nutrient content of the U.S. food supply, 1909–1990*. Hyattsville, Md: USDA, Home Economics Research Report No. 52.

49% in 1990. Fat availability ranged from a low of about 33% in 1909 to a high of about 43% in the 1970s. In recent years fat availability appears to have declined slightly to about 40% of total kilocalories in 1990.

Data from NHANES III for percent of kilocalories from carbohydrate, fat, protein, and alcohol are shown in Figure 4-8. Values for persons aged 2 months to 19 years are shown in part **A**, while values for persons aged 20 years and over are shown in part **B**. According to surveys conducted between 1965 and 1991 that measured actual food and nutrient intake, the percentage of kilocalories from fat has ranged from a high of 42% to a low of 34%.[35,36] These data are shown in Figure 4-9. Based on data from NHANES III, it appears that the percentage of kilocalories from fat in the U.S. diet may have slightly declined from previous years. However, given the difficulties of measuring dietary intake and the size of the apparent decrease (2%), conclusive evidence of a decline in kilocalories from fat may have to wait until future surveys corroborate this apparent decrease.

Factors other than a change in food consumption patterns could have influenced the percentage of kilocalories from fat. Among these are differences in how surveys collect dietary intake data, how foods are coded, and changes in nutrient composition databases. Compared with NHANES II, there was a greater percentage of 24-hour recalls collected for weekend days in

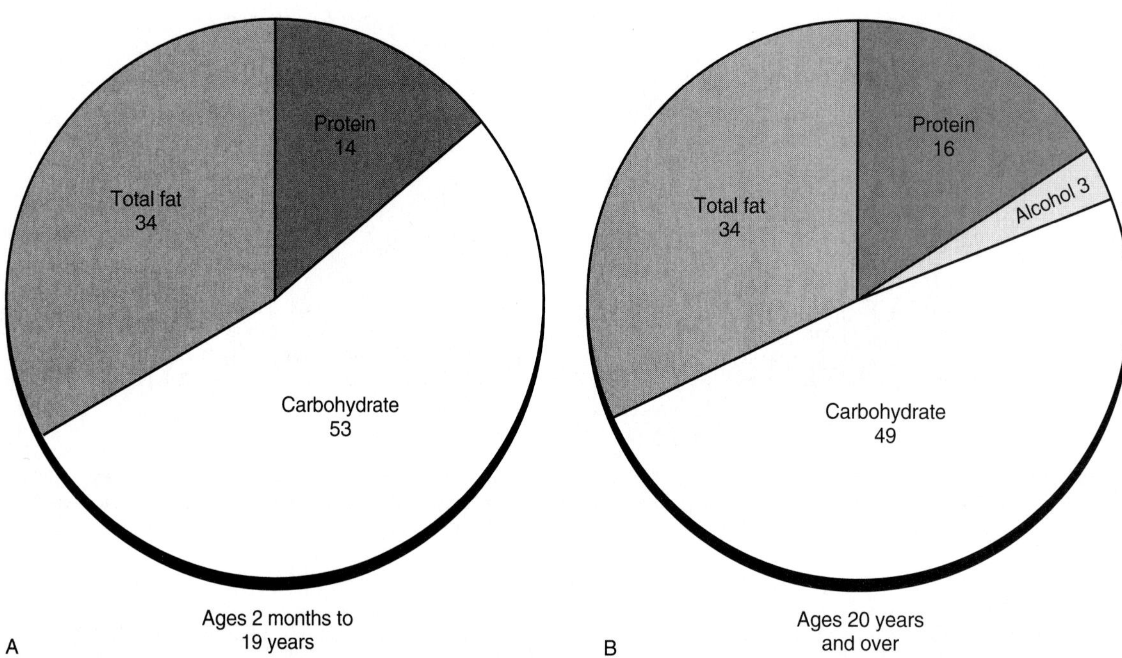

Figure 4-8 Percent of kilocalories from carbohydrate, fat, protein, and alcohol based on data from NHANES III. Values for persons aged 2 months to 19 years are shown in **A**. Values for persons aged 20 years and over are shown in **B**. Numbers may not add up to 100 due to rounding. Data from McDowell MA, Briefel RR, Alaimo K, Bischof AM, Caughman CR, Carroll MD, Loria CM, Johnson CL. 1994. Energy and macronutrient intakes of persons ages 2 months and over in the United States: Third National Health and Nutrition Examination Survey, Phase 1, 1988–1991. *Advance Data from Vital and Health Statistics*. No. 255. Hyattsville, Md; National Center for Health Statistics.

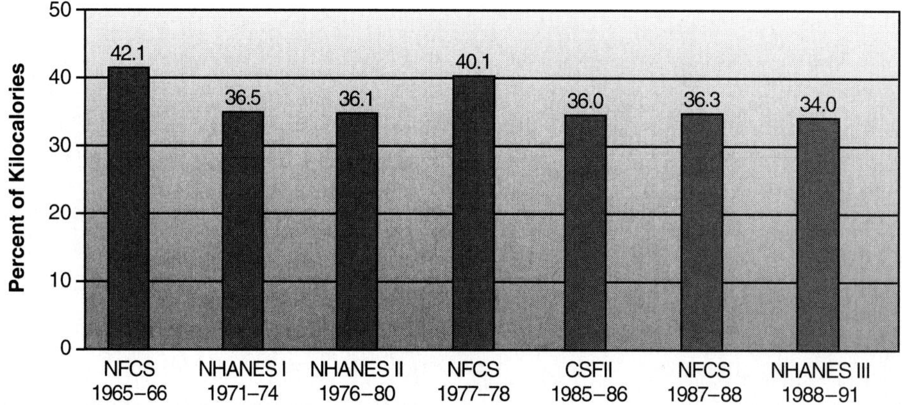

Figure 4-9 Percent of kilocalories from fat for selected years, 1965–1991. Data from the Nationwide Food Consumption Survey (NFCS) are for all age groups; data from the Continuing Survey of Food Intakes by Individuals (CSFII) are for children 1 to 5 years of age and men and women 19 to 50 years of age; data from the National Health and Nutrition Examination Survey (NHANES) are for individuals 20 to 74 years of age except for data from NHANES III, which are for all persons 20 years of age and over. Data from the USDA Human Nutrition Information Service and the USDHHS National Center for Health Statistics.

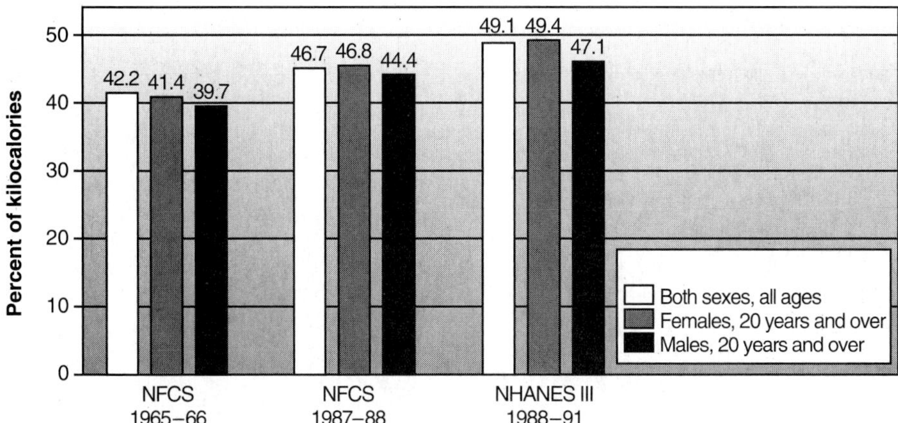

Figure 4-10 Percent of kilocalories from carbohydrate for males and females age 20 years and over and both sexes for all ages, 1977–78, 1987–88, 1988–91. Data from the USDA Human Nutrition Information Service and the Centers for Disease Control and Prevention, National Center for Health Statistics.

NHANES III. In NHANES II the 24-hour recalls were collected on paper forms and manually coded by dietary interviewers, whereas NHANES III used the Dietary Data Collection system discussed earlier in this chapter. In addition, the interviewers systematically probed for detailed information about all foods consumed and items added at the table. There were also differences between NHANES II and NHANES III in food coding and the nutrient composition databases used. As mentioned in Chapter 3, underreporting of food intake by as much as 25% frequently occurs, particularly in females, overweight persons, and those who are weight-conscious. In NHANES III this was addressed by comparing a participant's reported energy intake with his or her calculated resting energy expenditure. If the reported usual energy intake was < 1.2 times the participant's calculated resting energy expenditure, underreporting of energy intake, and therefore nutrient intake, was probable. Given the efforts made to ensure the collection of high quality data, the estimates of food and nutrient intake from NHANES III are probably among the best available to date.

Major dietary surveys of the past several decades indicate that the percentage of kilocalories from carbohydrate in the American diet is increasing. According to data from the 1977–78 NFCS, the 1987–88 NFCS, and NHANES III, percentage of kilocalories from carbohydrate (excluding alcoholic beverages) for all persons averaged 42%, 47%, and 49%, respectively. Percentage of energy from carbohydrate for males and females age 20 years and over and for all persons of both sexes are shown in Figure 4-10. Females tend to have a greater carbohydrate intake than males, as do children and adolescents compared with older persons. In contrast, the percentage of kilocalories from protein has changed little over the past several decades. Average protein intake for adults was approximately 17% of kilocalories according to the 1977–78 NFCS and the 1987–88 NFCS. Based on data from NHANES III, protein provided 16% of kilocalories.

Trends in Carbohydrates

Availability of total carbohydrates declined from about 488 g/day during 1909 to a low of about 370 g/day between 1963 and 1965. This decline was primarily due to decreased use of starches from grain products (flour and cereals), as shown in Figure 4-11.[37] Since the mid-1960s, availability of

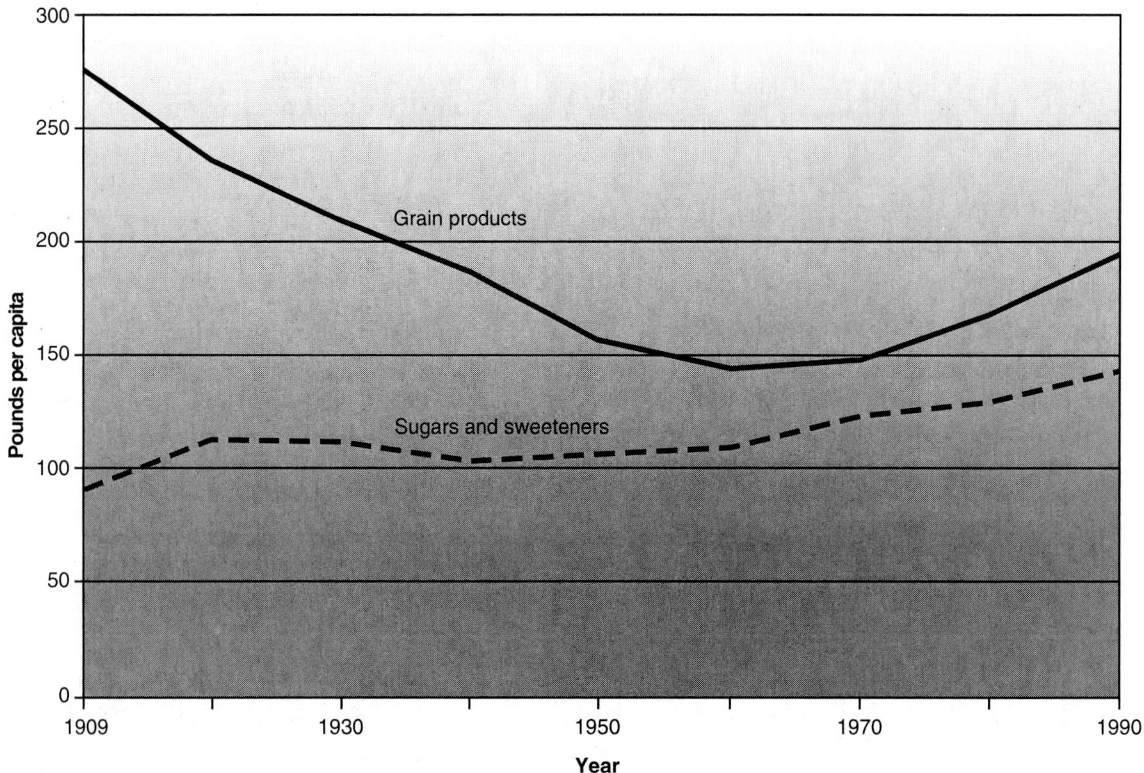

Figure 4-11 Annual per capita disappearance of grain products and sugars from the U.S. food supply from 1909 to 1990. Data from Gerrior SA, Zizza C. 1994. *Nutrient content of the U.S. food supply, 1909–1990.* Hyattsville, Md: U.S. Department of Agriculture, Home Economics Research Report No. 52.

carbohydrates has increased to about 452 g/day in 1990.[37] Figure 4-12 shows that between 1977–78 and 1987–88, consumption of cereals, other grain products, and mixed dishes containing grains has increased considerably.

Given the changes in carbohydrate availability, as shown in Figure 4-11, it is reasonable to assume that consumption of dietary fiber has declined since the early 1900s. Difficulties in measuring dietary fiber in foods has resulted in limited knowledge about fiber intake of the U.S. population.[39] Based on NHANES III data, mean dietary fiber intake for males and females of all ages is 17.0 g/day and 12.8 g/day, respectively.[38] This is

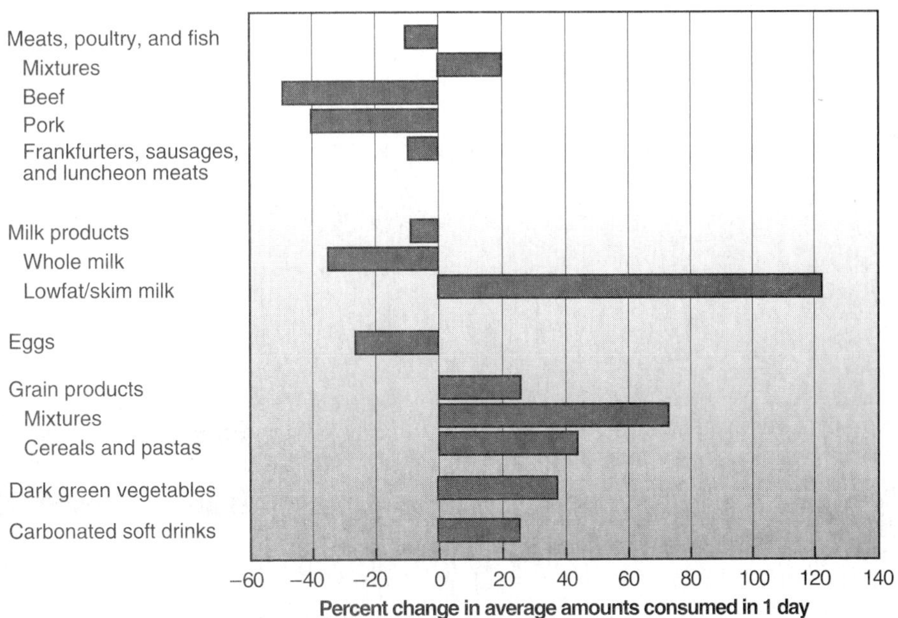

Figure 4-12 Dietary changes for selected foods between 1977–78 and 1989–90. Data from the 1977–78 Nationwide Food Consumption Survey and the 1989–90 Continuing Survey of Food Intakes by Individuals are for all age groups. The data represent changes in average intakes for all men, women, and children. Data from the USDA Human Nutrition Information Service.

greater than the estimate of 11 g/day based on data from NHANES II, but still less than the 20 to 35 g/day recommended by the Life Sciences Research Office's Expert Panel on Dietary Fiber.[39] According to NHANES III data, females consume more dietary fiber per 1000 kcal (7.36 g/1000 kcal) than males (6.86 g/1000 kcal).

Trends in Sugars

Estimates of sugar consumption come from two sources: food availability and food consumption data. Based on food disappearance data, the annual per capita availability of total sugars held relatively steady during the 1970s at about 125 lb but increased gradually to about 139 lb by 1991, as shown in Figure 4-13. These figures are sometimes reported as the average per-capita amount of sugars *consumed* in America. What may not be apparent, however, is that these estimates are based on *disappearance* data, not *consumption* data. Estimates of actual sugar consumption are considerably less. Estimated average U.S. consumption of all sugars (added and naturally occurring) is 95 g/day or about 76 lb/year.[42] This figure is based on 1977–78 NFCS food consumption data analyzed for sugar content using a specially created computerized database containing detailed information on the sugar content of foods. Table 4-5 shows that about 11% of the energy in the U.S. diet comes from sugars added to food. This is very close to that recommended by the U.S. Dietary Goals discussed in Chapter 2. An additional 10% of kilocalories comes from sugars that are naturally occurring in food. The 90th percentile represents a high sugar consumption. A person who is at the 90th

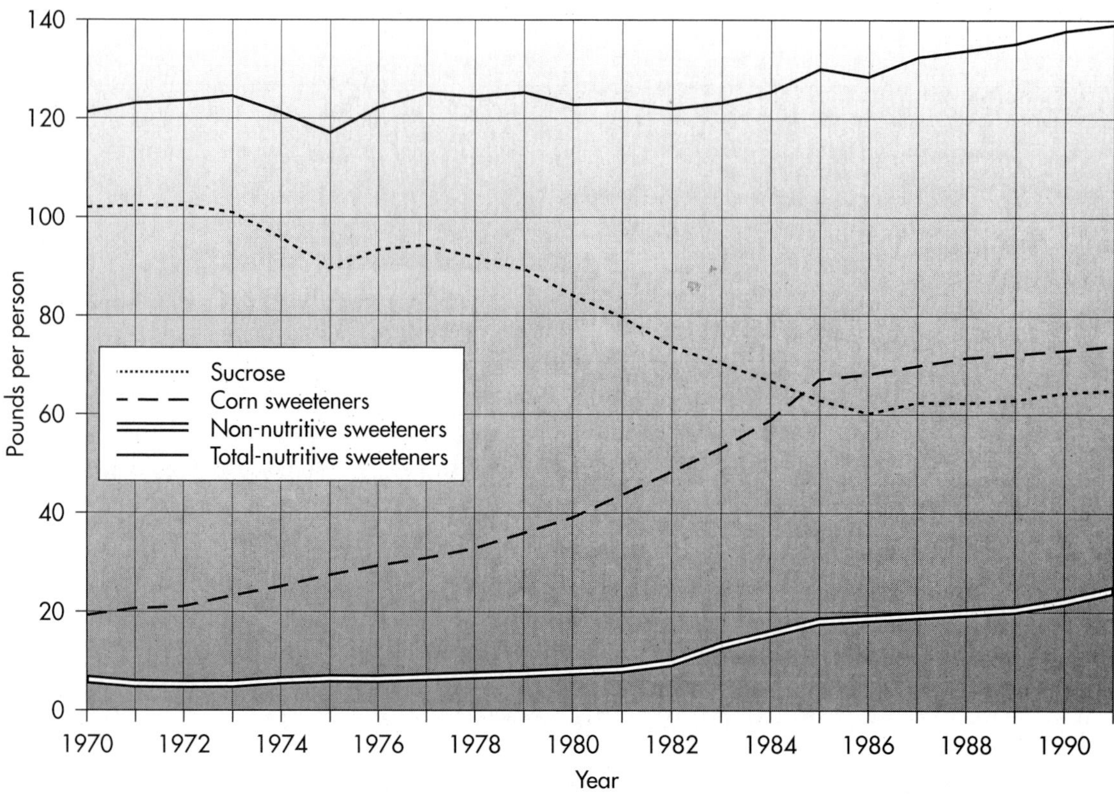

Figure 4-13 Trends in use of sweeteners, 1970–91, based on food disappearance. Values for sucrose include table sugar, honey, molasses, and maple syrup. Values for nonnutritive sweeteners are based on sugar-sweetness equivalence. Total nutritive sweeteners are corn and sucrose combined. Data from the USDA Economic Research Service.

percentile for sugar consumption eats more sugar than 90% of the population. According to Table 4-5, sugar consumption at the 90th percentile is about 130 lb/year, which represents 31% of all kilocalories coming from sugar.

How much sugar and sweeteners do Americans, on the average, actually consume each year? The value of 139 lb is an overestimation. Based on disappearance data, it fails to account for waste, spoilage, and nonfood uses of sugars (for example, in the production of alcoholic beverages). Estimates of sugar availability are based on shipments of sweeteners by refiners and importers to buyers such as food industries, wholesalers, and retailers. They are valuable for indicating trends in total sweetener use and use of specific sweeteners in the food supply.[40] The 76 lb estimate based on consumption data from the 1977–78 NFCS data is probably an underestimate. As noted earlier in this chapter, people tend to underreport their food consumption.[41–44] Actual per capita sugar consumption is somewhere between these two values. However, given the difficulties of measuring diet, we may never know the exact value.

The specific types of sweeteners consumed also have changed in recent years. In 1970, sucrose accounted for about 84% of all nutritive sweeteners that disappeared from the food distribution system, and corn sweeteners accounted for about 15%. By 1991, sucrose disappearance declined to 47% while that of corn sweeteners

TABLE 4-5 Summary of U.S. total sugar intake based on data from the 1977–78 Nationwide Food Consumption Survey

Sugars	Mean*		90th percentile†	
	Total population	Ranges for various groups by age/sex	Total population	Ranges for various groups by age/sex
	Daily intake (g/day)			
Added‡	53	10–84	104	30–155
Naturally occurring	42	33–59	74	60–99
Total minus lactose	80	31–116	139	65–193
Total	95	62–143	160	93–230
	Daily intake as percentage of calorie intake (%)			
Added‡	11	5–14	20	15–24
Naturally occurring	10	7–27	16	12–38
Total minus lactose	18	15–20	27	25–31
Total	21	18–32	31	27–43

From Glinsmann WH, Irausquin H, Park YK. 1986. Evaluation of health aspects of sugars contained in carbohydrate sweeteners: Report of sugars task force. *Journal of Nutrition* 116 (suppl):51–516.

* Total may not be equal to the sum of "added" and "naturally occurring" due to rounding.

† Data represent the 90th percentile value for each category of sugars. Thus, the values of added and naturally occurring sugars cannot be summed to give the 90th percentile value of total sugars.

‡ Excludes lactose added to infant formulas.

increased to 53%, primarily because of increased use of high fructose corn syrups, the predominant nutritive sweetener in soft drinks.[40] Figure 4-13 shows that by about 1985 corn sweetener disappearance had surpassed that of sucrose. The figure also shows that use of nonnutritive sweeteners has steadily increased since about 1981.

Trends in Dietary Fats

Because of its relation to coronary heart disease, cancer, and possibly obesity, fat consumption is of considerable public health significance. Intake of specific fatty acids also is related to coronary heart disease, as discussed in Chapter 9. Between 1909 and 1990, total fat disappearance increased from 124 to 165 g per capita per day.[37] This increase is primarily due to a 146% and 37% increase in the disappearance of polyunsaturated and monounsaturated fatty acids, respectively, while per capita amounts of saturated fat have remained relatively unchanged, as seen in Figure 4-14.[37] Although disappearance data indicate a shift away from animal fats to vegetable fats, monounsaturated and saturated fatty acids remain the predominate types of fat in the American diet.

The contribution of various fats and oils to per capita fat in the U.S. food supply between 1909 and 1985 is shown in Figure 4-15. The percent of fat available from butter, lard, and beef tallow has declined while that from margarine, vegetable shortening, and vegetable oils has increased.[37]

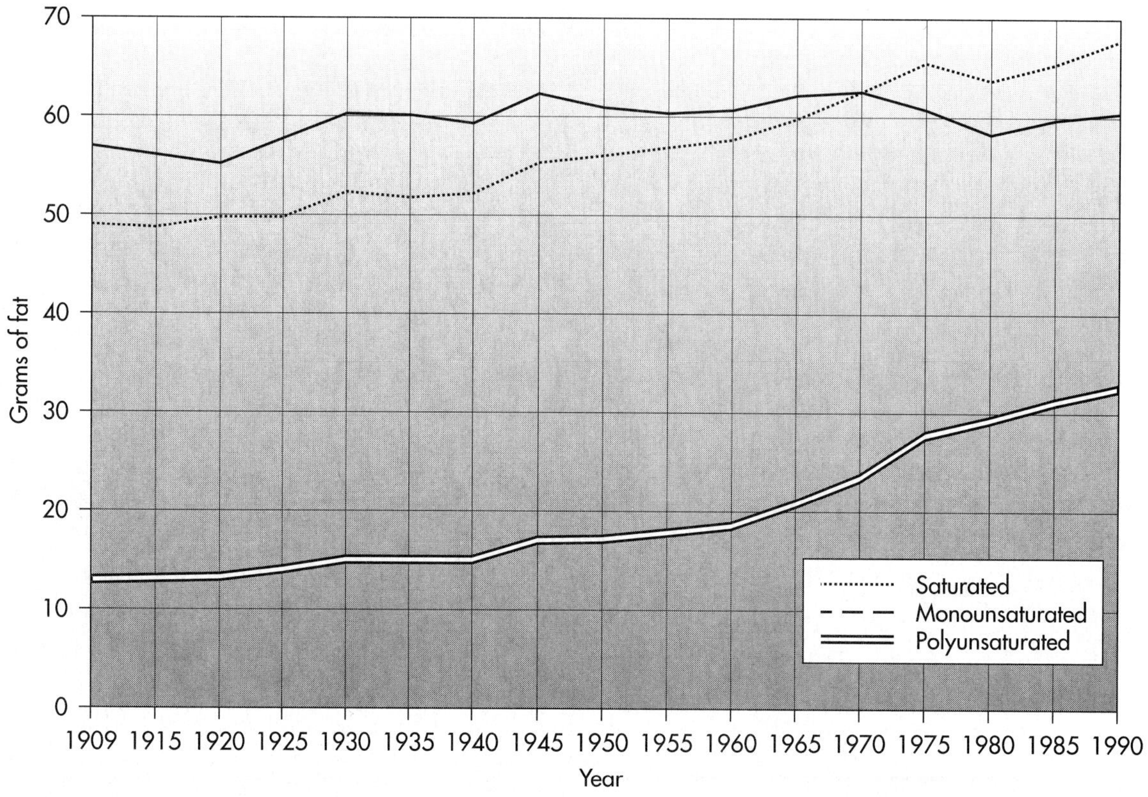

Figure 4-14 Trends in the disappearance of fatty acids from the U.S. food supply from 1909 to 1990. Data from Gerrior SA, Zizza C. 1994. *Nutrient content of the U.S. food supply, 1909–1990.* Hyattsville, Md: USDA, Home Economics Research Report No. 52.

Trends in Dairy Products

Americans have made substantial changes in the types of milk they are consuming. Disappearance of whole milk has decreased while that of lowfat and skim milk has increased markedly.[37] Between 1955 and 1990, for example, disappearance of whole milk fell from 123 to 61 quarts per person per year. During the same period, disappearance of low-fat and skim (nonfat) milk rose from 3 to 41 quarts per person per year. The gains in lowfat and skim milk have not offset the decline in whole milk, and overall, total milk disappearance is down. Changes in the disappearance of dairy products are summarized in Figure 4-16. According to food disappearance data, per capita egg usage has declined steadily since the end of World War II. Between 1970 and 1991 total annual per capita egg use decreased from 309 to 231 eggs, while annual per capita use of eggs in the form of egg products rose from 33 to 51 eggs. Figure 4-17 shows trends in the disappearance of eggs between 1970 and 1991. Some experts believe that the primary reason for these changes is concern about consuming too much cholesterol and saturated fat. Others point out that Americans are eating more meals away from home and are eating fewer cooked breakfasts at home.[45] See Figure 4-12 for the percent of change in consumption of dairy products and milk between the 1977–78 NFCS and the 1989–90 CSFII.

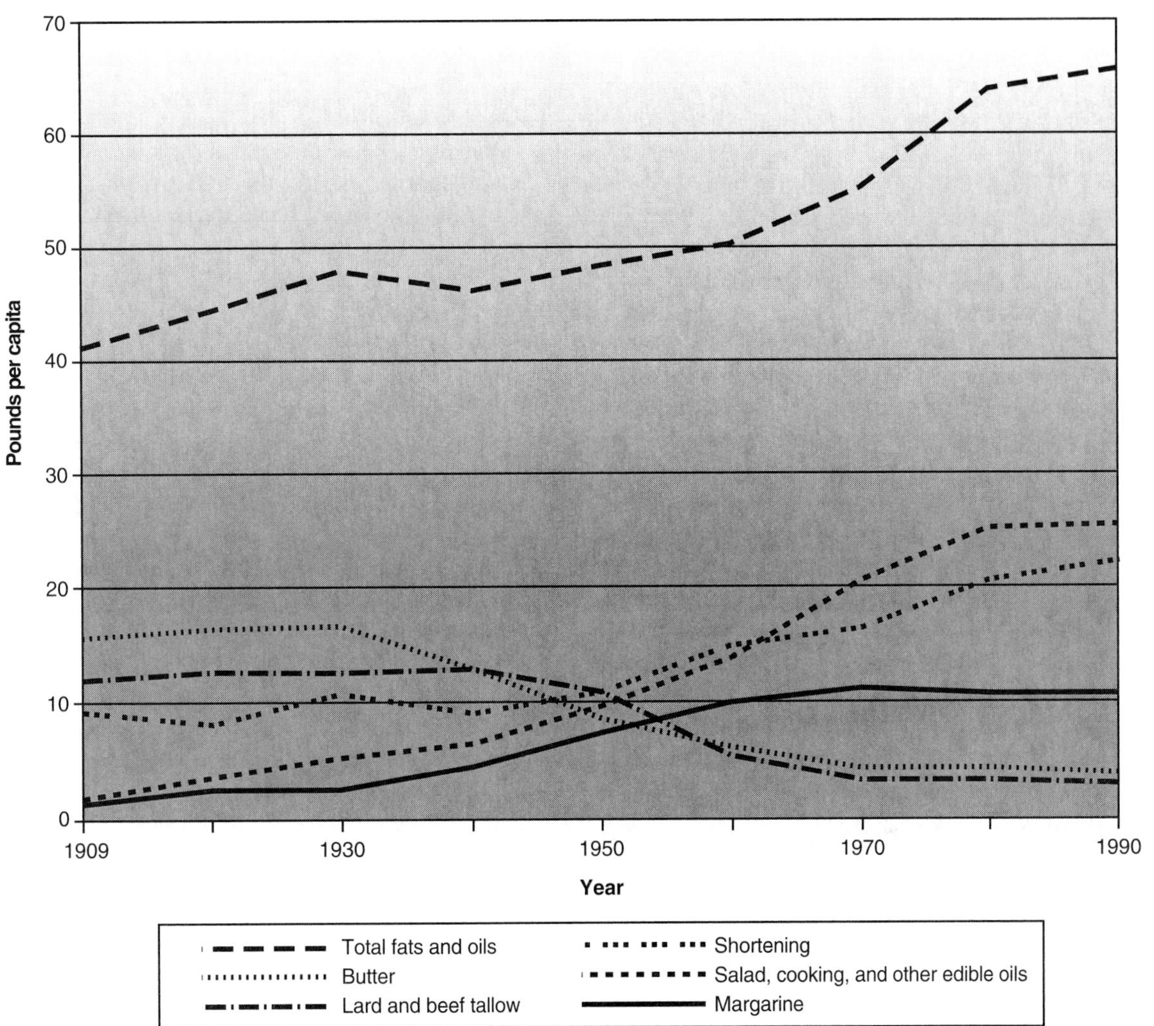

Figure 4-15 Disappearance of various fats and oils from the U.S. food supply from 1909 to 1990. Data from Gerrior SA, Zizza C. 1994. *Nutrient content of the U.S. food supply, 1909–1990.* Hyattsville, Md: U.S. Department of Agriculture, Home Economics Research Report No. 52.

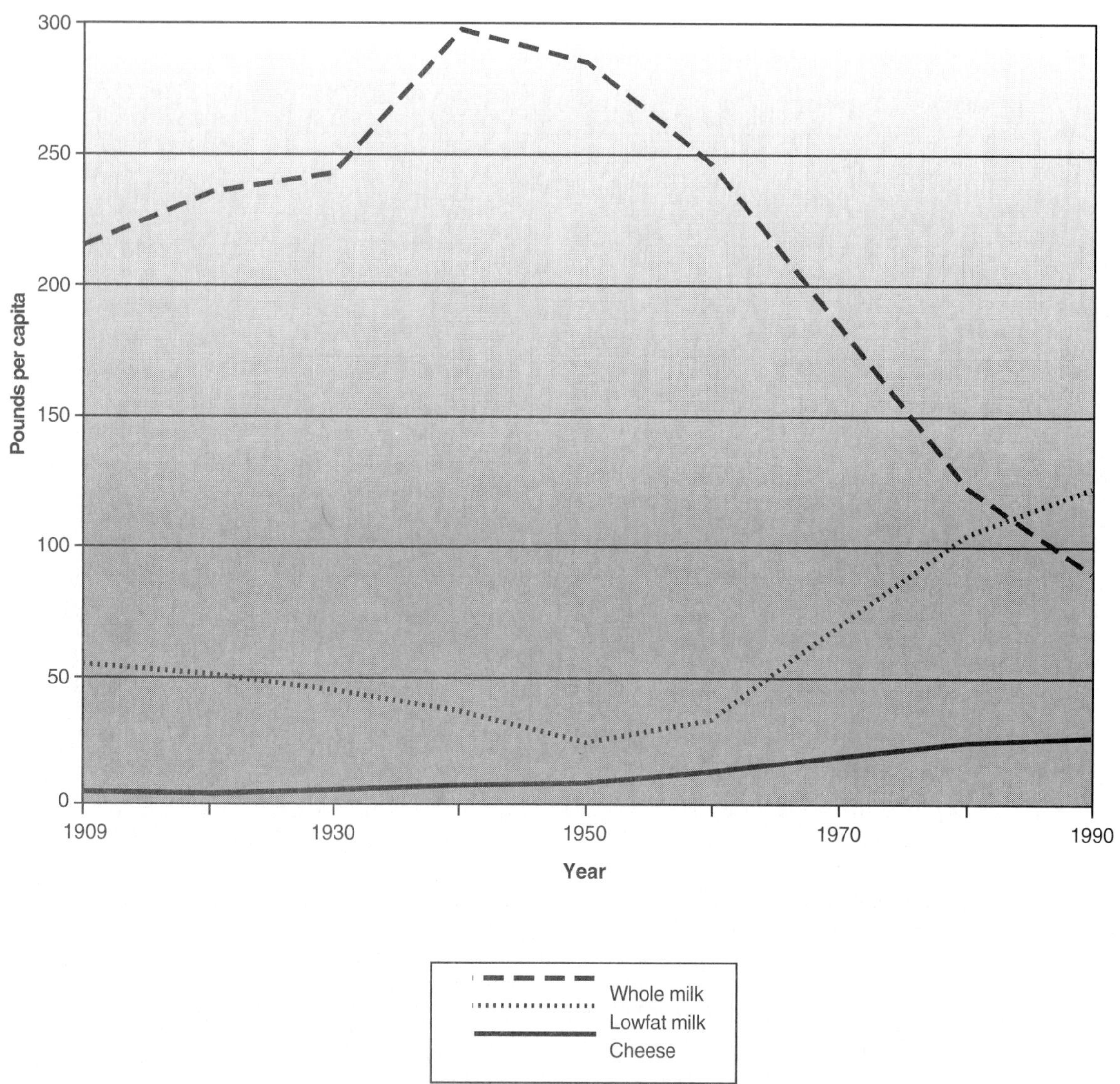

Figure 4-16 Trends in the disappearance of dairy products from the U.S. food supply from 1909 to 1990. Data from Gerrior SA, Zizza C. 1994. *Nutrient content of the U.S. food supply, 1909–1990.* Hyattsville, Md: U.S. Department of Agriculture, Home Economics Research Report No. 52.

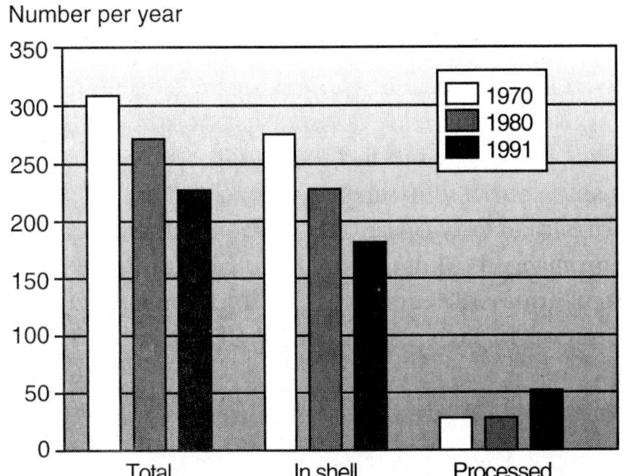

Figure 4-17 Trends in the disappearance of eggs from the U.S. food supply from 1970 to 1991. Data from the USDA Economic Research Service.

Trends in Beverages

Another factor in milk's drop in popularity is competition from other beverages, especially soft drinks, which are now America's favorite type of beverage. Coffee is the second most popular beverage, followed by milk, beer, bottled water, tea, and wine. However, as a group, alcoholic beverages—beer, wine, and distilled spirits, combined—surpass milk in per-capita consumption. Promotion and advertising of these beverages and greater preference for soft drinks while eating out also have contributed to declining milk consumption.[45] Figure 4-18 shows the percent change in per capita ethanol (ethyl alcohol) consumption from 1977 to 1989.

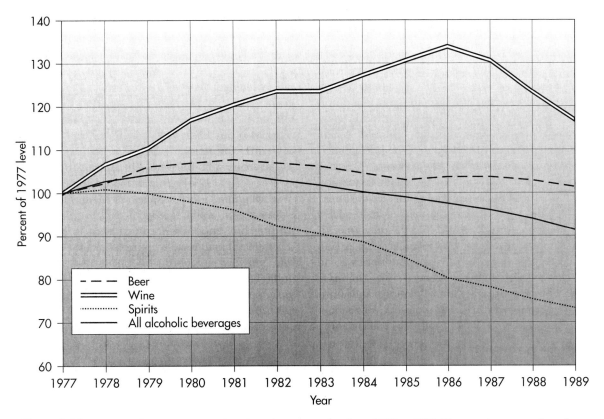

Figure 4-18 Percent change in per capita ethanol consumption from 1977 to 1989. These estimates are based on the total population 14 years of age and over. Data from the National Institutes of Health, National Institute on Alcohol Abuse and Alcoholism, Division of Biometry and Epidemiology, Alcohol Epidemiologic Data System.

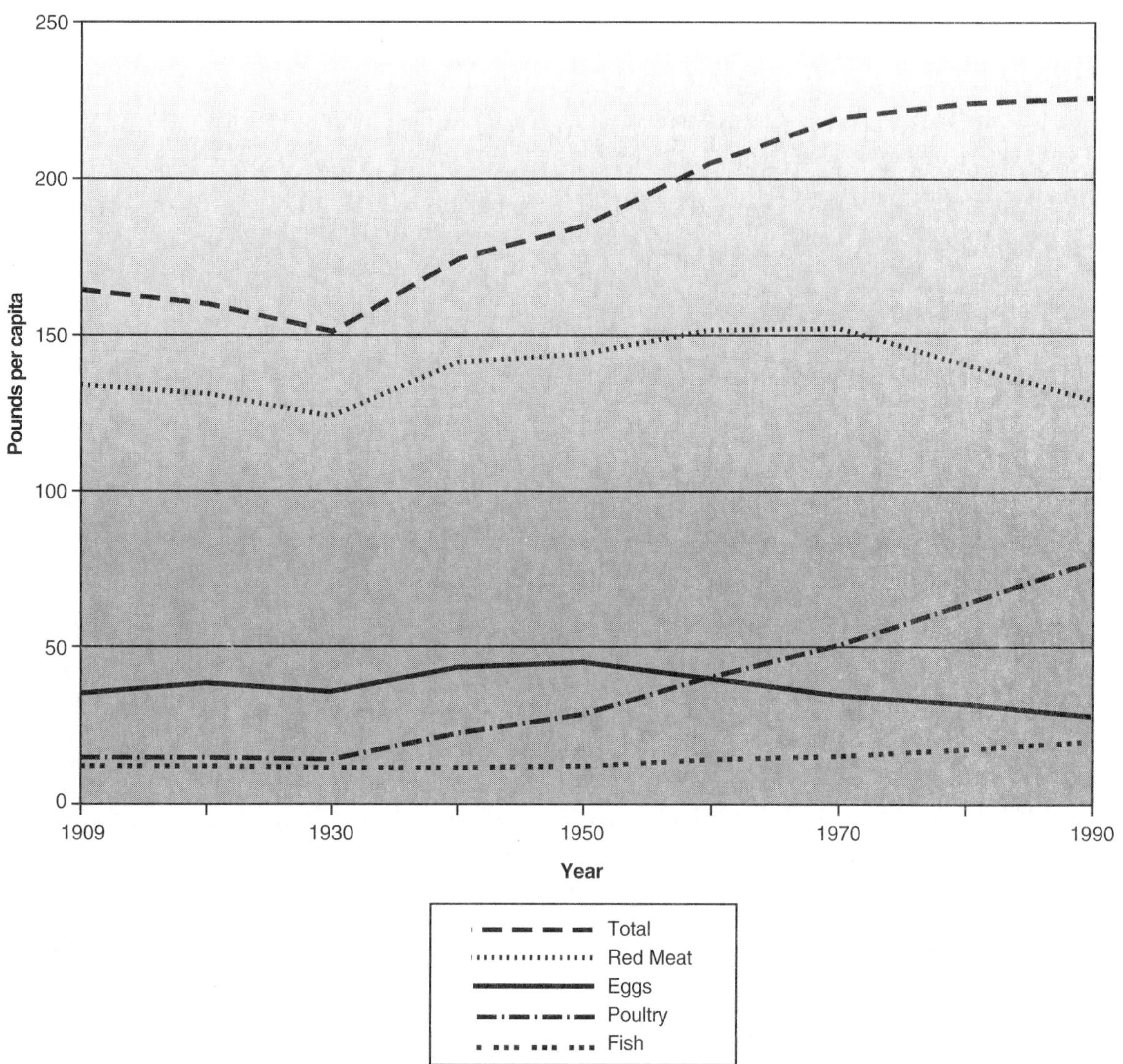

Figure 4-19 Trends in the disappearance of red meats (beef, pork, veal, lamb, mutton, and game meat), poultry (chicken and turkey), fish, and eggs from the U.S. food supply from 1909 to 1990. Data from Gerrior SA, Zizza C. 1994. *Nutrient content of the U.S. food supply, 1909–1990.* Hyattsville, Md: U.S. Department of Agriculture, Home Economics Research Report No. 52.

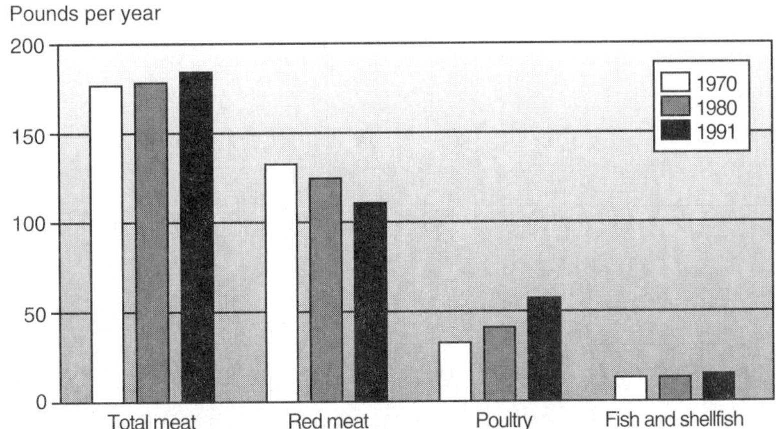

Figure 4-20 Trends in the disappearance of all meats, red meat (beef, pork, veal, lamb and mutton, and game meat), poultry (chicken and turkey), fish, and shellfish from 1970 to 1991. Data from the USDA Economic Research Service.

Trends in Red Meat, Poultry, and Fish

Figure 4-19 shows trends in the disappearance of red meats (beef, pork, veal, lamb and mutton, and game meat), poultry (chicken and turkey), and fish from 1909 to 1990. Although disappearance of total meat increased during this period, the disappearance of red meat has declined since 1970, and disappearance of poultry and fish—especially poultry—has increased significantly in recent years, as shown in Figure 4-20. The primary reasons for these changes seem to be lower prices for poultry due to technological advances and production efficiencies and aggressive marketing by the poultry industry.[46] Concerns about red meat consumption and risk of coronary heart disease may also play a role in these changes.

Comparing data from the 1977–78 NFCS with that from the 1989–90 CSFII, shown in Figure 4-12, it can be seen that consumption of beef, pork, frankfurters, sausages, and luncheon meats has decreased. During the same time Americans ate more meat and grain mixtures such as hamburgers on a bun, pizzas, and meat and rice mixtures. Fewer steaks and roasts were eaten separately and not in a mixture with grains.

Trends in Fruits and Vegetables

Figure 4-21 shows trends in the disappearance of certain fruits and vegetables from the U.S. food supply from 1909 to 1990. Figure 4-22 shows trends in fruit, vegetable, and potato disappearance between 1970 and 1990. After falling between 1909 and 1970, per capita use of fresh fruit increased from 96 lb in 1970 to 112 lb in 1990. This was due to sharp increases in use of noncitrus fruits.

Between 1970 and 1990, availability of vegetables increased 27%. Leading gainers were onions (up 6 lb per person), lettuce (up 5 lb), tomatoes (up 3 lb), and broccoli (up 3 lb).[36] Americans also used more artichokes, asparagus, carrots, cauliflower, cucumbers, eggplant, garlic, green peppers, and mushrooms, although use of cabbage, celery, corn, and green beans declined. Per capita use of fresh potatoes declined 26 percent between 1970 and 1990, but use of frozen potatoes nearly doubled to 25 lb per person in 1990.

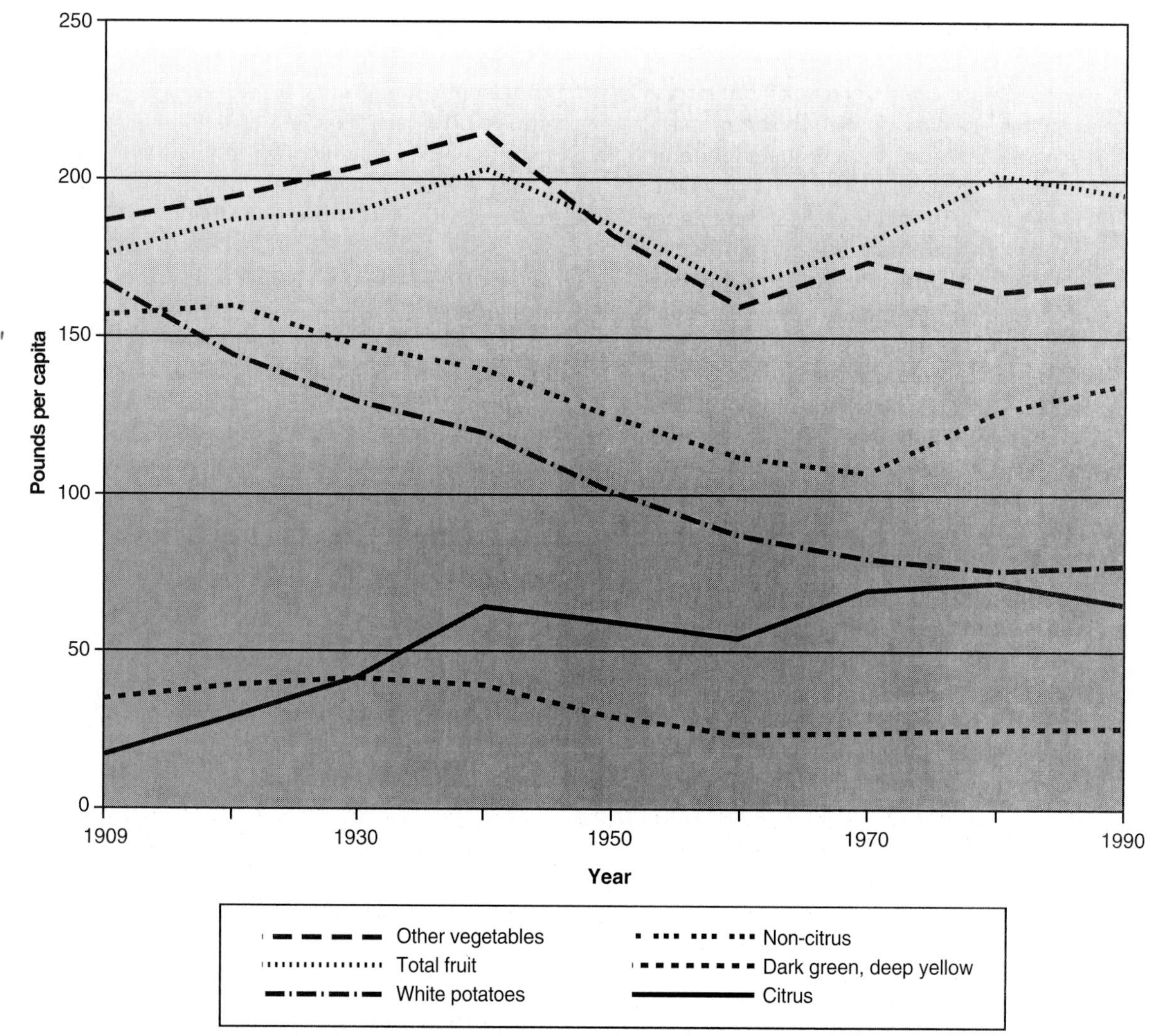

Figure 4-21 Trends in the disappearance of certain fruits and vegetables from the U.S. food supply from 1909 to 1990. Data from Gerrior SA, Zizza C. 1994. *Nutrient content of the U.S. food supply, 1909–1990.* Hyattsville, Md: U.S. Department of Agriculture, Home Economics Research Report No. 52.

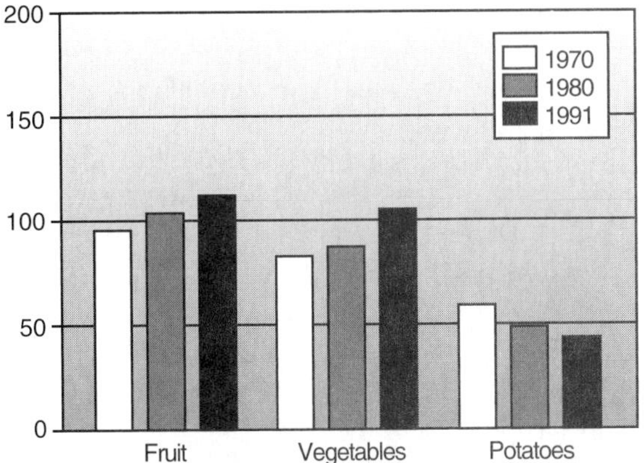

Figure 4-22 Trends in the disappearance of fruit, vegetables, and potatoes from 1970 to 1990. Data from the USDA Economic Research Services.

SUMMARY

1. National dietary and nutrition survey data are important in monitoring the nutritional status of a country's population, revealing the relationships between diet and health, identifying groups at nutritional risk and who may benefit from food assistance programs, and evaluating the cost effectiveness of food assistance and health education programs. These data can be used to track food consumption trends and monitor intakes of pesticides and other toxic substances.
2. Survey data provide a sound basis for agricultural policy and program development. They can provide an early warning of impending food shortages and indicate how such crises may be prevented or alleviated. Food balance sheets estimate the disappearance of food from the food distribution system and provide an indirect estimate of food consumption.
3. Nutritional monitoring is the assessment of dietary or nutritional status at intermittent times to detect changes in the dietary or nutritional status of a population. In the United States, this has been conducted by two federal agencies: the U.S. Department of Agriculture (USDA) and the U.S. Department of Health and Human Services (DHHS).
4. Passage of the National Nutrition Monitoring and Related Research Act of 1990 requires the USDA and DHHS to coordinate the nutrition monitoring activities of 22 federal agencies, which encompasses over 50 surveys and surveillance activities assessing the health and nutritional status of the U.S. population.
5. The USDA is involved in collecting data on food disappearance, individual food consumption, and household food consumption. Since 1909 the USDA has used the balance sheet approach to determine per capita disappearance of food from the food distribution system. Disappearance (or food availability) is not an actual measure of food consumption. It fails to account for losses resulting from spoilage, disposal of inedible parts, trimming by the consumer, and cooking. It is useful for examining food trends, making international comparisons, and studying the relationships between diet and disease.
6. The USDA began assessing individual food intake with the Household Food Consumption Survey, which had both an individual and a household component. This was later renamed the Nationwide Food Consumption Survey (NFCS) and was conducted during 1977–78 and 1987–88. The Continuing Survey of Food Intakes by Individuals replaces the NFCS. It provides timely information on U.S. diets, studies the dietary habits of persons at nutritional risk, provides data on "usual" diets by collecting several days of data over the course of a year, and demonstrates how diets vary over time.
7. The problem of low subject response rates in national surveys was illustrated in the 1987–88 NFCS. The response rate was so low that serious questions were raised about the usefulness of the survey's data. If the diets of nonrespondents are significantly different

from respondents, then a survey's results could be biased and not representative of the target population.

8. In 1936 the USDA began conducting the Household Food Consumption Surveys. In the household survey component, a food list-recall method was used to collect data from a nationally representative sample on the amounts and costs of foods used by households during a 7-day period.
9. Data from household consumption surveys indicate the kinds, quantities, money value, and nutrient content of food used at home by the nation's households. They provide data for determining the effects of income, household size, and other factors on total food and food group consumption. They show how diets on the household level conform to nutritional, budgeting, and other criteria.
10. Other nutrition monitoring activities of the USDA include development of food composition and nutrient databases, reporting of food and nutrient disappearance data, and oversight of the Diet and Health Knowledge Survey (DHKS). The DHKS studies how attitudes and knowledge about healthy eating affect actual dietary practices.
11. Surveys conducted by the DHHS include the National Health and Nutrition Examination Survey (NHANES), Hispanic Health and Nutrition Examination Survey (HHANES), Total Diet Study, Navajo Health and Nutrition Survey, Pediatric Nutrition Surveillance System, Pregnancy Nutrition Surveillance System, and the Health and Diet Survey.
12. The NHANES monitors overall nutritional status of the U.S. population through detailed interviews (using dietary, demographic, socioeconomic, and health-related questions) and comprehensive physical examinations, including medical and dental examination, anthropometric measurements, and diagnostic and laboratory tests.
13. NHANES III was conducted from 1988 to 1994. It provided data on the prevalence of compromised nutritional status and trends in nutrition-related risk factors; data on the relationships among diet, nutritional status, and health; prevalence estimates of overweight and obesity in the U.S. population; and anthropometric data on children and adolescents, allowing revision of the National Center for Health Statistics growth charts.
14. The HHANES was the largest and most comprehensive Hispanic health survey ever carried out in the United States. It collected health and nutritional data on the three largest subgroups of Hispanics living in the 48 continental states: Mexican-Americans residing in five Southwestern states, Cuban-Americans living in Dade County, Florida, and Puerto Ricans residing in the New York City metropolitan area.
15. Food availability data show that the percentage of kilocalories from protein has held fairly steady at 11% to 12% since 1909 to the present. During this same period, the percentage of kilocalories available from carbohydrate has decreased, while the percentage of energy available from fat has increased. Data from NHANES III indicate that adult Americans obtain about 16%, 49%, and 34% of their total energy from protein, carbohydrate, and fat, respectively.
16. Consumption of carbohydrates has declined because Americans now eat fewer grain and flour products and potatoes. Sugar consumption has increased, and estimated annual per capita sugar intake based on food consumption data is about 76 lb or about 11% of total kilocalories from sugars. Estimates based on food disappearance are considerably higher. Dietary fiber intake is estimated to average about 13 and 17 g/day for females and males, respectively.
17. The availability of kilocalories from fat has increased since the early 1900s because of increased consumption of polyunsaturated and monounsaturated fats. The percentage of kilocalories from saturated fat has remained relatively constant throughout the twentieth century.

18. Overall, Americans are drinking less milk and more soft drinks. Reasons for this include the popularity of soft drinks in restaurants and fast food outlets, more meals eaten away from home, concern about saturated fat intake in dairy products, and the heavy advertising of soft drinks. When Americans do drink milk, they are now more likely to drink lowfat or skim milk than whole milk.
19. The disappearance of red meat, poultry, and fish has increased steadily since 1909 to the present. In recent years, however, Americans have shown an increased preference for poultry because of its lower price.
20. After decreasing between 1909 and 1970, disappearance of fruits and vegetables has increased since 1970.

REFERENCES

1. U.S. General Accounting Office. 1994. Nutrition monitoring: Progress in developing a coordinated program. Washington, DC: United States General Accounting Office.
2. U.S. General Accounting Office. 1992. Early intervention: Federal investments like WIC can produce savings. Washington, DC: United States General Accounting Office, GAO/HRD-92–18.
3. National Research Council. 1989. *Diet and health: Implications for reducing chronic disease risk.* Washington, DC: National Academy Press.
4. Pao EM, Sykes KE, Cypel YS. 1989. *USDA methodological research for large-scale dietary intake surveys, 1975–88.* Washington, DC: U.S. Department of Agriculture, Human Nutrition Information Service.
5. Mason JB, Habicht JP, Tabatabai H, Valverde V. 1984. *Nutritional surveillance.* Geneva: World Health Organization.
6. Food and Agriculture Organization. 1990. *Bibliography of food consumption surveys.* Rome: Food and Agriculture Organization of the United Nations.
7. Life Science Research Office, Federation of American Societies for Experimental Biology. 1989. *Nutrition monitoring in the United States: An update report on nutrition monitoring.* Washington, DC: U.S. Government Printing Office.
8. Ostenso GL. 1984. National nutrition monitoring system: A historical perspective. *Journal of the American Dietetic Association* 84:1181–1185.
9. Brown GE. 1984. National nutrition monitoring system: A congressional perspective. *Journal of the American Dietetic Association* 84:1185–1189.
10. Brown GE. 1988. Remarks. *American Journal of Clinical Nutrition* 47:333–335.
11. U.S. Department of Health and Human Services, U.S. Department of Agriculture. 1993. Ten-year comprehensive plan for the national nutrition monitoring and related research program; notice. Federal Register. Vol. 58, No. 111, pp. 32751–32806.
12. Briefel RR. 1994. Assessment of the U.S. diet in national nutrition surveys: National collaborative efforts and NHANES. *American Journal of Clinical Nutrition* 59(suppl):164S-167S.
13. Kuczmarski MF, Moshfegh A, Briefel R. 1994. Update on nutrition monitoring activities in the United States. *Journal of the American Dietetic Association* 94:753–760.
14. Peterkin BB, Rizek RL, Tippett KS. 1988. Nationwide food consumption survey, 1987. *Nutrition Today* 23(1):18–24.
15. Nesheim RO. 1982. Measurement of food consumption—past, present, and future. *American Journal of Clinical Nutrition* 35:1292–1296.
16. Welsh SO, Martson RM. 1982. Review of trends in food use in the United States, 1909–1980. *Journal of the American Dietetic Association* 81:120–125.
17. Human Nutrition Information Service. 1987. Nationwide food consumption survey: CSFII, continuing survey of food intakes by individuals—1986. *Nutrition Today* 22(5):36–39.
18. Human Nutrition Information Service. 1989. Nationwide food consumption survey: CSFII, continuing survey of food intakes by individuals—1989. *Nutrition Today* 24(5):35–38.
19. United States General Accounting Office. 1991. Mismanagement of nutrition survey has resulted in questionable data. Washington, DC: United States General Accounting Office.
20. Human Nutrition Information Service. 1990. Unpublished data from the 1987–88 nationwide food consumption survey. Hyattsville, Md: U.S. Department of Agriculture, Human Nutrition Information Service.

21. Wright HS, Guthrie HA, Wang MQ, Bernardo V. 1991. The 1987–88 nationwide food consumption survey: An update on the nutrient intake of respondents. *Nutrition Today* 26(3):21–27.
22. Life Science Research Office, Federation of American Societies for Experimental Biology. 1991. *Impact of nonresponse on dietary data from the 1987–88 nationwide food consumption survey*. Bethesda, Md: Life Science Research Office, Federation of American Societies for Experimental Biology.
23. Rizek RL, Pao EM. 1990. Dietary intake methodology. I. USDA surveys and supporting research. *Journal of Nutrition* 120:1525–1529.
24. Yetley E, Johnson C. 1987. Nutritional applications of the health and nutrition examination surveys (HANES). *Annual Review of Nutrition* 7:441–463.
25. Citizens Board of Inquiry into Hunger and Malnutrition. 1968. *Hunger-USA*. Washington, DC: New Community Press.
26. Woteki CE, Hitchcock DC, Briefel RR, Winn DM. 1988. National health and nutrition examination survey—NHANES. *Nutrition Today* 23(1):25–27.
27. National Center for Health Statistics. 1994. *Plan and operation of the third national health and examination survey, 1988–94*. Hyattsville, Md: U.S. Department of Health and Human Services, Public Health Service, Centers for Disease Control and Prevention.
28. Lowenstein FW. 1976. Preliminary clinical and anthropometric findings from the first health and nutrition examination survey, USA, 1971–1972. *American Journal of Clinical Nutrition* 29:918–927.
29. Delgado JL, Johnson CL, Roy I, Treviño FM. 1990. Hispanic health and nutrition examination survey: Methodological considerations. *American Journal of Public Health* 80 (suppl):6–10.
30. Woteki CE. 1990. The Hispanic health and nutrition examination survey (HHANES 1982–1984): Background and introduction. *American Journal of Clinical Nutrition* 51:897S–901S.
31. Chumlea WC, Guo S, Kuczmarski RJ, Johnson CL, Leahy CK. 1990. Reliability for anthropometric measurements in the Hispanic health and nutrition examination survey (HHANES 1982–1984). *American Journal of Clinical Nutrition* 51(suppl):902S–907S.
32. Roche AF, Guo S, Baumgartner RN, Chumlea WC, Ryan AS, Kuczmarski RJ. 1990. Reference data for weight, stature, and weight/stature in Mexican Americans from the Hispanic health and nutrition examination survey (HHANES 1982–1984). *American Journal of Clinical Nutrition* 51(suppl):917S–924S.
33. Woteki CE, Briefel R, Hitchcock D, Ezzati T, Maurer K. 1990. Selection of nutrition status indicators for field surveys: The NHANES III design. *Journal of Nutrition* 120:1440–1445.
34. Woteki CE, Briefel RR, Kuczmarski R. 1988. Contributions of the National Center for Health Statistics. *American Journal of Clinical Nutrition* 47:320–328.
35. McDowell MA, Briefel RR, Alaimo K, Bischof AM, Caughman CR, Carroll MD, Loria CM, Johnson CL. 1994. Energy and macronutrient intakes of persons ages 2 months and over in the United States: Third national health and nutrition examination survey, phase 1, 1988–91. *Advance Data from Vital and Health Statistics*. No. 255. Hyattsville, Md: National Center for Health Statistics.
36. Interagency Board for Nutrition Monitoring and Related Research. 1993. *Nutrition monitoring in the United States, chartbook 1: Selected findings from the national nutrition monitoring and related research program*. Hyattsville, Md: Public Health Service.
37. Gerrior SA, Zizza C. 1994. *Nutrient content of the US food supply, 1909–1990*. Hyattsville, Md: U.S. Department of Agriculture, Home Economics Research Report No. 52.
38. Alaimo K, McDowell MA, Briefel RR, Bischof AM, Caughman CR, Loria CM, Johnson CL. 1994. Dietary intake of vitamins, minerals, and fiber of persons ages 2 months and over in the United States: Third national health and nutrition examination survey, phase 1, 1988–91. *Advance Data from Vital and Health Statistics*. No. 258. Hyattsville, Md: National Center for Health Statistics.
39. Life Science Research Office, Federation of American Societies for Experimental Biology. 1987. *Physiological effects and health consequences of dietary fiber*. Bethesda, Md: Life Science Research Office, Federation of American Societies for Experimental Biology.

40. Glinsmann WH, Irausquin H, Park YK. 1986. Evaluation of health aspects of sugars contained in carbohydrate sweeteners: Report of Sugars Task Force, 1986. *Journal of Nutrition* 116(suppl):S1–S16.
41. Mertz W, Tsui JC, Judd JT, Reiser S, Hallfrisch J, Morris ER, Steele PD, Lashley E. 1991. What are people really eating? The relation between energy intake derived from estimated diet records and intake determined to maintain body weight. *American Journal of Clinical Nutrition* 54:291–295.
42. Mertz W, Kelsay JL. 1984. Rationale and design of the Beltsville one-year diet study. *American Journal of Clinical Nutrition* 40(suppl):1323–1326.
43. Hallfrisch J, Steele P, Cohen L. 1982. Comparison of seven-day diet records with measured food intake of twenty-four subjects. *Nutrition Research* 2:263–273.
44. Schoeller DA. 1990. How accurate is self-reported dietary energy intake? *Nutrition Reviews* 48:373–379.
45. Rados B. 1985. Eggs and dairy foods: Dietary mainstays in decline. *FDA Consumer* 19(8):10–17.
46. Lecos C. 1985. Fish and fowl lure consumers from red meat. *FDA Consumer* 19(8):18–21.

FIVE

Computerized Dietary Analysis Systems

Outline

- Introduction
- Using Computers in Nutritional Assessment
- Factors to Consider in Selecting a Computerized Dietary Analysis System
    - Nutrient Database
    - Program Operation
    - System Output
- A Comparison of Eight Microcomputer Dietary Analysis Systems
    - How the Comparison Was Conducted
    - How the Systems Compare
        - Diet Balancer for Windows
        - DietMax Plus for Windows
        - Food Processor Plus
        - Counseling Nutrition Data System
        - Nutrient Analysis System 2 Plus 8
        - Nutritionist IV
        - Nutritional Software Library IV
        - Food/Analyst Plus
    - Why Systems Differ
- Summary
- References
- Assessment Activity 5-1: Using a Diet Analysis Program to Analyze a 3-day Food Record
- Assessment Activity 5-2: Dietary Analysis Program
- Assessment Activity 5-3: Cruising the Internet for Nutritional Information

INTRODUCTION

In Assessment Activity 3–1 you manually calculated your intake of kilocalories, protein, carbohydrate, total fat, calcium, and iron from a 24-hour recall form using nutrient data from Appendix L. Your first step was to find the appropriate food and then compare the amount you actually ate with the portion size listed for the food. If these differed, you had to mathematically adjust all of the nutrient values before listing them on a spreadsheet table. After doing this for all of the foods, you then added all of the values for each nutrient to calculate your final 24-hour intake. Quite an arduous process, wasn't it?

To alleviate the strain and reduce the time involved in dietary analysis, many scientists and nutrition professionals from around the world have developed dietary analysis software for personal microcomputers. Literally hundreds of programs are now available for all sorts of nutrition-related tasks.

The purpose of this chapter is to describe important characteristics of computerized dietary analysis systems to aid you in selecting an appropriate software package. Eight of the most popular programs are reviewed in detail as an example of the selection process.

USING COMPUTERS IN NUTRITIONAL ASSESSMENT

Before the computer era, nutrient analysis of food records, dietary recalls, food frequency forms, or diet histories was a tedious and cumbersome process. First, each food had to be located in a food composition table. Next the reported nutrient values had to be adjusted to match the actual serving size consumed. After all of the foods in the diet record or list had been processed in this

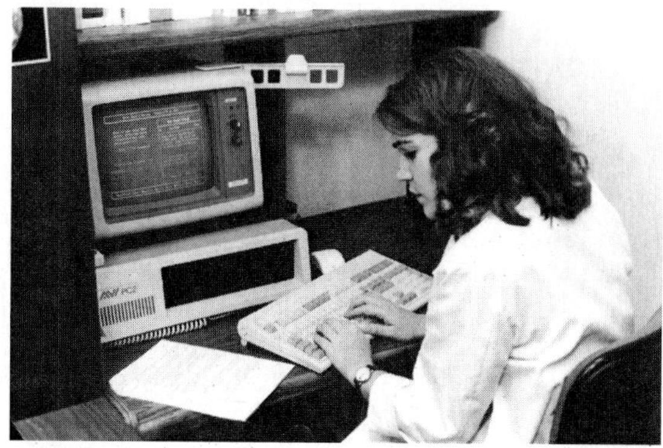

Figure 5-1 Computers are well suited to the task of nutrient analysis.

fashion, the data for each nutrient had to be summarized and then compared to a dietary standard such as the Recommended Dietary Allowances (RDA)[1]. Clearly, computers are perfectly suited to this task of nutrient analysis, which is nothing more than number crunching, and are useful in terms of saving time, labor, and expense while reducing error[2–5] (Figure 5-1).

Descriptions of computer applications in nutrition and dietetics first appeared in the literature in the late 1950s. Today there are many computer software programs available for delivering a wide variety of nutrition services including patient interviews, counseling, menu planning and forecasting, documentation of care, nutrition education, research, productivity assessment and employee scheduling, production scheduling and equipment use, nutritional assessment, and nutrient analysis[4,6]. Computer hardware cost is no longer the prohibitive factor it once used to be, and most hospitals, clinics, businesses, and educational facilities provide microcomputer work stations.

Nutrient intake analysis is one of the most widespread applications of computer technology in dietetics[7] (Box 5-1). Computerized dietary intake analysis has now become an important skill for dietitians and nutritionists to master. This chapter will review factors to consider in selecting computerized dietary analysis systems, with emphasis on the quality of the nutrient database, software program operation features, and important system output components. Eight popular microcomputer dietary analysis systems will be evaluated to help guide readers in their selection.

FACTORS TO CONSIDER IN SELECTING A COMPUTERIZED DIETARY ANALYSIS SYSTEM

During the 1980s and 1990s, the number of nutrient analysis software packages available for microcomputers proliferated. There are hundreds of these software packages, ranging from simplified programs designed for elementary school students to comprehensive programs designed for researchers. Unfortunately, not all of these software packages are reliable or accurate. The Nutrient Databank Directory contains information on more than 100 nutrient analysis software systems.[8] The information in the directory, presented in a tabular format, includes information on the names of the systems and vendors, the cost and availability of these systems, software features, hardware requirements, and the number of foods and nutrients in the database. This directory is currently available for $17 from the Department of Nutrition and Dietetics, Alison Hall, University of Delaware, Newark, Delaware 18715–3360.

The U.S. Department of Agriculture (USDA) Food and Nutrition Information Center (FNIC), which is located at the National Agriculture Library in Beltsville, Maryland (Room 304, 10301 Baltimore Blvd.), provides on-site review of more than 200 nutrient analysis software programs.[5] A description of the FNIC Microcomputer Software Collection is available on the Nutrient Databank Bulletin Board through the Internet in cooperation with the University of Maryland. To access the data, enter "telnet info.umd.edu" at your system prompt. The FNIC software information is also available from "ALF" (Agricultural Library Forum), which is an electronic bulletin board system produced by the National Agricultural Library of the USDA. To access ALF (with a computer, modem, and communications software), dial (301) 504–6510 or (301) 504–5111.

BOX 5-1

Five Categories of Computerized Nutrient Analysis Tasks

Category	Sample task
1. Clinical	Analyze patient intake against clinical standard
2. Educational	Produce nutrient intake profile that is easily understood by patient or lay person
3. Administrative	Analyze nutrient content of patient menus and make decisions regarding budget and inventory
4. Epidemiologic	Analyze intakes of large populations to identify diet-disease relationships
5. Metabolic/experimental	Develop precise test meals or menus for research subjects

From Frank GC, Pelican S. 1986. Guidelines for selecting a dietary analysis system. *Journal of the American Dietetic Association* 86:72–75.

In selecting a microcomputer system, the first step is to establish the major needs for obtaining the software, with specific tasks defined. Once this has been accomplished, the next step is to choose a dietary analysis system that is suitable to these needs and tasks. For example, a research professor in a nutrition department will probably need a completely different type of computerized dietary analysis system than a health educator working with minority groups in a public health department. In comparing software programs, dietitians and other health professionals should consider aspects of the database, program operation, and system output.[7]

Nutrient Database

The most important consideration to make when selecting a computerized diet analysis system is its nutrient database.[3,5] The database must be accurate, well documented, and large enough to meet all intended tasks. The USDA began publishing food composition values in 1896 and has continually revised and expanded their food composition tables ever since.[9,10] The USDA has also contributed to the development of food composition tables for other countries for many years and has participated in the International Network of Food Data Systems (INFOODS), organized first in 1983. INFOODS promotes worldwide acquisition and interchange of high quality food composition data.[9,11] The *International Directory of Food Composition Databases* is available from INFOODS Secretariat, Charles Street Station, Box 500, Boston, MA 02114–0500 (telephone (617) 227–8747).

Most software vendors begin development of their databases with data from the USDA. As part of its mission, the USDA's Nutrient Data Laboratory, Agricultural Research Service, operates the National Nutrient Databank, a computerized information system for storing and summarizing data on the composition of foods.[12] Data values are derived from many sources including the USDA Food Composition Laboratory and other government laboratories, the food industry, and university researchers. The USDA uses information from this databank to prepare tables on food composition for publication and for use with computers.

In Chapter 3, a description of the USDA Handbook No. 8, *Composition of Foods, Raw, Processed, Prepared* (revised series) was given.[13] This is the major printed source of USDA food composition data and includes information on over 60 different food components for more than 5200

BOX 5-2

Selected USDA Computerized Nutrition Databases

USDA nutrient database for standard reference

Updated versions are released periodically as new sections of the USDA *Handbook 8* are printed. Release 10 (1991) contains all the information from *Handbook 8–1* to *Handbook 8–21* plus additional imputed data where missing printed values occur.

USDA nutrient database for surveys of foods intakes by individuals

A nutrient database especially designed for nationwide government surveys (Continuing Survey of Food Intakes by Individuals, National Health and Nutrition Examination Survey). Complete data (no missing values) for energy and 28 food components for approximately 6500 food items. Three supporting computer files are included with this database, including (1) the Primary Nutrient Data Set for Food Consumption Surveys (includes all of the nutrient values), (2) the recipe file (designates recipe ingredients, their amounts, and any yield factors), and (3) a table of nutrient retention factors (for estimating recipe nutrient losses).

U.S. food supply

Contains data on the nutritional content of the U.S. food supply expressed on a per capita, per day basis for the years 1968 through 1988.

Provisional tables

Several separate files can be obtained on vitamin D, selenium, vitamin K, and sugar content of foods.

Adapted from data from Perloff BP. 1990. Analysis of dietary data. *American Journal of Clinical Nutrition* 501128–501132; and Perloff BP, et al. 1990. *Journal of Nutrition* 120:1530–1534.

food items.[9] The USDA Handbook 8 series has been organized into 21 food groups, each of which has been published separately beginning in 1976. The last two sections were released in 1991 (AH-8–19, *Snacks and Sweets*) and 1992 (AH-8–18, *Baked Products*). Future supplements from the USDA will be published on a regular basis to update Handbook 8 sections released earlier. For example, AH-8–13, *Beef Products,* was revised in 1990, and AH-8–10, *Pork Products,* was revised in 1992. Special supplements have been published on an annual basis since 1989. The USDA National Nutrient Databank will always be in a dynamic state, undergoing continual revision and improvement.

The USDA also publishes numerous **provisional tables** to complement the Handbook 8 series. The first provisional table was released in 1981 (nutrient content of bakery products and related items), and more than a dozen have been released since, giving valuable information on nutrient content of beverages and fast foods, dietary fiber, vitamin K, sugar, fatty acid, cholesterol, selenium, vitamin D, and amino acid content of selected foods.[9] (Tables of provisional values are available from USDA, Agricultural Research Service, Room 314, 4700 River Road, Riverdale, MD 20737).

Several different types of "machine-readable" or computerized data sets on food composition are maintained by the USDA. The major USDA computerized nutrition data sets are summarized in Box 5-2. The USDA Nutrient Database for Standard Reference (USDA NDB) is the computerized data set corresponding to the Handbook 8 series. Although the printed and computerized versions of the USDA database are nearly the same, the computerized versions contain additional and more current data and give imputed or estimated nutrient values where missing values appear in the printed form.[12]

Nationwide dietary surveys conducted within the federal government's National Nutrition Monitoring System use a nutrient database called the Nutrient Database for Surveys of Food Intakes by

Individuals (NDB-SFII), which was especially designed and maintained for this purpose by the Human Nutrition Information Service of the USDA.[14] Before NHANES III, 24-hour recalls were recorded on hard copy forms and manually coded by dietary interviewers. In 1986, the National Center for Health Statistics contracted with the University of Minnesota's Nutrition Coordinating Center to develop an automated, interactive dietary interview and coding system called the NHANES III Dietary Data Collection system, which uses the NDB-SFII. This database has values for energy and 28 food components for 6500 recipes and food items, with no missing values. A microcomputer version of the Survey Nutrient Database is available free through the Nutrient Databank Bulletin Board, which is sponsored by the USDA Nutrient Data Laboratory. It is operated as a public service to provide information about all current USDA publications and nutrient computer files. The information is presented in the form of bulletins that can be viewed directly or captured (saved) on a disk. Also available at no cost is the USDA's "Dietary Analysis Program," which contains 850 foods and 27 nutrients and food components and will analyze for up to 3 days of food intake.

To access the Nutrient Databank Bulletin Board, you need a computer, a modem, a telephone line, and communications software. The phone number is (301) 436–5635. You can call (301) 436–8491 for more information or contact Dr. David Haytowitz, Agricultural Research Service, USDA, 4700 River Road, Riverdale, MD 20737. As noted earlier in this chapter, the Nutrient Databank Bulletin Board is also available through the Internet (telnet info.umd.edu).

Developers of commercial computerized dietary analysis systems are faced with several challenges in formulating a high quality database.[15] The first challenge is to decide on how many foods and nutrients to include in the software program. Although the USDA has published values on more than 60 food components for over 5200 foods in the Handbook 8 series, few recipes and no name brand foods are included (except for ready-to-eat breakfast cereals and some types of candies). A surprising number of foods also have missing values for some nutrients. Although the USDA releases substantial amounts of new or updated information each year, the typical supermarket contains more than 20,000 brand name food products, and close to 13,000 new food items are introduced to consumers each year.[15] The best software vendors attempt to provide their customers with database updates at least once a year, and they use non-USDA sources to give information on certain brand name foods and to fill in missing data.

The total number of food items included in a database is important to ensure that substitution (choosing a similar food when the specific food is not in the database) is kept at a minimum. For example, if a patient in a cardiac rehabilitation program has given you a 3-day food record that includes several low-fat items not found in the database, you will have to make some less-than-ideal substitutions with other similar foods. However, more is not necessarily better.[2] As the database size increases, the difficulty in finding the right food and the processing time can increase. For some dietary analysis systems currently available (those with more than 10,000 foods and 50 nutrient components), the user may spend a lot of time waiting for the computer to search the database and process reports. The size of databases is sure to grow even more as computers improve in power and speed, and the user will be faced with the constant challenge of updating computer hardware to keep pace with software demands.

Some software packages report having more than 90 food components in their databases while others contain fewer than 30. Again, more is not necessarily better because values for certain trace minerals (e.g., chromium, selenium, molybdenum, manganese), amino acids, some fatty acids, and some vitamins (e.g., α-tocopherol, total tocopherol, vitamin D, vitamin K, biotin) are unknown for many foods.[2] Thus with an increasing number of food components, the software package developer has to cope with an expanding bank of missing values.[2] If missing data are entered as zero and not flagged (indicated by

BOX 5-3

Summary of Procedures to Impute Nutrient Values

1. Substitute one or more values from a similar or representative food (e.g., impute dietary fiber for pine nuts based on value for hickory nuts, which are similar in total carbohydrate content).
2. Calculate values from a different form of the same food based on moisture contents and/or retention factors (e.g., impute calcium for cooked horsemeat based on calcium in raw horsemeat using a retention factor [from the USDA] for calcium in roasted beef).
3. Calculate values for commercial products based on:
   a. a single major ingredient source of the missing nutrient(s) (e.g., impute fatty acids in split-pea soup based on the fatty acid profile of butter, which is the major type of fat in split-pea soup).
   b. estimation of ingredient amounts from product ingredient lists and nutrient profiles provided by manufacturers (e.g., missing nutrients in taco seasoning mix based on estimated amounts of each ingredient).
   c. a representative published recipe or product formula (e.g., missing nutrients in egg bagels calculated from a formula published in the scientific literature).

Adapted from Schakel SF, Sievert YA, Buzzard IM. 1988. Sources of data for developing and maintaining a nutrient database. *Journal of the American Dietetic Association* 88:1268–1271.

the software as missing), nutrient totals will appear lower than they actually are. During counseling sessions with patients or clients, some confusion can develop because for many of these nutrients, low values represent a "database deficiency," not a deficiency in the diet of the patient. The best software packages will give information on how many missing values are present for each nutrient or warn the dietitian or user about the issue.

One way to judge the quality of a computerized diet analysis system is to determine how the developer met the challenge of missing data in the management of their database. Some developers go to unusual lengths to ensure that missing values are substituted with either non-USDA data or imputed values. Many food companies provide information on the nutrient content of their products on request, but usually only for a small number of nutrients. Data on the composition of foods are frequently published in the scientific literature, with several journals (e.g., the *Journal of Food Science* and the *Journal of Food Composition*) specializing in reporting food composition data. Following published criteria, the nutrient content of mixed dishes and recipes can be estimated.[12] Calculations are also frequently used to impute values using data for another form of food or for a similar food.[5,16] (See Box 5-3 for procedures to impute nutrient values). Replacing missing values with imputed values is not an easy process and is especially difficult when only limited information exists for a certain nutrient (e.g., trace minerals). The process requires nutritionists with expertise in data evaluation and is a technique that is still evolving.

Other important measures for judging the vendor's quality are the strength of their service policy, the number of years the vendor and the software have been in business, the frequency with which their nutrient database is updated, the credentials of the database developers, and the cost of upgrades.

In summary, the content quality of nutrient databases from different software vendors may vary widely depending on the number of food items and nutrients included, whether or not the most recent USDA releases have been incorporated, and the degree to which non-USDA sources (food industry, scientific literature) or estimating calculations are used to fill in the missing values. Three questions to ask when evaluating a nutrient database for personal or professional use include[5] (1) Does the database contain all of the foods and nutrients of interest? (2) Is the database complete for the nutrients of interest? (3) Is the nutrient database kept up to date with the changing marketplace and the availability of new nutrient data?

Program Operation

General operating features of the computerized diet analysis system are extremely important, determining whether or not a software package is easy to use while generating the desired information.[2,3,12]

Important operating features include computer hardware requirements, cost of the software package, quality of help screens and user's manual, methods of searching for and entering foods to be analyzed (food codes, food names, and/or food groups), ability to preview single food nutrients while entering foods, ability to assign a variety of volume or weight measures for each food item, ease of editing the food list, food entry number limit, ease of averaging multiple days of dietary input, ability to compare results with a variety of dietary standards, and the quality and variety of printed reports. The ability to modify the database (adding new foods, deleting old ones, or altering the nutrient values) is another important concern. Another option that is meaningful for some nutritionists is the ability to enter dietary data from either the standard diet record approach or from a food frequency list.

Most of the modern computerized diet analysis systems have been developed for IBM or compatible personal computers, although several vendors also offer Macintosh versions.[17–26] The amount of conventional RAM (random access memory), required hard disk space, type of central process unit (CPU), and MS-DOS versions vary widely between software systems, and the user must carefully compare software requirements with hardware capabilities. Computer novices should seek the help of a local computer specialist before buying a diet analysis software program. Software package prices typically range from $200 to $600 for programs used by nutrition professionals and researchers. However, some research-based systems can cost much more than this.

Several of the best computerized diet analysis systems come with help screens that users can "pop up" during any segment of program operation (in other words, "context sensitive"). All software packages come with user's manuals, although the quality of these can vary widely. While many of the early computerized diet analysis systems were rather difficult to use, more recent versions tend to be user friendly. A user-friendly software package can usually be operated without use of the manual because the various menus and help-screens are simple to use and self-explanatory.

The method for searching and entering foods to be analyzed by the microcomputer is one of the most important program operation features. Most software programs allow users to search and enter foods by either full name, partial name, or code numbers.[7] However, diet analysis systems have different ways of accomplishing this task, with some requiring more effort and keystrokes than others. For example, some programs require the user to first choose a food group before selecting the specific food, a step that can slow down the food entry process. Users tend to prefer searching for the appropriate foods using food names rather than code numbers (which requires use of a food code manual) or food groups. Most of the best programs have near-instantaneous listing of foods after the user enters the food name. Some programs have a search capability that allows the user to find the food quickly and directly using only a few appropriate keystrokes (e.g., the first few letters of each word of the food description in any order).

While searching the database for the appropriate food from a patient or client diet record, substitutions (using a food that is as similar as possible) often have to be made, even with databases containing more than 5000 food items. Finding appropriate substitutes is much easier when the user is allowed to preview the nutrient breakdown of a certain food. Most of the top quality programs provide a "pop-up" window during food search and entry, summarizing the nutrient components for the specific amount of the food chosen.

Once the appropriate food has been located in the database, the user must assign a volume or weight measure for each food item. In comparison to earlier software programs, many modern diet analysis programs now allow users to assign a wide variety of such measures in an easy and accurate manner.

Often there is the need to edit the food list either during or following food search and entry. Ease of editing the food list is an important feature to evaluate when deciding on a software program. The best programs allow users to easily delete or insert foods, or allow the volume or weight measure to be changed with little additional effort.

Some of the earlier computerized diet analysis systems set low limits on the number of foods the user could enter before analysis. Although this wasn't a problem if only a 1-day food record was being analyzed, multiple-day food record analysis proved to be quite cumbersome, requiring multiple savings as separate meals and/or days before averaging. Many systems allow users to enter 200 or more food items, making it much easier to analyze multiple-day food records. For example, a typical 7-day food record may have 150 food items. All of these items can be entered into one list (without having to save each day separately), with nutrient values automatically divided by seven after designating this number as the divisor.

Software packages often include a wide variety of dietary standards against which individual nutrient intake can be compared. These dietary standards typically include both the U.S. Recommended Dietary Allowances (RDA) and the Canadian Recommended Nutrient Intakes (RNI). Additionally, many programs include "prudent diet" recommendations from the American Heart Association, the National Cancer Institute, the National Academy of Sciences, or the USDA. Often the user has the option to include automatic default or individualized values for both RDA and "prudent diet" recommendations, allowing tables and graphs to look complete and professional.

As stated previously, food composition data are continually being updated. Users need to ensure that they are using the most current data available and that their systems are operating accurately.[13] There are times when a user may want to add foods, delete old ones, or add nutrients to the database. Nearly all dietary analysis systems allow users to modify the database in this fashion.

As discussed in Chapter 3, there are both strengths and limitations in using dietary recall, dietary record, and food frequency nutrition assessment techniques. An important feature that is being included with some computerized dietary analysis systems is the option to enter foods by either the standard diet record approach (specific quantities of foods unique to each patient) or from a food frequency list. In the latter option, the number of specified portions of listed foods are entered according to frequency of use (per day, week, or month). The National Cancer Institute has developed dietary analysis software for the Health Habits and History Questionnaire. The dietary component consists of a quantitative food frequency questionnaire and associated food behavior questions from which estimates of 33 nutrients and up to 20 user-defined food groups can be produced. To request a copy of the software and accompanying documentation, send two formatted high-density 3.5-inch diskettes and a one- to three-sentence description of the study in which it is to be used to: Anne Hartman, Applied Research Branch, Division of Cancer Prevention and Control, National Cancer Institute, EPN Rm. 313, 9000 Rockville Pike, Bethesda, MD 20892.

System Output

Once the data have been entered into the computerized dietary analysis system, two important features are the software program's ability (1) to print out a variety of reports and (2) to export data to electronic files for further analysis.

Most software packages allow users to preview the output in both tabular and graphic form on the monitor before storage on a disk and/or printing. A variety of output formats are desirable to present the nutrient analysis data, including graphic and tabular comparisons with the RDA, RNI, or other nutrient standards, and a spreadsheet table that outlines the nutrient values for each food in the analysis. While some software programs print a spreadsheet table with all of the nutrients for each food after one or two keystrokes, others will print only two to five nutrients for each food at a time, requiring the user to print out a series of repeated reports.

A few computerized dietary analysis systems have unique features that greatly improve the value of printed information. As previously described in this chapter, very few nutrient databases have no missing values. To aid in the interpretation of results, some software programs list missing nutrient values. For example, if a nutritionist is analyzing a 3-day food record with 70 foods, the number of missing values for zinc, vitamin E, copper, and so on are listed separately beside each nutrient. Some software packages allow users to sort and print the analyzed diet for nutrients that may be of concern. For example, if a patient's diet is low in iron, the iron values for each food within the diet can be printed in descending order, allowing the nutritionist to make individualized recommendations. A few software packages also allow personal messages from the nutritionist to the client or patient to be included with each printed report through use of a text editor. Another feature that is extremely useful is the automatic calculation of food exchanges contained within the analyzed diet. This allows the nutritionist to counsel the client or patient about potential deficiencies from a food group perspective. The scope, content, and presentation of the information generated varies greatly from one program to another, and users should ensure that printouts are appropriate, meaningful, and useful for specific needs.[7]

Another system output feature that is useful to some nutritionists and most researchers is the ability of the software package to export the nutrient data to electronic files in a format that is useful for further statistical analysis. For example, if a researcher is analyzing the 7-day food records of 100 cancer patients, being able to electronically transport the nutrient summaries of each individual patient to a spreadsheet software program before performing a statistical analysis can save a tremendous amount of effort. The export file format most useful for this type of data transfer is called ASCII (American Standard Code for Information Interchange).

A COMPARISON OF EIGHT MICROCOMPUTER DIETARY ANALYSIS SYSTEMS

Although several nutrition periodicals and journals regularly review general features of microcomputer dietary analysis systems (e.g., *Nutrition Today, Journal of Nutrition Education, Food & Nutrition News,* and the *Journal of the American Dietetic Association*), very few comparative analyses have been published.[22,23,27–34] In general, the few reports in the literature demonstrate that use of different computerized dietary analysis systems may yield widely discrepant results.

Several problems exist, however, in generalizing these findings to the use of microcomputer dietary analysis systems that are now available to nutrition professionals. Most of these published reports either didn't identify the dietary analysis systems they used in their comparison,[30,32,34] or they used systems that are not readily available for use by dietitians on their own microcomputers.[28,29,31,33] Of those microcomputer dietary analysis systems identified, most are either outdated or no longer available. The focus of most of these reports has been to report variation between dietary analysis systems instead of using some standard as a guide to interpretation of results. Usually, only a limited number of nutrients were compared between systems, and more information is now needed because of the much larger databases that are currently available. Most vendors of computerized dietary analysis systems are constantly improving and expanding their programs. Because of the dynamic state of these software programs, periodic evaluations are necessary.

Annual nutrient database conferences have been held since 1976 to address issues that surround the development and use of computerized dietary analysis systems.[8,30] Participants at these conferences review data quality and analytical techniques, discuss methodologic issues concerned with dietary data collection and computers, and describe numerous applications for nutrient databases.[9] As noted earlier in this chapter, a *Nutrient Data Bank Directory* was compiled in 1980 and has been updated periodically to facilitate communication between developers and users of nutrient database systems.[8] Despite these efforts, there is still virtually no coordination between vendors, and dietitians are left with the task and responsibility of choosing among a bewildering array of systems.

Although development of most nutrient databases begins with data from the USDA, analysis of a standard food record or menu may still lead to substantial variation between dietary analysis systems because of several potential problems.* As discussed earlier in this chapter, variance can occur because of differences in the number of food items included in the database (leading to varying degrees of substitution), the recency of the nutrient data (whether or not the most recent USDA releases have been incorporated), and the number of missing values (the degree to which non-USDA sources or estimating calculations are used to fill in the blanks from the USDA). Other potential problems may include software program errors (incorrect adjustment of nutrients to specific portion sizes or random data entry error) or variation in yield or retention factors for calculating recipes.[36]

To enhance your understanding of microcomputer dietary analysis systems, we decided to compare the general features and nutrient data output of eight programs. The discussion that follows is written in a similar format to what you would find in a research journal. We hope this will allow each reader to compare dietary analysis systems from a scientific viewpoint and perhaps provide motivation for some of you to conduct similar research in the future.

*References 5,13,22,23,29,33,35

Each of the microcomputer systems met several selection criteria as follows: (1) the system must have a nutrient database of more than 5000 foods and 20 food components, (2) it must be readily available and marketed nationwide, and (3) the vendor must be willing to cooperate in the research project. In particular, dietary analysis systems were chosen that had been reviewed recently in professional journals or periodicals,[17–26] and/or had carried advertisements in the *Journal of the American Dietetic Association*. The eight systems chosen were (1) Diet Balancer for Windows, version 1.0; (2) DietMax Plus for Windows; (3) Food Processor Plus, version 6.0; (4) Counseling Nutrition Data System, version 2.6; (5) Nutrient Analysis System 2 Plus 8, version 1.0; (6) Nutritionist IV, version 3.5 (both DOS and Windows); (7) Nutritional Software Library IV; and (8) Food/Analyst Plus, CD-ROM version.*

How the Comparison Was Conducted

We prepared a 3-day food record with 73 basic food items similar to the record used in a previous study.[22] Foods were selected to create a diet that

*Diet Balancer for Windows from Nutridata Software Corporation, 1215 Route 9, Suite F, P.O. Box 769, Wappingers Falls, NY 12590; DietMax Plus for Windows from Positive Solutions, Inc., P.O. Box 267, Three Rivers, MI 49093; Food Processor Plus from ESHA Research, P.O. Box 13028, Salem, OR 97309; Counseling Nutrition Data System from the Nutrition Coordinating Center, University of Minnesota, Suite 300, 1300 South Second Street, Minneapolis, MN 55454–1015; Nutrient Analysis System 2 Plus 8 from DDA Software, P.O. Box 477, Long Valley, NJ 07853; Nutritionist IV from N-Squared Computing, First DataBank Division, The Hearst Corporation, 1111 Bayhill Dr., Suite 270, San Bruno, CA 94066; Nutritional Software Library IV from Computrition, 9121 Oakdale Avenue, Suite 201, Chatsworth, CA 91311; and Food/Analyst Plus from Hopkins Technology, 421 Hazel Lane, Hopkins, MN 55343–7116.

conformed to Step 2 guidelines published by the National Cholesterol Education Program (total fat less than 30% of calories, saturated fat less than 7% of calories, and dietary cholesterol less than 200 mg/day).[37] Foods were selected if they had a separate code number in the USDA Nutrient Database for Standard Reference, full version, release 10 (for microcomputers) (National Technical Information Service, 5285 Port Royal Road, Springfield, VA 22161). Brand-name foods and combination dishes were not included in our 3-day menu because these are not represented in the USDA NDB or incorporated in some of the microcomputer dietary analysis systems. Our purpose was to compare the nutrient output of eight dietary analysis systems with the USDA NDB, without confounding from a high degree of food item substitutions. The volume amount and specific gram weight of each food item are listed in Table 5-1.

General operating features of the eight selected microcomputer dietary analysis systems were summarized using information from the user's manual provided with each system and data collected during use of the software (see Table 5-2). In addition, each vendor was allowed to review the tables to confirm the accuracy of the information given for their system.

We entered foods from the 3-day food record, using the specific gram weight of each food item (except for Diet Balancer for Windows and DietMax Plus, which required volume measures for many foods). When the exact food was not available in a certain database system, the closest substitution was made using the preview option. Following food entry and a review of other specific attributes of each system, the operating features of each system were graded using a four-level grade system (excellent, good, fair, poor) (Table 5-3). Grades were assigned by comparing the eight systems with one another, with a grade of "excellent" given, for example, to those that best accomplished the task in our collective judgment. Microcomputers with a 486/33 MHz CPU and 8 MB RAM were used to test each of the dietary analysis systems.

Some 3-day nutrient summaries were printed and results tabled (Table 5-4). The nutrient data were compared with the USDA Nutrient Database for Standard Reference, full version, release 10. All of the nutrients listed in the USDA NDB were used, except for most of the fatty acids and amino acids (for which several representative components were selected). Percent differences were calculated by using the following formula:

$$\frac{\text{microcomputer value} - \text{USDA NDB value}}{\text{USDA NDB value}} \times 100$$

In that the USDA NDB is not being used as a "gold standard" in this study, but rather a point of reference, the presence of an asterisk is not meant to imply that there is necessarily something dissatisfactory about the microcomputer database. Instead, the asterisk is being used to draw attention to a nutrient summary value that may be higher or lower than the USDA NDB, followed by an appropriate discussion of these variances to help dietitians better understand the issues that are involved. Percent differences greater than 15% are noted with an asterisk in Table 5-4.

All of the nutrient values for each food from the USDA NDB and the individual dietary analysis systems were put into a spreadsheet format. The percent of missing values for each program was determined by counting the number of missing data for all nutrients listed in Table 5-4 for a particular program and dividing by the total number of potential data points (73 foods times the number of nutrients listed in Table 5-4 for the program). A dietary analysis system was not penalized for nutrients not present in its listing. For example, if a program did not include all of the 37 nutrients evaluated in this report (e.g., the five amino acids), the percent missing values was calculated by multiplying 73 × 32 and dividing this into the number of missing values and then multiplying by 100. The quality of the nutrient database was given an overall rating, and this was based on four factors: the total number of foods, the total number of nutrients, the percent of missing values, and the relative use of non-USDA and brand-name foods.

Text continued on p. 209

TABLE 5-1 Description of a 3-day menu using food items from the USDA Nutrient Database for Standard Reference (release 10) (USDA NDB).

USDA NDB Code # and Food Description		Volume	Weight (g)
Day 1	**Breakfast**		
09116	Grapefruit; raw, white, all areas	0.5 item	118
18290	Pancakes; plain, dry mix, complete, prepared	3 items	108
04130	Margarine; soft, unspecified oils, salt added	2 tsp	9.40
09019	Applesauce; canned, unsweetened	1 cup	244
02010	Spice; cinnamon, ground	0.25 tsp	0.58
01082	Milk; cow, lowfat, fluid, 1% fat	0.5 cup	122
14209	Coffee; brewed, prepared with tap water	8 fl oz	237
Day 1	**Lunch**		
15121	Fish/shellfish; tuna, canned, drained solids, light meat, canned in water	2 oz	56.7
18075	Bread; whole wheat, commercially prepared	2 slices	50.0
11252	Lettuce; iceberg, raw, leaf	1 piece	20.0
04025	Salad dressing; mayonnaise, soybean oil, with salt	2 tsp	9.20
11124	Carrots; raw	1 item	72.0
09003	Apple; raw, with skin	1 item	138
06463	Soup; tomato rice, with water	1 cup	247
18228	Crackers; saltines	6 items	16.5
09135	Grape juice; canned/bottled, unsweetened	0.75 cup	190
Day 1	**Dinner**		
13364	Beef; composite of trimmed retailed cuts, all grades, separated lean, cooked, 0 inches fat	3 oz	85.0
11363	Potato; baked, flesh, without salt	1 item	156
11093	Broccoli; frozen, chopped, boiled, drained, without salt	1 cup	184
11168	Corn; sweet, yellow, boiled, drained, without salt, kernels from one ear	1 item	77.0
04130	Margarine; soft, unspecified oils, salt added	3 tsp	14.1
09236	Peaches; raw	2 items	174
01082	Milk; cow, lowfat, fluid, 1% fat	1 cup	244
Day 2	**Breakfast**		
01121	Yogurt; fruit-flavored, lowfat	1 cup	227
18258	English muffin; plain, enriched, with calcium	1 item	57.0
09200	Orange; raw, all varieties	1 item	131
04130	Margarine; soft, unspecified oils, salt added	2 tsp	9.40
14209	Coffee; brewed, prepared with tap water	8 fl oz	237
Day 2	**Lunch**		
11455	Sauce; spaghetti, canned	0.75 cup	187
20121	Spaghetti; enriched, cooked, no sodium	1 cup	130
11252	Lettuce; iceberg, raw	1.5 cup	82.5
11529	Tomato; red, ripe, raw	0.5 item	61.5
11124	Carrots; raw, shredded	0.25 cup	27.5
11205	Cucumber; not pared, raw, sliced	0.25 cup	26.0
04021	Salad dressing; Italian, diet, with salt	2 tbsp	30.0
12036	Seeds; sunflower seed kernals, dried	1 tbsp	9.00

TABLE 5-1 Description of a 3-day menu using food items from the USDA Nutrient Database for Standard Reference (release 10) (USDA NDB)—cont'd

USDA NDB Code # and Food Description		Volume	Weight (g)
Day 2	**Lunch—cont'd**		
18030	Bread; French or Vienna, toasted	1.5 slices	35.0
04130	Margarine; soft, unspecified oils, salt added	1 tsp	4.70
02020	Spice; garlic powder	0.12 tsp	0.33
09132	Grapes; European type (adherent skin)	1 serving	160
14355	Tea; brewed	1 cup	237
Day 2	**Dinner**		
05064	Chicken; breast, meat only, roasted	3 oz	85.0
20037	Rice; brown, long, cooked, without salt	0.75 cup	146
11125	Carrots; boiled, drained, without salt	1 cup	156
18342	Roll; dinner, plain, commercially prepared	1 item	26.0
04130	Margarine; soft, unspecified oils, salt added	2 tsp	9.40
01082	Milk: cow, lowfat, fluid, 1% fat	1 cup	244
09316	Strawberries; raw	1 cup	146
18088	Cake; angelfood, dry mix, prepared	1 slice	53.0
Day 3	**Breakfast**		
08147	Cereals ready-to-eat; wheat, shredded, large biscuits	2 items	47.2
92290	Sugars; brown, pressed down	2 tsp	9.17
18076	Bread; whole wheat, commercially prepared, toasted	2 slices	42.0
09040	Banana; raw, without skin	1 item	114
12692	Nuts; peanut butter, with salt added	4 tsp	21.3
01082	Milk: cow, lowfat, fluid, 1% fat	1 cup	244
14209	Coffee; brewed, prepared with tap water	8 fl oz	237
Day 3	**Lunch**		
05186	Turkey; light, no skin, roasted	2 oz	56.7
01028	Cheese; natural, mozzarella, part skim	1 oz	28.4
18075	Bread; whole wheat, commercially prepared	2 slices	50.0
04025	Salad dressing; mayonnaise, soybean oil, with salt	2 tsp	9.20
11090	Broccoli; raw, chopped	0.5 cup	44.0
11135	Cauliflower; raw, one-inch pieces	0.5 cup	50.0
04023	Salad dressing; thousand island, diet, low calorie, with salt	2 tbsp	30.6
09252	Pears; raw	1 item	166
18184	Cookies; oatmeal, prepared from recipe, with raisins	3 items	39.0
14416	Carbonated beverage; low calorie, cola, with aspartame	1.5 cups	355
Day 3	**Dinner**		
10153	Pork products; cured, ham, whole, separated lean only, roasted	3 oz	85.0
11508	Sweet potato; baked, flesh only	1 item	114
11053	Beans; snap, green variety, boiled, drained, without salt	1 cup	125
04130	Margarine; soft, unspecified oils, salt added	2 tsp	9.40
09016	Apple juice; canned/bottled, unsweetened, without added ascorbic acid	1 cup	248
09181	Melons; cantaloupe, raw, cubed	1 cup	160
01065	Ice milk; vanilla, soft serve	0.5 cup	87.5

TABLE 5-2 General features of 8 selected microcomputer dietary analysis systems for collection and analysis of dietary data

Name of program	Diet Balancer for Windows	DietMax Plus for Windows	Food Processor Plus	Counseling Nutrition Data System	Nutrient Analysis System 2 Plus 8	Nutritionist IV	Nutritional Software Library IV	Food/Analyst Plus
Company	Nutridata Software Corporation	Positive Solutions Incorporated	ESHA Research	Nutrition Coordinating Center	DDA Software	N-Squared Computing	Computrition Incorporated	Hopkins Technology
Version analyzed	Windows	Windows	Version 6.0	Version 2.6	Version 1.0	Version 3.5		CD-ROM
List price (1994)	$50	$595	$495	$595	$290	$495	$495	$199
No. of other IBM programs	2	3	4	2	1	6	4	3
Year of first PC version	1988	1993	1984	1988	1982	1982	1986	1989
Computer requirements								
Hard drive space	3.0 MB	15 MB	6 MB	16.1 MB	3.2 MB	4.7 MB	5.5 MB	User files only
Memory (RAM)	4 MB	8 MB	2 MB	530K	512K	640K	640K	512K
Macintosh version?	Yes	No	Yes	No	Yes	Yes	No	No
No. of foods in database	5000	7100	>12,000	>23,000	8000	>12,000	>18,000	22,500
No. of nutrient components	26	54	94	32	79	75	24	84
proximates	6	9	12	9	11	8	5	10
vitamins	10	12	16	11	12	15	8	12
minerals	6	9	16	8	9	14	6	9
amino acids	0	18	18	0	18	18	0	18
fatty acids	4	6	29	4	29	9	4	24
sugars	0	0	3	0	0	7	1	11
ratios/percents/indexes	4	12	18	9	4	13	8	6
Data base sources								
USDA/Handbook #8	8–1 to 8–21	NDB Rel. #10	NDB Rel. #10	NDB Rel. #10	NDB Rel. #10	NDB Rel. #10	8–1 to 8–21	NDB Rel. #10
USDA Survey DATA	No	No	Yes	Yes	No	Yes	No	Yes
Canadian Nutrient Files	No	No	Available	No	No	Yes	Yes	Yes
Include brand-name foods	Yes	Yes	Yes	Yes	Yes	Yes	Yes	Yes
Imputed data	No	No	Extensive	Extensive	No	Extensive	No	No

TABLE 5-2 General features of 8 selected microcomputer dietary analysis systems for collection and analysis of dietary data—cont'd

Name of program	Diet Balancer for Windows	DietMax Plus for Windows	Food Processor Plus	Counseling Nutrition Data System	Nutrient Analysis System 2 Plus 8	Nutritionist IV	Nutritional Software Library IV	Food/Analyst Plus
Company	Nutridata Software Corporation	Positive Solutions Incorporated	ESHA Research	Nutrition Coordinating Center	DDA Software	N-Squared Computing	Computrition Incorporated	Hopkins Technology
Version analyzed	Windows	Windows	Version 6.0	Version 2.6	Version 1.0	Version 3.5		CD-ROM
Frequency of updates	1/yr	1/yr	1–2/yr	2/yr	½ yrs	2/yr	1/yr	⅓ yrs
Food search options								
Name search	No	No	Yes	Yes	Yes	Yes	Yes	Yes
Code search	No	No	Yes	No	Yes	Yes	No	No
Preview nutrients	Yes	Yes	Yes	No	Yes	Yes	Yes	No
Food entry no. limit	No limit	No limit	No limit	c. 200	40	No limit	No limit	20/meal
Modifiable database	Yes	Yes	Yes	No	Yes	Yes	Yes	Yes
Physical activity option	Yes	Yes	Yes	No	Yes	Yes	No	No
Food frequency option	No	No	No	Yes	No	Yes	No	No
Print/export options								
Graph RDA comparison	Yes	No	Yes	Yes	Yes	Yes	Yes	Yes
Print spreadsheet	Yes	No	Yes	Yes, 5/run	Yes	Yes	Yes, 20/run	Yes (one meal)
Single nutrient sort	Yes	No	Yes	Yes	Yes	Yes	Yes	Yes
Diabetic exchanges	No	Yes	Yes	No	No	Yes	No	No
Edit reports (text editor)	No	Yes	Yes	No	Yes	Yes	No	No
Export as ASCII file	No	No	Yes	No	Yes	Yes	Yes	Yes

TABLE 5-3 Rating of program operating features.* Based on data entry of 3-day menu (from Table 5-1).

Name of program	Diet Balancer	DietMax Plus	Food Processor Plus	Counseling Nutrition Data System	Nutrient Analysis System 2 Plus 8	Nutritionist IV	Nutritional Software Library IV	Food/ Analyst Plus
Version analyzed	Windows	Windows	Version 6.0	Version 2.6	Version 1.0	Version 3.5		CD-Rom
Quality of user's manual	G	E	E	E	G	E	E	G
Quality of help screens	E	E	E	G	G	G	G	E
Ease of food entry and search, previewing	G	P	E	G	F	G	G	G
Ease of editing food list	E	G	E	E	G	G	F	E
Utility of saving and averaging 3 days	G	E	E	F	P	E	E	E
Ease and quality of RDA comparison	E	G	E	E	E	E	E	E
Overall speed in entering foods, analyzing, and printing results	G	P	E	F	F	P	G	E
Quality and number of nutrient analysis options/printed reports	G	E	E	G	F	E	G	G
Overall ease of learning and using	G	P	E	F	F	G	F	E
Overall rating (based on process of entering/analyzing the 3-day food record)	G	F	E	G	F	G	G	E

E = excellent; G = good; F = fair, P = poor; NA not available with program

*Evaluation based on average grading conducted by three researchers.

TABLE 5-4 Average daily nutrient totals for a 3-day food record (from table 5-1) for eight selected microcomputer dietary analysis systems in comparison with the USDA Nutrient Database for Standard Reference (release 10).

Name of program	Diet Balancer	DietMax Plus	Food Processor Plus	Counseling Nutrition Data System	Nutrient Analysis System 2 Plus 8	Nutritionist IV	Nutritional Software Library IV	Food/Analyst Plus	USDA NDB
Version analyzed	Windows	Windows	Version 6.0	Version 2.6	Version 1.0	Version 3.5		CD-ROM	Release #10
Proximates									
Energy (kcal)	1977	2238	1979	1980	1976	1996	1972	2011	1984
Protein (g)	79.6	85.6	83.7	83.8	85.8	85.4	84.0	85.4	84.5
Total fat (g)	55.9	76.1*	54.1	52.9	53.0	56.2	52.3	55.4	53.7
Total carbohydrate (g)	304	319	306	309	305	303	305	309	307
Dietary fiber (g)	26.3	22.9*	29.3	30.1	30.8	24.4*	28.7	12.1*	30.7
Caffeine (mg)	174	170	170	170	170	172	—	170	170
Minerals									
Calcium (mg)	981	1072	998	974	1034	1022	1042	1018	999
Iron (mg)	12.7	19.7*	12.6	13.4	12.5	12.7	12.6	13.0	12.7
Magnesium (mg)	373	364	396	396	401	400	—	334*	397
Phosphorus (mg)	—	1350	1542	1412	1570	1534	1538	1497	1542
Potassium (mg)	4214	3834	4227	4266	4259	4216	4178	4229	4214
Sodium (mg)	3113	4128*	2756	3177	2844	2769	2799	2672	2822
Zinc (mg)	9.3	9.84	10.0	10.9	10.8	10.7	9.7	9.1	10.6
Copper (mg)	—	1.75	1.65	1.71	1.65	1.71	—	1.37*	1.65
Manganese (mg)	—	5.82	5.60	—	5.54	5.43	—	4.09*	5.62
Vitamins									
Ascorbic acid (mg)	212	226	200	219	212	200	210	204	200
Thiamin (mg)	2.22*	1.91	1.77	1.89	1.76	1.75	1.59	1.68	1.75
Riboflavin (mg)	2.12	2.42*	2.00	2.07	2.05	2.12	1.92	2.03	2.01
Niacin (mg)	25.4	25.9	25.6	25.4	25.3	25.0	24.1	24.4	25.2
Pantothenic acid (mg)	—	5.74	6.17	—	6.25	6.00	—	5.61	6.15
Vitamin B_6 (mg)	2.44	2.49	2.55	2.39	2.54	2.44	2.31	2.42	2.53
Folacin (μg)	298	346	305	291	310	294	247*	268	304
Vitamin B_{12} (μg)	3.25	4.17*	3.63	3.32	3.57	3.48	3.29	3.30	3.59
Total vitamin A (μg RE)	4108	3700	3998	3506	4106	4005	3993	3983	3999
Vitamin E-total tocopherol (mg)	25.5*	3.19*	13.1†	15.1	23.1*	—	15.7	16.0	
Vitamin E-α-tocopherol (mg)	—	—	—	—	2.99	11.0*	—	3.59	3.48

Continued

TABLE 5-4 Average daily nutrient totals for a 3-day food record (from table 5-1) for eight selected microcomputer dietary analysis systems in comparison with the USDA Nutrient Database for Standard Reference (release 10)—cont'd

Name of program	Diet Balancer	DietMax Plus	Food Processor Plus	Counseling Nutrition Data System	Nutrient Analysis System 2 Plus 8	Nutritionist IV	Nutritional Software Library IV	Food/Analyst Plus	USDA NDB
Version analyzed	Windows	Windows	Version 6.0	Version 2.6	Version 1.0	Version 3.5		CD-ROM	Release #10
Lipids									
Total SFA (g)	13.6	21.3*	13.1	14.5	13.2	13.4	8.83*	14.3	12.8
Total MFA (g)	18.8	25.4*	19.4	19.0	18.1	19.1	9.79*	16.3	18.3
Oleic FA (g)	—	23.3*	18.7	—	17.5	22.1*	—	18.8	17.7
Total PFA (g)	17.0	23.2*	17.2	14.7*	16.8	18.8	7.66*	15.7	17.6
Linoleic FA (g)	—	20.3*	15.6	—	15.4	17.2	—	15.6	16.1
Cholesterol (mg)	162*	152*	116	113	123	142*	121	126	122
Amino Acids									
Isoleucine (g)	—	3.35	3.79	—	3.88	3.88	—	3.42	3.82
Leucine (g)	—	5.67	6.34	—	6.49	6.48	—	5.68	6.40
Lysine (g)	—	4.96	5.55	—	5.68	5.68	—	5.31	5.60
Tryptophan (g)	—	0.86	0.97	—	0.97	0.99	—	0.84	0.97
Valine (g)	—	3.87	4.28	—	4.37	4.37	—	3.83	4.30
% Missing values ‡	0%	9.4%	0.3%	0%	7.9%	5.6%	7.9%	15.1%	7.9%
Overall rating of quality of database	G	F	E	E	G	E	G	G	

* More than 15% variance from USDA NDB (release 10)

† Vitamin E calculated as total α-tocopherol equivalents, instead of total tocopherol (USDA method).

‡ Based on analysis of 73 food items in 3-day food record in Table 5–1 and the number of missing values for each nutrient listed for each software package in this table.

E = excellent; G = good, F = fair; P = poor.

How the Systems Compare

Tables 5-2 and 5-3 summarize the general features of each microcomputer dietary analysis system, and Table 5-4 compares the nutrient output of each system with the USDA NDB. The eight software programs varied widely in cost ($50 to $595), number of foods (5000 to 23,000) and nutrient components in the database (24 to 94), use of non-USDA data and imputation of data for missing values, and the number of print/export options. As summarized in Table 5-3, the two operating features with the lowest grades among the eight systems were "overall speed" and "overall ease of learning and using," while features in which most of the programs did very well included "ease and quality of RDA comparison" and "quality of user's manual." Some of the programs took an inordinate amount of time to search for foods in the database or process reports.

In common with other reports,[23,29,33,30] we determined that despite the fact that the USDA database was the primary source of information for each of the dietary analysis systems we evaluated, substantial variation resulted when 73 foods from a 3-day food record were entered and analyzed by each program. One of the problems we encountered was that although most programs used the USDA NDB release 10, some foods were either deleted or the name changed enough to make finding the exact food difficult, forcing us to make food substitutions. Also, some systems did not allow us to enter specific gram amounts or even exact volume measurements, further contributing to error and variation from the USDA NDB standard.

In general, the dietary analysis systems tended to be similar to the USDA NDB for energy, protein, total fat, and total carbohydrates. For other nutrients, however, the number varying more than 15% from the USDA NDB varied considerably between programs. The food components from the eight dietary analysis systems that were most likely to vary from the USDA NDB included total tocopherols and α-tocopherols, dietary fiber, the various fatty acids, and cholesterol. Nutrients most likely to be absent from the databases of the eight systems included total tocopherols and α-tocopherols, manganese, the various amino acids and fatty acids, pantothenic acid, copper, magnesium, and caffeine.

A summary discussion of each system based on Tables 5-2 to 5-4 follows.

Diet Balancer for Windows

The Diet Balancer for Windows includes about 5000 foods and analyzes them for 26 nutrient components, for a low cost of just $50.

Foods are selected through food groups and lists, but this process is still quite straightforward because of the compact, attractive working screen. The user does have to go through a number of mouse and keystroke options, however, to search for and then select the food and portions size, which could be streamlined to make the process a bit quicker in future versions. For some of the larger food groups, the user has to wait longer than expected for the food list to appear on the screen, further slowing down the food search process.

Energy (or a nutrient of choice) is listed instantly after every food entry, and editing and nutrient sorting are easy. Unfortunately, specific gram amounts cannot be entered for all foods, but several other portion size options are usually available for each food (although they are not easy to select because of unnecessary use of the mouse). The Windows version is based primarily on USDA Handbook #8–1 to 8–21 and a relatively large number of brand name foods. Three nutrients (thiamin, vitamin E, and cholesterol) varied more than 15% from the USDA NDB standard, and this was probably due to food substitutions and imprecise portion size selection. Three-day averaging is basic and quite easy, a spreadsheet of the nutrient information can be viewed on the screen before printing, and an attractive graph with RDA comparison can also be viewed and then printed. For the price, the Diet Balancer for Windows is a great buy, and is a pleasure to use, with an attractive screen design.

DietMax Plus for Windows

DietMax Plus for Windows is a relatively new dietary analysis system and was developed for dietitians and other health professionals who analyze food intakes of patients or clients or who design recipes and institutional menu cycles.

DietMax Plus is a large and complicated program and is one of the few dietary analysis systems that currently runs on Windows. As a result, the program runs most effectively on a 486/33 MHz CPU (or faster) computer with 8 MB RAM. About 15 MB of hard drive space is required up front, with each large menu or diet requiring 1 to 3 MB more, and about 2 MB more needed on a temporary basis while running. The database includes about 7100 foods from many sources including the USDA, fast food outlets, and commercial name brands and analyzes them for 54 nutrient components. Feeling that "it makes no sense to place foods of all types into a single, large database," DietMax developers separated the database into base foods (for recipes), recipes, or meal items (for menus and client food intake). Unfortunately, only several hundred foods are available by default in the client food intake module. The user can stop and "define" new intake food items by identifying them from the "source" database and transferring them to the intake database. This is a lengthy process, but DietMax developers feel that this transfer is usually unnecessary because "most practitioners use intake analysis to roughly gauge a client's eating habits, and do not expect extreme accuracy." In other words, unless the user takes the time to define new intake food items, a relatively high number of food substitutions will have to be made.

Food selection from the small client intake database is through food groups, and once the food has been selected and highlighted, the user must first use the mouse to "copy" the food and then "paste" it to the client food listing. Another obstacle is selection of food portion size, which requires using the mouse to push an arrow tab that increases and decreases the portion size by set increments. Although the portion size increment arrows can be sidestepped by using the mouse to "click" in the box and then enter the exact volume measure, gram amounts cannot be entered. The working screen for all of this is compact and novel, and if the next version allows the user to search the entire database by name and enter portion sizes more easily, the entire process of food search and entry will be greatly improved. Switching from day-to-day food entry is easy, 3-day averaging is automatic, and previewing nutrients for single foods or the total diet is simple. Although the processing time for producing reports is lengthy and a spreadsheet cannot be printed, the basic reports are well designed and attractive and include food exchange groups. DietMax for Windows is one of the few programs to provide printed reports in color. Missing data (which were calculated at 9.4% for our 3-day menu) are flagged by placing a small asterisk next to the nutrient value. The user manual and help screens are excellent. As shown in Table 5-4, DietMax had more than one third of the nutrients analyzed that exceeded 15% variance from the USDA NDB standard, more than any of the programs analyzed. This was primarily due to the large number of food substitutions, difficulty in choosing exact portion sizes, and the substantial number of missing data.

Food Processor Plus (version 6.0)

Food Processor Plus, version 6.0 includes over 12,000 foods and analyzes them for 94 nutrient components and a large variety of nutrient ratios, percents, and other indexes.

The nutrient database is based on the USDA NDB (release 10) and complemented by over 1000 sources, including the USDA Survey Database, USDA provisional data, scientific literature, food manufacturers, and foreign food composition tables. Values are imputed where similar data are available. As a result there are very few missing data (only 0.3% for our 3-day food record). The data are updated continuously, and food manufacturers are contacted on a regular basis to keep name brand food data current and to expand the database for emerging products. Cooking and preparation yields are also calculated so that the user can enter foods as raw with bone, or in dry uncooked form, with skin or shells, and the program will calculate the cooked and prepared yield of the edible portion.

Food search and entry and editing of the food list are quick and easy, and nutrient values for individual food items can be previewed while searching. Food retrieval is very fast, and the "smart search" system allows the user to look up foods by name, a key word, a partial name, or food code number. The printed reports are excellent and include a variety of unique features including food exchange groups and a graph of protein quality. A complete spreadsheet with all nutrients listed for each food can be printed in a compressed format. Personalized messages can be included with each printed report through a text editor, and results compared to American or Canadian standards. Data can be imported from other programs or results exported in the ASCII format. Two excellent manuals accompany the software. Help messages automatically appear during use of all phases of the software program, helping the user to gain a basic understanding of what keystrokes are necessary.

The Food Processor Plus received our highest number of "excellents" because of the quality of their operating features and database. Only one nutrient varied more than 15% from the USDA NDB (total tocopherol) and that was because the Food Processor is one of the few programs to provide total α-tocopherol–equivalent data (which the RDA are based on). The USDA NDB provides only total tocopherol data and does not adjust the data by the various activity levels of the different tocopherols and tocotrienols. Additionally, the USDA NDB has a large number of missing total tocopherol data (86% of our 3-day food menu). The Food Processor Plus developers have gone to extraordinary lengths to provide users with nearly complete vitamin E data in total α-tocopherol equivalent format.

Counseling Nutrition Data System (version 2.6)

The Nutrition Data System (NDS) was originally developed for use in two major research projects, the Lipid Research Clinics and the Multiple Risk Factor Intervention Trial, by the Nutrition Coordinating Center, University of Minnesota. The program has been modified for use on microcomputers and customized for use in the ongoing National Health and Nutrition Examination Survey (NHANES)[16,38–42].

Several versions of the NDS are available, including the NDS 93 ($8000), NDS 32 ($2550), and the Counseling NDS, version 2.6 ($595). While the majority of users are medical researchers in the United States and Canada, the NDS is also used by other nutrition professionals who desire research-quality results. The program includes over 23,000 food items and brand name foods (although additional prompts allow the user to describe over 160,000 possible variants of the foods). The nutrient database for the Counseling NDS provides complete information on 32 nutrient components and 9 nutrient ratios/percents for each food item and is updated on a continual basis using current information from the USDA, scientific literature, food manufacturers, and foreign food composition tables. (The nutrient database for the NDS 93 includes 93 nutrient components.) Values are imputed when none are available using published procedures[42]. Missing values are only tolerated when no information is available to indicate whether or not a nutrient is present in a food, the value is believed to be negligible, or the food is usually eaten in very small amounts (all of the 32 nutrients have less than 3% missing values, and for the 3-day food record, no missing data were found). More than 350 food manufacturers are contacted by the Nutrition Coordinating Center each year to obtain updated nutrient and ingredient information for over 7000 products.

Prompts, messages, and "help" screens guide the user through all phases of the program. The chief characteristic of the software program is the extensive interactive system that prompts the user to select appropriate answers regarding specific quantities and qualities of the food and methods of preparation. Although this increases the amount of time it takes to enter a food record, the user is ensured of research-quality nutrient results. Editing of the food list is very easy, but with version 2.6 the NDS does not allow previewing of nutrient information during food search and entry, and the spreadsheet can print only five nutrients at a time. The software program is designed for analyzing 1-day food records, recalls, recipes, and diet histories. Analysis of multiple-day food records is cumbersome in that a separate software module is used for this purpose. The program would benefit by using a master menu that controls all of the various functions of the software package, and the Nutrition Coordinating Center is currently rewriting the software operating features to make it more user-friendly.

As with the Food Processor Plus, the NDS is one of the few systems that provides total tocopherol and α-tocopherol equivalent data so that nutrient output can be compared directly with the RDA. Vitamin A values for NDS tended to be lower than the USDA standard because values for raw carrot were 45% lower (1112 versus 2025 μg RE, respectively, for 72 g raw carrot). However, the NDS has chosen to use non-USDA data that are based on an analysis technique that gives more valid, but lower, vitamin A values for carrots and other vegetables[43]. This is an excellent example as to why variance from the USDA NDB should not necessarily be construed as negative, in that it may represent effort by the developer (in this case, the Nutrition Coordinating Center) to provide more accurate or additional information.

In summary, the Counseling NDS has one of the most comprehensive food lists and complete databases of all the programs reviewed and is suitable for research-quality dietary analysis. The software is a bit difficult to use but has an excellent user's manual, series of "help screens," and a unique probing system to ensure proper data input.

Nutrient Analysis System 2 Plus 8 (version 1.0)

The Nutrient Analysis System 2 Plus 8 (NAS2+8), version 1.0, has about 8000 foods in the database and analyzes them for 79 nutrient components. NAS2 has all of the basic features expected in a dietary analysis system including tabular and spreadsheet printouts, comparison with RDA and other dietary standards in graphic form, nutrient sorting, and the ability to expand the database. The database uses nutrient data from every food item listed in the USDA NDB release #10 but also includes name brand foods, combination foods, fast foods, infant formulas, nutrient supplements, and other food items. The NAS2+8 actually uses the same code numbers as the USDA NDB, and as a result, the 3-day nutrient summary varied little from the USDA NDB standard (except for some error introduced because of inexact gram portion size selection and mathematical rounding).

Editing of the food list (especially through a listing of the code numbers) was easy. NAS2 did have several problems, however, with other program operating features, especially food search and entry, and averaging 3 days worth of food records. Food search is through food groups, is limited to 40 foods, and more keystrokes than normal are required to complete each selection. Three-day averaging is cumbersome and difficult, requiring the use of the manual to figure it out, and extensive line-by-line deleting and then adding. Once the 3-day average table is obtained, it can be viewed on the screen but not printed out except in graphic form (with most weight summary values deleted). Although nutrients can be viewed on the screen by groups, 3-day nutrient summaries could not be obtained for all of the nutrients. For these reasons, NAS2 received only a "fair" rating for program operation.

Nutritionist IV (version 3.5)

Nutritionist IV, version 3.5, includes more than 12,000 foods and analyzes them for 75 nutrient components. The nutrient data are based primarily on all available USDA data and are complemented by information from a large variety of journal and industry sources. The database is continuously revised by three full-time dietitians, and updates are released approximately twice a year. Nutritionist IV, version 3.5, is now available for MS-DOS and Windows. Although both programs use the same database, program operating features and printed reports differ in ease of use and quality.

Nutritionist IV (MS-DOS) has a large number of special features such as the ability to calculate the number of food exchanges for the diet record data, print the Food Guide Pyramid with food group recommendations, print default or personalized reports using a text editor, analyze food frequency lists, and print a wide variety of nutrient sorts. The printed reports are very attractive. The software program is accompanied by an excellent user's manual and good help screens. The food search process is made easier through use of a "smart search" technique.

Although the database is quite extensive, we did find 5.6% missing data for the 3-day food record and more than 15% variance from the USDA NDB for dietary fiber, total and α-tocopherol, oleic fatty acid, and cholesterol. This was largely due to missing data and differences in nutrient values for some of the foods.

Nutritionist IV received a "poor" rating for processing speed. The system takes an excessive amount of time to process reports and graphs. (The Windows version is slower than the MS-DOS version, and we found producing, viewing, and printing reports to be a laborious process). Editing was cumbersome, difficult to figure out (requiring the use of the manual), and irksome because the cursor would jump to different positions on the food list after making insertions or deletions. Although the user can preview nutrients for a default portion size during food search and entry, previewing of nutrients for the exact portion size entered is not possible until the spreadsheet is printed.

We encountered difficulty freeing enough conventional RAM to avoid memory drains during operation. Even though we used a computer with 8 MB RAM, the MS-DOS version of Nutritionist IV only uses conventional RAM. About 560 conventional RAM is recommended, and with many newer systems, this is difficult to achieve. The system comes with a built-in memory "optimizer," but we found this helped very little. The Windows version did not have these RAM memory problems.

Overall, Nutritionist IV has some very unique features and a large database. However, the program has become so large and complicated that processing speed is slow and memory drain problems are common. Nutritionist V will correct many of these problems, according to company representatives.

Nutritional Software Library IV

The Nutritional Software Library IV by Computrition, Inc. includes more than 18,000 foods and analyzes them for 24 nutrient components. A number of programs are included within the software library, including "dietplan" (to plan a balanced menu), "intake" (to analyze nutrient content of diets), "nutribld" (to build an index or recipes), "nutrirec" (to determine the nutritional content of recipes), and "profile" (to establish a plan for weight loss or weight gain).

The database has a relatively large number of missing values (7.9% for the 3-day food record), and as a result, values for folacin and three fatty acids varied more than 15% from the USDA NDB standard. For example, values for saturated, monounsaturated, and polunsaturated fatty acids were missing for pancakes, margarine, some salad dressings, and cured ham, explaining the unusually low values. The program has only a limited number of print options, and the spreadsheet (which displays 20 nutrients at a time) must be printed on a wide-carriage printer or in landscape format on a laser or ink jet printer.

Program operating procedures are cumbersome, requiring the use of the manual and help screens to know what words to type in to move through various command structures. Editing is also difficult, requiring an unusually high number of keystrokes to accomplish the task. Food search is by name only, with the user then required to type a number corresponding to the food list on the screen. Previewing of nutrients for each food, however, is simple and adjusted to the exact portion size entered. Averaging 3 days of intake required more keystrokes than most programs, and it was not readily apparent how to accomplish this task.

Overall, the Nutritional Software Library has a huge food list but only 24 nutrient components and a relatively high number of missing values. The program operating features could also be more user friendly.

Food/Analyst Plus (CD-ROM)

Food/Analyst Plus from Hopkins Technology is one of the few dietary analysis systems that takes advantage of CD-ROM technology. The database contains 22,500 foods, divided separately into the USDA NDB release #10, the USDA Survey database, and the Canadian Nutrient File (in both French and English). Also included are over 8000 brand name foods from about 160 food manufacturers and restaurants. Overall, 84 nutrients are analyzed, although the number varies from one database to the other. The Santé CD-ROM program ($60) is also available from Hopkins Technology and contains 18,000 foods and 30 nutrients.

We found the Food/Analyst Plus to be user-friendly, extremely fast, and fun to use. Food search and entry is easy, although previewing of nutrients is not available. Editing and averaging of 3-day food records is simple. The number of print options is limited, and printing of RDA graphs is difficult. Food lists, spreadsheets for entire meals, and tables of all nutrients with RDA percent comparisons can be printed with ease, however. Although the entire database can be sorted by specific nutrients, diets that have been entered cannot be sorted.

Missing data are not imputed or substituted for, and as a result, the database has a relatively high number of missing values (15.1% for the 3-day menu). Dietary fiber and three minerals were more than 15% below the USDA NDB standard, and this was traced to an unusually high number of missing data for bakery items.

The Food/Analyst Plus CD-ROM dietary analysis system received an overall "excellent" rating for program operating features, although there still are areas for improvement (especially previewing and more print options). The database, although the largest of all the systems compared in this chapter, was searched quickly and easily by taking advantage of CD-ROM technology.

Why Systems Differ

This comparison has demonstrated that microcomputer dietary analysis systems vary widely in general operating features, system output, and nutrient database content. Some programs were difficult to use and took an inordinate amount of time to search for foods or process reports. Other problems included software program deficiencies such as an inability to adjust food portion sizes to specific gram or volume amounts. Some programs placed a heavy demand on computer hardware requirements, or required Windows or a CD-ROM drive.

Variance between programs for 3-day food record nutrient values occurred because of differences in the number of food items included in the database (leading to varying degrees of substitution), the recency of the nutrient data (whether or not the most recent USDA releases had been incorporated), and the number of missing values (the degree to which non-USDA sources or estimating calculations were utilized to fill in the blanks from the USDA standard).

There are several limitations in this type of comparison. The 3-day food record for this study consisted primarily of common, basic food items, and we purposely avoided using recipes or food items not found in the USDA NDB. Obviously, much greater variation between dietary analysis systems would have occurred had combination foods, recipes, and brand name products not found in the USDA NDB been used.

Reasons for variance from the USDA standard are based on several factors. The USDA standard itself had 7.9% missing values, primarily because of incomplete nutrient information for certain nutrients (especially total tocopherol, α-tocopherol, copper, manganese, amino acids, and some fatty acids). For example, the USDA gave vitamin E values only for mayonnaise, margarine, salad dressings, and a limited number of fruits and vegetables. Thus the USDA NDB is incomplete and cannot be regarded as a "gold standard." While some dietary analysis system developers attempted to fill in the missing data using other sources or imputed values, others were less energetic in going beyond the basic USDA standard.

Developers of dietary analysis software programs will continue to be challenged as the USDA publishes new releases or updates of earlier releases, the food industry experiences rapid change (in terms of mergers and acquisitions, new product introductions, nutrient and health claims for new products, and development of new ingredients and technologies), and consumers change their food attitudes and behavior (especially toward low-fat and healthy foods)[15]. During the mid-1980s, about 6000 new food products were introduced each year, a figure that has now risen to about 13,000[15]. Food categories that have had the most aggressive change are condiments, candy/gum/snacks, beverages, bakery products, and dairy products. The best software vendors attempt to provide their customers with database updates at least once a year to keep pace with the rapid changes that are occurring. They also have developed relationships with a network of food companies to receive current brand name food data and use a wide variety of non-USDA sources to give information on missing data. For these reasons, until there is a nutrient database that is adopted as the "standard" and made available to all vendors, microcomputer dietary analysis system databases will continue to vary widely, and the dietitian is left with the responsibility of carefully choosing a dietary analysis system that is suitable to specific needs and tasks.

The task of analyzing the nutrient intake of individuals or groups from dietary records or lists has been greatly simplified and streamlined by microcomputers. However, as discussed in Chapter 3, measurement of the diet has many limitations (i.e., food composition values are average approximates, influenced by soil type, weather, season, geographic area, genetic make-up, harvesting conditions, processing methods, storage conditions, cooking methods, and so on). This chapter has shown that dietary analysis systems vary in their estimates of the nutrient content of a standard 3-day menu. Unfortunately, both nutrition professionals and patients tend to view computerized printouts as precise descriptions of nutrient intake. Computerized diet analysis systems can be a problem unless everyone involved learns to view these software packages as nothing more than tools that facilitate and expedite the unwieldy task of analyzing nutrient intake.

This chapter was written during the fall of 1994. The reader should realize that newer versions for each of the microcomputer dietary analysis systems have been released since then, and may be substantially different from the versions reviewed in this chapter. Nonetheless, the principles reviewed in this chapter remain the same.

SUMMARY

1. Computers are perfectly suited to the task of nutrient analysis, which is one of the most widespread applications of computer technology in dietetics. Computerized nutrient analysis tasks include clinical, educational, administrative, epidemiologic, and metabolic/experimental applications.
2. There are many factors to consider in selecting computerized dietary analysis systems. The first step is to establish the major needs for obtaining the software, with specific tasks defined. Once this has been

accomplished, the next step is to choose a dietary analysis system that is suitable to these needs and tasks. There are three characteristics of software programs that dietitians and other health professionals can use to compare programs. These include (1) aspects of the database, (2) software program operation, and (3) system output.

3. The most important consideration to make when selecting a computerized diet analysis system is the nutrient database. The database must be accurate, verified, and large enough to meet all intended tasks. The USDA National Nutrient Databank is the most important source of nutrient data for developers of diet analysis systems. The USDA provides both printed and computerized versions of their database.
4. Developers of commercial computerized dietary analysis systems are faced with several challenges in formulating a high quality database. These include deciding on how many foods and nutrients to include in the software program and use of non-USDA sources to give information on certain brand name foods and to fill in the missing data. The contents of nutrient databases from different software vendors may vary widely depending on the number of food items and nutrients included, whether or not the most recent USDA releases have been incorporated, and the degree to which non-USDA sources (food industry, scientific literature) or estimating calculations are used to fill in the missing values.
5. The general operating features of the computerized diet analysis system are extremely important, determining whether a software package is easy to use while generating the desired information. These features include everything from search and entry of food items to the comparison of results with a variety of dietary standards.
6. Once the data have been entered into the computerized dietary analysis system, two important features are the software program's ability to (1) print out a variety of printed reports and (2) export the data to a variety of electronic files for further analysis.
7. General operating features and nutrient databases of eight microcomputer dietary analysis systems were compared. A 3-day food record with 73 food items was entered into each program, with nutrient averages compared with the USDA NDB.
8. The eight programs were found to vary widely in cost, number of foods and nutrients in the database, use of non-USDA data and imputation of data for missing values, the number of print/export options, time to analyze the 3-day food record, and overall ease of use.
9. Although the dietary analysis systems tended to be similar to the USDA NDB for energy, protein, total fat, and total carbohydrates, the number of other nutrients varying more than 15% from the USDA NDB varied considerably between programs. The food components from the eight dietary analysis systems that were most likely to vary from the USDA NDB included total tocopherols and α-tocopherols, dietary fiber, the various fatty acids, and cholesterol. Nutrients most likely to be absent from the databases of the eight systems included total tocopherols and α-tocopherols, manganese, the various amino acids and fatty acids, pantothenic acid, copper, magnesium, and caffeine. These results demonstrate the importance of each dietitian carefully choosing a microcomputer dietary analysis system that is suitable to specific and predetermined needs.

REFERENCES

1. National Research Council. 1989. *Recommended Dietary Allowances,* 10th edition Washington, D.C: National Academy Press.
2. Byrd-Bredbenner C. 1988. Computer nutrient analysis software packages: Considerations for selection. *Nutrition Today* 23(5):13–21.
3. Thompson FE. 1994. Dietary assessment resource manual. *Journal of Nutrition* 124:2245S–2317S.
4. Gregoire MB, Nettles MF. 1994. Is it time for computer-assisted decision making to improve the quality of food and nutrition services? *Journal of the American Dietetic Association* 94:1371–1374.
5. Buzzard IM, Price KS, Warren RA. 1991. Considerations for selecting nutrient-calculation software: Evaluation of the nutrient database. *American Journal of Clinical Nutrition* 54:7–9.
6. Thompson JK, Dwyer JT. 1987. Computer applications in out-patient nutrition services: Fostering the computer connection. *Clinical Nutrition* 6:185–191.
7. Frank GC, Pelican S. 1986. Guidelines for selecting a dietary analysis system. *Journal of the American Dietetic Association* 86:72–75.
8. Smith JL. 1993. *Nutrient data bank directory* (9th ed). Newark, Del: University of Delaware Press.
9. Pao EM, Sykes KE, Cypel YS. 1989. *USDA methodological research for large-scale dietary intake surveys, 1975–88.* Human Nutrition Information Service. USDA Home Economics Research Report No. 49. Available from HNIS, USDA, 6505 Belcrest Rd, Room 338, Hyattsville, MD 20782.
10. Pao EM, Sykes KE, Cypel YS. 1990. Dietary intake—large scale survey methods. *Nutrition Today* 25(6):11–17.
11. Rand WM. 1985. Food composition data: Problems and plans. *Journal of the American Dietetic Association* 85:1081–1083.
12. Perloff BP. 1989. Analysis of dietary data. *American Journal of Clinical Nutrition* 50:1128–1132.
13. United States Department of Agriculture. *Composition of foods, raw, processed, prepared.* Washington, DC: US Government Printing Office, 1976–1990. [Agriculture Handbook 8:AH-8–1, Dairy and Egg Products, 1976; AH-8–2, Spices and Herbs, 1977; AH-8–3, Baby Foods, 1978; AH-8–4, Fats and Oils, 1979; AH-8–5, Poultry Products, 1979; AH-8–6, Soups, Sauces, and Gravies, 1980; AH-8–7, Sausages and Luncheon Meats, 1980; AH-8–8, Breakfast Cereals, 1982; AH-8–9, Fruits and Fruit Juices, 1982; AH-8–10, Pork Products, 1992 (revised); AH-8–11, Vegetables and Vegetable Products, 1984; AH-8–12, Nut and Seed Products, 1984; AH-8–13, Beef Products, 1990 (revised); AH-8–14, Beverages, 1986; AH-8–15, Finfish and Shellfish Products, 1987; AH-8–16, Legumes and Legume Products, 1986; AH-8–17, Lamb, Veal, and Game Products, 1989; AH-18, Baked Products, 1992; AH-19, Snacks and Sweets; AH-8–20, Cereal Grains and Pasta, 1989; AH-8–21, Fast Foods, 1988.]
14. Perloff BP, RL Rizek, DB Haytowitz, PR Reid. 1990. Dietary intake methodology II. USDA's Nutrient Database for Nationwide Dietary Intake Surveys. *Journal of Nutrition* 120:1530–1534.
15. Stillings BR. 1994. Trends in foods. *Nutrition Today* 29(5):6–13.
16. Schakel SF, Sievert YA, Buzzard IM. 1988. Sources of data for developing and maintaining a nutrient database. 1988. *Journal of the American Dietetic Association* 88:1268–1271.
17. Mitchell DC, Shacklock F. 1991. The Minnesota nutrition data system. *Nutrition Today* 26(1):52–53.
18. Matzkin J. 1989. Nutrition databases: Changing your diet to improve your health. *PC Magazine* January 31, pp. 364, 366.
19. Somer E. 1994. Computer dining. *Shape* September, 1994, pp. 41–44.
20. Marecic M, Bagby R. 1988. Nutrient analysis system 2. *Nutrition Today* 23(4):38–37.
21. Marecic M, Bagby R. 1988. Computer software review. *Nutrition Today* 23(1):40; *Nutrition Today* 23(2):38.
22. Nieman DC, Butterworth DE, Nieman CN, Lee KE, Lee RD. 1992. Comparison of six microcomputer dietary analysis systems with the USDA Nutrient Data Base for Standard Reference. *Journal of the American Dietetic Association* 92:48–56.

23. Nieman DC, Nieman CN. 1987. A comparative study of two microcomputer nutrient databases with the USDA nutrient database for standard reference. *Journal of the American Dietetic Association* 87:930–932.
24. Orta J. 1991. Software scan: Scanning recent nutrition computer software. *Food Nutrition News* 63(2):10.
25. Manore MM, Vaughan LA, Lehman W. 1989. Development and testing of a statistical and graphics-enhanced nutrient analysis program. *Journal of the American Dietetic Association* 89:246–250.
26. Orta J. 1994. Nutritionist IV for Windows. *Journal of the American Dietetic Association* 94:937–938.
27. Marecic M, Bagby R. 1988. Computer software review. *Nutrition Today* 23(4):38.
28. Eck LH, Klesges RC, Hanson CL, Baranowski T, Henski J. 1988. A comparison of four commonly used nutrient database programs. *Journal of the American Dietetic Association* 88:602–604.
29. Shanklin D, Endres JM, Sawicki M. 1985. A comparative study of two nutrient databases. *Journal of the American Dietetic Association* 85:308–313.
30. Hoover LW. 1983. Computerized nutrient databases: I. Comparison of nutrient analysis systems. *Journal of the American Dietetic Association* 83:501–510.
31. Frank GC, Farris RP, Hyg MS, Berenson GS. 1984. Comparison of dietary intake by 2 computerized analysis systems. *Journal of the American Dietetic Association* 84:818–820.
32. Adelman MO, Dwyer JT, Woods M, Bohn E, Otradovec CL. 1983. Computerized dietary analysis systems: A comparative view. *Journal of the American Dietetic Association* 83:421–429.
33. Dwyer J, Suitor CW. 1984. Caveat emptor: Assessing needs, evaluating computer options. *Journal of the American Dietetic Association* 84:302–312.
34. Taylor ML, Kozlowski BW, Baer MT. 1985. Energy and nutrient values from different computerized data bases. *Journal of the American Dietetic Association* 85:1136–1138.
35. Block G. 1989. Human dietary assessment: Methods and issues. *Preventive Medicine* 18:653–660.
36. Powers PM, Hoover LW. 1989. Calculating the nutrient composition of recipes with computers. *Journal of the American Dietetic Association* 89:224–232.
37. Expert Panel on Detection, Evaluation, and Treatment of High Blood Cholesterol in Adults. 1993. Summary of the second report of the National Cholesterol Education Program Expert Panel on Detection, Evaluation, and Treatment of High Blood Cholesterol in Adults (Adult Treatment Panel II). *Journal of the American Medical Association* 269:3015–3023.
38. Woteki CE, Briefel RR, Kuczmarski R. 1988. Contributions of the National Center for Health Statistics. *American Journal of Clinical Nutrition* 47:320–328.
39. Buzzard IM, Feskanich D. 1987. Maintaining a food composition database for multiple research studies: The NCC food table. In Rand WM, Windham CT, Wyse BW, Young VR (eds). *Food composition data: A user's perspective.* The United Nations University.
40. Sievert YA, Schakel SF, Buzzard IM. 1989. Maintenance of a nutrient database for clinical trials. *Controlled Clinical Trials* 10:416–425.
41. Feskanich D, Sielaff BH, Chong K, Buzzard IM. 1989. Computerized collection and analysis of dietary intake information. *Computer Methods and Programs in Biomedicine* 30:47–57.
42. Feskanich D, Buzzard IM, Welch BT, Asp EH, Dieleman LS, Chong KR, Bartsch GE. 1988. Comparison of a computerized and a manual method of food coding for nutrient intake studies. *Journal of the American Dietetic Association* 88:1263–1267.
43. Bureau JL, Bushway RJ. 1986. HPLC determination of carotenoids in fruits and vegetables in the United States. *Journal of Food Science* 51:28–130.

Assessment Activity 5-1

USING A DIET ANALYSIS PROGRAM TO ANALYZE A 3-DAY FOOD RECORD

In Assessment Activity 3-2 you collected a 3-day food record of your personal food intake. In this activity, you are to enter all the foods from this 3-day food record into a computerized diet analysis program and determine your average nutrient intake over the three days.

1. How does your 3-day average nutrient intake compare with the Recommended Dietary Allowances? List all the nutrients that fall below 70% of the RDA.
2. What are some of the possible reasons why your intake of certain nutrients as reported by the computer may be less than 70% of the RDA?
3. List the strengths and weaknesses of using computerized dietary analysis programs to analyze a 3-day food record such as the one you prepared in Assessment Activity 3-2.
4. How does your 3-day average intake of kilocalories, protein, carbohydrate, total fat, calcium, and iron compare with the values for these nutrients from the 24-hour recall you analyzed using the food composition table in Appendix L? What are some possible reasons for differences between these two methods? (See Chapter 3).

Assessment Activity 5-2

DIETARY ANALYSIS PROGRAM

You can obtain a free copy of the *Dietary Analysis Program* from the USDA's Human Nutrition Information Service (HNIS). It can be downloaded from the HNIS Nutrient Data Bank Bulletin Board to a personal computer (see Using the Nutrient Data Bank Bulletin Board below for instructions).

The *Dietary Analysis Program* is capable of analyzing up to 3 days of food intake for food energy and 27 nutrients and food components. It is designed for IBM-compatible computers and is menu driven and easy to use. Foods are selected from common food groups, and quantities are estimated using household measures. The database contains 850 of the most commonly reported foods in the USDA's food consumption surveys, and data are from the USDA's National Nutrient Data Bank.

The program's printout includes a list of reported foods and quantities; bar graphs showing how reported intake for 15 nutrients compare with the 1989 Recommended Dietary Allowances; the percent of toal kilocalories from protein, carbohydrate, fat, and alcohol; and amounts of 27 nutrients and food components in reported foods.

Using the Nutrient Data Bank Bulletin Board

To access the Nutrient Data Bank Bulletin Board and obtain the Dietary Analysis Program, you need the following:

- A computer
- A modem connected to a telephone line
- The communication software that accompanied your modem

Set the following parameters on your modem or through your communications software:

- No parity
- 8 bits
- Stop bit = 1 (n/8/1)

Because the file contains 631 kilobytes, you will need two low-density (370 kilobyte) diskettes or one high-density (1.2 megabyte or 1.4 megabyte) diskette. The name of the file to download is DAPZ.EXE. The telephone number to call is (301) 436-5078. It takes about 22 minutes to download the file using a 2400 baud modem, less time if you have a faster modem.

Once you have connected with the bulletin board, it will prompt you for your first and last names. If they are not located in a list of previous users, a welcome message will appear on your screen explaining the purpose of the bulletin board. Next, it will ask you if you want to register or exit. By pressing "R" for register, you will be asked to enter your own password and your city and state. *Be sure to remember your password; you will need it for successive log-ons.*

After signing on, you will be shown a list of the available bulletins. A menu of appropriate responses will always appear on the screen, and additional help is available by selecting the question mark "?" or the letter "h." However, if you wish to capture or download files and you are unsure how to proceed, you will need to consult the instructions for your communications software.

The computer is on line 24 hours a day, 7 days a week, with a few hours a month set aside for performing maintenance work on the computer and files. For further information, contact:

Human Nutrition Information Service
U.S. Department of Agriculture
6505 Belcrest Road, Room 315
Hyattsville, Maryland 20782
(301) 436-5635

The program also can be ordered. For pricing and ordering information, contact:

U.S. Department of Commerce
National Technical Information Service
Springfield, Virginia 22161
(703) 487-4650
FAX (703) 321-8547

Assessment Activity 5-3

CRUISING THE INTERNET FOR NUTRITION INFORMATION

In addition to obtaining information through electronic bulletin boards as mentioned in Assessment Activity 5-2, you can obtain a variety of nutrition information through the Internet. The Internet provides easy access to libraries and universities throughout the world, is a valuable source of information, and is usually available 24 hours a day, 7 days a week. Users have access to thousands of documents containing valuable information from remote areas that otherwise may not be accessible. With electronic-mail (e-mail), the Internet becomes a powerful communication tool for collaboration with colleagues and other health professionals. It is easy to get distracted using the Internet if you do not have a clearly defined topic for which you are searching and do not stay focused. Because there are few restrictions on the type of information appearing on the Internet, users should carefully scrutinize the scientific merit of available information and the credentials of authors.

One especially valuable source of nutrition information is the USDA's Human Nutrition Information Service. Here you can get information on upcoming USDA conferences, the availability of food composition data sets from the USDA's Human Nutrition Information Service, a list of current publications from the USDA, how to download nutrient composition data, and the names of USDA staff and how to contact them by phone or e-mail. You can access these through the University of Maryland's Gopher by entering "gopher info.umd.edu" at your system prompt. Choose the following line items at various menus:

- Educational Resources
- Academic Resources and Topics
- Agriculture and Environmental Resources
- United States Department of Agriculture (USDA)
- USDA Food Composition Data

  Keep in mind that these menu selections will change from time-to-time.

Many other organizations provide information on food, diet, and nutrition. A good source of information about on-line food and nutrition resources is the journal *Nutrition Reviews,* which publishes detailed directions on accessing nutrition information from sources such as government, universities, and private organizations.

If you haven't had much experience using a computer, the thought of getting on the Internet may be intimidating. It isn't that hard and it can be educational, exciting, and fun. Climb on board! You'll be glad you did.

SIX

ANTHROPOMETRY

OUTLINE

INTRODUCTION

Anthropometry is of considerable interest to scientists and the public. It is a valuable adjunct in assessing nutritional status. Concerns about the health implications of overweight and obesity have led many people to question the appropriateness of their weight, body composition, and body image. This has resulted in debate and confusion about which methods and standards should be used in assessing body weight and composition. Unfortunately, in some people it has led to such a preoccupation with body weight that their eating habits and body image have become disordered.

The effect of nutrition on human growth and development has made accurate measurement of the body's dimensions and weight indispensable to the practice of nutritional assessment. Properly assessing growth and development requires that standardized methods be followed for measuring the body. Assessment of the body's protein and muscle stores is fundamental to the diagnosis and treatment of malnutrition and to the evaluation of a patient's response to nutritional and other therapy. Nutritional research often depends on methods of accurately assessing changes in body growth and composition.

This chapter describes the available techniques for measuring the body's dimensions and composition. Some of these techniques will be used daily by practitioners, and others will be limited to nutritional research. This chapter establishes an essential foundation for applying the principles for assessing growth and development, nutritional status, and response to nutritional and other therapy, which are discussed in later chapters.

Mastering and intelligently applying the techniques and information in this chapter will provide you with skills that will be invaluable to your work in the field of nutrition.

WHAT IS ANTHROPOMETRY?

Anthropometry is the measurement of body size, weight, and proportions.[1–3] Measures obtained from anthropometry can be sensitive indicators of health, development, and growth in infants and children.[2] Anthropometric measures can be used to evaluate nutritional status, whether it be obesity caused by overnutrition or emaciation resulting from protein-energy malnutrition. They are valuable in monitoring the effects of nutritional intervention for disease, trauma, surgery, or malnutrition.[1,4] Anthropometry also is considered the method of choice for estimating body composition in a clinical setting.[5]

MEASURING LENGTH, STATURE, AND HEAD CIRCUMFERENCE

Measurements of length, stature (or height), weight, and head circumference are among the most fundamental and easily obtained anthropometric measurements. Among infants and children, these measurements are the most sensitive and commonly used indicators of health. A child's growth and development can be assessed by comparing height for age, weight for age, and weight for height with standards obtained from studies of large numbers of healthy, normal children. The measurement of stature is important for calculating certain indices such as weight for stature, weight divided by stature, and the creatinine height index, and for estimating basal energy expenditure.[6]

In measurements of length and stature, reference will be made to positioning the head in the **Frankfort horizontal plane**. As shown in Figure 6-1, this plane is represented by a line between the lowest point on the margin of the orbit (the bony socket of the eye) and the *tragion* (the notch above the tragus, the cartilaginous projection just anterior to the external opening of the ear). With the head in line with the spine, this plane should be horizontal.[7]

In all anthropometric measurements, consistency in technique and units of measurement (feet/inches, centimeter/millimeter, and so on) will help eliminate potential sources of error.[1,2]

Length

Length (also referred to as **recumbent** length) is obtained with the subject lying down and gener-

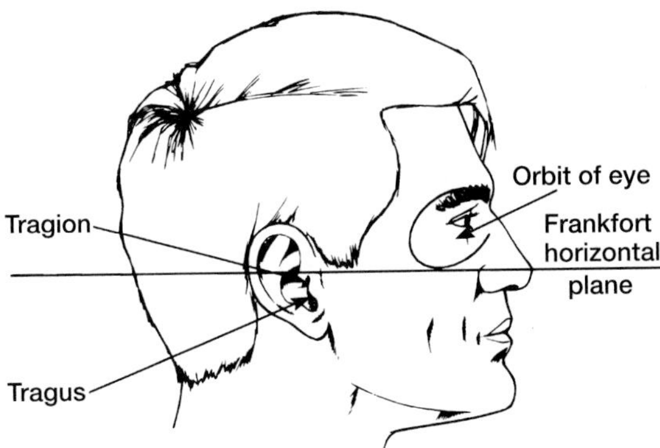

Figure 6-1 Length and stature are measured with the head in the Frankfort horizontal plane. This plane is represented by a line between the lowest point on the margin of the orbit (the bony socket of the eye) and the tragion (the notch above the tragus, the cartilaginous projection just anterior to the external opening of the ear).

ally is reserved for children less than 24 months of age or for children between 24 and 36 months of age who cannot stand erectly without assistance.[2,7] The growth charts used for persons birth to 36 months of age are based on recumbent length, whereas the growth charts for those age 2 to 18 years are based on stature.[8] Measurement of recumbent length requires a special measuring device (Figure 6-2) with a stationary headboard and moveable footboard that are perpendicular to the backboard. The device's measuring scale (in millimeters or inches) should have its zero end at the edge of the headboard and allow the child's length to be read from the footboard.[2]

Two persons are required to measure recumbent length, as shown in Figure 6-2. With the child in the supine position (lying on his or her back), one person holds the child's head against the backboard, with the crown securely against the headboard and with the Frankfort plane perpendicular to the backboard. This person also keeps the long axis of the child's body aligned with the center line of the backboard, the child's shoulders and buttocks securely touching the backboard, and the shoulders and hips at right angles to the long axis of the body. The other person keeps the child's legs straight and against the backboard, slides the footboard against the bottom of the feet (without shoes or socks) with the toes pointing upward, and reads the measurement. The footboard should be pressed firmly enough to compress the soft tissues of the soles but without diminishing the vertebral column length. Length should be recorded to the nearest 0.1 cm or ⅛ in. using a consistent unit over repeated measurements.[2,7] Gentle restraint is often required to keep a squirming infant properly positioned during measuring.[8] When this is not possible, the best estimate should be recorded with a notation of the circumstances.[2]

Stature

Stature or standing height can be measured for subjects 2 to 3 years of age and older who are cooperative and able to stand without assistance.[2,7] Stature can be measured in several ways. The simplest is to fasten a measuring stick or nonstretchable tape measure to a flat, vertical surface (for example, a wall) and use a right-angle headboard for reading the measurement. If a wall is used, it should not have a thick baseboard, and the subject should not stand on carpet, which could affect the accuracy of measurements.[7] Using the moveable rod on a platform scale is not recommended because it often lacks rigidity, the headboard is not always correctly aligned, there is no rigid surface against which to position the body, and the platform height will vary depending on the subject's weight.[9]

Another approach is to use a **stadiometer** such as the Holtain or the Accustat© Ross Stadiometer (see list of suppliers in Appendix N). The Holtain stadiometer is considered by many to be the best instrument for measuring stature, but its cost may be prohibitive. Equally reliable but less expensive is the Accustat© stadiometer.[9] Plans for building a stadiometer are available to health professionals by writing the Nutrition Services Section, Division of Health Promotion and Screening, Illinois Department of Public Health, 535 West Jefferson Street, Springfield, Illinois 62761.

When being measured with the stadiometer, the subject should be barefoot and wear minimal

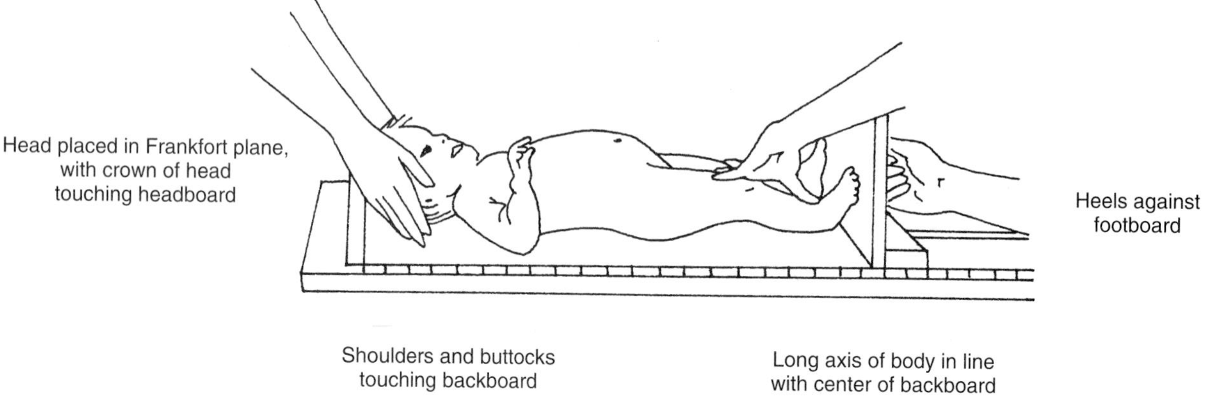

Figure 6-2 Special device for measuring the length of children who cannot stand erectly without assistance. The device has a stationary headboard and a moveable footboard. (Drawing by William Gagnon, Jr.)

clothing to facilitate correct positioning of the body. The subject should stand with heels together, arms to the side, legs straight, shoulders relaxed, and head in the Frankfort horizontal plane ("look straight ahead"). Heels, buttocks, scapulae (shoulder blades), and back of the head should, if possible, be against the vertical surface of the stadiometer, as shown in Figure 6-3. Some people may not be able to touch all four points against the stadiometer because of obesity, protruding buttocks, or curvature of the spine. Rather than creating an embarrassing situation by trying to force a subject into a physically impossible position, have the subject touch two or three of the four points to the vertical surface of the stadiometer or estimate height from knee height, as is discussed in Chapter 7.

Just before the measurement is taken, the subject should inhale deeply, hold the breath, and maintain an erect posture ("stand up tall") while the headboard is lowered on the highest point of the head with enough pressure to compress the hair.[1,2,7] The measurement should be read to the nearest 0.1 cm or ⅛ in. and with the eye level with the headboard to avoid errors caused by **parallax**, which is a difference in the apparent reading of a measurement scale or a skinfold caliper's needle when these are viewed from various points not in a straight line with the eye.[1,2,7] Hair ornamentation may have to be removed if this interferes with the measurement.

Nonambulatory Persons

In nonambulatory persons (those unable to walk) or those who have such severe spinal curvature that measurement of height would be inaccurate, stature can be estimated from knee height.[1,6] This and other recumbent measures and their application in nutritional assessment of older persons are discussed in Chapter 7.

Head Circumference

Head circumference measurement is an important screening procedure to detect abnormalities of head and brain growth, especially in the first year of life. Although these conditions may or may not be related to nutritional factors, discussion of head circumference measurement is included here for convenience.[2,10] Head circumference increases rapidly during the first 12 months of life but by 36 months, growth is much slower.[11] Therefore, it is recommended that head circumference should be measured routinely on infants and young children up to age 36 months.[2]

Head circumference is most easily measured when the infant or child is sitting on the lap of the

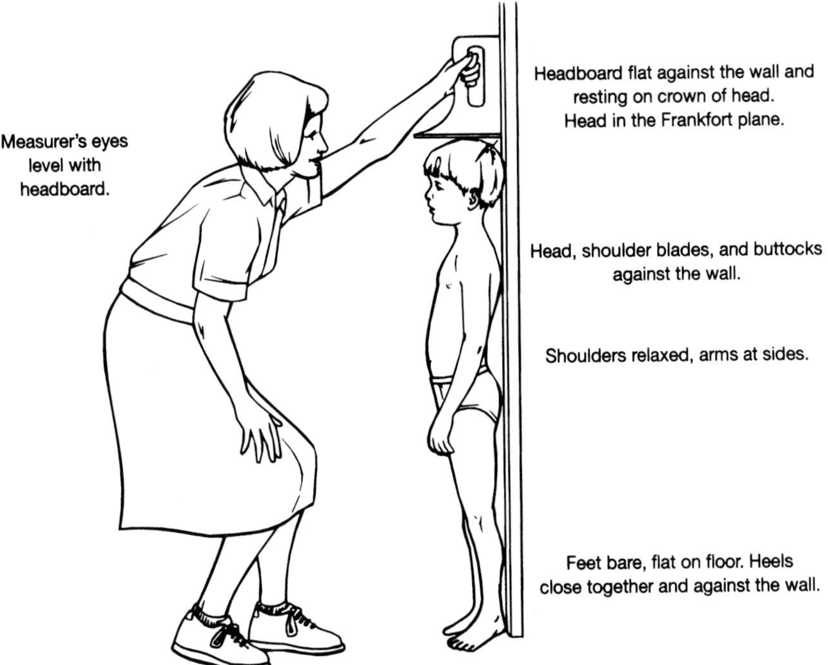

Figure 6-3 Body position when measuring stature.

caregiver, although older children can be measured when they are standing.[2,7] A flexible, nonstretchable measuring tape is required. Objects such as pins should be removed from the hair. As shown in Figure 6-4, the lower edge of the tape should be positioned just above the eyebrows, above (not over) the ears, and around the back of the head so that the maximum circumference is measured. The tape should be in the same plane on both sides of the head and pulled snug to compress the hair. The measurement is read to the nearest 0.1 cm or ⅛ in. and written in the infant's file. Reliability of the measurement should be verified with a second reading.[2,7]

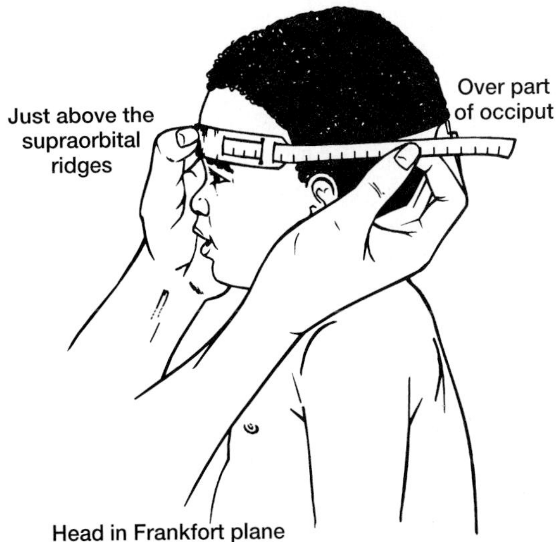

Figure 6-4 When measuring head circumference, the lower edge of the tape should be just above the eyebrows and ears, around the occipital prominence of the head, tight enough to compress the hair.

MEASURING WEIGHT

One of the most important measurements in nutritional assessment is body weight. Weight is an important variable in equations predicting caloric expenditure and in indices of body composition.[12]

Body weights should be obtained using an electronic scale or a balance-beam scale with nondetachable weights, as shown in Figure 6-5. Compared with balance beam scales, electronic scales tend to be lighter in weight, somewhat more portable, and faster and easier to use. They provide easy-to-read digital output in either metric or English units and, when properly calibrated, are highly accurate. Errors are commonly made in reading scale, dials, and rulers. The large, easily-read digital output from electronic scales can help reduce this error. Digital scales can record a subject's weight quickly. This can be an advantage in weighing infants who tend to resist lying still for very long.

Scales should be placed on a flat, hard surface that will allow them to sit securely without rocking or tipping. The zero weight on the scale's horizontal beam should be checked periodically and after the scale has been moved.[1,2] On balance beam scales this can be done by sliding the main and fractional weights to their respective zero positions and adjusting the zeroing weight until the beam balances at zero. Two or three times a year the accuracy of the scales should be further assured by using standard weights or by a professional dealer. Because spring-type bathroom scales may not provide the required accuracy after repeated use, they are not recommended.[1,2,7] Balance-beam scales with wheels that are moved from one location to another are not recommended either because scales must be recalibrated every time they are moved.

Infants

Infants should be weighed on a pan-type pediatric electronic or balance-beam scale that is accurate to within 10 g (0.01 kg) or ½ oz, as shown in Figure 6-5.[2,7] Any cushion (for example, a towel or diaper) used in the pan either should be in place when the zero adjustments are made on the scale or its weight should be subtracted from the infant's weight. Whatever practice is used, it must be uniformly followed and noted in the infant's file. Infants can be weighed nude, or the weight of the infant's diaper can be subtracted from the infant's weight. The infant should be set lying down in the middle of the pan. The average of two or three weighings is recorded numerically in the infant's file to the nearest 10 g (0.01 kg) or ½ oz and then is plotted on the growth chart in the presence of the subject's care giver. If, on comparison with previous data, the current values appear unusual, the measurements should be repeated.[2,7]

Excessive infant movement can make it difficult to obtain an accurate weight, in which case the weighing can be deferred until later in the examination. When too active to weigh on a baby scale, an infant can be weighed on a platform scale while being held by an adult with the weight derived by difference. Because this weight will be less accurate than desired (but still better than no weight), the method should be noted in the infant's chart.

Children and Adults

Children and adults who can stand without assistance are weighed on a platform electronic or balance-beam scale that is accurate to 100 g (0.1 kg) or ¼ lb, as shown in Figure 6-5.[1,2,7] The subject should stand still in the middle of the scale's platform without touching anything and with the body weight equally distributed on both feet. The weight should be read to the nearest 100 g (0.1 kg) or ¼ lb and recorded. Two measurements taken in immediate succession should agree to within 100 g (0.1 kg) or ¼ lb.[1] The weight of children then can be plotted on their growth charts. As with infants, if there seems to be any discrepancy between the current and past values, the measurement should be repeated for verification. Diurnal variations (cyclical changes occurring throughout the day) in weight of about 1 kg in children and 2 kg in adults are known to occur.[7,12] For this reason, it is a good practice to also record the time weight was measured.

Ideally, subjects should be weighed nude after voiding.[2] Although nude weighing is practical for infants, it often is not for children and adults.

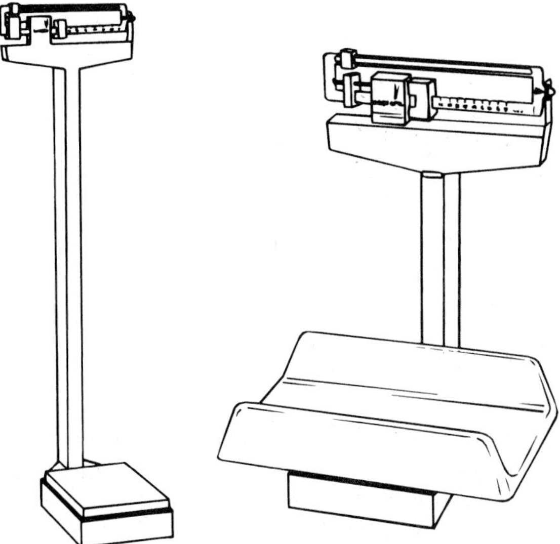

Figure 6-5 Balance beam scales (platform on the left and pan type on the right) are used in weighing subjects. The zero weight on the horizontal beam of the scale should be checked periodically and after the scale has been moved.

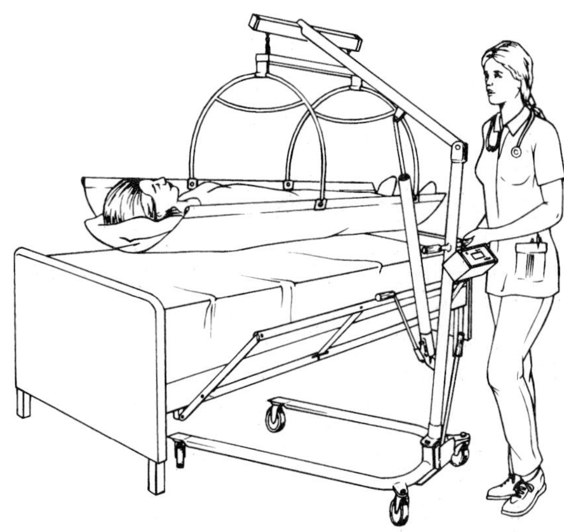

Figure 6-6 A bed scale can be used to weigh bedridden patients.

Therefore, minimal underclothing or an examination gown can be worn, and scales should be placed where adequate privacy is provided.[1,2,7] Should the weight of clothing be subtracted from the subject's weight? It depends on the purpose for which measurements are obtained and how accurate they need to be. In settings requiring a high degree of accuracy, subjects can be clothed in an examination gown of known weight for which consideration can be easily made. In situations having somewhat less stringent requirements, a reasonable estimate of clothing weight can be subtracted from a subject's weight.[1,7]

Nonambulatory Persons

Persons who cannot stand unassisted on a scale can be weighed in a bed scale or chair scale.[1,7] The subject to be weighed in the bed scale (shown in Figure 6-6) is comfortably positioned in the weighing sling, which then is gently raised until the subject is suspended off the bed. In a chair scale, the subject sits upright in the center of the chair while leaning against the backrest. Using either method, once the subject is still, weight can be read and recorded to the nearest 100 g (0.1 kg) or ¼ lb. Reliability of the measurement can be verified with a second reading, which should agree to within 100 g or ¼ lb.[1]

Body weight also can be computed from knee height, calf circumference, midarm circumference, and subscapular skinfold thickness.[1,12] Descriptions of these anthropometric measurements and computational formulas for computing body weight are given in Chapter 7.

NCHS GROWTH CHARTS

The National Center for Health Statistics (NCHS) has developed growth charts for comparing the size of an infant or child with other infants or children in the United States of comparable age and sex. The charts allow comparisons based on weight for age, length or stature for age, weight for length or stature, and head circumference for age. Charts have been developed for both males and females for two age intervals: birth to 36 months, and 2 to 18 years. One page of a chart is shown in Figure 6-7. The entire set of charts is shown in Appendix M. The charts are available to health professionals through Ross Laboratories, Columbus, Ohio. For the charts for birth to 36 months, percentiles are provided for body weight for age, length for age, body weight for length, and head circumference for age. The charts for 2 to 18 years provide percentile curves for body weight for age, stature for age, and weight for stature. When using the birth-to-36-month chart, length should be measured in the recumbent position (lying down). When using the 2-to-18-year chart, height should be measured with the child standing. The median difference between length and stature at 2 to 3 years of age is about 0.2 in (0.5 cm).[13] Head circumference, a variable included in the birth-to-36-month chart, is omitted in the 2-to-18-year chart. All other variables are the same between the two charts.

These charts were developed in 1976 using anthropometric data (weight, length or stature, and head circumference) collected from two sources. Reference data used in the birth-to-36-months charts were collected between 1929 and 1974 by researchers at Wright State University as part of the Fels Longitudinal Study. Children in the Fels Study were from a predominantly white, middle-class population in southwestern Ohio and thus were not representative of the general U.S. population. Reference data used to create the 2-to-18-year charts were collected between 1963 and 1974 as part of the National Health Examination Survey cycles II and III and the first National Health and Nutrition Examination Survey (NHANES I). Data from these surveys are representative of the general U.S. population.[13]

The values displayed in the charts are called "reference data" rather than "standards." Reference data represent a cross-sectional description of a population and describe "what is." Standards, on the other hand, describe "what should be" and imply that the values are "ideals" or "goals" associated with maximum health and longevity.[13] Since the development of the charts in 1976, new anthropometric data (from NHANES II and III) and improved statistical techniques have become available that are being used to revise the charts.

Using the Charts

To properly use the charts, measurements for length, stature, head circumference, and weight must be carefully taken following the standardized methods originally used in collecting the data from which the charts were developed. The approaches outlined in this book conform to those standardized methods and therefore are appropriate. Because chronological age is the most influential variable in rapidly growing children, it is essential that the subject's exact age be known before plotting age-dependent variables (for example, weight for age).[2,8] Age should be calculated to the nearest month when using the birth-to-36-month chart and to the nearest quarter year when using the 2-to-18-year chart.[2]

To plot the data, first locate the subject's age on the chart's horizontal axis (see Figure 6-7). Then locate the subject's length, stature, weight, or head circumference on the vertical axis. Draw a small circle on the chart where the lines representing these two values intersect. Check to make sure that the circle you have drawn is at the correct point in reference to the two variables. Use of a Ross Laboratories Accuplot™ Growth Plotting Aid can make plotting easier and reduce the possibility of errors.[2] A complete growth chart should include data that are both recorded numerically and plotted on the chart. If you plot the data while the subject is still present, you may repeat the measurements if unusual or changed values appear.[2]

Variables on the chart are presented as seven **percentile** curves: 5, 10, 25, 50, 75, 90, and 95. A 6-year-old girl's stature for age would be considered average when, once it was plotted, it was on or near the 50th percentile curve. In other words, the 50th percentile is considered the average or **median** value for the specific population of interest. If her plotted stature for age was on the 75th percentile curve, 75% of girls her age would

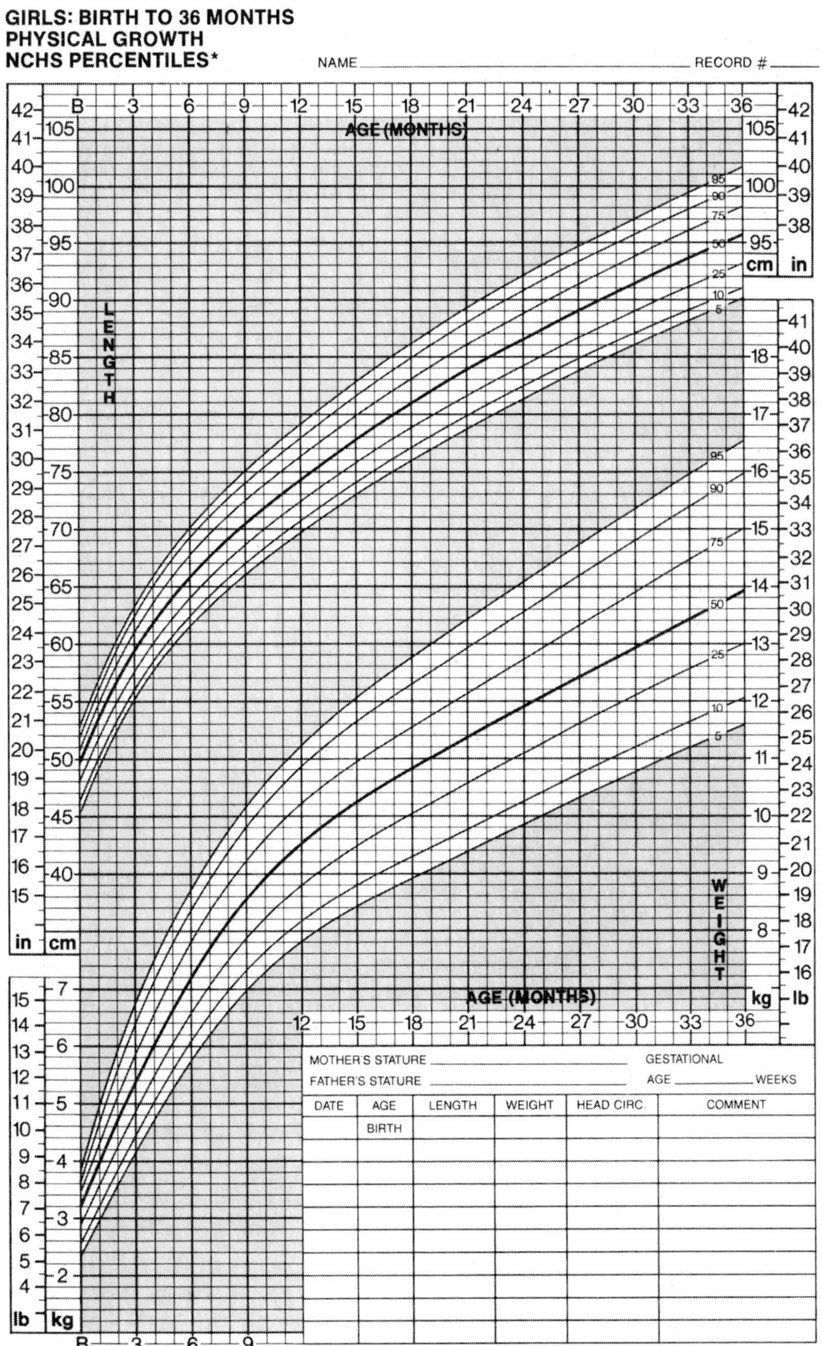

Figure 6-7 Example of a growth chart developed by the National Center for Health Statistics. This one is for females from birth to age 36 months. Additional growth charts are shown in Appendix M. Adapted from Hamill PVV, Drizd TA, Johnson CL, Reed Rb, Roche AF, Moore WM. 1979. Physical growth: National Center for Health Statistics Percentiles, *American Journal of Clinical Nutrition* 32:607–629. Data from the Fels Longitudinal Study, Wright State University School of Medicine, Yellow Springs, Ohio. 1982.

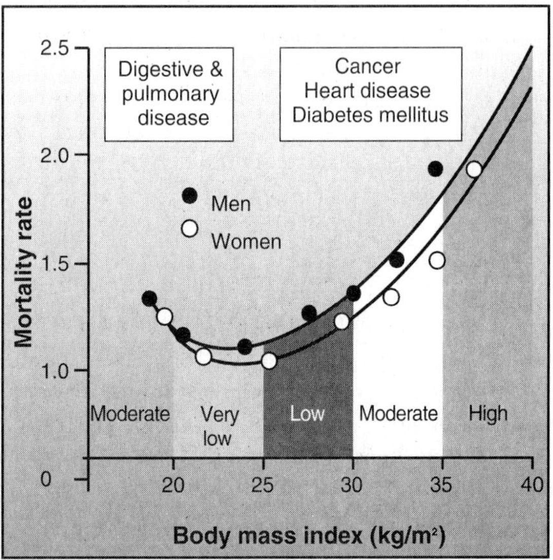

Figure 6-8 Risk of death from certain cancers, coronary heart disease, and diabetes mellitus increases as body mass index increases. Digestive disease and pulmonary diseases increase risk of death and often result in marked weight loss. Data from the American Cancer Society (adapted from Lew and Garfinkel).

be shorter than she would. If a child's height for age was at the 10th percentile, only 10% of children of the same age and sex would be shorter. Ranking persons this way is appropriate if they are part of the reference population from which the data were obtained. Plotted values between the 15th and 85th percentiles are generally considered within normal limits. Values less than the 15th percentile and greater than the 85th percentile warrant evaluation. If, over time, a person's plotted values change markedly (i.e., cross two percentile lines), the reasons for that change should be investigated.

WEIGHT STANDARDS

Overweight is defined as a body weight above some reference point of acceptable weight that usually is defined in relation to height.[14] **Obesity** is defined as an excess of body fat in relation to lean body mass.[15,16] There is good evidence that overweight persons, as a group, tend to die sooner than average-weight persons, especially those who are overweight at younger ages. As seen in Figure 6-8, risk of death increases as body mass index (a weight-height index discussed later in this chapter) increases above about 25 kg/m^2.[16] Some researchers believe that the lowest mortality rates in the United States (and many other Western nations) is associated with body weights somewhat below the average weight of the population under consideration.[17–21] In other words, the "average" body weights of middle-aged Americans may not necessarily be the most healthy.

At the same time, however, dietitians and nutritionists should be cautioned against encouraging weight loss when it is not indicated. There is no question that a body weight that is too low is unhealthy and increases risk of death. This is seen in persons suffering starvation or anorexia nervosa. A person whose BMI is $<$ 25 kg/m^2 probably does not have a weight problem and probably does not need to lose weight. Figure 6-8 shows the relationship between body mass index (BMI) and risk of death to be curvilinear instead of linear. It suggests that as BMI falls below about 20 kg/m^2, risk of death increases. This relationship is referred to as a "J-shaped" curve. But what actually increases risk of mortality in persons with low BMI? Is it low body weight itself or certain diseases (e.g., chronic obstructive pulmonary disease, cancers of the gastrointestinal tract, and lung cancer) that, in addition to markedly increasing risk of death, often causes marked weight loss? A recent 26-year mortality study of nearly 9000 nonsmoking, nondrinking men did not show this curvilinear relationship, even among the 5% of men whose BMI was $<$ 20kg/m^2.[22]

A variety of approaches exist for determining a person's recommended body weight. A very simple one frequently used by dietitians in the clinical setting is to allow 100 lb (45.5 kg) for the first 60 in (152 cm) of height for females and then add 5 lb (2.3 kg) for each additional 1 in (2.54 cm). For males, allow 106 lb (48 kg) for the first 60 in (152 cm) of height and then add 6 lb (2.7 kg) for each additional 1 in (2.54 cm). By creating a range of ±10%, allowance for the effects of frame size can be made. Consider, for example, a female who is 68 in tall. Based on this approach, her recommended body weight range would be 126 to 154 lb (140 lb ±10%).

Height-Weight Tables

Body weight can be assessed through the use of height-weight tables and the use of **relative weight** and **height-weight indices**. Height-weight tables are convenient, quick and easy to use, and understood by practically every adult, but they do have their limitations.

The life insurance industry has been in the forefront of developing height-weight tables because of its access to the data necessary for generating them. The tables were developed by comparing the heights and weights of life insurance policyholders with statistical data (known as actuarial data) on mortality rates and/or longevity of policyholders. Actuarial data were compiled on literally millions of insured persons in the United States and Canada in an attempt to define weights associated with the greatest longevity and lowest mortality rates.[15,17,18,23] The insurance industry has used data from the tables to help screen applicants to avoid insuring persons who are poor risks.[23] Good reviews of the topic have been published by Weigley,[23] Harrison,[14] and Manson and coworkers.[24]

The Metropolitan Life Insurance Company published the Ideal Weight Tables in 1942 and 1943,[25,26] the Desirable Weight Tables in 1959,[27] and the Height-Weight Tables in 1983.[28] Table 6-1 is the 1959 Metropolitan Life table. Table 6-2 is the 1983 Metropolitan Life table. Table 6-3 compares the 1959 and 1983 Metropolitan tables with average weights from several studies.[24] The 1959 and 1983 Metropolitan tables were based on data from the Build and Blood Pressure Study 1959 and Build Study 1979, respectively. The American Cancer Society Study examined data on body weight and longevity on about 750,000 adult males and females from 1959 to 1973. In this study, the lowest mortality rates occurred among nonsmokers weighing 80% to 89% of average weight.[24] Data from the first National Health and Nutrition Examination Survey show average weights for a representative sampling of the U.S. population between 1971 and 1974.

For a given stature, the weights defined by the Metropolitan tables as recommended were *less than the average* weights of the population under study. Although limitations with much of the existing data preclude a valid assessment of optimal weight, it appears that minimum mortality occurs at weights approximately 10% below the U.S. average.[24] Such terms as "ideal" or "desirable" were used to identify those weights, for a given stature, that were associated with greatest longevity or the least mortality from diabetes and diseases of the gallbladder, heart, kidneys, and blood.[17,23,24,29]

Another source of information about weight and height has come from the NCHS. Over the last several decades, the NCHS has collected weight, stature, and other health data on a representative sample of tens of thousands of Americans.[15] In formulating its height-weight tables, the NCHS has arbitrarily defined *overweight* and *severely overweight* persons as those at and above the 85th and 95th percentiles of weight for height, respectively. Those persons whose weight would rank them in the upper 15% to 5% were classified as overweight. Those whose weight would rank them in the very top 5% of weights for their sex and stature were considered severely overweight. In addition, the NCHS used the weights of persons 20 to 29 years of age as a reference, reasoning that weights at this age would be "desirable" for all subsequent ages.[15,17,20]

Age-Specific Weight Standards

Some researchers believe that weight in early adulthood should not be used as a standard of "desirable" or "healthy" weight throughout the remainder of life. They believe that data on body weight and morbidity and mortality suggest that overweight during early adult life is more dangerous than a similar degree of overweight in later adult life.[19] Some of the same researchers think that weight standards should be more liberal for older adults than for younger adults. To support

TABLE 6-1 1959 Metropolitan Life Insurance Company desirable weights for persons age 25 years and older (height without shoes, weight without clothing*)

Height		Small frame		Medium frame		Large frame	
in	cm	lb	kg	lb	kg	lb	kg
MEN							
61	155	105–113	48–51	111–122	50–55	119–134	54–61
62	157	108–116	49–53	114–126	52–57	122–137	55–62
63	160	111–119	50–54	117–129	53–59	125–141	57–64
64	163	114–122	52–55	120–132	55–60	128–145	58–66
65	165	117–126	53–57	123–136	56–62	131–149	60–68
66	168	121–130	55–59	127–140	58–64	135–154	61–70
67	170	125–134	57–61	131–145	60–66	140–159	64–72
68	173	129–138	59–63	135–149	61–68	144–163	65–74
69	175	133–143	60–65	139–153	63–70	148–167	67–76
70	178	137–147	62–67	143–158	65–72	152–172	69–78
71	180	141–151	64–68	147–163	67–74	157–177	71–80
72	183	145–155	66–70	151–168	69–76	161–182	73–83
73	185	149–160	68–73	155–173	70–79	166–187	75–85
74	188	153–164	70–75	160–178	73–81	171–192	78–87
75	191	157–168	71–76	165–183	75–83	175–197	80–90
WOMEN							
57	145	90–97	41–44	94–106	43–48	102–118	46–54
58	147	92–100	42–45	97–109	44–49	105–121	48–55
59	150	95–103	43–47	100–114	45–51	108–124	49–56
60	152	98–106	45–48	103–115	47–52	111–127	50–58
61	155	101–109	46–50	106–118	48–54	114–130	52–59
62	157	104–112	47–51	109–122	49–55	117–134	53–61
63	160	107–115	49–52	112–126	51–57	121–138	55–63
64	163	110–119	50–54	116–131	53–59	125–142	57–65
65	165	114–123	52–56	120–135	54–61	129–146	59–66
66	168	118–127	54–58	124–139	56–63	133–150	60–68
67	170	122–131	55–60	128–143	58–65	137–154	62–70
68	173	126–136	57–62	132–147	60–67	141–159	64–72
69	175	130–140	59–64	136–151	62–68	145–164	66–75
70	178	134–144	61–65	140–155	64–70	149–169	68–77

Adapted from Metropolitan Life Insurance Company. 1959. New weight standards for men and women, *Statistical Bulletin of the Metropolitan Life Insurance Company* 4:1–3. Courtesy of the Metropolitan Life Insurance Company.

*Height without shoes obtained by subtracting 1 in. and 2 in. from height with shoes for males and females, respectively. Weight without clothes obtained by subtracting 7 lb and 4 lb from weight with clothes for males and females, respectively.

TABLE 6-2 1983 Metropolitan Life Insurance Company height-weight table for persons age 25 to 59 years (height without shoes, weight without clothing*)

Height		Small frame		Medium frame		Large frame	
in	cm	lb	kg	lb	kg	lb	kg
MEN							
61	155	123–129	56–59	126–136	57–62	133–145	60–66
62	157	125–131	57–60	128–138	58–63	135–148	61–67
63	160	127–133	58–60	130–140	59–64	137–151	62–69
64	163	129–135	59–61	132–143	60–65	139–155	63–70
65	165	131–137	60–62	134–146	61–66	141–159	64–72
66	168	133–140	60–64	137–149	62–68	144–163	65–74
67	170	135–143	61–65	140–152	64–69	147–167	67–76
68	173	137–146	62–66	143–155	65–70	150–171	68–78
69	175	139–149	63–68	146–158	66–72	153–175	70–80
70	178	141–152	64–69	149–161	68–73	156–179	71–81
71	180	144–155	65–70	152–165	69–75	159–183	72–83
72	183	147–159	67–72	155–169	70–77	163–187	74–85
73	185	150–163	68–74	159–173	72–79	167–192	76–87
74	188	153–167	70–76	162–177	74–80	171–197	78–90
75	191	157–171	71–78	166–182	75–83	176–202	80–92
WOMEN							
57	145	99–108	45–49	106–118	48–54	115–128	52–58
58	147	100–110	45–50	108–120	49–55	117–131	53–60
59	150	101–112	46–51	110–123	50–56	119–134	54–61
60	152	103–115	47–52	112–126	51–57	122–137	55–62
61	155	105–118	48–54	115–129	52–59	125–140	57–64
62	157	108–121	49–55	118–132	54–60	128–144	58–65
63	160	111–124	50–56	121–135	55–61	131–148	60–67
64	163	114–127	52–58	124–138	56–63	134–152	61–69
65	165	117–130	53–59	127–141	58–64	137–156	62–71
66	168	120–133	55–60	130–144	59–65	140–160	64–73
67	170	123–136	56–62	133–147	60–67	143–164	65–75
68	173	126–139	57–63	136–150	62–68	146–167	66–76
69	175	129–142	59–65	139–153	63–70	149–170	68–77
70	178	132–145	60–66	142–156	65–71	152–173	69–79
71	180	135–148	61–67	145–159	66–72	155–176	70–80

Adapted from 1983 Metropolitan Height and Weight Tables. 1983. *Statistical Bulletin of the Metropolitan Life Insurance Company* 64 (Jan.–June):3. Courtesy of the Metropolitan Life Insurance Company.

*Height without shoes obtained by subtracting 1 in. from heights with shoes for males and females. Weight without clothes obtained by subtracting 5 lb and 3 lb from weight with clothes for males and females, respectively.

■ **TABLE 6-3** Comparison of Metropolitan desirable weights with average weights from U.S. cohorts

Height (without shoes), cm (ft, in.)	Metropolitan tables* (medium frame), weight in kilograms (pounds) (without clothing)		Average weight for age 40–49 yr, kg (lb)			
			Insured lives			
	1959	1983	Build and Blood Pressure Study 1959† (1935–1953)‡	Build Study 1979† (1950–1971)‡	American Cancer Society Study 1979§ (1959)‡	National Health and Nutrition Examination Survey (HNANES I, 1979)‖ (1971–1974)‡
Men						
156 (5 1)	50–55 (111–122)	57–62 (126–136)	60 (133)	61 (135)	—	—
159 (5 2)	52–57 (114–126)	58–63 (128–138)	62 (137)	63 (139)	67 (148)	66 (145)#
162 (5 3)	53–59 (117–129)	59–64 (130–140)	64 (141)	65 (144)	68 (149)	68 (150)#
164 (5 4)	54–60 (120–132)	60–65 (132–143)	66 (145)	68 (149)	69 (153)	73 (162)
167 (5 5)	56–62 (123–136)	61–66 (134–146)	68 (149)	69 (153)	71 (156)	72 (159)
169 (5 6)	58–64 (127–140)	62–68 (137–149)	70 (154)	72 (158)	73 (160)	75 (166)
172 (5 7)	59–66 (131–145)	64–69 (140–152)	72 (158)	73 (162)	74 (163)	78 (173)
174 (5 8)	61–68 (135–149)	65–70 (143–155)	73 (162)	76 (167)	77 (169)	79 (174)
177 (5 9)	63–69 (139–153)	66–72 (146–158)	76 (167)	78 (171)	78 (173)	79 (175)
179 (5 10)	65–72 (143–158)	68–73 (149–161)	78 (171)	80 (176)	80 (177)	83 (184)
182 (5 11)	67–74 (147–163)	69–75 (152–165)	80 (176)	82 (181)	83 (182)	85 (188)
185 (6 0)	68–76 (151–168)	70–77 (155–169)	82 (180)	85 (187)	85 (187)	88 (194)
187 (6 1)	70–78 (155–173)	72–78 (159–173)	84 (185)	87 (192)	87 (192)	92 (203)
190 (6 2)	73–81 (160–178)	73–80 (162–177)	86 (190)	90 (198)	90 (198)	92 (203)#
192 (6 3)	75–83 (165–183)	75–83 (166–182)	89 (196)	92 (203)	92 (203)#	—
Women						
146 (4 9)	43–48 (94–106)	48–54 (106–118)	54 (120)	52 (115)	—	58 (127)#
149 (4 10)	44–49 (97–109)	48–54 (106–120)	56 (123)	54 (118)	52 (115)	59 (131)#
151 (4 11)	45–51 (100–112)	50–56 (110–123)	57 (126)	54 (120)	55 (121)	62 (136)
154 (5 0)	47–52 (103–115)	51–57 (112–126)	59 (129)	56 (124)	57 (126)	64 (141)
156 (5 1)	48–54 (106–118)	52–59 (115–129)	60 (132)	57 (126)	58 (128)	63 (138)
159 (5 2)	49–55 (109–122)	54–60 (118–132)	62 (136)	59 (130)	60 (132)	64 (141)
162 (5 3)	51–57 (112–126)	55–61 (121–135)	63 (139)	60 (133)	62 (136)	67 (148)
164 (5 4)	53–59 (116–131)	56–63 (124–138)	65 (143)	62 (136)	63 (139)	68 (151)
167 (5 5)	54–61 (120–135)	58–64 (127–141)	67 (147)	64 (140)	64 (142)	71 (156)
169 (5 6)	56–63 (124–139)	59–65 (130–144)	68 (151)	65 (144)	66 (146)	71 (156)
172 (5 7)	58–65 (128–143)	60–67 (133–147)	70 (155)	67 (147)	68 (150)	72 (158)
174 (5 8)	60–67 (132–147)	62–68 (136–150)	73 (160)	70 (152)	71 (156)	78 (172)
177 (5 9)	62–68 (136–151)	63–69 (139–153)	75 (165)	70 (155)	73 (161)	—
179 (5 10)	64–70 (140–155)	64–71 (142–156)	77 (170)	72 (159)	75 (165)	—

Used with permission from Manson JE, Stampfer MJ, Henniker CH, and Willett WC. 1987. Body weight and longevity: A reassessment. *Journal of the American Medical Association* 257:353–358. Copyright 1987, American Medical Association.

*Not age specific: 1959 tables recommended for ages 25 years and older, 1983 tables for ages 25 to 59 years.

†Without shoes or clothing.

‡Years when measurements were taken.

§Values are means for age groups 40 to 44 years and 45 to 49 years. Self-reported heights without shoes and weights with indoor clothing.

‖Values are means for age groups 35 to 44 years and 45 to 54 years. Measured without shoes; clothing ranged from 0.20 to 0.62 lb (not deducted from weights shown).

#Estimated values obtained from linear regression equations.

TABLE 6-4 Suggested weights for adults

Height* (in)	Weight (lb) † 19 to 34 years	35 years and older
60	97–128‡	108–138
61	101–132	111–143
62	104–137	115–148
63	107–141	119–152
64	111–146	122–157
65	114–150	126–162
66	118–155	130–167
67	121–160	134–172
68	125–164	138–178
69	129–169	142–183
70	132–174	146–188
71	136–179	151–194
72	140–184	155–199
73	144–189	159–205
74	148–195	164–210
75	152–200	168–216
76	156–205	173–222
77	160–211	177–228
78	164–216	182–234

Nutrition and your health: Dietary guidelines for Americans, ed 3, US Department of Agriculture and US Department of Health and Human Services, 1990.

*Without shoes.

†Without clothes.

‡The higher weights in the ranges generally apply to men, who tend to have more muscle and bone; the lower weights more often apply to women, who have less muscle and bone.

this view, they cite statistics showing that as people age from their 20s to their 60s, the body weight associated with lowest mortality tends to increase about 4.5 kg or 10 lb per decade.[20,30,31]

Table 6-4 shows the height-weight table published in the 1990 revision of the *Dietary Guidelines for Americans.* Note that the suggested weights are considered applicable to both male and female adults and no reference is made to frame size. Also unique is the greater allowable weight range for persons 35 years of age or older compared with those 19 to 34 years old. This represents a substantial increase over earlier weight recommendations. For example, compare the upper weight limit for a 68-in. female from Table 6-4 with the upper weight limit for a 68-in. female with medium frame from the 1959 Metropolitan table (Table 6-1). The maximum suggested weight from the 1990 *Dietary Guidelines for Americans* allows this person to weigh 17 lb more (if age 19 to 34 years) and 31 lb more (if 35 years or older) than the 1959 Metropolitan table. The appropriateness of higher allowable weights for older persons is discussed in the next section.

Limitations of Height-Weight Tables

Height-weight tables have several limitations, which are summarized in Box 6-1.[14,21,24,29] Because tables are formulated from data drawn from specific groups or populations, they may not be applicable to other groups or populations. This is especially true of tables based on insurance industry data, which are derived from people who apply for life insurance—predominantly white, middle-class adults. African Americans, Asians, Native Americans, Hispanics, and low-income persons are not proportionally represented.[11]

The quality of the data on height and weight is variable.[14] The same care in obtaining the NHANES data was not used in collecting data for the Metropolitan tables, where approximately 10% of the heights and weights were self-reported. Self-reporting of height and weight has been shown to be inaccurate, and the error is influenced by such factors as sex, actual height, and actual weight.[32–34] Rowland,[33] for example, showed that errors in self-reported weight were directly related to a person's overweight status and increased directly with the magnitude of overweight. The frequency of overreporting height increases with increasing height and is more common in males than females.[35]

There is often inadequate documentation and control of certain variables known to confound

BOX 6-1

Strengths and Limitations of Height-Weight Tables

Strengths

Weight is an important distinguishing feature of identification.

Weight and height can be accurately measured.

Height-weight tables are easily understood and used by many.

Height-weight tables are a part of our culture.

Limitations

The data upon which height-weight tables are based are not representative of the entire population.

Quality of the data is variable.

Some of the data are cross-sectional and do not allow associations between weight and mortality to be drawn.

There is inadequate control of potential confounding variables, especially smoking.

It is not always clear how frame size was determined.

Tables do not provide information on body composition.

the relationships between weight and mortality.[14,24] Most important among these confounding variables is cigarette smoking. Smokers tend to weigh less than nonsmokers but have higher mortality rates because of smoking-related diseases. Including data on smokers in height-weight tables tends to make lower weights appear less healthy and higher weights appear more healthy.[18,20,36] Because the 1959 Metropolitan tables are less affected by the cumulative exposure to smoking among Americans than are the 1983 tables, many authorities believe the 1959 tables are more valid than and should be used in preference to the more liberal 1983 tables.[24,36,37]

People with serious chronic or acute disease are likely to be refused life insurance. Many of these diseases (for example, hypertension, coronary heart disease, and diabetes) are related to obesity, and exclusion of these individuals from actuarial data, again, results in bias toward higher apparent optimal weights.[36]

There have been problems associated with frame measurements.[21,29] The 1959 Metropolitan tables never defined how frame size was determined. The frame size measurements used in the 1983 Metropolitan tables are based on NHANES I and NHANES II data and are so devised that 25% of the population is classified as having a small frame, 50% as having a medium frame, and 25% as having a large frame. Within the range of body weights considered acceptable for a given height and sex, the lower end of the weight range was assumed to be for small-framed persons, the middle of the range for medium-framed persons, and the upper end of the range for large-framed persons. This practice may not be appropriate because data on height/weight and frame size were obtained from two distinct population groups.[21]

The weight measurements used in compiling the data were only those taken when the subjects initially applied for life insurance.[29] If weight changed between issuance of the policy and death, this was not taken into account. Age also was not taken into account.[20,21]

Finally, weight tables fail to provide information on actual body composition—the proportions of fat and lean tissue—or on the distribution of body fat.[21] This is a critical weakness because the quantity of weight (a person's actual weight) is considerably less important than the quality of weight (how much of that weight is fat and how much is lean tissue). An unusually muscular person with a low body fat content (for example, a football player or weight lifter) may be overweight according to a height-weight table but not obese.[15,38,39] Body composition can be estimated from measurements of skinfolds, densitometry (hydrostatic or underwater weighing), and other methods discussed later in this chapter.

The more liberal suggested weights for older persons have been called into question by several leading authorities on the health consequences of obesity and overweight.[36,40] Based on the limitations of height-weight tables, Willett and coworkers[36] regard the height-weight standards in the 1990 revision of the *Dietary Guidelines for Americans* as "fundamentally invalid" and state that there is "no biologic rationale for recommending that persons increase their weight as they grow older; indeed, there is much evidence to the contrary." The height-weight standards suggest an average weight gain of approximately 16 lb between early and later adulthood. A weight gain of this magnitude has been shown to be associated with a 50% increase in risk of diabetes and a 30% increase in coronary heart disease risk.[41,42] Higher blood pressure and lower concentrations of high-density lipoprotein also would likely result. The researchers suggest that the only probable benefit would be increased bone density and reduced risk of hip fracture.[36] In the study of nearly 9000 nonsmoking, nondrinking men mentioned earlier, there was no evidence for a "J-shaped" relationship between BMI and mortality in these males. Although the protective effect associated with a lower BMI decreased somewhat with increasing age, persons with a lower BMI still had a lower risk of death than persons with a higher BMI at all ages.[22]

Although all the major height-weight tables are biased toward higher-than-optimal weights, Willett et al.[36] state that "the 1959 Metropolitan Life tables are probably least biased because the distorting impact of cigarette smoking was less at this earlier period."

Strengths of Height-Weight Table

Despite these limitations, height-weight tables have some definite strengths.[14] Body weight is an important concept, and next to age, sex, and race, it is regarded as the most distinguishing feature of identification. Height and weight are easily measured, and most adults and many adolescents and children are able to understand and use height-weight tables. The tables have become ingrained in the medical and nonmedical culture of North America.[14]

Thus, although height-weight tables have their shortcomings, they are useful as a health education tool but should be regarded as only a rough guide in helping persons determine in what range their weight should fall.[18,29]

MEASURING FRAME SIZE

The classification of subjects on the basis of frame size has been a common feature of the Metropolitan height-weight tables. However, it was not until the 1983 tables that a technique for determining frame size (elbow breadth) was even specified. Additionally, the data on which the 1983 tables were based included no physical measurements of frame size.[17] In preparing the Metropolitan tables, classification of frame size apparently relied as much on subject self-appraisal as on any other method.[43]

Several approaches to determining frame size have been proposed,[44] including biacromial breadth (distance between the tips of the biacromial processes at the top of the shoulders) and bitrochanteric breadth (distance between the most lateral projections of the greater trochanter of the two femurs),[43,45–47] the ratio of stature to wrist circumference,[48] breadth of the chest based on chest x-rays,[49] knee and wrist breadth,[50] and elbow breadth.[51] Measuring elbow breadth appears to be the most practical way of determining frame size and was taken into consideration when the 1983 Metropolitan tables were developed.[17,43,44,51] The other methods are limited by

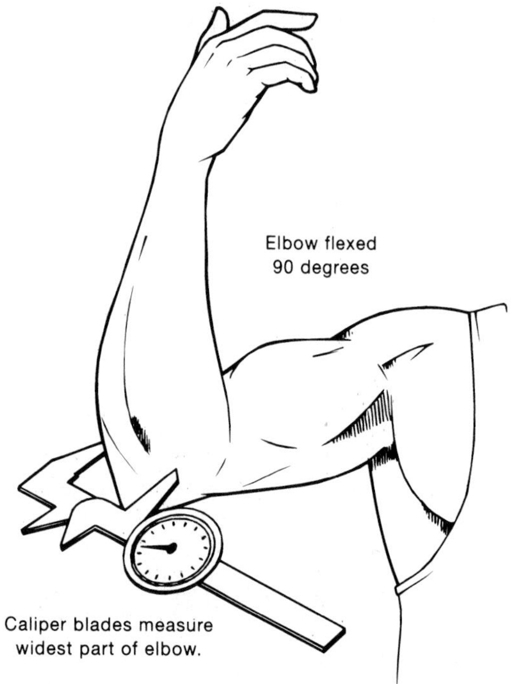

Figure 6-9 Elbow breadth is sometimes used for determining frame size. With the arm and hand in this position, a sliding caliper can be used to measure the widest point at the elbow.

such factors as lack of population norms, difficulty in obtaining measurements, and the influence of adiposity.[17,29,43]

When measuring elbow breadth, the subject stands erectly, with the right upper arm extended forward perpendicular to the body, as shown in Figure 6-9. The forearm is then flexed until the elbow forms a 90-degree angle, with fingers up, palm facing the subject. The measurer then should feel for the widest bony width of the elbow and place the heads of a flat-blade sliding caliper at those points. Pressure should be firm enough to compress soft tissues. The measurement should be read to the nearest 0.1 cm or ⅛ in.[45] A low-cost plastic caliper for measuring elbow breadth is available from the Metropolitan Life Insurance Company, Health and Safety Division, One Madison Avenue, New York, New York 10010. Elbow breadth classifications for males and females of various stature are given in Table 6-5. Some data suggest that frame measurements do not materially improve the ability to predict body fat from body weight.[50,52] Other researchers suggest avoiding frame-adjusted tables because of the lack of data on the relationship of frame size to body weight.[20]

The following formula can be used to determine frame size from the ratio of body height to wrist circumference,[48]

$$r = \frac{H}{C}$$

where r = the ratio of body height to wrist circumference; H = body height in centimeters; and C = circumference of the right wrist in centimeters. Compare the value for r with those in Table 6-6 to determine frame size.[48]

To measure the right wrist circumference, the arm should be flexed at the elbow with the palm facing upward and the hand muscles relaxed. Place the measuring tape around the wrist crease just distal to (beyond) the styloid processes of the radius and ulna (the two bony prominences at the wrist). The measuring tape must be no wider than 0.7 cm so that it can fit into the depressions between the styloid processes and the bones of the hand. The tape should be perpendicular to the long axis of the forearm. The tape should be touching the skin but not compressing the soft tissues. Record the measurement to the nearest 0.1 cm.[53]

HEIGHT-WEIGHT INDICES

In view of the shortcomings of height-weight tables, particularly their inability to provide information on actual body composition, investigators have sought better approaches to assessing body weight and fatness that can be derived from easily obtainable anthropometric measures such as weight and stature.[54] This has led to the development of various height-weight indices or body mass indices, the most common of which are shown in Table 6-7. An index is simply a ratio of one dimension (e.g., weight) to another dimension (e.g., height). The height-weight indices are of two types: relative weight and the power-type indices.[55]

TABLE 6-5 Elbow breadth classifications for males and females of various stature

Height*		Small frame		Medium frame		Large frame	
in	cm	in	mm	in	mm	in	mm
Males							
61–62	155–158	<2½	<64	2½–2⅞	64–73	>2⅞	>73
63–66	159–168	<2⅝	<67	2⅝–2⅞	67–73	>2⅞	>73
67–70	169–178	<2¾	<70	2¾–3	70–76	>3	>76
71–74	179–188	<2¾	<70	2¾–3⅛	70–90	>3⅛	>79
≥75	≥189	<2⅞	<73	2⅞–3¼	73–83	>3¼	>83
Females							
57–58	145–148	<2¼	<57	2¼–2½	57–64	>2½	>64
59–62	149–158	<2¼	<57	2¼–2½	57–64	>2½	>64
63–66	159–168	<2⅜	<60	2⅜–2⅝	60–67	>2⅝	>67
67–70	169–178	<2⅜	<60	2⅜–2⅝	60–67	>2⅝	>67
≥71	≥179	<2½	<64	2½–2¾	64–70	>2¾	>70

Courtesy of the Metropolitan Life Insurance Company.

*Table adapted to represent height without shoes.

TABLE 6-6 Determining frame size from the ratio of body height to the circumference of the right wrist

Frame size	r Value	
	Women	Men
Small	>10.9	>10.4
Medium	10.9–9.9	10.4–9.6
Large	<9.9	<9.6

Adapted from Grant JP, Custer PB, Thurlow J. 1981. Current techniques of nutritional assessment. *Surgical Clinics of North America* 61:437–463.

Relative Weight

Relative weight is a person's *actual weight* divided by some *reference weight* for that person's height and multiplied by 100 so that it can be expressed as a percentage. The Framingham Heart Study, for example, used an index called Metropolitan relative weight, which uses as its reference weight the midpoint of the "desirable" weight range for a person of medium frame as given in the 1959 Metropolitan tables.[17,18]

To calculate the Metropolitan relative weight (MRW), take as an example a 35-year-old male whose stature is 70 in or 179 cm and who weighs 181 lb or 82 kg. The midpoint of the weight range for a 70-in person with a medium frame from the 1959 Metropolitan height-weight table would be 151 lb or 69 kg. The MRW for this person would be calculated as follows:

$$\frac{181\text{ lb (actual weight)}}{151\text{ lb (reference weight)}} \times 100 = 120\%\text{ MRW}$$

Thus this man's MRW is 120%, or his weight is 20% greater than the reference weight. Depending as it does on height-weight tables, relative weight is subject to the same limitations of height-weight tables discussed previously. A relative weight within the range of 90% to 120% is generally considered acceptable.

Power-Type Indices

Of the several power-type indices available (Table 6-7), authorities disagree on the preferred one to use for assessing obesity among adults. Most investigators agree that the preferred index should be maximally correlated with body mass

TABLE 6-7 Height-weight indices*

Relative weight:	$\frac{\text{Actual weight}}{\text{Reference weight}} \times 100$
Weight/height ratio:	$\frac{\text{Weight}}{\text{Height}}$
Quetelet's index:	$\frac{\text{Weight}}{\text{Height}^2}$
Khosla-Lowe index:	$\frac{\text{Weight}}{\text{Height}^3}$
Ponderal index:	$\frac{\text{Height}}{\text{Weight}^{1/3}}$
Benn's index:†	$\frac{\text{Weight}}{\text{Height}^p}$

Data from Lee J, Kolonel LN, and Hinds MW. 1981. Relative merits of the weight-corrected-for-height indices. *American Journal of Clinical Nutrition* 34:2521–2529.

*The numerical values of the indices depend on the values used (for example, kilograms and meters or pounds and inches).

†"p" is a population-specific exponent derived from height-weight data of the population sample. Consequently, its value changes from sample to sample.

(weight) and should be minimally correlated with stature. In other words, it should be equally good at indicating body mass no matter how tall or short a person is.[56] However, some researchers question this qualification.[52] Much of the debate has centered around the Quetelet's index (W/H^2) and Benn's index (W/H^p).[56–59] The argument has primarily dealt with the degree that the two indices are influenced by stature and how important this may be, and how well body mass index correlates with estimates of body fatness.

Quetelet's Index

The most widely used height-weight index is the **Quetelet's index** (W/H^2), which is more commonly known as **body mass index BMI.**[18,21,59,60] Because all the power-type indices are body mass indices, the more technically correct name for W/H^2 is Quetelet's index. Quetelet's index is obtained by dividing weight in kilograms by height in meters squared. Consider a male weighing 70 kg (154 lb) and standing 178 cm or 1.78 m (70 in) tall. His body mass index would be:

$$\frac{70 \text{ kg (weight in kilograms)}}{3.17 \text{ m}^2 \text{ (height in meters squared)}} = 22 \text{ kg/m}^2$$

Body mass index has a relatively high correlation with estimates of body fatness and a low correlation with stature.[18,21] Garrow and Webster,[59] for example, showed that Quetelet's index correlated well with estimates of body composition from three methods—body density, total body water, and total body potassium (these will be discussed later in this chapter)—and concluded that Quetelet's index "is both a convenient and reliable indicator of obesity." The National Institutes of Health[21] has recommended that physicians use Quetelet's index in evaluating patients. Roche and coworkers[61] have found Quetelet's index to be the best single indicator of total body fat in girls and adults and the best single indicator of percent body fat in men. Of the other height-weight indices, Quetelet's index has shown the closest correlation with estimates of body fatness by skinfold measurements and densitometry.[62,63]

Frisancho and Flegel[64] have shown Quetelet's index to correlate well with estimates of body fatness based on skinfold measurements, and they recommend combining Quetelet's index with skinfold measurements whenever possible. Investigators have suggested combining Quetelet's index with the rather easily obtained waist-to-hip ratio (the circumference measurement of the waist divided by the circumference measurement of the hips, discussed later in this chapter) as an improved means of assessing risk for heart disease, stroke, diabetes mellitus, and premature death.[65,66]

A **nomogram** for determining Quetelet's index is shown in Figure 6-10. To use the nomogram, place a straightedge on the point of the height scale that corresponds to height in centimeters or inches and on the point of the weight scale that

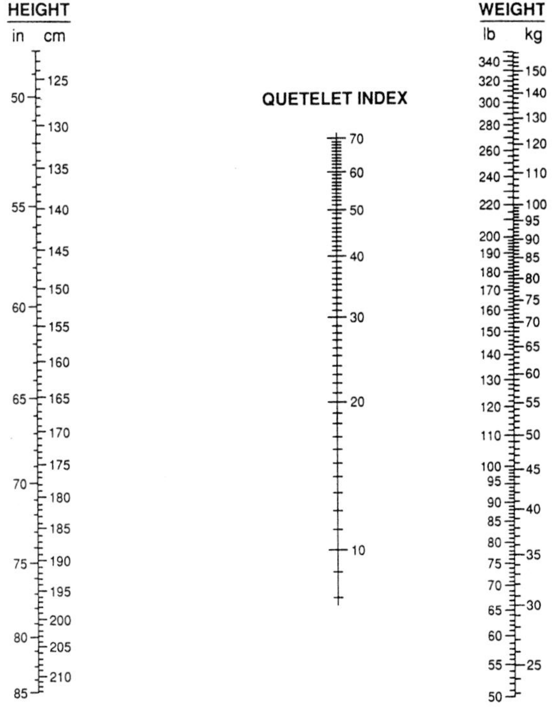

Figure 6-10 The Quetelet index (kg/m²) is calculated from this nomogram by placing a straightedge on the measurements for height and body weight and reading the point at which the straightedge intersects the central scale. Adapted with permission from Nieman DC. 1995. *Fitness and sports medicine: A health-related approach,* ed 3. Palo Alto: Bull Publishing Co.

TABLE 6-8 Recommended classifications of body mass for adults using Quetelet's index

Quetelet's index (kg/m²)	Classification
<16	Too lean (may indicate an eating disorder)
16–19.9	Lean, underweight
20–24.9	Desirable
25–29.9	Grade I obesity
30–40	Grade II obesity
>40	Grade III obesity

Data from Jéquier E. 1987. Energy, obesity, and body weight standards. *American Journal of Clinical Nutrition* 45:1035–1047.

corresponds to weight in kilograms or pounds. Then read the Quetelet's index on the center scale. Use nomograms with caution. In some publications, nomograms may be inadvertently modified and thus rendered inaccurate.[67] This occurred in two highly respected reports: *The Surgeon General's Report on Nutrition and Health* and the National Research Council's *Diet and Health.* Recommended classifications of body mass using Quetelet's index adapted from The Panel on Energy, Obesity, and Body Weight Standards are shown in Table 6-8.[68] Several studies have shown a Quetelet's index of between 20 and 25 kg/m² to be associated with the least mortality. Above 25 kg/m² mortality and morbidity slowly increase, but above 30 kg/m², there is a rapid increase in mortality.[52] A BMI $<$ 20 kg/m² is considered underweight or lean, and a BMI 16 kg/m² is indicative of a possible eating disorder.

An alternate equation for calculating body mass index is shown below. You may find this one easier to use than the conventional formula. In this equation, lb = weight in lb; in. = height in inches.

$$\text{BMI (kg/m}^2\text{)} = \text{lb} \div \text{in.} \div \text{in.} \div 0.0014192$$

How do the BMIs of Americans compare with these standards? Table 6-9 shows mean BMIs of Americans based on four different national surveys; NHES I, NHANES I, NHANES II, and NHANES III. Using 25 kg/m² as the point above which morbidity and mortality increase, it can be seen that the mean BMI for Americans age 20 to 74 years has been above this point since NHANES I was conducted between 1971 and 1974. Looking at the NHANES III column it can be seen that mean BMIs are greater than 25 kg/m² for every age group except 20 to 29 years. Again, this illustrates the concept that "average" is not necessarily acceptable or healthy.[69]

Although height-weight indices tend to be better predictors of obesity than height-weight

TABLE 6-9 Mean body mass index for Americans age 20 to 74 years from 1960 to 1991 by race, sex, and age

Population group	NHES I (1960–62)	NHANES I (1971–74)	NHANES II (1976–80)	NHANES III (1988–91)
Age 20 to 74 years	24.8	25.2	25.3	26.3
White males	25.1	25.6	25.5	26.3
White females	24.4	24.6	24.8	26.1
Black males	24.8	25.7	25.5	26.6
Black females	26.8	27.3	27.5	28.3
Males				
20–74 years	25.0	25.5	25.5	26.3
20–29 years	24.3	24.5	24.3	24.9
30–39 years	25.2	26.1	25.6	26.1
40–49 years	25.6	26.2	26.4	27.3
50–59 years	25.6	26.0	26.2	27.6
60–74 years	24.9	25.4	25.7	26.9
Females				
20–74 years	24.7	24.9	25.1	26.3
20–29 years	22.2	23.0	23.2	24.1
30–39 years	24.1	24.7	24.9	24.4
40–49 years	25.2	25.7	25.7	26.7
50–59 years	26.4	26.2	26.5	28.5
60–74 years	27.2	26.5	26.5	27.2

Data from Kuczmarski RJ, Flegal KM, Campbell SM, Johnson CL. 1994. Increasing prevalence of overweight among US adults. *Journal of the American Medical Association* 272:205–211.

NHES = National Health Examination Survey; NHANES = National Health and Nutrition Examination Survey

tables or relative weight (they are more closely associated with percent of body fat than height-weight tables or relative weight), they still do not distinguish between overweight resulting from obesity and that resulting from muscular development. This requires the use of indirect and direct measurements of body composition such as densitometry, total body water, and total body potassium. These measurements and the concept of body composition are discussed in the next sections.

BODY FAT DISTRIBUTION

Body fat distribution is an important concept in considering the health implications of obesity.[16] Where fat is placed or distributed within the body may actually be more important than quantity of body fat. Body fat distribution can be classified into two types: upper body, android, or male type; and lower body, gynoid, or female type.[16] Obese persons having a greater proportion of fat within the upper body, especially within the abdomen, compared with that within the hips and thighs, have **android obesity**. Obese persons with most of their fat within the hips and thighs have **gynoid obesity**. Android obesity is generally (but not always) seen in obese males, whereas females generally carry a greater proportion of their body fat on the hips and thighs.[16]

Numerous studies have shown that risk of insulin resistance, hyperinsulinemia (elevated blood insulin levels), noninsulin-dependent (Type II) diabetes mellitus, hypertension, hyperlipidemia (elevated blood cholesterol and triglyceride levels), and stroke, as well as risk of death are increased in persons with android obesity. Although the approaches used to assess fat distribution varied somewhat among these studies, they consistently showed that disease risk is associated with upper-body placement of body fat.[16,70] They also showed that fat distribution is a more important risk factor for morbidity and mortality than obesity per se.[16,71] In obese adolescent females, android obesity tends to be associated with elevated levels of triglyceride, serum cholesterol, and low-density lipoprotein (LDL) cholesterol. Android obesity in adolescent males tends to be associated with lower levels of high-density lipoprotein (HDL) cholesterol, a higher ratio of total cholesterol to HDL-cholesterol, and higher levels of LDL cholesterol.[72]

Waist-to-Hip Ratio

Determining the ratio of the waist or abdominal circumference to the hip or gluteal circumference is an easy way to assess body fat distribution. The **waist-to-hip ratio (WHR)** provides an index of regional body fat distribution and is a valuable guide in assessing health risk.[16]

The waist circumference is measured at the most narrow area below the rib cage and above the umbilicus as viewed from the front.[29,53] The subject stands erectly, abdominal muscles relaxed, arms at the side, and feet together. The measurer faces the subject and places an inelastic, flexible tape measure in a horizontal plane and measures the area of least circumference. If there is no apparent area of least circumference, the measurement should be taken at the level of the umbilicus. The measurement should be taken at the end of a normal expiration.[53]

The hip circumference is the point of greatest circumference around the hips or buttocks with the subject standing.[16,29,53] The measurer should squat beside the subject to see the maximum extension of the buttocks. The tape should be placed in a horizontal plane around the hips at the point of greatest circumference, and the measurement should be taken with the tape in close contact with the skin but without indenting the soft tissues. The measurement should be recorded to the nearest 0.1 cm.[53]

In taking both measurements, an assistant may be necessary to help properly position the tape in a horizontal plane. Measurements should not be taken over street clothing. The subject should be undressed to light underwear to allow proper positioning of the tape and should wear a gown or smock.[53]

The WHR is calculated by dividing the waist circumference by the hip circumference. A nomogram for easily determining the WHR (sometimes called the abdominal-to-gluteal ratio, or AGR) is shown in Figure 6-11. As previously noted, nomograms should be used with caution.[67] Figure 6-12 shows preliminary norms for the WHR in males and females based on age. The risk of disease rises steeply when the WHR rises above 0.9 in males and above 0.8 in females.

BODY COMPOSITION

Interest in human body composition has grown over the past several decades, largely because obesity has been associated with such diseases as diabetes mellitus, hypertension, and coronary heart disease.[21,73,74] Overweight is one of the most prevalent diet-related problems in the United States. As shown in Figure 6-13, the prevalence of overweight among Americans has been increasing in recent decades. For example, during the interval between NHANES II (1976–1980) and Phase 1 of NHANES III (1988–1991), the prevalence of overweight increased 8%. During this interval, mean body weight for males and females age 20 to 74 years increased 8 lb (3.6 kg). Based on 1990 population estimates, approximately 58 million Americans are currently overweight (26 million men and 32 million women). It is unlikely that this increase is due to methodologic or procedural artifacts in measuring height and weight.[69]

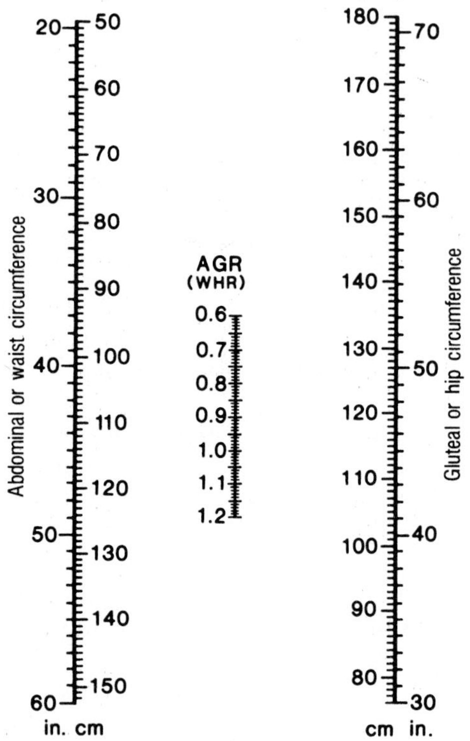

Figure 6-11 The abdominal (waist) to gluteal (hip) ratio (AGR or WHR) can be determined by placing a straightedge on the measurement for waist circumference and the measurement for hip circumference and reading the ratio from the point where this straightedge crosses the AGR or WHR line. The waist or abdominal circumference is the smallest circumference below the rib cage and above the umbilicus, and the hip or gluteal circumference is taken as the largest circumference at the posterior extension of the buttocks. From Bray GA, Gray DS. 1988. Obesity, part I: Pathogenesis. *Western Medical Journal* 149:429–441.

Figure 6-14 compares the prevalence of overweight between 1976 and 1991 among Americans adults based on sex, race, and Hispanic origin. Among Americans 12 to 19 years of age, 20% of males and 22% of females are considered overweight (Figure 6-15).[75] Measurements of body fat are important in studying the nature of obesity and the obese person's response to treatment.[4,65] As previously mentioned, the percent of body fat, as well as its placement, can have profound effects on health.[17,65,76]

Estimating fat and protein reserves is a common practice in assessing a patient's nutritional status. During nutritional deprivation, these stores are depleted, leading to increased morbidity and mortality caused at least in part by nutrition-related impairment of the body's immune system.[77,78] Simple techniques to screen fat and protein reserves of patients are critical in the light of reports that malnutrition is seen in as many as half of all hospitalized patients in the United States, Canada, and other industrialized countries.[79,80,81]

Body composition can be an important factor in certain athletic events. For example, carrying excess fat can be detrimental to the performance of runners and gymnasts. Body composition measurements can help these athletes maintain body fat at levels that are neither too high nor too low.[4] Too low a percent body fat can adversely affect metabolism and health. Female athletes will experience oligomenorrhea and amenorrhea when their percent body fat is too low. This, in turn, can result in bone demineralization and increased risk of osteoporosis and bone fractures. Inadequate body fat may indicate disease, starvation, or an eating disorder such as anorexia nervosa.

The perspective that the body consists of two chemically distinct compartments forms the model on which most body composition methods are based.[82] In the two-compartment model, the body can be divided into fat mass and fat-free mass, or, according to an alternative approach, into adipose tissue and lean body mass. In the former view, developed by Keys and Brozek,[83] the fat mass includes all the solvent-extractable lipids contained in both adipose tissue and other tissues, and the residual is the fat-free mass. The fat-free mass is composed of muscle, water, bone, and other tissues devoid of fat and lipid. For example, the solvent ether could be used to extract all the fat and lipid from a minced animal carcass. That remaining after all the fat and lipid were extracted would be the fat-free mass. The lean body

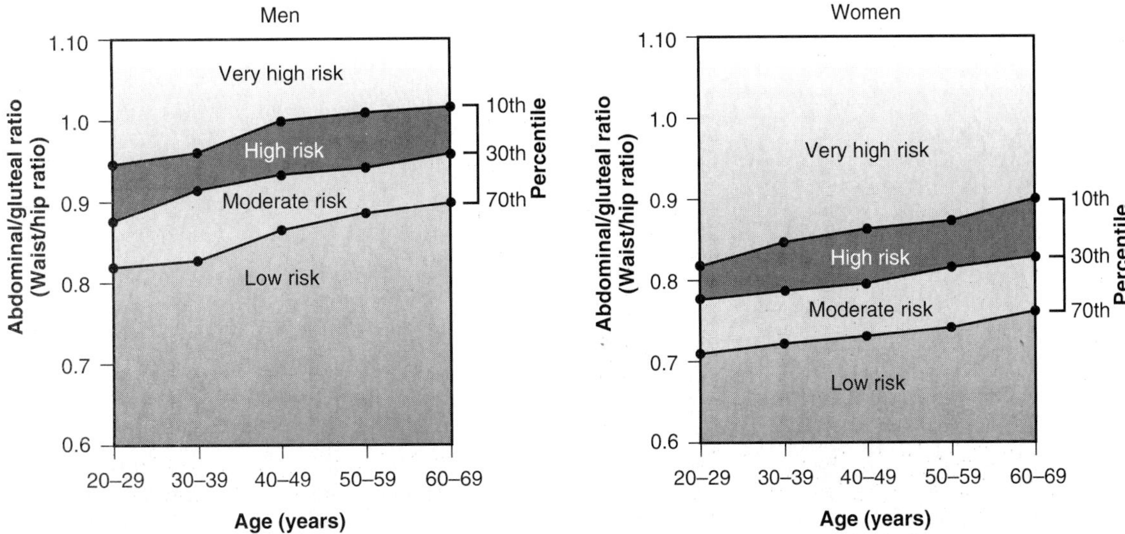

Figure 6-12 The percentage of males (left) and females (right) at risk for disease based on their waist to hip ratios or abdominal to gluteal ratios. From Bray GA, Gray DS, 1988. Obesity, part I: Pathogenesis. *Western Medical Journal* 149:429–441.

mass of the latter approach is similar to the fat-free mass except that lean body mass includes a small amount of lipid that our bodies must have—for example, lipid that serves as a structural component of cell membranes or lipid contained in the nervous system.[84] This essential lipid constitutes about 1.5% to 3% of the weight of the lean body.

Body composition often is defined as the *ratio of fat to fat-free mass* and frequently is expressed as a percentage of body fat.[4,29] Adipose tissue contains about 14% water, is nearly 100% free of the electrolyte potassium, and is assumed to have a density of 0.90 g/cm^3.[4,82] The less homogenous *fat-free compartment* is primarily composed of bone, muscle, other fat-free tissue, and body water. Its chemical composition is assumed to be relatively constant, with a water content of 72% to 74%, a potassium content of 60 to 70 mmol/kg in males and 50 to 60 mmol/kg in females, and a density of 1.10 g/cm^3 at normal body temperature.[82] However, several factors can affect the density of the fat-free compartment. Among these are age (the fat-free compartment in children is less dense than that of middle-aged persons, and bone density is decreased in elderly persons, especially those with osteoporosis), the degree of fitness (athletes have denser bone and muscle), and the body's state of hydration.[4] The use of anthropometry (measures of skinfold thicknesses, bone dimensions, and limb circumferences), determination of whole-body density (most commonly by underwater weighing), electrical conductance and impedance, and other methods to estimate body composition are based on the two-compartment model.[82]

An alternative approach to the two-compartment model is the four-compartment model, which views the human body as composed of four chemical groups: water, protein, mineral, and fat.[82] Methods for estimating body composition based on the four-compartment model include neutron activation analysis, isotope dilution techniques, bioelectrical impedance, total body electrical conductivity, and absorptiometry.[82]

A variety of methods exist for estimating body composition, and each has its strengths and limitations. Except for cadaveric studies, all of the following techniques are *indirect* measures.

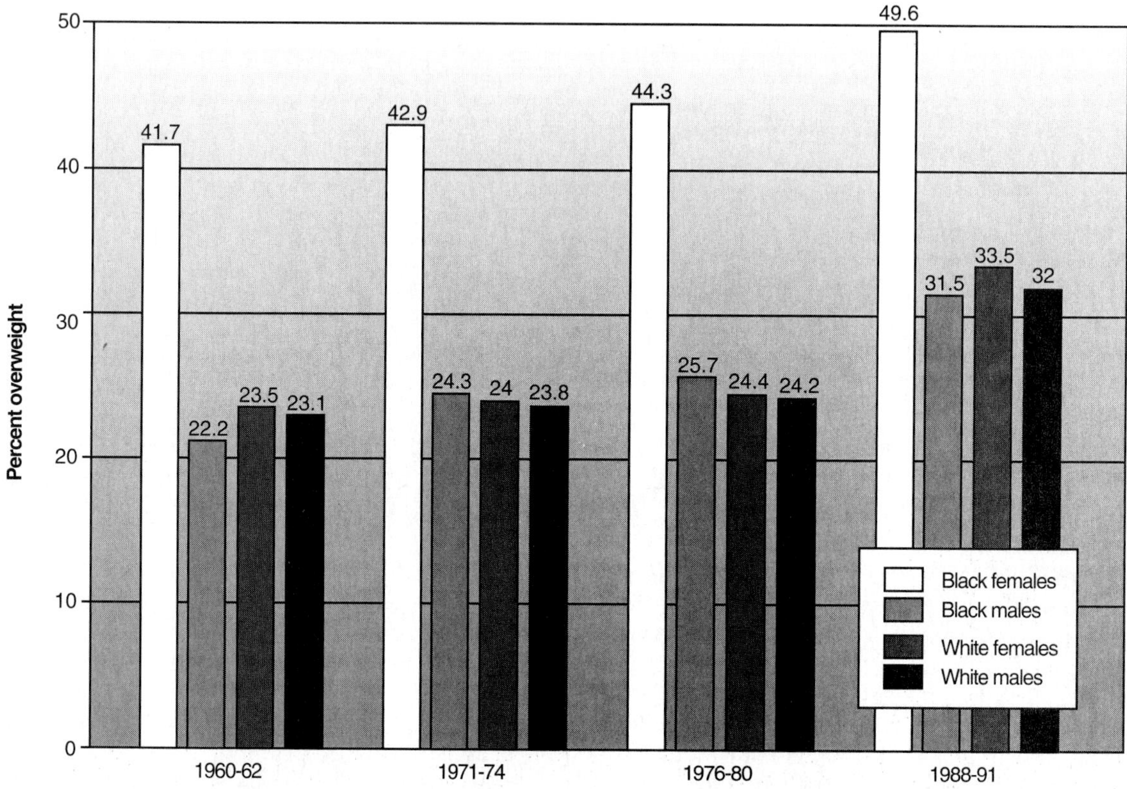

Figure 6-13 One out of every three American adults is considered overweight. In recent decades, the prevalence of overweight among Americans has increased. Overweight is defined as a body mass index ≥ 27.8 kg/m² and ≥ 27.3 kg/m² for males and females, respectively. These values represent the sex-specific 85th percentiles for persons 20 to 29 years of age in NHANES II. Data from the National Center for Health Statistics.

CADAVERIC STUDIES

Only by analyzing cadavers can direct measurement of human body composition be made.[4] The most comprehensive direct study of body composition was the Brussels Cadaver Analysis Study (CAS) in which more than 30 cadavers were studied from 1979 to 1983.[85] The CAS helped validate various in vivo methods for estimating body composition and collected data for developing new anthropometric models for determining body composition.[85] Recumbent length, hydrostatic (underwater) weight, numerous girths and breadths, and skin surface area were measured. Skinfolds were measured at 14 standard sites. The skin and subcutaneous tissue then were cut open and carefully measured so that skinfold measurements could be directly compared with measurements of skin and subcutaneous adipose tissue thickness. The skin, adipose tissue, skeletal muscle, bone, and viscera were dissected out and weighed in air and under water to determine density of the organs and tissues. The CAS allowed examination of several assumptions underlying the use of skinfold measurements and hydrostatic weighing to determine body composition, which will be discussed in later sections. A major assumption of the CAS was that anthropometric measures and body composition in cadavers were similar to those of living subjects.[85,86]

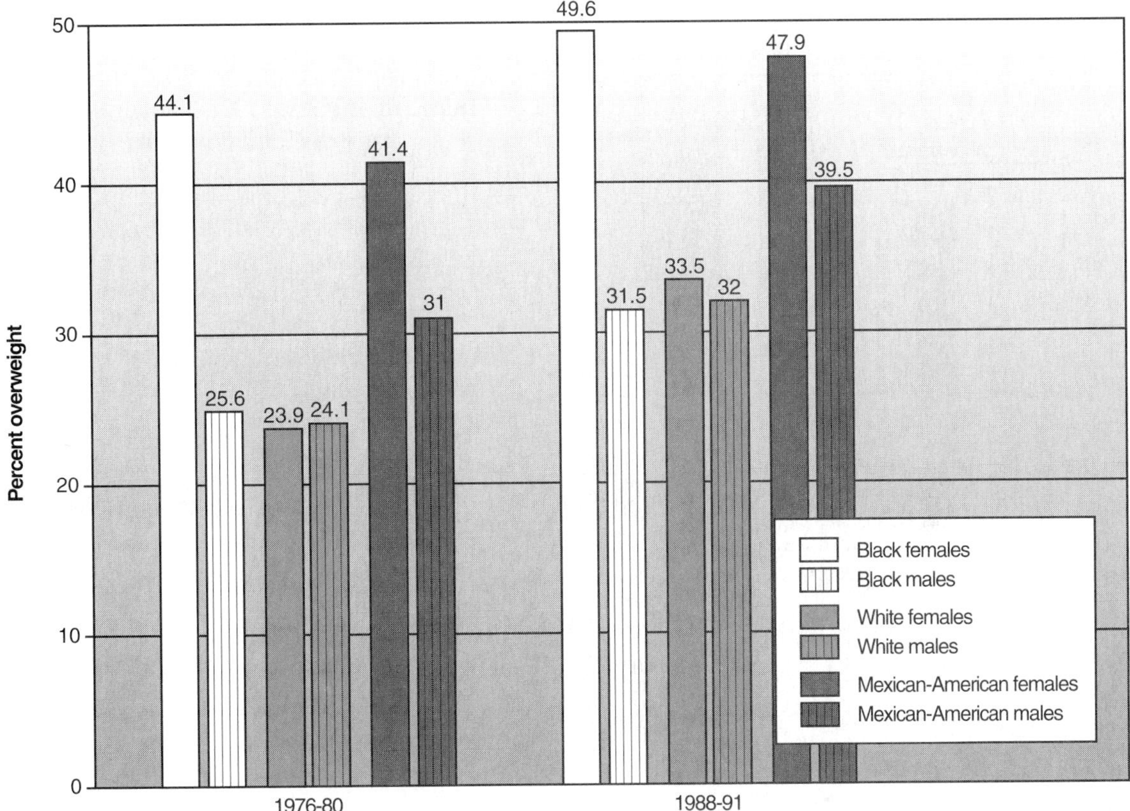

Figure 6-14 The prevalence of overweight among Americans age 20 to 74 years based on sex, race, and Hispanic origin, 1976–1991. Data from the National Center for Health Statistics.

SKINFOLD MEASUREMENTS

The most widely used method of indirectly estimating percent body fat in clinical settings is to measure skinfolds—the thickness of a double fold of skin and compressed subcutaneous adipose tissue (Figure 6-16).[5,29,86] Although more accurate methods for assessing percent body fat exist, skinfold measurement has these advantages: the equipment needed is inexpensive and requires little space; measurements are easily and quickly obtained; and when correctly done, skinfold measurement provides estimates of body composition that correlate well with those derived from hydrostatic weighing, the most widely used laboratory method for determining body composition.[5,29,88]

Assumptions in Using Skinfold Measurements

Estimating body fat from skinfold thickness measurements involves several assumptions, outlined in Box 6-2, that may not always hold true.[86] When a caliper is initially applied to a skinfold, the caliper reading decreases as its tips compress the fold of skin and subcutaneous adipose tissue. Thus it is recommended to read the caliper dial about 4 seconds after the caliper tips have been applied to the skinfold.[89] Research has shown significant differences in skinfold compressibility at a particular site among individuals (interindividual variation) and at different sites on one individual (intraindividual variation).[86,90] Even after

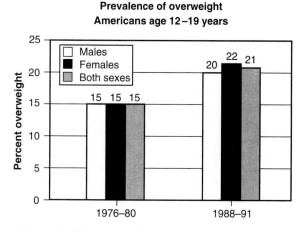

Figure 6-15 Between 1976–80 (NHANES II) and 1988–91 (NHANES III) the prevalence of overweight rose 5% and 7% for American males and females age 12–19 years, respectively. In this figure, overweight is defined as a body mass index greater than the age- and sex-specific 85th percentile in NHANES II. Data from the National Center for Health Statistics.

BOX 6-2

Assumptions Involved in Using Skinfold Thickness Measurements to Predict Body Fat

1. The double thickness of skin and subcutaneous adipose tissue has a constant compressibility.
2. Thickness of the skin is negligible or a constant fraction of the skinfold.
3. The thickness of subcutaneous adipose tissue is constant or predictable within and between individuals.
4. The fat content of adipose tissue is constant.
5. The proportion of internal to external fat is constant.
6. Body fat is normally distributed.

Adapted from Martin AD, Ross WD, Drinkwater DT, and Clarys JP. 1985. Prediction of body fat by skinfold caliper: Assumptions and cadaver evidence. *International Journal of Obesity* 9 (Suppl 1):31–39.

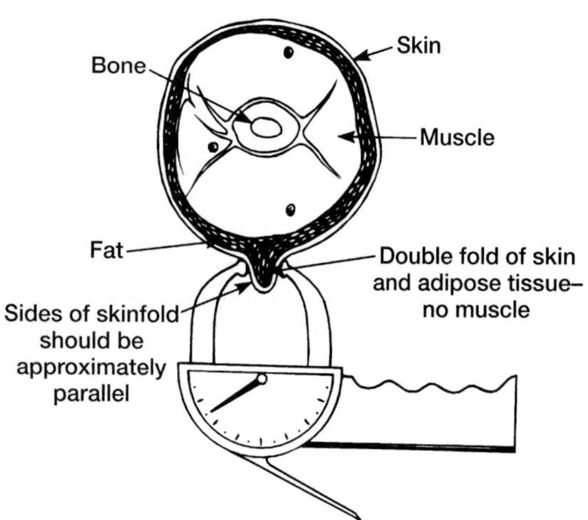

Figure 6-16 The double fold of skin and adipose tissue between the tips of the skinfold caliper should be large enough to form approximately parallel sides. Care should be taken to elevate only skin and adipose tissue and not muscle.

the timing of caliper readings has been standardized, similar thicknesses of adipose tissue may yield different caliper readings because of differences in compressibility.[86] Alternatively, compressibility differences may result in skinfolds of different thicknesses yielding similar caliper readings.[43] Of all the assumptions considered in this section, this probably has the greatest potential for being a significant source of error in estimating body composition from skinfold measurements.[86]

The CAS showed that skin thickness as a percent of total caliper reading varies at different sites and that "while the contribution of skin to total skinfold thickness is generally not large, it may lead to significant error especially in lean subjects."[86]

Thickness of subcutaneous adipose tissue varies widely among different skinfold sites within individuals and for the same skinfold site between individuals.[85,86,91] Consequently, overall subcutaneous adipose tissue is best assessed by measuring multiple skinfold sites. A minimum of three is recommended. Proper site selection is critical because subcutaneous fat layer thickness can vary significantly within a 2- to 3-cm proximity of certain sites.[82,92] Research has shown that certain skinfold sites are highly correlated to total subcutaneous adipose tissue and that sites from the lower limbs should be included in body composition prediction formulas.[86,93]

Adipose tissue can be divided into external or subcutaneous (what lies directly under the skin) and internal portions (that within and around muscles and surrounding organs).[92] The only direct data on the relationship of external-to-internal adipose tissue comes from the CAS. These data show that each kilogram of subcutaneous adipose tissue is associated with approximately 200 g of internal adipose tissue and that skinfolds are significantly correlated with total adiposity.[85]

Although estimating body composition by skinfold measurement fails to meet all the assumptions of Box 6-2, it is preferred over use of other anthropometric variables and is certainly better than height-weight indices.[94] Thus skinfold measurement is the most widely used method of indirectly estimating percent body fat in clinical settings.

Measurement Technique

Proper measurement of skinfolds requires careful attention to site selection and strict adherence to the following protocol that is standard among researchers who have developed the prediction equations for determining body fatness from skinfold measurements.

1. Most North American investigators (including those conducting large national surveys from which reference data are derived) take skinfold measurements on the right side of the body. European investigators typically perform measurements on the left side.[95] From a practical standpoint, it matters little on which side measurements are taken. However, the authors suggest that North American students be taught to take all measurements on the right side (except where indicated otherwise) to coincide with the efforts of most U.S. and Canadian researchers.
2. As a general rule, those with little experience in skinfold measurement should mark the site to be measured once it has been carefully identified. A flexible, nonstretchable tape measure can be used to locate midpoints on the body.[89]
3. The skinfold should be firmly grasped by the thumb and index finger of the left hand about 1 cm or ½ in. **proximal** to the skinfold site and pulled away from the body. This is usually easy with thin people, but it may be difficult with the obese and may be somewhat uncomfortable. The amount of tissue grasped must be enough to form a fold with approximately parallel sides. The thicker the fat layer under the skin, the wider the necessary fold.
4. The caliper is held in the right hand, perpendicular to the long axis of the skinfold and with the caliper's dial facing up and easily readable. The caliper tips should be placed on the site and should be about 1 cm or ½ in. **distal** to the fingers holding the skinfold, so that pressure from the fingers will not affect the measured value, as shown in Figure 6-17.
5. The caliper should not be placed too deeply into the skinfold or too close to the tip of the skinfold. The measurer should try to visualize where a true double fold of skin thickness is and place the caliper tips there. It is a good practice to position the caliper arms one at a time on the skinfold.
6. The dial is read approximately 4 seconds after the pressure from the measurer's hand has been released on the lever arm of the caliper. If caliper tips exert force for longer than 4 seconds, the reading will gradually become smaller as fluids are forced from the compressed tissues. The measurer's eyes and caliper dial should be positioned to avoid errors caused by parallax. Readings should be recorded to the nearest 1 mm.

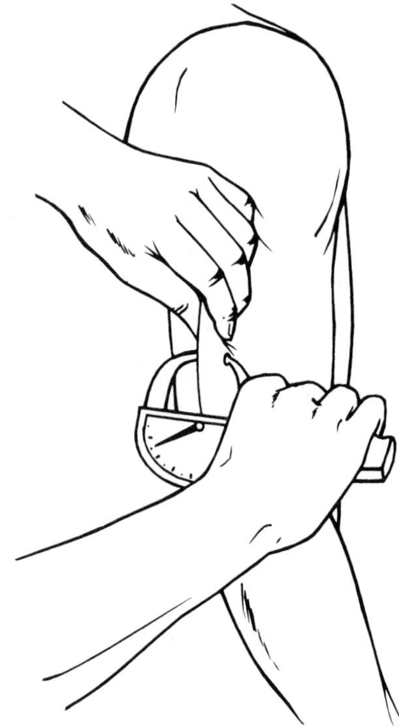

Grasp a double fold of skin and subcutaneous adipose tissue with the thumb and index finger of the left hand.

Place the caliper tips on the site where the sides of the skinfold are approximately parallel and 1 cm distal to where the skinfold is grasped.

Position the caliper dial so that it can be read easily. Obtain the measurement about 4 sec after placing the caliper tips on the skinfold.

Figure 6-17 Accurate skinfold measurements require careful site selection and proper technique in placing and reading the caliper.

7. A minimum of two measurements should be taken at each site. Measurements should be at least 15 seconds apart to allow the skinfold site to return to normal. If consecutive measurements vary by more than 1 mm, more should be taken until there is consistency.
8. The measurer should maintain pressure with the thumb and index finger throughout each measurement.
9. When measuring the obese, it may be impossible to elevate a skinfold with parallel sides, particularly over the abdomen. In this situation, the measurer should use both hands to pull the skinfold away while a partner attempts to measure the width. If the skinfold is too wide for the calipers, underwater weighing or another technique will have to be used.
10. Measurements should not be taken immediately after exercise or when the person being measured is overheated because the shift in body fluid to the skin will inflate normal skinfold size.
11. It takes practice to consistently grasp skinfolds at the same location every time. Accuracy can be tested by having several technicians take the same measurements and comparing results. It may take up to 20 to 50 practice sessions to become proficient in measuring skinfolds.

Several types of skinfold calipers are available (see Figure 6-18). The Lange skinfold caliper is most popular among U.S. researchers, whereas the Harpenden and Tanner are commonly used in Great Britain and Europe. Several less expensive plastic calipers are available, such as the Slim Guide, Fat-O-Meter, and the Fat-Control Caliper, which also is marketed by Ross Laboratories under the trade name Adipometer™. Some of the

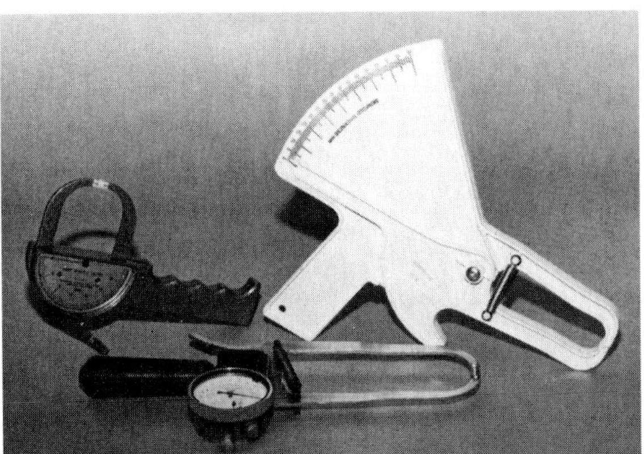

Figure 6-18 Left to right: the Lange, Harpenden, and Slim Guide skinfold calipers. From Nieman DC. 1995. *Fitness and sports medicine: A health-related approach,* ed 3. Palo Alto: Bull Publishing Co.

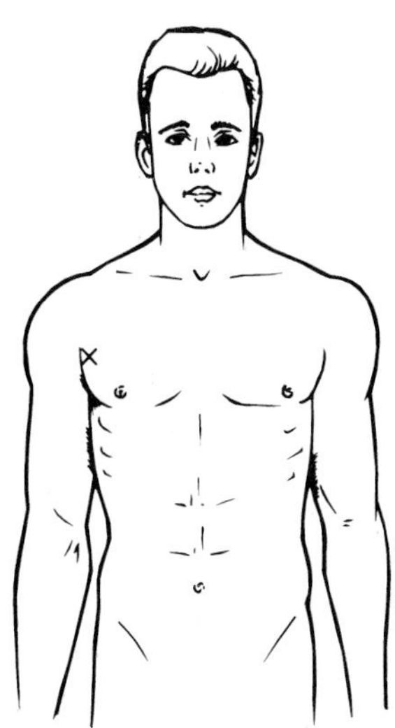

Figure 6-19 The location of the pectoral or chest skinfold site is the same for males and females.

plastic calipers have been shown to give results comparable to the more expensive calipers.[96,97] The Slim Guide, which is being used increasingly, may be an acceptable caliper for those who cannot afford a more expensive instrument. Currently, the Lange and Harpenden calipers are highly recommended because these were used in developing prediction equations and reference values. Whatever the caliper is used, the jaw tips should exert a pressure of 10 g/mm^2 throughout the caliper's full measurement range. The calipers should be calibrated periodically (for example, before measuring skinfolds on groups of subjects) by checking the dial reading against a graduated calibration block. Caliper readings should be within at least ±1 mm at each 5-mm interval from 5 to 50 mm.[98]

Site Selection

This section describes eight of the most commonly used skinfold sites following the Airlie Consensus Conference protocol as outlined in the *Anthropometric Standardization Reference Manual.*[93]

Chest

The chest or pectoral skinfold site is measured using a skinfold with its long axis running from the top of the anterior axillary fold to the nipple. The skinfold is grasped as high as possible on the anterior axillary fold, and the thickness of the fat fold is measured 1 cm or 1/2 in below the fingers along the axis, as shown in Figures 6-19 and 6-20. The skinfold site is the same for males and females. Other than to help determine the long axis of the skinfold, the nipple is not used as a landmark for either males or females. This site can be measured on a female wearing a brassiere or two-piece bathing suit.

Triceps

Because of its accessibility, the triceps is the most commonly measured site. The triceps skinfold site is on the posterior aspect of the right arm, over the triceps muscle, midway between the lateral projection of the acromion process of the scapula and the inferior margin of the olecranon process of the ulna. These bony landmarks are shown in Figure 6-21. The midpoint between the acromion

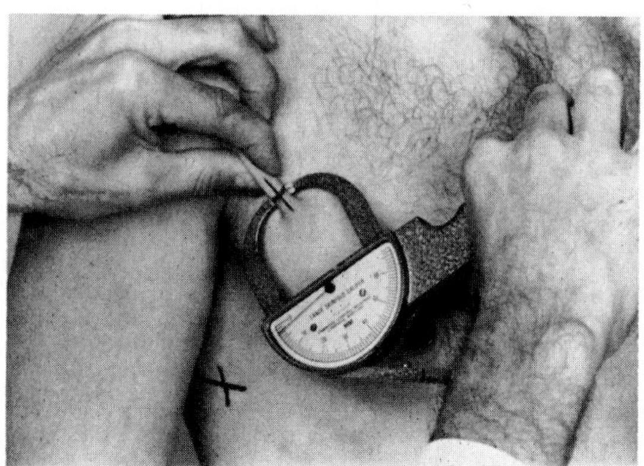

Figure 6-20 Measurement of the pectoral or chest skinfold. Note that the caliper is held perpendicular to the long axis of the skinfold. The blade tips are approximately 1 cm distal to the fingers grasping the skinfold. From Nieman DC. 1995. *Fitness and sports medicine: A health-related approach,* ed 3. Palo Alto: Bull Publishing Co.

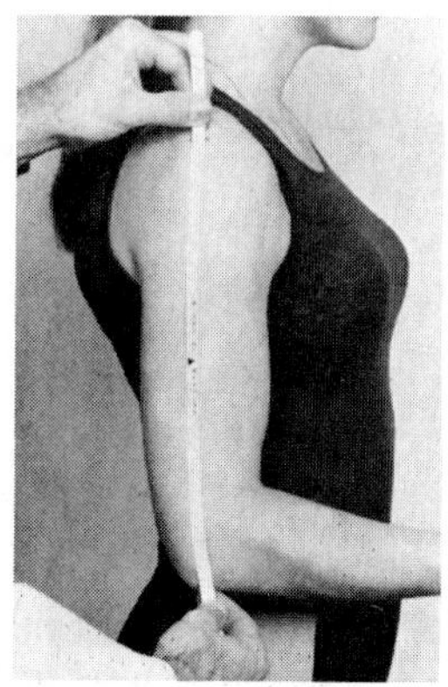

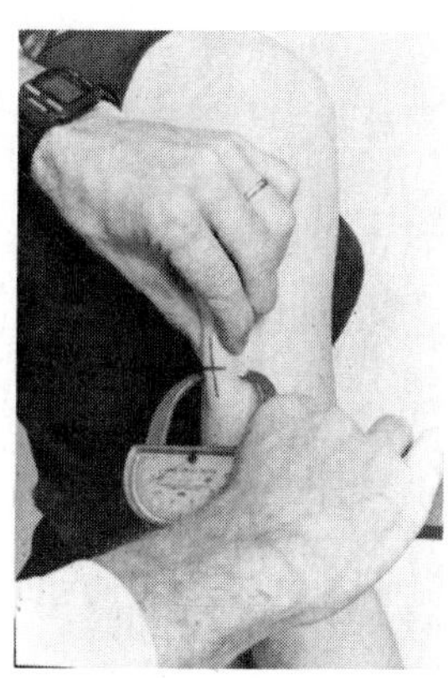

Figure 6-22 Measurement of the triceps skinfold. From Nieman DC. 1995. *Fitness and sports medicine: A health-related approach,* ed 3. Palo Alto: Bull Publishing Co.

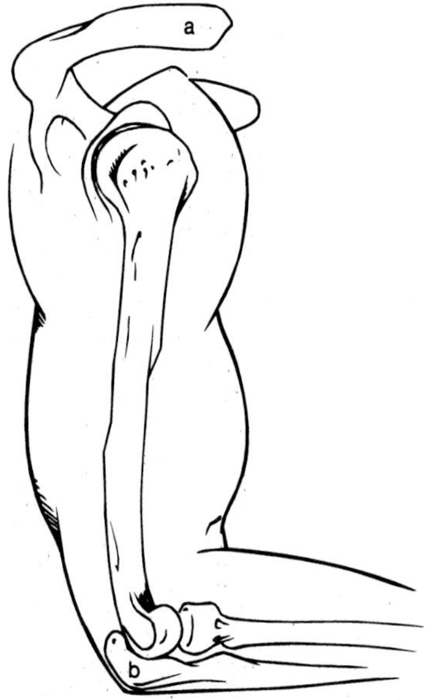

Figure 6-21 The triceps skinfold site is located midway between the lateral projection of the acromion process of the scapula, **A**, and the olecranon process of the ulna, **B**, with the elbow flexed 90 degrees.

and olecranon processes should be marked along the *lateral* side of the arm with the elbow flexed 90 degrees, as shown in Figure 6-22. The subject's arm should now hang loosely at the side with the palm of the hand facing *anteriorly* to properly determine the posterior midline. The skinfold site should be marked along the posterior midline of the upper arm at the same level as the previously marked midpoint. The measurer should stand behind the subject, grasp the skinfold with the thumb and index finger of the left hand about 1 cm or ½ in. proximal to the skinfold site, as shown in Figure 6-22. Again, notice in Figure 6-22 that the caliper tips are about 1 cm or ½ in. from the thumb and finger, the caliper is perpendicular to the long axis of the skinfold, and the dial can be easily read.

Subscapular

This site is 1 cm below the lowest or inferior angle of the scapula, as shown in Figure 6-23. The long axis of the skinfold is on a 45-degree angle directed down and to the right side. The site can be located by gently feeling for the inferior angle of the scapula or by having the subject place his or her right arm behind the back. It is measured with the subject standing with arms relaxed to the sides. The skin is grasped 1 cm above and medial to the site along the axis (see Figure 6-24).

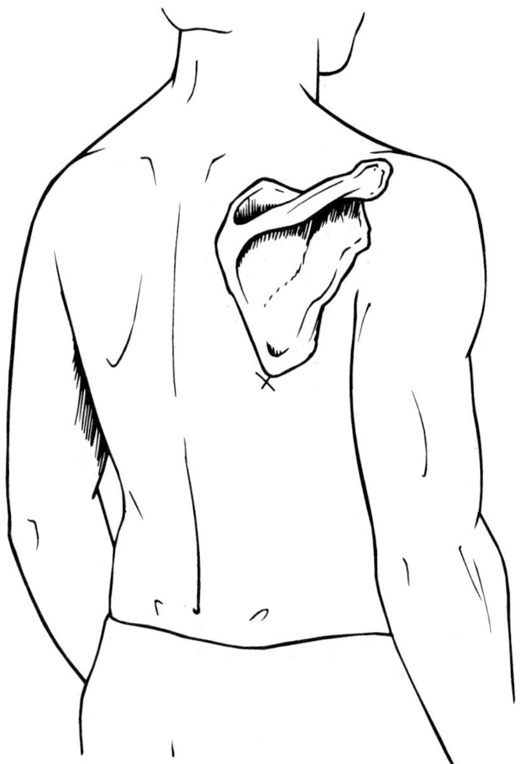

Figure 6-23 The subscapular skinfold site is just below the inferior border of the scapula. The long axis of the site runs at 45 degrees of horizontal.

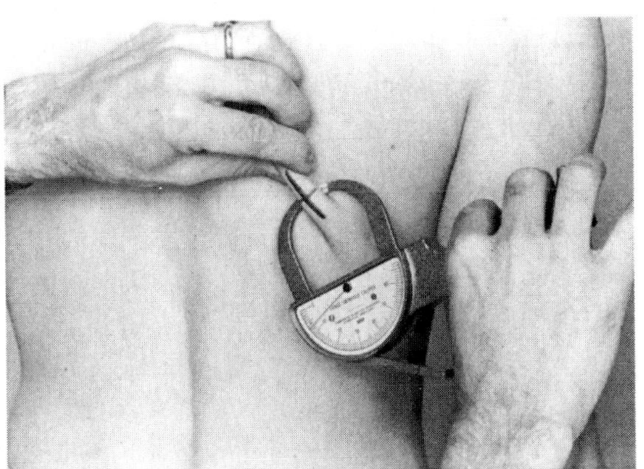

Figure 6-24 Measurement of the subscapular skinfold site. From Nieman DC. 1995. *Fitness and sports medicine: A health-related approach*, ed 3. Palo Alto: Bull Publishing Co.

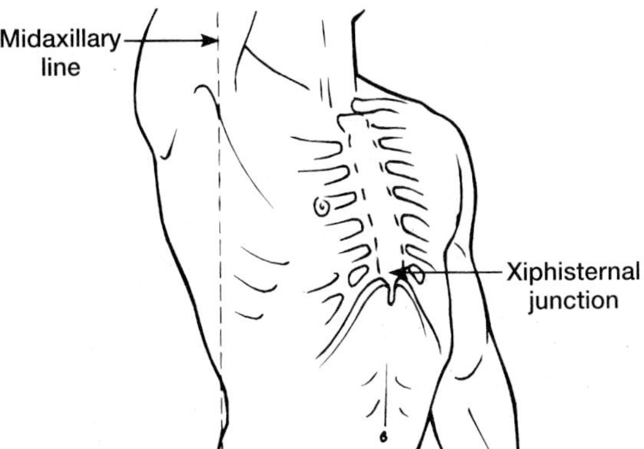

Figure 6-25 The midaxillary site is a horizontal skinfold along the midaxillary line at the level of the xiphisternal junction.

Midaxillary

As shown in Figure 6-25, this site is at the right midaxillary line (a vertical line extending from the middle of the axilla) level with the xiphisternal junction (at the bottom of the sternum where the xiphoid process begins). It is measured with the subject standing erectly and with the right arm slightly abducted (moved away from center of the body) and flexed (bent posteriorly) as in Figure 6-26.

Suprailiac

This skinfold is measured just above the iliac crest at the midaxillary line (see Figure 6-27 and Figure 6-28). The long axis follows the natural cleavage lines of the skin and runs diagonally. The subject should stand erectly with feet together and arms hanging at the sides, although the right arm can be abducted and flexed slightly to improve access to the site. The measurer should grasp the skinfold about 1 cm posterior to the midaxillary line and measure the skinfold at the midaxillary line.

Abdomen

The subject stands erectly with the body weight evenly distributed on both feet, abdominal muscles

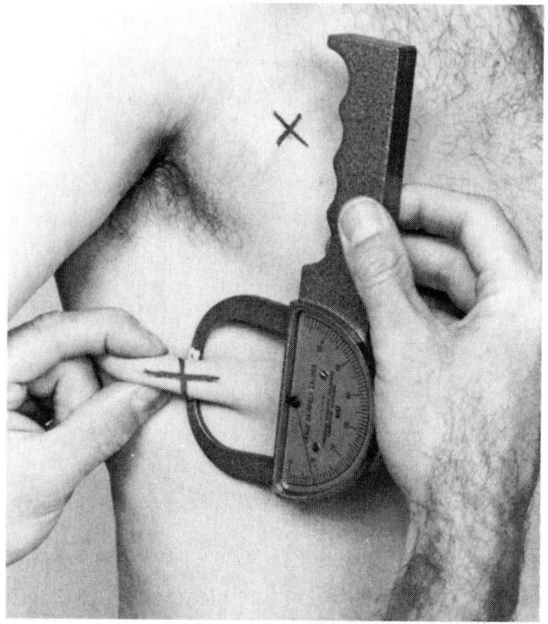

Figure 6-26 Measurement of the midaxillary skinfold. From Nieman DC. 1995. *Fitness and sports medicine: A health-related approach,* ed 3. Palo Alto: Bull Publishing Co.

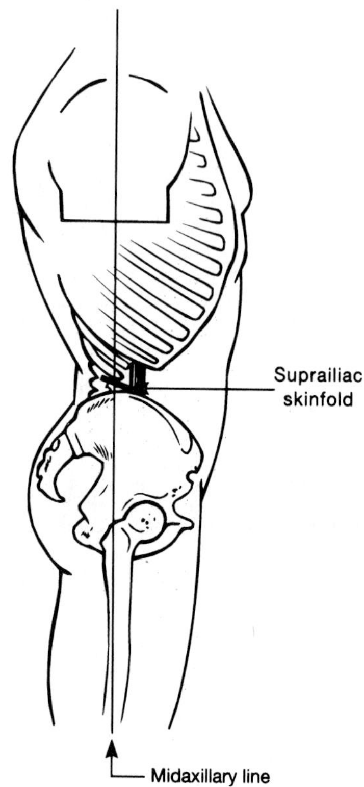

Figure 6-27 The suprailiac skinfold is measured just above the iliac crest at the midaxillary line. The long axis of the skinfold follows the natural cleavage lines of the skin.

relaxed, and breathing quietly. A horizontal skinfold 3 cm to the right of and 1 cm below the midpoint of the umbilicus is measured (Figure 6-29).

Thigh

This site is a vertical skinfold along the midline of the anterior aspect of the thigh midway between the junction of the midline and the inguinal crease and the proximal (upper) border of the patella or knee cap (Figure 6-30). Flexing the subject's hip helps to locate the inguinal crease. The subject shifts the weight to the left foot and relaxes the leg being measured by slightly flexing the knee with the foot flat on the floor. The skinfold is measured as shown in Figure 6-31.

Medial Calf

With the subject sitting, the right leg is flexed about 90 degrees at the knee with the sole of the foot flat on the floor. The measurement also may be taken with the subject standing with the foot resting on a platform so that the knee and hip are flexed about 90 degrees. The point of maximum calf circumference is marked at the medial (inner) aspect of the calf. A vertical skinfold is grasped about 1 cm proximal to the marked site and measured at the site (Figure 6-32).

Single-Site Skinfold Measurements

The triceps is the most commonly used single site for assessing body composition.[29] The ease by which it is accessed and measured has made it popular in large population studies such as NHANES. Although single-site skinfold measurements cannot be used to estimate percent body

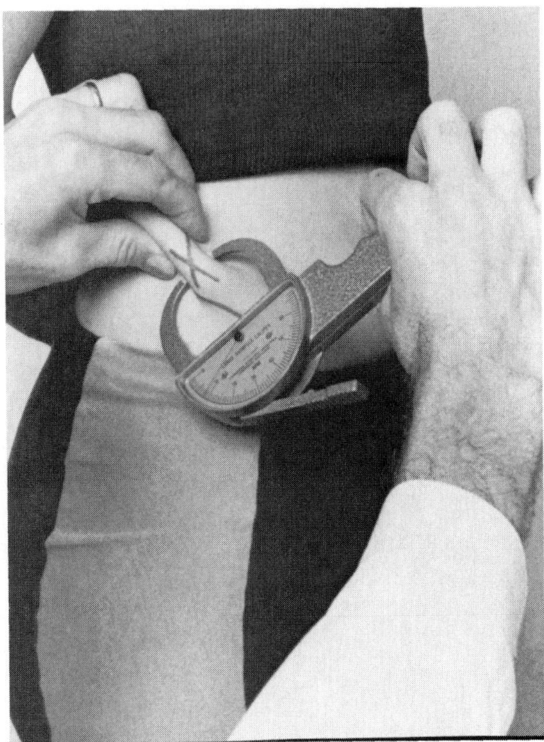

Figure 6-28 Measurement of the suprailiac skinfold. From Nieman DC. 1995. *Fitness and sports medicine: A health-related approach*, ed 3. Palo Alto: Bull Publishing Co.

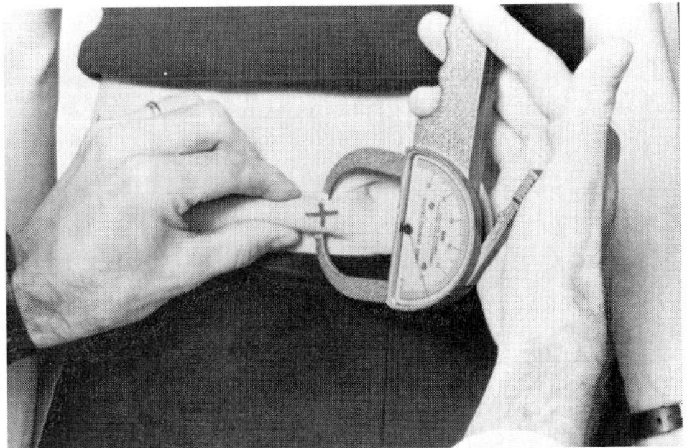

Figure 6-29 Measurement of the abdominal skinfold. From Nieman DC. 1995. *Fitness and sports medicine: A health-related approach*, ed 3. Palo Alto: Bull Publishing Co.

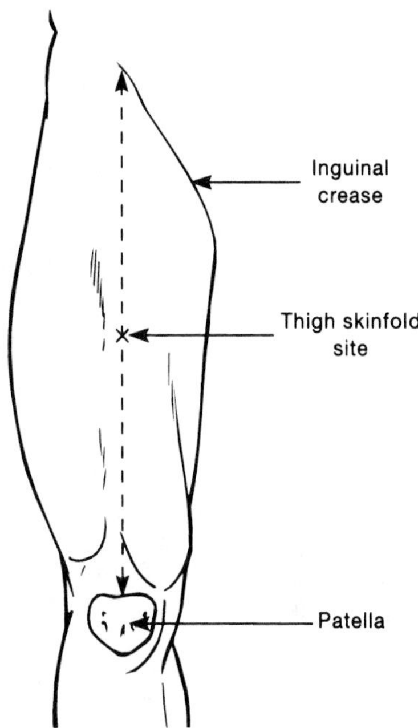

Figure 6-30 The thigh skinfold lies along the anterior midline of the thigh halfway between the inguinal crease and the proximal border of the patella.

fat, they are useful for making comparisons among subjects for which reference data are available. For example, the triceps skinfold measurements of a child can be compared with reference data on triceps skinfolds taken from a large group of children of a similar sex and age. Reference data derived from NHANES II are shown in Appendixes O and P. Using the tables, the 50th percentile represents the median value for each age/sex group. If a subject had a skinfold thickness at the 85th percentile for his or her age/sex group, 85% of the subjects studied in that group would have smaller measurements and only 15% would have larger measurements.

Using single skinfold measurements has certain limitations: investigators disagree about what is the best single site to use as an index of body composition;[55] no equations exist for estimating body fat using just the triceps skinfold measurement; and multiple anthropometric measures are required to achieve reasonably accurate body

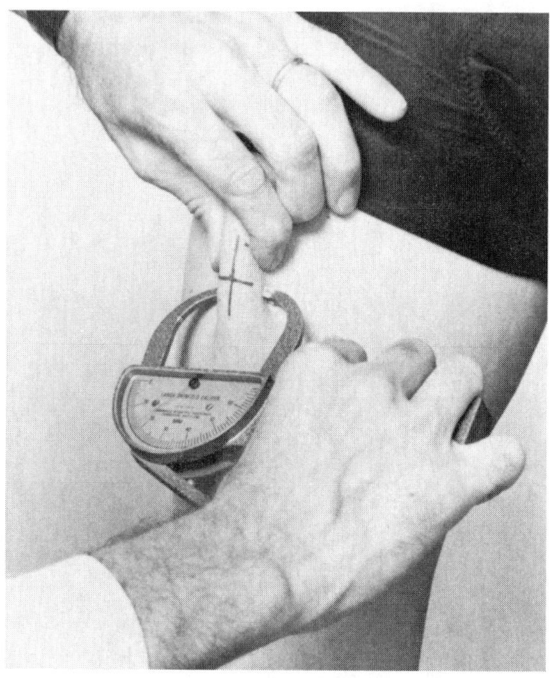

Figure 6-31 Measurement of the thigh skinfold. From Nieman DC. 1995. *Fitness and sports medicine: A health-related approach,* ed 3. Palo Alto: Bull Publishing Co.

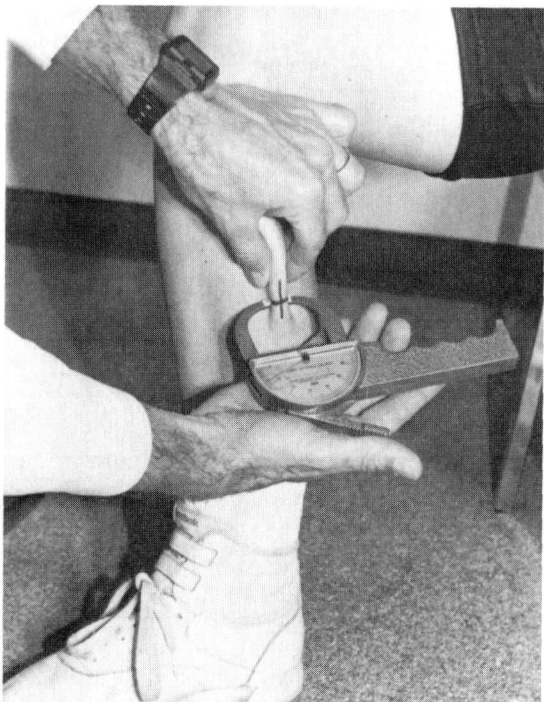

Figure 6-32 Measurement of the medial calf skinfold. From Nieman DC. 1995. *Fitness and sports medicine: A health-related approach,* ed 3. Palo Alto: Bull Publishing Co.

composition estimates because of variations in subcutaneous adipose tissue distribution. Therefore, single-site skinfold measurements must be interpreted with caution and should be used only as a rough approximation of total body fat percentage or to compare individuals for which reference data exist.[29]

Two-Site Skinfold Measurements

The most commonly used approach to assessing body composition for young people age 6 years through the mid-20s uses the sum of the triceps and subscapular sites.[98,99] These sites have the following advantages: they are highly correlated with other measures of body fatness; they are more reliably and objectively measured than most other sites; and national norms are available for them.[29] Figure 6-33 outlines skinfold and body fat standards developed for persons age 6 to 17 years using the sum of the triceps and subscapular skinfolds.[99]

Because measurement of the subscapular skinfold may be embarrassing to some children and youth or may raise ethical questions about male teachers touching female students, norms using the sum of the triceps and medial calf skinfold measurements have been developed.[29,99–101] This sum has proved to be a reasonably valid and reliable indicator of body composition. The medial calf site is easily accessible and can be measured without raising concerns about modesty. In some persons, the skin at the site may be quite taut, making it difficult to measure the site. Figure 6-34 provides standards based on the sum of triceps and medial calf skinfold measurements for persons 6 to 17 years old.[99] Using Figures 6-33 and 6-34, obesity for 6- to 17-year-old males and females is greater than 25% body fat and greater

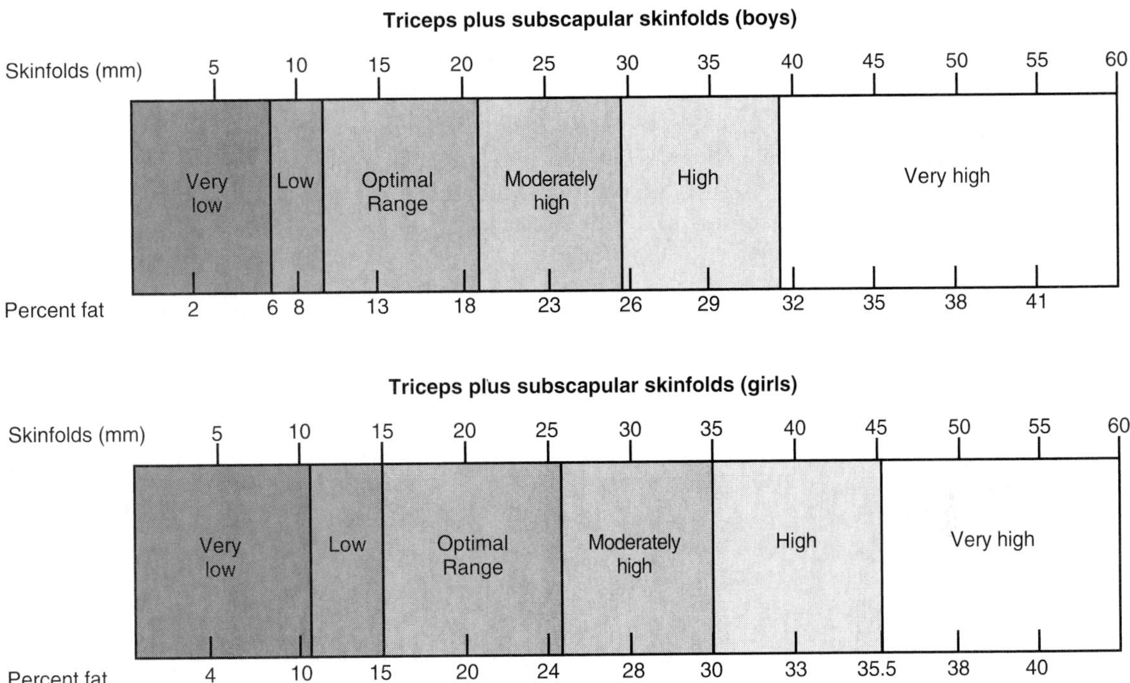

Figure 6-33 Body fat standards for persons 6 to 17 years old based on the sum of triceps and subscapular skinfold measurements. From the *Journal of Physical Education, Recreation & Dance,* November–December 1987, pp. 98–102.

than 32% body fat, respectively. An alternate approach for estimating percent body fat in children is to calculate the sum of biceps, triceps, subscapular, and suprailiac skinfold measurements (discussed in the next section).

Multiple-Site Skinfold Measurements

Predicting body density and then percent of body fat from skinfold measurements requires regression equations. These formulas have been developed by comparing a variety of skinfold and other anthropometric measures with measurements of body density (usually by hydrostatic weighing) to see which anthropometric measures are best at predicting body density. A statistical process called multiple-regression analysis is used.[4,94,102–104] The measure or combinations of measures most highly correlated with body density as determined by a separate method are then used in the regression equation.

The more than 100 different regression equations that have been developed can be classified as either population-specific equations or generalized equations.[92,94] Population-specific equations are derived from data on groups of people sharing certain characteristics such as age and gender. The first valid regression equations, for example, were developed in 1951 for young and middle-aged men.[105] Numerous other population-specific equations have been developed since then, but their use is limited. Equations developed from data on middle-aged females, for example, may not be valid for females of other ages.

More recently, generalized equations have been developed that are applicable to persons varying greatly in age and body fatness. The primary advantage of this approach is that one generalized equation can replace several population-specific equations with no loss in prediction accuracy.[5,94] Table 6-10 shows several generalized prediction equations for calculating

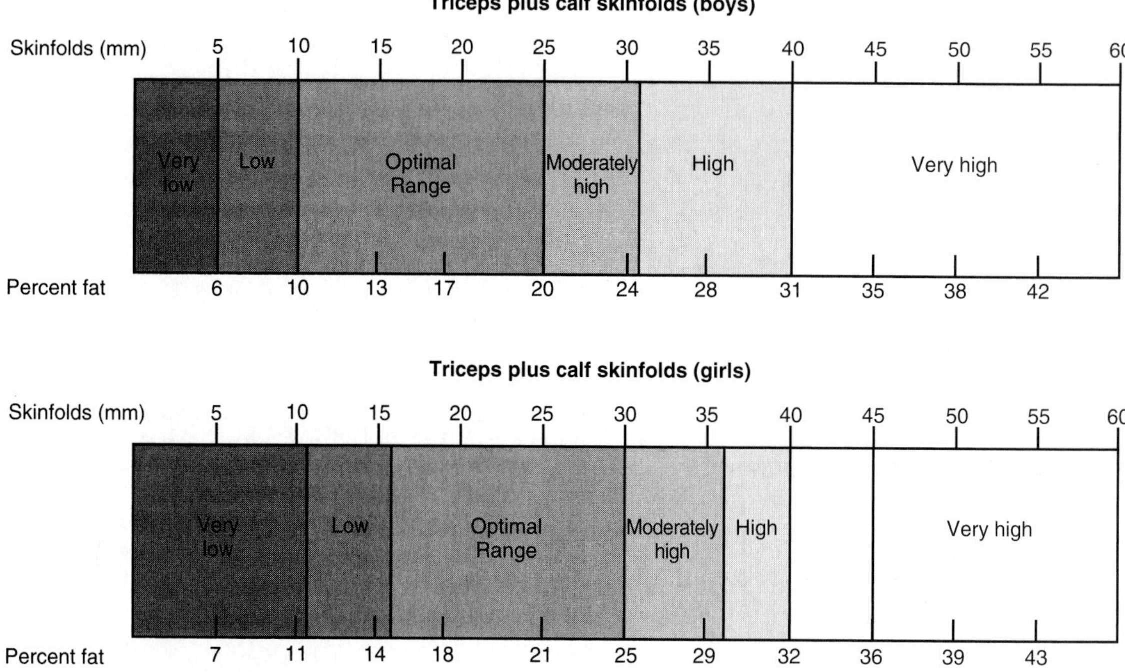

Figure 6-34 Body fat standards for person 6 to 17 years old based on the sum of triceps and medial calf skinfold measurements. From the *Journal of Physical Education, Recreation & Dance,* November–December 1987, pp. 98–102.

body density or percent body fat. Because fat placement differs between males and females, separate equations are given for each sex.

Table 6-11 shows equations for estimating body density developed by Durnin and Womersley.[106] These have been used by many researchers and differ according to sex and age. The equations are based on the logarithm of the sum of four skinfolds—triceps, subscapular, suprailiac, and biceps. The biceps skinfold is a vertical fold on the anterior aspect of the arm, over the belly of the biceps muscle, directly opposite the triceps skinfold site.[89]

The equations in Table 6-10 and Table 6-11 predict either body fat percent or body density. Body density formulas require an additional calculation to estimate percent body fat. Two formulas are available for this step: the Brozek and the Siri equations.[29]

Brozek: Percent body fat = $(457 - \text{body density}) - 414$

Siri: Percent body fat = $(495 \div \text{body density}) - 450$

A programmable calculator will help in the use of these equations. The nomogram shown in Figure 6-35 greatly simplifies calculating percent body fat from the sum of three skinfold thicknesses.[107] For males, the sum of the chest, abdomen, and thigh skinfold measurements should be used. For females, the sum of the triceps, suprailiac, and thigh skinfold measurements should be used. The nomogram was developed from data on males from 18 to 61 years old and females 18 to 55 years old, with the sum of skinfold measurements ranging from 14 to 118 mm and 16 to 126 mm for males and females, respectively.[107] The nomogram should be used with caution for subjects outside these ranges.

TABLE 6-10 Generalized body composition equations for male and female adults*

Males

Body density = $1.11200000 - 0.00043499(X_1) + 0.00000055\ (X_1)^2 - 0.00028826\ (X_8)$

Percent body fat = $0.29288\ (X_2) - 0.00050\ (X_2)^2 + 0.15845\ (X_8) - 5.76377$

Body density = $1.1093800 - 0.0008267\ (X_3) + 0.0000016\ (X_3)^2 - 0.0002574\ (X_8)$

Body density = $1.1125025 - 0.0013125\ (X_4) + 0.00000055\ (X_4)^2 - 0.0002440\ (X_8)$

Percent body fat = $0.39287\ (X_5) - 0.00105\ (X_5)^2 + 0.15772\ (X_8) - 5.18845$

Females

Body density = $1.0970 - 0.00046971\ (X_1) + 0.00000056\ (X_1)^2 - 0.00012828\ (X_8)$

Percent body fat = $0.29699\ (X_2) - 0.00043\ (X_2)^2 + 0.02963\ (X_8) + 1.4072$

Percent body fat = $0.41563\ (X_6) - 0.00112\ (X_6)^2 + 0.03661\ (X_8) + 4.03653$

Body density = $1.0994921 - 0.0009929\ (X_7) + 0.0000023\ (X_7)^2 - 0.0001392\ (X_8)$

Data from Jackson AS and Pollock ML. 1985. Practical assessment of body composition, *Physician and Sportsmedicine* 13(5):76–90; Golding LA, Myers CR, and Sinning WE. 1989. *The Y's way to physical fitness,* 3d ed. Champaign, Ill. Human Kinetics Books.

*X_1 = sum of chest, midaxillary, triceps, subscapular, abdomen, suprailiac, and thigh skinfolds; X_2 = sum of abdomen, suprailiac, triceps, and thigh skinfolds; X_3 = sum of chest, abdomen, and subscapular skinfolds; X_4 = sum of chest, triceps, and subscapular skinfolds; X_5 = sum of abdomen, suprailiac, and triceps skinfolds; X_6 = sum of triceps, abdomen, and suprailiac skinfolds; X_7 = sum of triceps, suprailiac, and thigh skinfolds; X_8 = age in years.

TABLE 6-11 Age- and sex-specific body composition equations developed by Durnin and Womersley.

Age range (years)	Equation
Males	
17–19	Body density = $1.1620 - 0.0630 \times (\log \Sigma)$*
20–29	Body density = $1.1631 - 0.0632 \times (\log \Sigma)$
30–39	Body density = $1.1422 - 0.0544 \times (\log \Sigma)$
40–49	Body density = $1.1620 - 0.0700 \times (\log \Sigma)$
50+	Body density = $1.1715 - 0.0779 \times (\log \Sigma)$
Females	
17–19	Body density = $1.1549 - 0.0678 \times (\log \Sigma)$
20–29	Body density = $1.1599 - 0.0717 \times (\log \Sigma)$
30–39	Body density = $1.1423 - 0.0632 \times (\log \Sigma)$
40–49	Body density = $1.1333 - 0.0612 \times (\log \Sigma)$
50+	Body density = $1.1339 - 0.0645 \times (\log \Sigma)$

Equations from Durnin JVGA, Womersley J. 1974. Body fat assessment from total body density and its estimation from skinfold thickness: Measurements on 481 men and women aged 16–72 years. *British Journal of Nutrition* 32:77–97.

*Σ = sum of the triceps, subscapular, suprailiac, and biceps skinfolds.

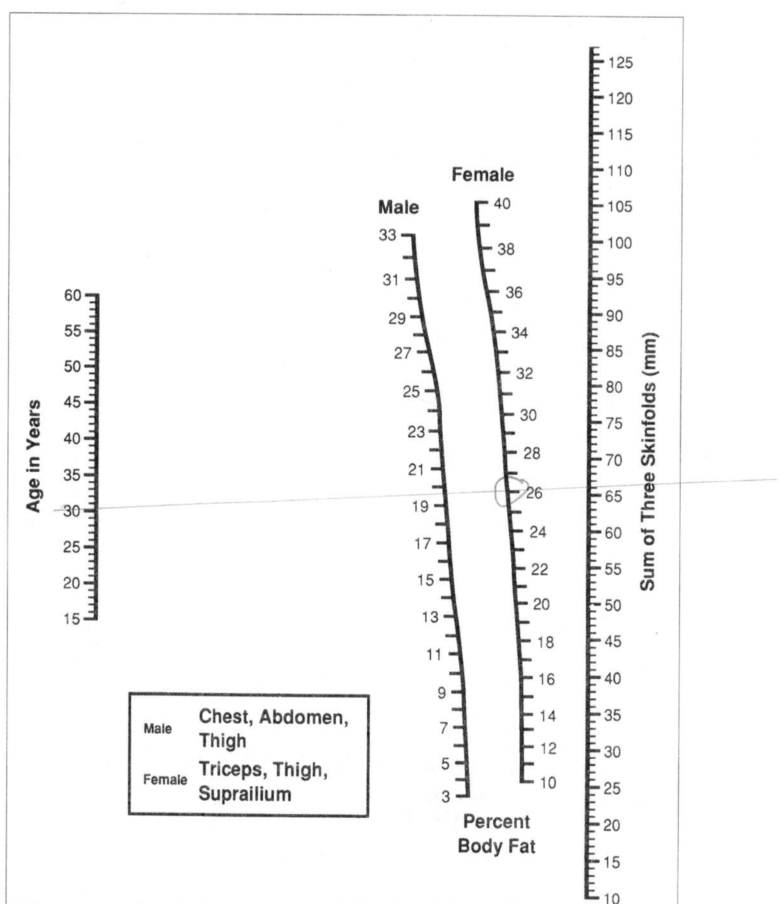

Figure 6-35 Nomogram for calculating percent of body fat from the sum of three skinfolds. Use a straightedge to connect the subject's age (left axis) with the skinfold value (right axis). The percent body fat is read where the straightedge crosses the line representing the subject's sex. From the *Research Quarterly for Exercise and Sport* 52(3), 1981.

Investigators in the Netherlands have proposed regression equations for estimating body density and percent body fat in persons from infancy to age 18 years.[108] Based on their equations, they have formulated a table (Table 6-12) allowing the estimation of percent body fat of persons in this age range from the sum of biceps, triceps, subscapular, and suprailiac skinfold measurements.

What Is a Desirable Level of Fatness?

Determining with certainty just what constitutes a desirable level of body fatness is difficult. However, suggested percent body fat norms are given in Table 6-13. Note that the values are given in a range. This allows for error in measurement and for individual differences; what may be appropriate for one person may not be appropriate for another.[84,94]

Using the values in Table 6-13, the form shown in Figure 6-36, and the following formulas, a person can calculate a target weight necessary to achieve a certain percent body fat.[29]

Weight of fat = Total body weight × Percent body fat
Fat-free weight = Total body weight − Fat weight
Target weight = Present fat-free weight
÷ (100 − desired percent body fat)

TABLE 6-12 Percent body fat estimated from the sum of skinfold thickness measurements* in persons from infancy to age 18 years

	Percent body fat				
Age (years)	15%	20%	25%	30%	35%
Male					
0†	17	22	30	40	52
1‡	18	24	32	43	58
2	18	25	34	45	60
4	20	27	37	51	68
6	22	30	41	57	78
8	32	33	46	64	88
10	25	36	51	72	101
12	27	40	57	81	115
14	27	44	63	92	132
16	32	48	71	104	152
18	34	52	79	117	175
Female					
0†	17	22	30	40	52
1‡	18	24	32	43	58
2	18	25	34	45	60
4	18	25	34	46	62
6	19	25	35	47	63
8	19	26	35	48	65
10	19	27	37	51	69
12	21	30	42	58	80
14	23	33	47	66	92
16	25	37	53	75	106
18	27	40	58	85	122

From Westrate JA, Deurenberg P. 1989. Body composition in children: Proposal for a method for calculating body fat percentage from total body density or skinfold-thickness measurements, *Am J Clin Nutr* 50:1104–1115.

*Sum of biceps, triceps, subscapular, and suprailiac skinfold measurements, given in millimeters. See reference 88 for measurement of the biceps skinfold site.

†Mean age used was 6 months.

‡Mean age used was 18 months.

For example, take a subject who weighs 200 lb, has 25% body fat, and desires to have a 15% body fat:

Weight of fat = 200 lb × 0.25 = 50 lb
Fat-free weight = 200 lb − 50 lb = 150 lb
Target weight = 150 lb − 0.85 = 176 lb

DENSITOMETRY

Densitometry is assessing body composition by measuring the density of the entire body.[82] Density is expressed as mass per unit volume and usually is obtained through **hydrostatic** or

TABLE 6-13 Suggested percent body fat standards for adults

Classification	Males	Females
Lean	<8%	<13%
Optimal	8%–15%	13%–23%
Slightly overfat	16%–20%	24%–27%
Fat	21%–24%	28%–32%
Obese (overfat)	≥25%	≥33%

Adapted from Nieman DC. 1995. *Fitness and sports medicine: A health-related approach*, ed 3. Palo Alto: Bull Publishing Co.

Skinfold Measurements

Name ______________________ Date ______

Age ______ Sex ____ Height ______ Weight ______

Measurements (mm)

________	Chest	________	Suprailiac
________	Triceps	________	Abdominal
________	Subscapular	________	Thigh
________	Midaxillary	________	Medial calf

Calculations
(Use appropriate formula)

________________ Sum of skinfolds (mm)

________________ Percent body fat

________________ Fat weight
(Body weight x Percent body fat)

________________ Lean body weight
(Body weight – Fat weight)

________________ Classification

________________ Desired body weight
LBW + (100% – Desired % body fat)

Figure 6-36 Skinfold recording and calculation form.

underwater weighing, although other methods have been developed as described later in this section.[109]

Underwater Weighing

The most widely used technique of determining whole-body density is hydrostatic or underwater weighing.[82] The technique is based on **Archimedes' principle**, which states that the volume of an object submerged in water equals the volume of water the object displaces. Thus if the mass and the volume of a body are known, the density of that body can be calculated. Using another formula, percent body fat can be calculated from body density.

This approach is based on the two-compartment model of body composition: the fat and fat-free mass. The fat-free mass is assumed to have a constant level of hydration and a constant proportion of bone mineral to muscle. The approach also assumes a constant fat mass density of 0.90 g/cm^3 and a density of the fat-free mass of 1.10 g/cm^3.[82] The densities of bone and muscle tissue are greater than the density of water (density of distilled water = 1.00 g/cm^3), whereas fat is less dense than water. Thus muscular subjects having a low percentage of body fat will tend to weigh more submerged in water than will subjects having a higher percentage of body fat.[29]

Body density can be calculated from the following formula:[4]

$$\text{Body density} = \frac{WA}{\dfrac{(WA - WW)}{DW} - (RV + VGI)}$$

where WA = body weight in air; WW = body weight submerged in water; DW = density of water; RV = residual lung volume; VGI = volume of gas in the gastrointestinal tract.

Equipment

The necessary equipment for underwater weighing includes a tank, tub, or pool of water of sufficient size for total body submersion, a scale

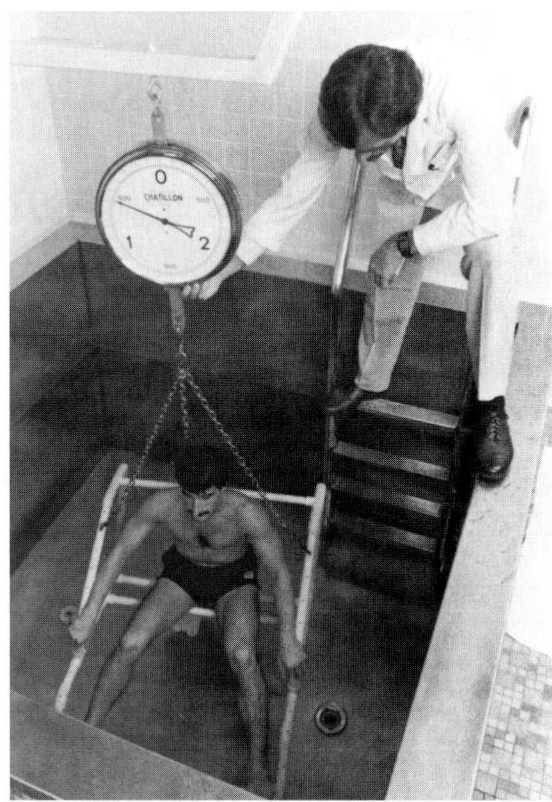

Figure 6-37 Equipment for underwater weighing includes a tank of sufficient size and shape for total human submersion, an accurate scale for measuring weight with 10-gram divisions, a method of measuring water temperature, and a chair that is weighted to prevent flotation. From Nieman DC. 1995. *Fitness and sports medicine: A health-related approach*, ed 3. Palo Alto: Bull Publishing Co.

or other method of determining the subject's underwater weight, and, attached to the scale, a chair or frame lowered into the water on which the subject sits (Figure 6-37).

The water should be comfortably warm, filtered, chlorinated, and undisturbed by wind or other activity in the water during testing.[29] A method of underwater weighing in a swimming pool using a wooden shell placed within the pool to reduce water movement that can adversely affect weighing has been described.[109]

The chair should be constructed so that the subject can sit under the water with legs slightly bent and the water at neck level, as shown in Figure 6-37. Weights should be attached to the chair so that its empty or tare weight while under water is at least 3 kg for subjects of moderate body fatness and at least 4 to 6 kg for obese subjects.[11] Some researchers use a frame on which the subject lies submerged in the prone (face down) position while breathing through a snorkel.[4,109] They think that this position results in less up-and-down movement of the body in the water, thus resulting in fewer fluctuations of the scale.

Typically an autopsy scale (such as the 9-kg capacity Chatillon autopsy scale shown in Figure 6-37) is used in underwater weighing. A strain gauge or force cell gives more precise measurements.[4,82,110] These instruments can be interfaced with a computer which, with the appropriate software, can easily determine the midpoint of fluctuations and use that as the basis for further calculations.[4]

Procedure[4,29]

1. Obtaining basic data: Name, date, age, sex, stature, and weight (in kilograms) in air should be collected and recorded on a form such as the one shown in Figure 6-38. The tester should record the tare weight—the underwater weight of the chair (and any attached weights)—before the subject sits in it. The subject should be several hours **postprandial**, clean, and wearing only a swim suit, and should have urinated and defecated immediately before weighing. Carbonated beverages and flatus-causing foods should be avoided before the procedure because gastrointestinal tract gas will decrease the subject's underwater weight, resulting in erroneously low measurements of body density.
2. Measuring skinfolds: Skinfold measurements can help verify results from underwater weighing. These can be recorded on the form shown in Figure 6-38.

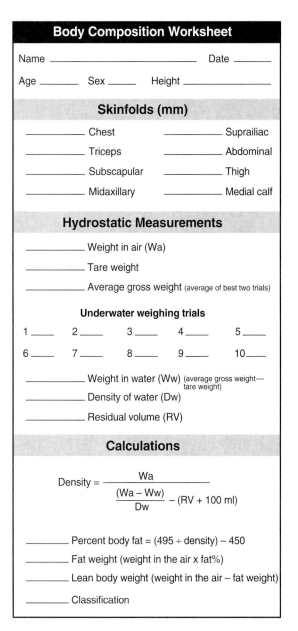

Body Composition Worksheet

Name ____________________ Date ______

Age ______ Sex ______ Height ______________

Skinfolds (mm)

________	Chest	________	Suprailiac
________	Triceps	________	Abdominal
________	Subscapular	________	Thigh
________	Midaxillary	________	Medial calf

Hydrostatic Measurements

________ Weight in air (Wa)

________ Tare weight

________ Average gross weight (average of best two trials)

Underwater weighing trials

1____	2____	3____	4____	5____
6____	7____	8____	9____	10____

________ Weight in water (Ww) (average gross weight—tare weight)

________ Density of water (Dw)

________ Residual volume (RV)

Calculations

$$\text{Density} = \frac{\text{Wa}}{\dfrac{(\text{Wa} - \text{Ww})}{\text{Dw}} - (\text{RV} + 100\text{ ml})}$$

________ Percent body fat = (495 ÷ density) – 450

________ Fat weight (weight in the air x fat%)

________ Lean body weight (weight in the air – fat weight)

________ Classification

Figure 6-38 Body composition worksheet.

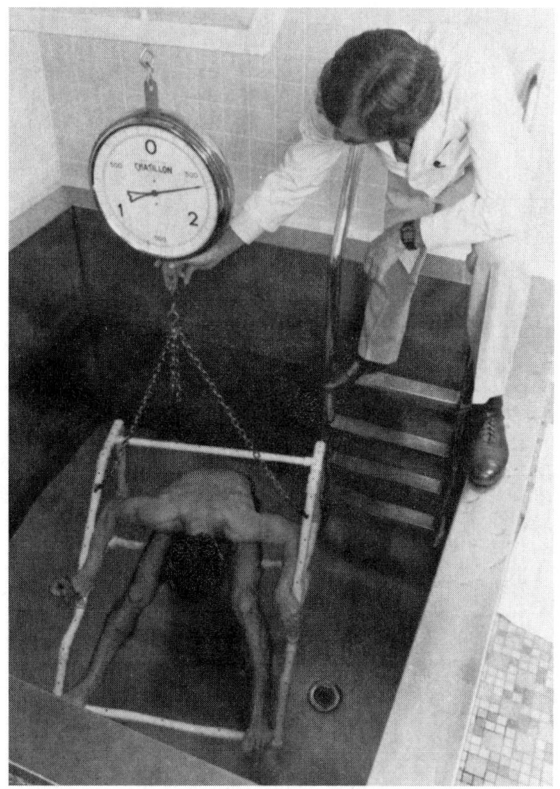

Figure 6-39 Subject's body position while he is submerged during underwater weighing. The water should be kept as calm as possible to get a good reading on the scale. Note how the tester is steadying the scale with his hand. Once the scale is relatively steady, he should remove his hand and take the reading. From Nieman DC. 1995. *Fitness and sports medicine: A health-related approach*, ed 3. Palo Alto: Bull Publishing Co.

3. Submerging: While comfortably seated in the chair, the subject exhales as fully as possible and slowly leans forward until the head is completely under the water, as shown in Figure 6-39. The subject continues to press as much air from the lungs as possible. After exhaling fully, the subject remains motionless and counts for 5 to 7 seconds before coming up for air. This will allow the tester time to read the scale. While in the water, the subject should move slowly and deliberately to prevent water turbulence that can make the subject bob up and down and make scale reading difficult. When the subject submerges, the tester can keep one hand on the scale to steady it, as shown in Figure 6-39.
4. Recording underwater weight: Several trials usually are necessary before the subject becomes accustomed to the procedure and consistent readings are obtained. Katch and coworkers[109] weighed subjects nine to ten

times and took the average of the last three underwater readings as the "true" underwater weight. Underwater weight should be recorded on the Body Composition Worksheet (Figure 6-38) as the gross weight in water. The net body weight in water is the gross weight in water minus the tare weight. The temperature of the water should be measured, and water density should be determined from standard tables.

5. Determining residual volume: Residual volume (RV) is the amount of air remaining in the lungs after a maximal exhalation.[87] All other things being equal, a subject with a large RV will be more buoyant (have a lower underwater weight) than one with a smaller RV. Although RV often is estimated, whenever possible it should be measured directly. When RV is estimated, hydrostatically determined percent body fat is no more accurate than when derived from skinfold measurements.[29] Techniques for measuring RV include nitrogen washout,[111] helium dilution,[112] and oxygen dilution.[113] The choice of technique is generally a matter of which is available to the investigator.[4] Whether RV should be measured at the same time as underwater weighing or immediately before or after is a point of contention among investigators.[4] Currently, there seems to be no clear advantage of one approach over the other.

   If equipment for measuring RV is not available, it can be estimated from vital lung capacity.[114] RV is approximately 24% of vital lung capacity, provided the vital capacity is measured while the subject is in water.[4] Another approach is to use the following sex-specific formulas:[115]

   Male RV $= 0.017\,A + 0.06858\,S - 3.477$
   Female RV $= 0.009\,A + 0.08128\,S - 3.900$
   Where A $=$ age in years; S $=$ stature in inches.

   Because measuring gastrointestinal tract gas is impossible using conventional methods, it is nearly always estimated to be 100 ml in adults.[4,82] The value is likely smaller in children and larger in subjects who consumed flatus-producing foods or carbonated beverages before being measured.[4] The volume of gastrointestinal gas can range from 50 to 300 ml.[82]

6. Calculating density and percent body fat: Using the formulas on the Body Composition Worksheet (Figure 6-38), estimates of body density and percent body fat can be calculated. The remainder of the calculations on the Body Composition Worksheet are the same as those discussed previously under skinfold measurements (see the section entitled "What is a Desirable Level of Fatness?").

Weaknesses of Underwater Weighing

Underwater weighing has several weaknesses. It is not practical for testing large numbers of people. Subjects must be willing and able to remain submerged and motionless long enough for an accurate measurement of weight to be made. This requires considerable subject cooperation and training.[82,116] Consequently, about 10% to 20% of subjects find it difficult to be weighed under water. The technique requires some special equipment, experience, and financial investment. In many situations, skinfold measurements may be more practical.[29]

Densitometry is based on several assumptions. Perhaps the most tenuous of these is a constant density of the fat-free compartment.[4,82,85] As already mentioned in this chapter, a number of factors can affect the density of the fat-free mass, and these can influence the accuracy of body density measurement by 3% to 4%.[11] Athletes, for example, tend to have denser bone and muscle tissue, which may result in underestimation of body fat (possibly even *negative* body fat values), whereas the tendency of older persons to have less-dense bones will likely result in overestimation of body fat.[4] Fat-free tissue density values for adults are probably not appropriate for use with children. Another concern is gas trapped in the gut, the amount of which can only be estimated.[116] Other factors affecting the accuracy of body density measurements include the consumption of food and carbonated beverages shortly before underwater weighing, fluid loss during intensive training, fluid retention before menstruation, and the degree of forcible exhalation while submerged.[4] Despite these weaknesses, underwater weighing remains the standard laboratory technique for determining body density and percent body fat.[29,116]

Other Densitometry Approaches

Several approaches have been developed to measure body volume (and consequently body density and percent body fat) without requiring the subject to be totally immersed in water. The most practical of these uses a **plethysmograph** to measure body volume. Diethelm and coworkers[117,118] have developed a plethysmograph fashioned from a tank in which the subject stands immersed in water to the neck. A clear plastic lid is sealed over the top of the tank, and the volume of air displaced by the subject's head is determined by measuring air pressure changes produced by a pump of known stroke volume.[82,117] The procedure takes only a few moments, and the tester is able to communicate with the subject via intercom. Total body volume is the sum of the water displaced by the immersed body and the volume of air displaced by the head and neck above the water's surface. The technique compares favorably with other methods of measuring body composition and may be the most accurate method for estimating body fat.[116,117]

More recently, investigators in the Netherlands have developed a whole-body plethysmograph.[119] The system consists primarily of a cylindrically shaped measuring chamber vertically cut in half. The two halves are hinged so the chamber can open to allow a subject to step in. When closed, it is airtight. The chamber is of a known volume and connected to a piston of known stroke volume. While in the chamber, the subject can breathe freely and communicate with the tester via intercom.

The measuring chamber is first closed and sealed, the piston is actuated, and the increased pressure is recorded. The measuring chamber is then opened, and the subject steps into it. It is closed and sealed during the measurement period lasting about 10 seconds. The piston is again actuated, momentarily increasing pressure within the chamber, which also is recorded. The rise in pressure caused by the subject's presence within the chamber is used, along with other values, to calculate the subject's body volume.[119]

Both methods appear to yield density measurements as accurate as those from underwater weighings performed on the most cooperative subjects by the best-trained testers. Because plethysmography is better tolerated by subjects than underwater weighing and requires considerably less subject cooperation, it should have superior validity and reproducibility.[116,119] Although the equipment for plethysmography is more complex and costly than that needed for underwater weighing, plethysmography has the advantage that it does not require measurement of residual volume because air within the subject's lungs and gut does not contribute to subject volume.[4,82,116,119]

TOTAL BODY WATER

Water is normally the largest component of the human body. It composes approximately 60% and 50% of the weight of the adult male and female body, respectively. As much as 80% to 90% of the weight of neonates is water.[4,116] Because fat is free of water, all the water in the body is found in the fat-free mass. It has been assumed that fat-free tissue has an average water content of approximately 73.2%. Based on this assumption, a measure of total body water (TBW) should allow calculation of total body fat from the following formula:[52,82]

Total body water is measured indirectly using **dilution techniques** where a known concentration and volume of a certain substance (a tracer) is given orally or parenterally to a subject, time is allowed for the tracer to equilibrate with water in the subject's body, and the concentration of the tracer in a sample of the subject's blood, urine, or saliva is analyzed. From this data, TBW is measured using the following relationship:

$$C_1V_1 = C_2V_2$$

where C_1 and V_1 = the concentration and volume, respectively, of tracer given to the subject; C_2 = the concentration of tracer in the body fluid sample taken from the subject; and V_2 = the volume of water in the body, or TBW.[82]

Of the numerous tracers used throughout the years, three are currently in common use: water labeled with either **tritium** (^3H_2O), **deuterium** (^2H_2O), or the stable isotope of oxygen ($H_2{}^{18}O$). Of these three, the tritium and deuterium isotopes of water are the most frequently used.[4,52,82,116] A tracer at a specified concentration and volume is either ingested orally or injected intravenously. This is followed by an equilibration period and then a sampling period.[82]

Deuterium is a stable isotope of hydrogen (does not emit radiation) that has a mass twice that of ordinary hydrogen. Lukaski and coworkers[120] have described TBW measurement using deuterium-labeled water (deuterium oxide, or D_2O). After a subject had fasted 10 hours overnight, blood and saliva samples were obtained. A 10-g oral dose of D_2O in fruit juice or deionized water was given to each subject. During the next 4 hours, the subjects remained in a quiet state. Blood and saliva samples were taken at 30, 60, 90, 120, 180, and 240 minutes following the dose. Concentrations of D_2O in samples were determined by infrared absorption.

The concentration of D_2O in blood or saliva also can be determined by gas chromatography and mass spectrometry.[82] The use of D_2O has been found to be simple, accurate, noninvasive (if saliva collections are used), and suitable for field studies.[4] In healthy subjects, the tracer equilibrates in the body's water within 2 hours after ingestion and remains at a constant concentration for the next 3 hours. In subjects experiencing edema, ascites, or some other form of water accumulation, 4 to 6 hours may be required for the D_2O to equilibrate.[81] Because deuterium is a stable isotope, its use is safe and ethical, even with children and females of childbearing age. Major drawbacks of the method are the cost of the equipment necessary to measure the D_2O in samples and the tedious work involved in preparing samples for analysis.[4,116]

Tritium (^3H) is a radioactive isotope of hydrogen with a mass three times that of ordinary hydrogen. Its use in measuring TBW is similar to that of deuterium oxide. Its radioactivity, however, makes it unsuitable in research involving children and females of childbearing age, or in studies requiring repeated administration of the tracer over a short period (for example, every 2 weeks or less).[82] The concentration of the isotope in body fluids is determined by a liquid scintillation counter that measures the radioactive emission from the sample.[52,116]

The use of water labeled with the heavy isotope of oxygen (^{18}O) as a tracer in dilution studies is gaining popularity among researchers. It has the advantage of being a stable (nonradioactive) isotope, and exhaled carbon dioxide in the form of $C^{18}O_2$ is in isotopic equilibrium with body water and can be used as the sample for easy analysis by mass spectrometry.[52,116] These advantages are offset somewhat by the higher cost of $H_2{}^{18}O$ compared with that of the hydrogen isotopes.[52]

Garrow has pointed out three main sources of error in measuring total body water: failure to administer an accurately measured dose; consumption of beverages by subjects during the equilibration period, which may prevent equilibration from being reached; and contamination of the samples by atmospheric water before analysis.[116] As mentioned previously, calculation of the fat mass from TBW is based on the assumption that fat-free tissue has a constant water content that averages approximately 73%. This average value is based on analyses of a limited number of cadavers with actual values ranging from 67.4% to 77.5%. These variations can result in considerable error in calculating total body fat from TBW.[52] It also appears that fatter subjects tend to have a higher water content in their fat-free tissues. Failure to account for this will lead to an underestimation of fat mass based on TBW.[116]

TOTAL BODY POTASSIUM

Two factors make measurements of total body potassium of interest to those studying body composition. More than 90% of all the body's potassium is located within fat-free tissues (as an intracellular cation), and 0.012% of all potassium is the naturally occurring potassium-40 (^{40}K) isotope, which emits a very small yet detectable amount of high-energy gamma radiation.[4,52,82,116]

Measurement of total body potassium (TBK) requires a specially constructed counter fitted with multiple gamma-ray detectors that are interfaced with a computer for data collection and processing. Because of the low levels of gamma radiation emitted from a subject, very sensitive detectors are required. The counter must be large enough to admit a subject and be screened from external radiation (cosmic and local sources of ionizing radiation) by massive shields of lead or steel, thus making it very expensive.[52] The counting process requires about 30 minutes. Recently developed counters will yield an estimate of TBK with a precision of about ±3%.[52]

A major assumption of TBK measurement is that fat-free tissue has a known and constant potassium content. Researchers disagree on the concentration of potassium in fat-free tissue and whether there is a difference between the sexes.[4,52] The most widely published estimates are 66 and 60 mmol/kg of potassium in men and women, respectively.[52,116] It has been reported that the fat-free tissues of obese subjects tend to have a lower potassium content than the tissues of lean subjects. This may be due to actual differences in potassium content between obese and lean subjects. Another explanation may be that obese subjects have a thicker layer of potassium-poor fat surrounding a potassium-rich core of fat-free tissue, absorbing some of the radiation and thus leading to an underestimation of actual TBK and an overestimation of fat content in the obese.[52,116] It also has been reported that the potassium content of fat-free tissues decreases with increasing age.[52] Another factor affecting the performance of the counters is the presence of radioactive contamination on the subject's body and clothing from atmospheric radon gas.[4,82] Therefore, it is recommended that subjects shower, wash their hair, and wear clean clothes before undergoing TBK measurements.[82]

Despite the reported precision of ±3%, the high cost and inherent limitations of the technique limit its use in estimating body composition. However, the technique does have value when used in conjunction with other measures. As Garrow[116] points out, combining the use of TBW measurements (which tend to underestimate body fat in obese subjects) with TBK measurements (which tend to overestimate body fat in the obese) may lead to more reliable estimates of body fat than either method alone.

NEUTRON ACTIVATION ANALYSIS

Neutron activation analysis allows measurement of the body's content of calcium, iodine, hydrogen, sodium, chloride, phosphorus, carbon, and nitrogen.[4,82,121,122] Also known as in vivo neutron activation analysis, the method delivers a beam of neutrons to the subject, which interacts with the body's elements in several characteristic ways. In the most important of these (in terms of neutron activation analysis), atoms of target elements are activated, creating unstable isotopes such as calcium-49 (^{49}Ca), nitrogen-15 (^{15}N), and sodium-24 (^{24}Na).[121] As these unstable isotopes revert back to their stable forms, gamma radiation of a characteristic energy is emitted from each. This is received by the system's detectors and analyzed by its computers. The unique energy level of the γ radiation identifies the element, and the radiation's level of activity represents its abundance.[82,122] Gamma-ray emission can occur almost immediately (in which case the technique is referred to as *prompt γ analysis*) or over a several-minute period (in which case it is known as *delayed γ analysis*).[121]

Because a major component of muscle is nitrogen, the ability to measure nitrogen using neutron activation analysis allows the body's muscle and nonmuscle mass to be estimated.[82,123]

The precision of repeated nitrogen determinations in healthy humans has been 2% and 3%.[82]

Bone mineral content is of considerable interest to those studying osteoporosis, and neutron activation analysis is useful in measuring total body calcium, which is then used to quantitate total body bone mineral. The precision of repeated calcium measurements in healthy adults using neutron activation analysis has been 2.5%, making the method suitable for longitudinal studies of bone mass.[82] A more recent study of calcium content in phantoms (representations of the human body used for precision and accuracy testing) as measured by neutron activation analysis resulted in values within 3.6% of their known composition.[124]

Neutron activation analysis has been recently used successfully in clinical studies to assess the time required for body nitrogen to return to preoperative levels following aortic reconstruction surgery and to assess nutritional status in patients receiving continuous ambulatory peritoneal dialysis.[125,126] The accuracy and precision of the method are as good as, if not better than, those of other methods. It is preferable to isotope dilution techniques in patients requiring continuous intravenous fluid therapy and in those with large increases in body water. It is noninvasive and is not based on certain assumptions concerning ratios of major body compartments or their density, as are some of the methods used to assess body fat.[121]

The method has several drawbacks. It exposes subjects to ionizing radiation, is costly, and requires skilled operators. In addition, the units are not mobile and are not widely available.[82]

CREATININE EXCRETION

The amount of creatinine excreted in the urine over a 24-hour period can be used in estimating body muscle mass.[4,82] Creatinine is the only metabolite of creatine, a nitrogenous compound synthesized from amino acids in the liver and taken up by many tissues, but primarily by muscle. Ninety-eight percent of the body's creatine is found in muscle, primarily in the form of creatine phosphate (bound to adenosine triphosphate, where it serves as an immediate source of energy).[4,82] Creatine spontaneously dehydrates to form creatinine, which is then excreted unaltered in the urine. Therefore, measurement of creatinine in a 24-hour urine collection should reflect the level of total body creatinine and consequently total body muscle mass.[4]

Several problems are associated with this approach. The most notable of these are the influence of meat consumption on urinary creatinine levels and the large intraindividual variability in daily urinary creatinine excretion (about ±11%) in persons consuming a meat-free diet.[82] Dietary creatine can influence urinary creatinine independently of muscle mass. Therefore, the diets of subjects undergoing urinary creatinine measurements should be meat free or be of a constant composition.[4] Urine collections must be complete because an error of 15 minutes in the timing of 24-hour urine collections can affect results of creatinine measurements by 1%.[4,82] Some researchers advise making three consecutive 24-hour urine collections to assure a representative creatinine excretion for an individual.[82] The precision of automated procedures for determining creatinine concentration in urine is approximately 1% to 2%, introducing further error.[82]

Despite these potential sources of error, estimates of fat-free mass based on 24-hour urinary excretion of creatinine have been shown to correlate reasonably well with those derived from measurements of body density, total body nitrogen, and total body potassium.[127,128] More accurate estimates of fat-free mass can be obtained from measurement of body density, total body nitrogen, and total body potassium. However, when the necessary facilities or resources are unavailable or when subjects are too ill to undergo such testing, urinary creatinine may be the most acceptable approach. Another urinary metabolite that appears better correlated with densitometrically determined fat-free mass is 3-methylhistidine.

3-METHYLHISTIDINE

3-Methylhistidine is an amino acid found in actin and myosin, the contractile proteins of muscle. 3-Methylhistidine is a *derived amino acid;* it is formed by the addition of methyl groups to histidine present in actin and myosin after these contractile proteins have been synthesized. When these proteins are catabolized, the 3-methylhistidine is released, not reutilized for protein synthesis, but excreted quantitatively in the urine.[129] Assuming that muscle protein synthesis and degradation are balanced during steady-state periods, urinary 3-methylhistidine should be proportional to muscle mass.[4]

Lukaski and coworkers[127] have shown 24-hour urinary excretion of 3-methylhistidine to be well correlated to fat-free mass determined by densitometry in healthy males age 23 to 52 years consuming a meat-free diet. In a later study, Lukaski and coworkers[128] assessed skeletal muscle mass in 14 healthy adult males on a meat-free diet using measurements of 3-methylhistidine, total body nitrogen, and total body potassium. Urinary excretion of 3-methylhistidine was significantly related to skeletal muscle mass and appeared to be a valid index of muscle and fat-free mass.

Measurement of urinary 3-methylhistidine excretion is subject to the same potential errors as are possible in measurement of urinary creatinine excretion.[4,82] Intraindividual variability is reported to range from 10% to 20%. Subjects should refrain from eating meat during the measurement period. Twenty-four-hour urine collections should be accurately timed and complete.[82] Before 3-methylhistidine can be used as a routine indicator of muscle mass, however, the effects of sex, age, maturity, fitness status, recent intense exercise, disease, and injury on 3-methylhistidine levels must be better understood.[55]

ELECTRICAL CONDUCTANCE

The use of electrical conductance to assess body composition is based on the marked difference in electrolyte content between fat and fat-free tissue.[130,131] Electrolytes such as sodium, chloride, potassium, and bicarbonate are found primarily in the fat-free tissues, whereas concentrations of these ions in adipose tissue are very low. Because electrolytes in body water are capable of conducting electricity, the body's fat-free mass has a greater electrical conductivity than its fat mass. This difference in conductivity is the basis of two body assessment methods: bioelectrical impedance and total body electrical conductivity.

Bioelectrical Impedance

When an electrical current is passed through the body, it is opposed by the nonconducting tissues (principally fat and cell membranes) and transmitted by electrolytes dissolved in water (largely found in the fat-free tissues, although adipose tissue contains about 14% water).[4,82,130,131] This opposition to an alternating current is called impedance, which is composed of two elements: resistance and reactance. In bioelectrical impedance analysis (BIA), an electronic instrument (Figure 6-40) generates an alternating current, which is passed through the body by means of four electrodes placed on the hand and foot. The current (50 kHz, 800 ÌA) is harmless and cannot be felt by the subject. The body's resistance to this current is measured by the instrument. Some BIA instruments simply provide the operator with a value for resistance, which is then used (along with the subject's stature, weight, and sex) to manually calculate total body water, fat-free mass, and percent of body fat. More sophisticated BIA instruments contain a computer and printer and are capable of automatically performing these calculations and providing a printed record.

Bioelectrical impedance analysis yields values for TBW that are very close to those obtained by dilution techniques.[130,132] One of the primary weaknesses of BIA, however, is estimating fat-free mass and percent of body fat from the value for TBW using regression equations. Because BIA relies upon regression equations for calculating

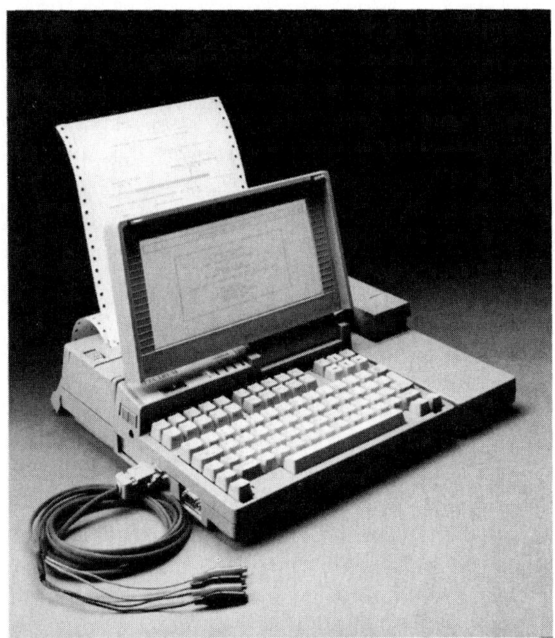

Figure 6-40 Bioelectrical impedance offers a convenient, rapid, noninvasive, and safe method for assessing body composition, that correlates well with more cumbersome methods. Photo courtesy of RJL Systems, Mount Clemens, MI.

fat-free mass and percent of body fat, the method is only as good as the equation used.[133] Earlier equations tended to give inaccurate estimates of fat-free mass and percent of body fat; more recent equations are considerably better. Another weakness is that BIA assumes that subjects are normally hydrated. Dehydration caused by insufficient water intake, excessive perspiration, heavy exercise, or caffeine or alcohol use (which stimulates urine production possibly leading to dehydration) will result in overestimation of fat mass. To prevent this, subjects are advised to drink plenty of water, refrain from consuming caffeine and alcohol the day before testing, and avoid heavy exercise 12 hours before testing.

Multiple BIA measurements of 14 subjects over 5 consecutive days yielded a precision of less than 2%, showing good reliability.[134] When compared with estimates of percent body fat derived from underwater weighing, BIA was shown to be as good as (if not slightly better than) skinfold measurements in predicting percent body fat.[130,131] The method has the advantage of being safe, convenient to use, portable, rapid, and noninvasive. Bioelectrical impedance was among the procedures used in NHANES III. The only drawback is the instrument's cost, which can range from $2500 to $8000.

Total Body Electrical Conductivity

The degree to which an object placed in an electromagnetic field will tend to disrupt that field depends on the quantity of conducting material in the object. Because electrolytes within the fat-free mass are capable of conducting electricity, the degree to which a body placed in an electromagnetic field (EMF) disrupts that field is closely related to the amount of fat-free mass.[133] The instrument for measuring total body electrical conductivity consists of a large solenoid coil driven by an oscillating radio-frequency current that generates an EMF. The subject is placed on a table, which is slowly rolled into the coil. Changes in the EMF are measured between the condition when the subject is inside the coil and when the coil is empty.[135,136] These changes are proportional to the total electrical conductivity of the subject's body. Using the statistical process of multiple-regression analysis, regression equations have been developed allowing TBW, TBK, fat-free mass, and percent of body fat to be predicted from these changes.[137]

Total body electrical conductivity (TOBEC) originally was developed to quantify lean tissue in meat and live animals and has proved valuable for this purpose.[82] As a method for assessing body composition, TOBEC has been shown to compare favorably with other assessment methods such as underwater weighing, TBW determined by deuterium dilution, and TBK.[137–139] It has been shown to be an acceptable technique for body composition assessment in teenagers[136] and in adults.[137] Like BIA, the accuracy of TOBEC in estimating

TBW can be affected by dehydration.[82] TOBEC appears to be safe because the body is subjected to the EMF for only a 3-minute interval and the level of energy exposure is less than one thousandth of the established regulatory limits for continuous exposure to radio-frequency waves.[82] A serious limiting factor is the high cost of the units (approaching $100,000).

INFRARED INTERACTANCE

A recently developed approach to estimating body composition is infrared interactance (also known as nearinfrared interactance). When a material is exposed to infrared light, the light is absorbed, reflected, or transmitted, depending on the scattering and absorption properties of the material.[82] For example, water, protein, and fat have specific infrared absorption characteristics because of the stretching and bending of hydrogen bonds associated with the carbon, oxygen, and nitrogen they contain.[140] Information about the chemical composition (for example, water, protein, and fat content) of a material is contained in the infrared light reflected from the material.[82] Infrared instruments have been used successfully since about 1965 to determine the amount of moisture, protein, fat, and starch in grains and oil seeds.[82,140]

In human body composition analysis, a battery-powered, computerized infrared spectrophotometer marketed as the Futrex-5000 is used. A probe or "light wand," which acts as both an infrared transmitter and detector, is attached to the unit by an electrical cord. The probe is placed on the subject's skin, and infrared light of two wavelengths is transmitted through the skin from the probe. Infrared light reflected from the skin and underlying tissues is detected by the probe. Estimates of body composition are made by analyzing certain characteristics of the reflected light (the shape of the interactance spectrum).[82,140,141] The instrument does not provide a measurement of fat thickness.[142]

As an approach to estimating body composition, infrared interactance is safe, noninvasive, rapid, and convenient to use.[141] These advantages have made infrared interactance a popular body composition technique at some hospitals, health clubs, and weight-loss clinics.[142] Some researchers have reported "excellent reliability and good validity" in using infrared interactance to estimate body composition.[143] Recent validation studies, however, have raised questions about its accuracy.[142,144–148] When compared with other body composition methods (underwater weighing, skinfold measurements, and bioelectrical impedance analysis), infrared interactance overestimated percent body fat in lean subjects (<8% body fat) and underestimated body fat in obese subjects (>30% body fat).[142] The tendency of infrared interactance to underestimate percent body fat in obese subjects has been shown by other researchers as well.[144–146,148]

As a method for estimating body composition, most researchers report that infrared interactance is inferior to skinfold measurements.[142,145–148] At this time, it is not a recommended approach for determining body composition.

ULTRASOUND

Ultrasound is a widely used medical imaging method and has been studied as a possible tool in nutritional assessment. The heart of the technique is the transducer.[149] The transducer converts electrical energy into high-frequency sound and then converts that sound back into electric energy; in other words, it acts both as a transmitter and a receiver. When the transducer is applied to the body surface, the ultrasound is transmitted into the body in the form of short pulses. As the ultrasound perpendicularly strikes the interface between two tissues differing in density (for example, adipose tissue and muscle), some of the sound is reflected and received by the transducer. The first reflection occurs at the transducer-skin interface. Each succeeding tissue interface results in a reflection, the intensity of which is reduced by the depth of the patient's tissues. This reflected sound is visually displayed on a video screen.[4,82,149]

In most published studies, ultrasonography has been compared with use of skinfold calipers. The results have been mixed and may be due to differences in instrumentation, technique, and interpretation.[150–152] Considerable skill is required in using the method and interpreting its results. The transducer must be applied to the skin surface with uniform and constant pressure to prevent differences in adipose and other soft tissue compression.[82,153] Differences in study populations could partly explain the conflicting results. For example, ultrasound may be preferable to skinfold calipers in measuring very obese individuals because of difficulty in accurately measuring skinfolds on them.[133,153]

Ultrasound has several advantages. It is noninvasive, nonradioactive, safe, and relatively portable, although less so than skinfold calipers. It may be a more appropriate technique for assessing persons whose skinfolds are thick and/or difficult to measure. Compared with the use of skinfold calipers, ultrasound is much more expensive and requires more training for its operation and interpretation.[82,133]

COMPUTED TOMOGRAPHY

Computed tomography (CT) is an imaging technique producing highly detailed cross-sectional images of the body resulting from differences in the transmission of an x-ray beam through body tissues of differing density.[133] Although its role in medicine is primarily for diagnostic purposes, it has proved to be a valuable research tool in assessing body composition and nutritional status. The CT system consists of an x-ray source aligned opposite an array of radiation detectors. In some CT scanners, the beam and detectors rotate in a plane perpendicular to the subject. However, in the latest models (so-called fourth-generation scanners) the detectors are stationary, and only the x-ray source moves.[149]

As the x-ray beam passes through the subject, it is weakened or attenuated by the body's tissues and eventually picked up by the detectors. The response of the detectors is then transmitted to a computer, which also considers the spatial arrangement of the subject and x-ray beam. From this data, the computer reconstructs the subject's cross-sectional anatomy using mathematic equations adapted for computer processing.[149]

CT has been particularly useful in studying the relative deposition of subcutaneous and intraabdominal fat.[154–156] This is of particular interest because, as discussed earlier in this chapter, not only does the total amount of body fat affect health, but the placement of that fat is important as well. Estimates of subcutaneous and intraabdominal fat from CT have been shown to compare very closely with direct measurements in cadavers and laboratory animals.[157,158] CT scans at three sites—lower chest, abdomen, and midthigh—have been shown effective in estimating body fat mass in premenopausal obese women.[159]

The potential for using CT in assessing body composition and nutritional status is limited by problems of radiation exposure and the high cost and limited availability of the instrument.[82,160] Multiple scans of the same individual, whole-body scans, and use of CT with children and women of childbearing age are not encouraged because of the exposure to ionizing radiation. The use of the technology in nutritional assessment is restricted, for the most part, to special research applications.

MAGNETIC RESONANCE IMAGING

Magnetic resonance imaging (MRI) is a technology that allows both imaging of the body and in vivo chemical analysis without hazard to the subject.[160] Originally referred to as nuclear magnetic resonance, this approach is based on the fact that the nucleus of an atom acts like a magnet; it has a north and south pole and is said to be a *magnetic dipole*. Ordinarily nuclei or magnetic dipoles are oriented randomly. However, if a subject is placed in a large bore magnet generating a very strong magnetic field, the magnetic dipoles become aligned in relation to the magnetic field. If a radio-frequency wave is then directed into the subject's body, some of the nuclei will absorb energy from the radio wave and change their orientation with respect to the magnetic field. When the radio wave is discontinued, the nuclei gradually return to their equilibrium state (relaxation) and emit a signal that can be received by the system. These data are then processed by computer to generate an image much the same way as in CT.[82,133,149,160]

The hydrogen nucleus is particularly well suited for analysis because of its high concentration and abundance in the body and its easy detection by MRI. Tissue levels of phosphorus also can be detected in tissues using MRI. This allows investigators to quantify the relative amounts of ATP, phosphocreatine, and inorganic phosphorus in the body's tissues.[160] MRI allows researchers to monitor the metabolic functions of certain tissues and organs in response to certain treatments including various nutritional regimens.[160]

MRI has been used successfully to measure the amount and distribution of intraabdominal fat.[161] The reproducibility of measurements was less than 3% for total body areas, less than 5% for subcutaneous fat areas, and less than 10% for internal fat areas. Reproducibility was better for individuals with higher percent total body fat. Researchers in the United Kingdom estimated total body fat from 28 transaxial MRI scans (perpendicular to the long axis of the body) taken of a group of lean and obese women.[162] The correlation of total body fat estimated by MRI with the average of six methods used simultaneously was 0.99. When the number of transaxial scans was reduced to four, the correlation was reduced to 0.97. MRI was used to measure TBW in baboons.[163] These values were similar to those obtained by direct measurements. In contrast, the tritium dilution technique performed on the same animals was found to generally overestimate TBW.

The advantages of MRI are several. It is totally noninvasive, uses no ionizing radiation (thus it is safe for children, females of childbearing age, and multiple studies on the same subject), produces high-quality images of the body, allows the amount and distribution of body fat to be studied, and can be used to study the metabolic activity of tissues or organs. MRI currently can image hydrogen and phosphorus, and future developments will allow imaging of carbon, nitrogen, sodium, and chloride.[82] The low-contrast resolution of MRI is much better than that of CT.[147] Drawbacks of the method are its restricted availability and high cost.[82]

DUAL-ENERGY X-RAY ABSORPTIOMETRY

Dual-energy x-ray absorptiometry (DEXA) is discussed in Chapter 7 as a means of assessing bone mineral density, an area in which it is particularly well suited because of its high precision in measuring bone mineral density. In recent years, considerable attention has been given to using DEXA to measure fat and nonbone lean tissue.[164] DEXA has the advantage of being safe (because of the low-radiation dose subjects receive) and relatively quick (a whole-body scan takes 20 to 35 minutes). The fact that the procedure requires little cooperation from patients makes it an attractive body composition assessment method for the very young, the very old, and the sick. The use of effective and user-friendly software allows personnel with minimal training to operate the instrument and produce high-quality output.[164] Estimates of percent body fat from DEXA have been found to be highly correlated with those from underwater weighing.[165,166]

As with any relatively new technology, DEXA has some limitations. Marked differences in the hydration of lean tissue from that seen in healthy adults may adversely affect the accuracy of body composition measures. Consequently, concerns have been raised about the appropriateness of using DEXA for assessing body composition in infants (who tend to have a higher degree of lean tissue hydration than adults) and persons with acute or chronic alterations in body water. Body composition measurements may be affected by the thickness of the body part being scanned, possibly resulting in systematic differences between thin and obese persons or affecting the accuracy of serial measurements in persons losing or gaining weight. The accuracy of regional soft tissue measurements can be adversely affected by the presence of bone (especially by ribs in the thorax) and the calcification of soft tissues (as is seen in the aortas of older people).[164]

Dual-energy x-ray absorptiometry has considerable promise as a body composition assessment technique, but further research and development is necessary before it can be considered a "gold standard."[164]

SUMMARY

1. Anthropometry is the measurement of body size, weight, and proportions. Adherence to proper technique is critical to obtaining accurate and precise measurements. Among children, length, stature, weight, and head circumference are the most sensitive and commonly used anthropometric indicators of health.
2. Body weight, one of the most important measurements in nutritional assessment, should be obtained using an electronic of balance beam scale with nondetachable weights that is appropriate for the subject. Attention must be given to regular calibration of balance beam scales, especially after they have been moved.
3. Standards for assessing physical growth of persons from birth to age 18 years have been developed by the National Center for Health Statistics. These growth charts allow a child's development to be easily categorized relative to the development of other children of similar age and sex.
4. Overweight is a body weight above some reference weight, which usually is defined in relation to stature. Obesity is an excess of body fat in relation to lean body mass. Overweight persons tend to die sooner than average-weight persons, especially those who are overweight at younger ages. The lowest mortality in the United States is associated with body weights that are somewhat below average for a given group based on sex and stature.
5. Approaches to assessing body weight include height-weight tables, relative weight, and height-weight indices. The life insurance industry, a leader in the development of height-weight tables, has attempted to define body weights for a given sex and stature that are associated with the lowest mortality.
6. Height-weight tables fail to provide information on body composition. Their data are not drawn from representative population samples and are sometimes self-reported. They inadequately control for confounding variables, such as cigarette smoking, that tend to make lower body weights appear less healthy.
7. Relative weight is a person's actual weight divided by some reference weight for that person's height, multiplied by 100, and expressed as a percentage of reference weight. Relative weights between 90% and 120% are considered within normal limits.
8. Of the various body mass indices available, the most common is Quetelet's index—weight in kilograms divided by height in meters squared. Although body mass indices tend to be better predictors of obesity than height-weight tables or relative weight, they still do not distinguish between overweight resulting from obesity and that resulting from unusual muscular development.
9. The distribution of body fat may be as important a consideration as total quantity of fat. Body fat distribution can be classified into two types: upper body (android or male type) and lower body (gynoid or female type). Android obesity is associated with increased risk of insulin resistance, hyperinsulinemia, non-insulin-dependent (Type II) diabetes mellitus, hypertension, hyperlipidemia, stroke, and death. The waist-to-hip ratio is a valuable index of regional body fat distribution.
10. Body composition analysis can provide estimates of the body's reserves of fat, protein, water, and several minerals. The two-compartment model divides the body into fat and

fat-free masses. The four-compartment model views the human body as composed of four chemical groups: water, protein, mineral, and fat. Most approaches to determining body composition are indirect measures.

11. Measurement of skinfolds is the most widely used method of indirectly estimating percent body fat. What is actually measured is the thickness of a double fold of skin and compressed subcutaneous adipose tissue.
12. Skinfold measures have several advantages. The equipment is inexpensive and portable. Measurements can be easily and quickly obtained, and they correlate well with body density measurements. Proper measurement of skinfolds requires careful site selection and strict adherence to the standardized techniques outlined in this chapter.
13. The triceps is the most commonly used single skinfold site. Single-site skinfold measurements must be interpreted with caution and should only be used as a rough approximation of total body fat percentage. Results should be compared with reference data derived from large population surveys, such as NHANES III.
14. For assessing body composition of young people, the sum of two sites (triceps and subscapular or triceps and medial calf) often is used. These sites correlate with other measures of body fatness and are more reliably and objectively measured than most other sites, and reference data are available.
15. Regression equations allow body density and percentage of body fat to be estimated from multiple skinfold measures. These equations were developed by seeing which combination of anthropometric measures best predicted body density. Generalized equations can be applied to groups varying greatly in age and body fatness and can replace several population-specific equations with little loss in prediction accuracy.
16. Densitometry involves measuring the density of the entire body, usually by hydrostatic (underwater) weighing. If mass and volume of the body are known, its density can be calculated. However, hydrostatic weighing is not practical for testing large groups. It requires considerable subject cooperation, special equipment, experience, and financial investment.
17. Despite its weaknesses, underwater weighing remains the standard laboratory technique for determining body density and percent body fat. Compared with other body density methods and more sophisticated body composition techniques, the costs are low.
18. Body plethysmography measures body density without requiring subjects to be totally immersed in water. Subjects better tolerate this method than underwater weighing. It requires less subject cooperation, and residual lung volume measurements are not needed. It appears as accurate and precise as underwater weighing, but the equipment is considerably more complex and costly.
19. Total body water is measured indirectly using dilution techniques where a tracer of known concentration and volume is given to a subject, time is allowed for the tracer to equilibrate with the subject's body water, and the concentration of the tracer in a sample of the subject's blood, urine, or saliva is analyzed. Commonly used tracers include deuterium oxide and water labeled with the heavy isotope of oxygen.
20. Measurement of total body potassium can also be used to evaluate body composition. More than 90% of body potassium is located within fat-free tissues, and 0.012% of potassium is potassium-40 isotope, which emits gamma radiation.
21. Neutron activation analysis is based on the response of elements (e.g., nitrogen, calcium, and carbon) to neutron beam irradiation and is particularly useful in estimating total body muscle. The method's drawbacks include ionizing radiation exposure, high cost, and limited availability.
22. Measurement of creatinine in a 24-hour urine collection reflects total body muscle mass.

Despite limitations by such factors as dietary creatine, intraindividual variation, and timing of urine collections, estimates of fat-free mass based on urinary creatinine correlate reasonably well with estimates derived from measurements of body density, total body nitrogen, and total body potassium.

23. 3-Methylhistidine is an amino acid found in the contractile proteins actin and myosin. When these proteins are catabolized, 3-methylhistidine is released and excreted in the urine. Urinary excretion has been shown to be a valid index of muscle and fat-free mass. However, its measurement is subject to the same potential errors as those in measurements of urinary creatinine excretion.
24. The marked difference in electrolyte content between fat and fat-free tissues is a basic principle behind body composition estimates from bioelectrical impedance analysis (BIA) and total body electrical conductivity (TOBEC). In BIA, the body's resistance to a minute electrical current is used to calculate total body water, from which the percentages of body fat and fat-free mass are calculated using various formulas.
25. In TOBEC, the degree to which a body placed in an electromagnetic field (EMF) disrupts that field is closely related to the amount of fat-free mass. TOBEC uses an instrument consisting of a large solenoid coil driven by an oscillating radio-frequency current that generates an EMF. Like BIA, the accuracy of total body water estimates can be affected by dehydration. It appears to be an acceptable technique for body composition assessment, but its use is limited by high cost.
26. When infrared light is projected through the skin, some of the energy is reflected from the skin and underlying tissues. Estimates of body composition are made by analyzing certain characteristics of this reflected energy. The approach tends to overestimate percent body fat in lean subjects and underestimate percent body fat in obese subjects. It is an inferior method to skinfold measurements and is not recommended for determining body composition.
27. In ultrasound, high-frequency sound waves are transmitted into the body from a transducer applied to the skin surface. As ultrasound strikes the interface between two tissues differing in density (for example, adipose tissue and muscle), some of it is reflected and received by the transducer. The time lag between reflections allows tissue layer depth to be calculated. Ultrasound compares favorably to skinfold measurements but may be preferable to skinfold measurements when evaluating very obese people.
28. Computed tomography is an imaging technique producing highly detailed cross-sectional images of the body caused by differences in the transmission of an x-ray beam through body tissues of differing density. Magnetic resonance imaging is a technology allowing both imaging of the body and in vivo chemical analysis without radiation hazard to the subject.
29. Body composition estimates derived from dual-energy x-ray absorptiometry (DEXA) compare favorably with those from underwater weighing. DEXA has the advantage of requiring little subject cooperation, being relatively quick, and having a low radiation dose. Differences in hydration and the presence of bone or calcified soft tissues may affect the accuracy of body composition measurements.

REFERENCES

1. Chumlea WC, Roche AF, Mukherjee D. 1987. *Nutritional assessment of the elderly through anthropometry*. Columbus, Ohio: Ross Laboratories.
2. Moore WM, Roche AF. 1983. *Pediatric anthropometry*, 2nd ed. Columbus, Ohio: Ross Laboratories.

3. Heymsfield SB, Casper K. 1987. Anthropometric assessment of the adult hospitalized patient. *Journal of Parenteral and Enteral Nutrition* 11:36S–41S.
4. Brodie DA. 1988. Techniques of measurement of body composition. Part I. *Sports Medicine* 5:11–40.
5. Pollock ML, Jackson AS. 1984. Research progress in validation of clinical methods of assessing body composition. *Medicine and Science in Sports and Exercise* 16:606–613.
6. Chumlea WC, Roche AF, Steinbaugh ML. 1985. Estimating stature from knee height for persons 60 to 90 years of age. *Journal of the American Geriatrics Society* 33:116–120.
7. Gordon CC, Chumlea WC, and Roche AF. 1988. Stature, recumbent length, and weight. In Lohman TG, Roche AF, Martorell R, eds. *Anthropometric standardization reference manual*. Champaign, Ill. Human Kinetics Books.
8. Hamill PVV, Drizd TA, Johnson CL, Reed RB, Roche AF, Moore WM. 1979. Physical growth: National Center for Health Statistics percentiles. *American Journal of Clinical Nutrition* 32:607–629.
9. Roche AF, Shumei G, Baumgartner RN, and Falls RA. 1988. The measurement of stature. *American Journal of Clinical Nutrition* 47:922.
10. Winick M, Rosso P. 1969. Head circumference and cellular growth of the brain in normal and marasmic children. *Journal of Pediatrics* 74:774–778.
11. Roche AF, Himes JH. 1980. Incremental growth charts. *American Journal of Clinical Nutrition* 33:2041–2052.
12. Chumlea WC, Guo S, Roche AF, Steinbaugh ML. 1988. Prediction of body weight for the nonambulatory elderly from anthropometry. *Journal of the American Dietetic Association* 88:564–568.
13. National Center for Health Statistics. 1993. *Executive summary of the growth chart workshop, 1992*. Hyattsville, Md: U.S. Department of Health and Human Services, Public Health Service, Centers for Disease Control.
14. Harrison GG. 1985. Height-weight tables. *Annals of Internal Medicine* 103:989–994.
15. Food and Nutrition Board, National Research Council. 1989. *Diet and health: Implications for reducing chronic disease risk*. Washington, DC: National Academy Press.
16. Bray GA, Gray DS. 1988. Obesity. Part I: Pathogenesis. *Western Medical Journal* 149:429–441.
17. Simopoulos AP, VanItallie TB. 1984. Body weight, health, and longevity. *Annals of Internal Medicine* 100:285–295.
18. Simopoulos AP. 1985. The health implications of overweight and obesity. *Nutrition Reviews* 43:33–40.
19. VanItallie TB. 1985. Health implications of overweight and obesity in the United States. *Annals of Internal Medicine* 103:983–988.
20. Andres R. 1985. Mortality and obesity: The rationale for age-specific height-weight tables. In Andres R, Bierman EL, and Hazzard WR, eds. *Principles of geriatric medicine*. New York: McGraw Hill.
21. National Institutes of Health. 1985. Consensus Development Conference Statement. Health implications of obesity. *Annals of Internal Medicine* 103:1073–1077.
22. Lindsted K, Tonstad S, Kuzma JW. 1991. Body mass index and patterns of mortality among Seventh-day Adventist men. *International Journal of Obesity*. 15:397–406.
23. Weigley ES. 1984. Average? Ideal? Desirable? A brief overview of height-weight tables in the United States. *Journal of the American Dietetic Association* 84:417–423.
24. Manson JE, Stampfer MJ, Hennekens CH, Willett WC. 1987. Body weight and longevity: A reassessment. *Journal of the American Medical Association* 257:353–358.
25. Ideal weights for women. 1942. *Statistical Bulletin of the Metropolitan Life Insurance Company* 23(October):6–8.
26. Ideal weights for men. 1943. *Statistical Bulletin of the Metropolitan Life Insurance Company* 24(June):6–8.
27. New weight standards for men and women. 1959. *Statistical Bulletin of the Metropolitan Life Insurance Company* 40(November-December): 1–3.
28. Metropolitan Height and Weight Tables. 1983. *Statistical Bulletin of the Metropolitan Life Insurance Company* 64(January-June):2.

29. Nieman DC. 1990. *Fitness and sports medicine: An introduction*. Palo Alto, Calif: Bull.
30. Andres R, Elahe D, Tobin JD, Muller DC, Brant L. 1985. Impact of age on weight goals. *Annals of Internal Medicine* 103:1030–1033.
31. Waaler HT. 1984. Height, weight, and mortality: The Norwegian experience. *Acta Medica Scandinavica* Supplementum 679:1–56.
32. Pirie P, Jacobs D, Jeffery R, Hannan P. 1981. Distortion in self-reported height and weight data. *Journal of the American Dietetic Association* 78:601–606.
33. Rowland ML. 1991. Self-reported weight and height. *American Journal of Clinical Nutrition* 52:1125–1133.
34. Schlichting PF, Hoilund-Carlsen PF, Quaade F, Lauritzen SL. 1981. Comparison of self-reported height and weight with controlled height and weight in women and men. *International Journal of Obesity* 5:67–76.
35. DelPrete LR, Caldwell M, English C, Banspach SW, Lefebvre C. 1992. Self-reported and measured weights and heights of participants in community-based weight loss programs. *Journal of the American Dietetic Association* 92:1483–1486.
36. Willett WC, Stampfer M, Manson J, VanItallie T. 1991. New weight guidelines for Americans: Justified or injudicious? *American Journal of Clinical Nutrition* 53:1102–1103.
37. Robinett-Weiss N, Hixson ML, Keir B, Sieberg J. 1984. The Metropolitan height-weight tables: Perspectives for use. *Journal of the American Dietetic Association* 84:1480–1481.
38. Behnke AR, Feen BG, Welham WC. 1942. The specific gravity of healthy men. *Journal of the American Medical Association* 118:495–498.
39. Welham WC, Behnke AR. 1942. The specific gravity of healthy men. *Journal of the American Medical Association* 118:498–501.
40. Marwick C. 1993. Obesity experts say less weight still best. *Journal of the American Medical Association* 269:2617–2618.
41. Colditz GA, Willett WC, Stampfer MJ, Manson JE, Hennekens CH, Arky RA, Speizer FE. 1990. Weight as a risk factor for clinical diabetes in women. *American Journal of Epidemiology* 132:501–513.
42. Manson JE, Colditz GA, Stampfer MJ, Willett WC, Rosner B, Monson RR, Speizer FE, Hennekens CH. 1990. A prospective study of obesity and risk of coronary heart disease in women. *New England Journal of Medicine* 322:882–889.
43. Frisancho AR. 1990. *Anthropometric standards for the assessment of growth and nutritional status*. Ann Arbor, Mich: University of Michigan Press.
44. Novascone MA, Smith EP. 1989. Frame size estimation: A comparative analysis of methods based on height, wrist circumference, and elbow breadth. *Journal of the American Dietetic Association* 89:964–966.
45. Wilmore JH, Frisancho RA, Gordon CC, Himes JH, Martin AD, Martorell R, Seefeldt VD. 1988. Body breadth equipment and measurement techniques. In Lohman TG, Roche AF, Martorell R, eds. *Anthropometric standardization reference manual*. Champaign, Ill: Human Kinetics Books.
46. Katch VL, Freedson PS. 1982. Body size and shape: Derivation of the HAT frame size model. *American Journal of Clinical Nutrition* 36:669–675.
47. Katch VL, Freedson PS, Katch FI, Smith L. 1982. Body frame size: Validity of self-appraisal. *American Journal of Clinical Nutrition* 36:676–679.
48. Grant JP, Custer PB, Thurlow J. 1981. Current techniques of nutritional assessment. *Surgical Clinics of North America* 61:437–463.
49. Garn SM, Pesick SD, Hawthorne VM. 1983. The bony chest breadth as a frame size standard in nutritional assessment. *American Journal of Clinical Nutrition* 37:315–318.
50. Baecke JAH, Burema J, Deurenberg P. 1982. Body fatness, relative weight and frame size in young adults. *British Journal of Nutrition* 48:1–6.
51. Frisancho AR, Flegel PN. 1983. Elbow breadth as a measure of frame size for U.S. males and females. *American Journal of Clinical Nutrition* 37:311–314.
52. Garrow JS. 1983. Indices of adiposity. *Nutrition Abstracts and Reviews* 53:697–708.
53. Callaway CW, Chumlea WC, Bouchard C, Himes JH, Lohman GT, Martin AD, Mitchell CD, Mueller WH, Roche AF, Seefeldt VD. 1988. Circumferences. In Lohman TG, Roche AF, Martorell R, eds. *Anthropometric standardization reference manual*. Champaign, Ill: Human Kinetics Books.

54. Roche AF. 1984. Anthropometric methods: New and old, what they tell us. *International Journal of Obesity* 8:509–523.
55. Gibson RS. 1990. *Nutritional Assessment.* New York: Oxford University Press.
56. Lee J, Kolonel LN, Hinds MW. 1981. Relative merits of the weight-corrected-for-height indices. *American Journal of Clinical Nutrition* 34:2521–2529.
57. Lee J, Kolonel LN, Hinds MW. 1982. Relative merits of old and new indices of body mass: a commentary. *American Journal of Clinical Nutrition* 36:727–728.
58. Lee J, Kolonel LN. 1983. Body mass indices: A further commentary. *American Journal of Clinical Nutrition* 38:660–661.
59. Garrow JS, Webster J. 1985. Quetelet's index (w/h^2) as a measure of fatness. *International Journal of Obesity* 9:147–153.
60. Smalley KJ, Knerr AN, Kendrick ZV, Colliver JA, Owen OE. 1990. Reassessment of body mass indices. *American Journal of Clinical Nutrition* 52:405–408.
61. Roche AF, Siervogel RM, Chumlea WC, Webb P. 1981. Grading body fatness from limited anthropometric data. *American Journal of Clinical Nutrition* 34:2831–2838.
62. Keys A, Fidanza F, Karvonen MJ, Kimura N, Taylor HL. 1972. Indices of relative weight and obesity. *Journal of Chronic Diseases* 25:329–343.
63. Norgan NG, Ferro-Luzzi A. 1982. Weight-height indices as estimators of fatness in men. *Human Nutrition: Clinical Nutrition* 36C:363–372.
64. Frisancho AR, Flegel PN. 1982. Relative merits of old and new indices of body mass with reference to skinfold thickness. *American Journal of Clinical Nutrition* 36:697–699.
65. Björntorp P. 1987. Classification of obese patients and complications related to the distribution of surplus fat. *American Journal of Clinical Nutrition* 45:1120–1125.
66. Health and Welfare Canada. 1988. *Canadian guidelines for Healthy Weights. Report of an Expert Committee Convened by Health Promotion Directorate.* Ottawa: Health and Welfare, Health Services and Promotion Branch.
67. Kahn HS. 1991. A major error in nomograms for estimating body mass index. *American Journal of Clinical Nutrition* 54:435–437.
68. Jéquier E. 1987. Energy, obesity, and body weight standards. *American Journal of Clinical Nutrition* 45:1035–1047.
69. Kuczmarski RJ, Flegal KM, Campbell SM, Johnson CL. 1994. Increasing prevalence of overweight among U.S. adults. *Journal of the American Medical Association* 272:205–211.
70. Kaye SA, Folsom AR, Prineas RJ, Potter JD, Gapstur SM. 1990. The association of body fat distribution with lifestyle and reproductive factors in a population study of postmenopausal women. *International Journal of Obesity* 14:583–591.
71. Troisi RJ, Weiss ST, Segal MR, Cassano PA, Vokonas PS, Landsberg L. 1990. The relationship of body fat distribution to blood pressure in normotensive men: The normative aging study. *International Journal of Obesity* 14:515–525.
72. Zwiauer K, Widhalm K, Kerbl B. 1990. Relationship between body fat distribution and blood lipids in obese adolescents. *International Journal of Obesity* 14:271–277.
73. US Department of Health and Human Services. 1988. *The Surgeon General's Report on Nutrition and Health.* Washington, DC: US Government Printing Office.
74. US Department of Health and Human Services. 1991. *Healthy people 2000: National health promotion and disease prevention objectives.* Washington, DC: US Government Printing Office.
75. National Center for Health Statistics. 1994. Prevalence of overweight among adolescents: United States, 1988–1991. *Morbidity and Mortality Weekly Report* 43:818–821.
76. Björntorp P. 1985. Regional patterns of fat distribution. *Annals of Internal Medicine.* 103:994–995.
77. Chandra RK. 1981. Immunodeficiency in undernutrition and overnutrition. *Nutrition Reviews* 39:225–231.
78. Chandra RK. 1991. 1990 McCollum Award lecture. Nutrition and immunity: Lessons from the past and new insights into the future. *American Journal of Clinical Nutrition* 53:1087–1101.
79. Bistrian BR, Blackburn GL, Hallowel E, Heddle R. 1974. Protein status of general surgical patients. *Journal of the American Medical Association* 230:858–860.

80. Bistrian BR, Blackburn GL, Vitale J, Cochran D, Naylor J. 1976. Prevalence of malnutrition in general medical patients. *Journal of the American Medical Association* 235:1567–1570.
81. Coats KG, Morgan SL, Bartolucci AA, Weinsier RL. 1993. Hospital-associated malnutrition: A reevaluation 12 years later. *Journal of the American Dietetic Association* 93:27–33.
82. Lukaski HC. 1987. Methods for the assessment of human body composition: Traditional and new. *American Journal of Clinical Nutrition* 46:537–556.
83. Keys A, Brozek J. 1953. Body fat in adult man. *Physiological Reviews* 33:245–325.
84. Wilmore JH, Buskirk ER, DiGirolamo M, Lohman TG. 1986. Body composition: A round table. *Physician and Sportsmedicine* 14:144–162.
85. Clarys JP, Martin AD, Drinkwater DT, Marfell-Jones MJ. 1987. The skinfold: Myth and reality. *Journal of Sports Sciences* 5:3–33.
86. Martin AD, Ross WD, Drinkwater DT, Clarys JP. 1985. Prediction of body fat by skinfold caliper: Assumptions and cadaver evidence. *International Journal of Obesity* 9:31–39.
87. Pollock ML, Wilmore JH, Fox SM. 1984. *Exercise in health and disease*. Philadelphia: Saunders.
88. Katch FI, McArdle WD. 1973. Prediction of body density from simple anthropometric measurements in college-age men and women. *Human Biology* 45:445–454.
89. Harrison GG, Buskirk EB, Carter JEL, Johnston JE, Lohman TG, Pollock ML, Roche AF, Wilmore J. 1988. Skinfold thicknesses and measurement technique. In Lohman TG, Roche AF, Martorell R, eds. *Anthropometric standardization reference manual*. Champaign, Ill: Human Kinetics Books.
90. Himes JH, Roche AF, Siervogel RM. 1979. Compressibility of skinfolds and the measurement of subcutaneous fatness. *American Journal of Clinical Nutrition* 32:1734–1740.
91. Siervogel RM, Roche AF, Himes JH, Chumlea WC, McCammon R. 1982. Subcutaneous fat distribution in males and females from 1 to 39 years of age. *American Journal of Clinical Nutrition* 36:162–171.
92. Lohman TG. 1981. Skinfolds and body density and their relation of body fatness: A review. *Human Biology* 53:181–225.
93. Lohman TG. 1988. Anthropometry and body composition. In Lohman TG, Roche AF, Martorell R, eds. *Anthropometric standardization reference manual*. Champaign, Ill: Human Kinetics Books.
94. Jackson AS, Pollock ML. 1985. Practical assessment of body composition. *Physician and Sportsmedicine* 13(5):76–90.
95. Martorell R, Mendoza F, Mueller WH, Pawson IG. 1988. Which side to measure: Right or left? In Lohman TG, Roche AF, Martorell R, eds. *Anthropometric standardization reference manual*. Champaign, Ill: Human Kinetics Books.
96. Leger LA, Lambert J, Martin P. 1982. Validity of plastic skinfold caliper measurements. *Human Biology* 54:667–675.
97. Burgert SL, Anderson CF. 1979. A comparison of triceps skinfold values as measured by the plastic McGaw caliper and Lange caliper. *American Journal of Clinical Nutrition* 32:1531–1533.
98. Ross JG, Pate RR, Delpy LA, Gold RS, Svilar M. 1987. New health-related fitness norms. *Journal of Physical Education, Recreation, and Dance* 58:(9)66–70.
99. Lohman TG. 1987. The use of skinfolds to estimate body fatness on children and youth. *Journal of Physical Education, Recreation, and Dance* 58(9):98–102.
100. AAHPERD. 1980. *Health Related Physical Fitness Test Manual*. Reston, Va: American Alliance for Health, Physical Education, Recreation, and Dance.
101. AAHPERD. 1985. *Norms for college students: health-related physical fitness test*. Reston, Va: American Alliance for Health, Physical Education, Recreation, and Dance.
102. Jackson AS, Pollack ML, Ward A. 1980. Generalized equations for predicting body density of women. *Medicine and Science in Sports and Exercise* 12:175–182.
103. Pollock ML, Laughridge EE, Coleman B, Linnerud AC, Jackson A. 1975. Prediction of body density in young and middle-aged women. *Journal of Applied Physiology* 38:745–749.
104. Jackson AS, Pollock ML. 1978. Generalized equations for predicting body density in men. *British Journal of Nutrition* 40:497–504.
105. Brozek J, Keys A. 1951. The evaluation of leanness-fatness in man: norms and intercorrelations. *British Journal of Nutrition* 5:194–205.

106. Durnin JVGA, Womersley J. 1974. Body fat assessment from total body density and its estimation from skinfold thickness: Measurements on 481 men and women aged 16–72 years. *British Journal of Nutrition* 32:77–97.
107. Baun WB, Baun MR, Raven PB. 1981. A nomogram for the estimate of percent body fat from generalized equations. *Research Quarterly for Exercise and Sport* 52:380–384.
108. Westrate JA, Deurenberg P. 1989. Body composition in children: Proposal for a method for calculating body fat percentage from total body density or skinfold-thickness measurements. *American Journal of Clinical Nutrition* 50:1104–1115.
109. Katch F, Michael ED, Horvath SM. 1967. Estimation of body volume by underwater weighing: Description of a simple method. *Journal of Applied Physiology* 23:811–813.
110. Akers R, Buskirk ER. 1969. An underwater weighing system utilizing "force cube" transducers. *Journal of Applied Physiology* 26:649–652.
111. Wilmore JH. 1969. The use of actual, predicted and constant residual volumes in the assessment of body composition by underwater weighing. *Medicine and Science in Sports and Exercise* 1:212–216.
112. Beauchamp RK. 1994. Pulmonary function testing procedures. In Barnes TA, ed. *Respiratory care practice*. St. Louis: Mosby.
113. Wilmore JH, Vodak PA, Parr RB, Girandola RN, Billing JE. 1980. Further simplification for a method for determination of residual lung volume. *Medicine and Science in Sports and Exercise* 12:216–218.
114. Wilmore JH. 1969. A simplified method for determination of residual volumes. *Journal of Applied Physiology* 27:96–100.
115. Goldman HI, Becklake MR. 1959. Respiratory function tests: Normal values at median altitudes and the prediction of normal results. *American Review of Tuberculosis and Pulmonary Diseases* 79:457–467.
116. Garrow JS. 1982. New approaches to body composition. *American Journal of Clinical Nutrition* 35:1152–1158.
117. Diethelm R, Garrow JS, Stalley SF. 1977. An apparatus for measuring the density of obese patients. *Journal of Physiology* 267:14P–15P.
118. Garrow JS, Stalley S, Diethelm R, Pittet P, Hesp R, Halliday D. 1979. A new method for measuring the body density of obese adults. *British Journal of Nutrition* 42:173–183.
119. Gundlach BL, Visscher GJW. 1986. The plethysmometric measurement of total body volume. *Human Biology* 58:783–799.
120. Lukaski HC, Johnson PE, Bolonchuk WW, Lykken GI. 1985. Assessment of fat-free mass using bioelectrical impedance measurements of the human body. *American Journal of Clinical Nutrition* 41:810–817.
121. Beddoe AH, Hill GL. 1985. Clinical measurement of body composition using *in vivo* neutron activation analysis. *Journal of Parenteral and Enteral Nutrition* 9:504–520.
122. Cohn SH, Ellis KJ, Wallach S. 1974. In vivo neutron activation analysis. *The American Journal of Medicine* 57:683–686.
123. Cohn SH, Vartsky D, Yasumura S, Sawitsky A, Zanzi I, Vaswani A, Ellis KJ. 1980. Compartmental body composition based on total-body nitrogen, potassium, and calcium. *American Journal of Physiology* 239:E524-E530.
124. Ryde SJ, Morgan WD, Compston J, Evans CJ. 1990. Measurements of total body calcium by prompt-gamma neutron activation analysis using a 252Cf source. *Biological Trace Element Research* 26–27:429–437.
125. Fletcher JP, Allen BJ, Blagojevic N. 1990. Changes in body protein composition following aortic reconstruction. *Australian and New Zealand Journal of Surgery* 60:209–211.
126. Pollock CA, Allen BJ, Warden RA, Caterson RJ, Blagojevic N, Cocksedge B, Mahoney JF, Waugh DA, Ibels LS. 1990. Total body nitrogen by neutron activation in maintenance dialysis. *American Journal of Kidney Diseases* 16:38–45.
127. Lukaski HC, Mendez J. 1980. Relationship between fat free weight and urinary 3-methylhistidine excretion in man. *Metabolism* 29:758–761.
128. Lukaski HC, Mendez J, Buskirk ER, Cohn SH. 1981. Relationship between endogenous 3-methylhistidine excretion and body composition. *American Journal of Physiology* 240:E302–307.
129. Munro HN, Crim MC. 1994. The proteins and amino acids. In Shils ME, Olson JA, Shike M, eds. *Modern nutrition in health and disease,* 8th ed. Philadelphia: Lea & Febiger.

130. Segal KR, Gutin B, Presta E, Wang J, VanItallie TB. 1985. Estimation of human body composition by electrical impedance methods: a comparative study. *Journal of Applied Physiology* 58:1565–1571.
131. Lukaski HC, Bolonchuk WW, Hall CB, Siders WA. 1986. Validation of tetrapolar bioelectrical impedance method to assess human body composition. *Journal of Applied Physiology* 60:1327–1332.
132. Kushner RF, Schoeller DA. 1986. Estimation of total body water by bioelectrical impedance analysis. *American Journal of Clinical Nutrition* 44:417–424.
133. Brodie DA. 1988. Techniques of measurement of body composition. Part II. *Sports Medicine* 5:74–98.
134. Lukaski HC, Johnson PE. 1985. A simple, inexpensive method of determining total body water using a tracer dose of D_2O and infrared absorption of biological fluids. *American Journal of Clinical Nutrition* 41:363–370.
135. Presta E, Wang J, Harrison GG, Björntorp P, Harker WH, VanItallie TB. 1983. Measurement of total body electrical conductivity: A new method for estimation of body composition. *American Journal of Clinical Nutrition* 37:735–739.
136. Van Loan M, Mayclin P. 1987. A new TOBEC instrument and procedure for the assessment of body composition: Use of Fourier coefficients to predict lean body mass and total body water. *American Journal of Clinical Nutrition* 45:131–137.
137. Van Loan MD, Segal KR, Bracco EF, Mayclin P, VanItallie TB. 1987. TOBEC methodology for body composition assessment: A cross-validation study. *American Journal of Clinical Nutrition* 46:9–12.
138. Van Loan MD. 1990. Assessment of fat-free mass in teenagers: Use of TOBEC methodology. *American Journal of Clinical Nutrition* 52:586–590.
139. Horswill CA, Geeseman R, Boileau RA, Williams BT, Layman DK, Massey BH. 1989. Total-body electrical conductivity (TOBEC): Relationship to estimates of muscle mass, fat-free weight, and lean body mass. *American Journal of Clinical Nutrition* 49:593–598.
140. Conway JM, Norris KH. 1987. Noninvasive body composition in humans by near infrared interactance. In Ellis KJ, Yasumura S, Morgan WD, eds. *In Vivo Body Composition Studies*. London: Institute of Physical Sciences in Medicine.
141. Conway JM, Norris KH, Bodwell CE. 1984. A new approach for the estimation of body composition: Infrared interactance. *American Journal of Clinical Nutrition* 40:1123–1130.
142. Mclean KP, Skinner JS. 1992. Validity of Futrex-5000 for body composition determination. *Medicine and Science in Sports and Exercise* 24:253–258.
143. Davis PO, Dotson CO, Manny PD. 1988. NIR evaluation for body composition analysis. *Medicine and Science in Sports and Exercise* 20:8S.
144. Heyward VH, Cook KL, Hicks VL, Jenkins KA, Quatrochi JA, Wilson WL. 1992. Predictive accuracy of three field methods for estimating relative body fatness of nonobese and obese women. *International Journal of Sport Nutrition* 2:75–86.
145. Hortobágyi T, Isreal RG, Houmard JA, O'Brien KF, Johns RA, Wells JM. 1992. Comparison of four methods to assess body composition in black and white athletes. *International Journal of Sport Nutrition* 2:60–74.
146. Elia M, Parkinson SA, Diaz E. 1990. Evaluation of near infrared interactance as a method for predicting body composition. *European Journal of Clinical Nutrition* 44:113–121.
147. Isreal RG, Houmard JA, O'Brien KF, McCammon MR, Zamora BS, Eaton AW. 1989. Validity of a near-infrared spectrophotometry device for estimating human body composition. *Research Quarterly for Exercise and Sport* 60:379–383.
148. Davis PG, Van Loan M, Holly RG, Krstich K, Phinney SD. 1989. Near infrared interactance vs. hydrostatic weighing to measure body composition in lean, normal, and obese women. *Medicine and Science in Sports and Exercise* 21:S100.
149. Bushong SC. 1993. *Radiologic science for technologists: physics, biology, and protection,* 5th ed. St. Louis: Mosby.

150. Borkan GA, Hults DE, Cardarelli JC, Burrows BA. 1982. Comparison of ultrasound and skinfold measurements in assessment of subcutaneous and total fatness. *American Journal of Physical Anthropology* 58:307–313.
151. Fanelli MT, Kuczmarski RJ. 1984. Ultrasound as an approach to assessing body composition. *American Journal of Clinical Nutrition* 39:703–709.
152. Chiba T, Lloyd DA, Bowen A, Condon-Meyers A. 1989. Ultrasonography as a method of nutritional assessment. *Journal of Parenteral and Enteral Nutrition* 13:529–534.
153. Booth RAD, Goddard A, Paton A. 1966. Measurement of fat thickness in man: A comparison of ultrasound, Harpenden calipers and electrical conductivity. *British Journal of Nutrition* 20:719–725.
154. Weits T, van der Beek EJ, Wedel M, Hubben MW, Koppeschaar HP. 1989. Fat patterning during weight reduction: A multimodal investigation. *Netherlands Journal of Medicine* 35:174–184.
155. Seidell JC, Bakker CJG, van der Kooy K. 1990. Imaging techniques for measuring adipose-tissue distribution—a comparison between computed tomography and 1.5-T magnetic resonance. *American Journal of Clinical Nutrition* 51:953–957.
156. Grauer WO, Moss AA, Cann CE, Goldberg HI. 1984. Quantification of body fat distribution in the abdomen using computed tomography. *American Journal of Clinical Nutrition* 39:631–637.
157. Rössner S, Bo WJ, Hiltbrandt E, Hinson W, Karstaedt N, Santago P, Sobol WT, Crouse JR. 1990. Adipose tissue determinations in cadavers—a comparison between cross-sectional planimetry and computed tomography. *International Journal of Obesity* 14:893–902.
158. Weingand KW, Hartke GT, Noordsy TW, Ledeboer DA. 1988. A minipig model of body adipose tissue distribution. *International Journal of Obesity* 13:347–355.
159. Ferland M, Despres JP, Tremblay A, Pinault S, Nadeau A, Moorjani S, Lupien PJ, Theriault G, Bouchard C. 1989. Assessment of adipose tissue distribution by computed axial tomography in obese women: Association with body density and anthropometric measurements. *British Journal of Nutrition* 61:139–148.
160. Heymsfield SB, Rolandelli R, Casper K, Settle R, Koruda M. 1987. Application of electromagnetic and sound waves in nutritional assessment. *Journal of Parenteral and Enteral Nutrition* 11:64S–69S.
161. Staten MA, Totty WG, Kohrt WM. 1989. Measurement of fat distribution by magnetic resonance imaging. *Investigative Radiology* 24:345–349.
162. Fuller MF, Fowler PA, McKeill G, Foster MA. 1990. Body composition: the precision and accuracy of new methods and their suitability for longitudinal studies. *Proceedings of the Nutrition Society* 49:423–436.
163. Lewis DS, Rollwitz WL, Bertrand HA, Masoro EJ. 1986. Use of NMR for measurement of total body water and estimation of body fat. *Journal of Applied Physiology* 60:836–840.
164. Roubenoff R, Kehayias JJ, Dawson-Hughes B, Heymsfield SB. 1993. Use of dual-energy x-ray absorptiometry in body composition studies: Not yet a "gold standard." *American Journal of Clinical Nutrition* 58:589–591.
165. Going SB, Massett MP, Hall MC, Bare LA, Root PA, Williams DP, Lohman TG. 1993. Detection of small changes in body composition by dual-energy x-ray absorptiometry. *American Journal of Clinical Nutrition* 1993. 57:845–850.
166. Wellens R, Cameron W, Guo S, Roche AF, Reo NV, Siervogel RM. 1994. Body composition in white adults by dual-energy x-ray absorptiometry, densitometry, and total body water. *American Journal of Clinical Nutrition* 59:547–555.

Assessment Activity 6-1

COMPARISON OF ANTHROPOMETRIC AND BODY COMPOSITION METHODS

This chapter has discussed a variety of anthropometric measures and different approaches for determining body composition. These vary widely in ease of use, cost, equipment required, precision, and accuracy. This Assessment Activity will give you an opportunity to use and compare some of the more simple techniques.

We recommend that you review how each measurement is performed before taking it. Ideally, your instructor should demonstrate the techniques and give you an opportunity to practice them in a class laboratory under experienced supervision. We also recommend that you perform these measurements on three or more classmates or friends to get more practice; some of these techniques cannot be fully mastered without practice. You might want to photocopy Figure 6-41 so that you can adequately record the data you collect. When appropriate, remember to use the correct unit of measure (for example, use millimeters for the skinfold measurements).

FIGURE 6-41 Anthropometric and body composition worksheet

Name ______________________ Date ________ / ________ / ________

Age ______________________ Stature ________ (in.) ________ (cm)

Sex M F Weight ________ (lb) ________ (kg)

Method	Measurement	Classification
Relative weight (use 1959 Metropolitan table)	________	________
Quetelet's index	________	________
Waist-hip ratio	________	________
Triceps skinfold	________	________
Percent body fat (from three-site skinfold)	________	________

________ Fat weight Fat weight = Body weight × Percent body fat

________ Fat-free weight Fat-free weight = Body weight − Fat weight

________ Target weight Target weight = Fat-free weight ÷ (100% − desired fat %)

Assessment Activity 6-2

COMPARING METHODS OF ASSESSING BODY COMPOSITION

As would be expected, different methods of estimating body composition will yield different results. Some of this difference will be due to errors made by the tester. Even if the technique is performed "perfectly" by the tester, there will still be some difference because each method has a limited accuracy and precision. Accuracy, you'll remember, describes how close a measurement comes to its true value. Precision is the ability of a method to arrive at the same value on two or more times of measurement.

This Assessment Activity will allow you to compare results from several different approaches for estimating body composition. If possible, have as many of these different body composition measurements done on yourself and a classmate. Record the results in Figure 6-42. If facilities or class size limit the number of students who can be tested, your instructor can select several students to be measured, and their results can be compared.

If your class does not have access to any of these methods, consider going to another laboratory where you and your classmate can have measurements taken, or your instructor may be able to arrange a laboratory session at another facility where the measurements can be demonstrated and taken for several class members.

FIGURE 6-42 Comparing methods of assessing body composition

Method	Percent body fat
Three-site skinfold measurement	__________
Seven-site skinfold measurement	__________
Bioelectrical impedance analysis	__________
Underwater weighing	__________
Infrared interactance	__________
Ultrasound	__________

SEVEN

ASSESSMENT OF THE HOSPITALIZED PATIENT

OUTLINE

INTRODUCTION

In today's cost-conscious health care environment, the desire to control health care costs supports the assessment of the nutritional status of hospitalized patients. Many patients are at nutritional risk. Consequently, they are at increased risk of morbidity and mortality than comparable, well-nourished patients. They will likely require hospitalizations that are longer and more expensive. Appropriate nutritional support of these patients can result in faster recovery and shorter hospital stays, which translate into reduced health care expenditures. Another reason that nutritional assessment of hospitalized patients is important is our increasing capability to provide nutritional support to these patients through enteral and parenteral routes.

This chapter discusses approaches to assessing the nutritional status of hospitalized patients. It brings together many of the various assessment techniques discussed in previous chapters (e.g., anthropometric and dietary) and shows how they are used to evaluate nutritional status in hospitalized patients. It also builds on the previous chapter by introducing several new anthropometric techniques that are unique to the acute care setting.

ASSESSING NUTRITIONAL STATUS

Assessing the nutritional status of the hospitalized patient involves four goals.[1,2] First, patients who are nutritionally at risk need to be identified through a process known as *nutritional screening*. Once a patient is shown to be at nutritional risk, a nutritional assessment should be done to determine the severity and causes of the patient's nutritional impairment. Although both undernutrition and overnutrition can negatively affect health, most frequently it is undernutrition (particularly protein-energy malnutrition) that is of greatest concern in hospitalized patients. The risk of the patient's undernutrition worsening his or her condition, causing a related disease, or possibly resulting in death, should then be ascertained. Finally, the patient should be monitored to ensure an appropriate response to nutritional support.

Nutritional Screening

Nutritional screening "is the process of identifying characteristics known to be associated with nutrition problems. Its purpose is to pinpoint individuals who are malnourished or at nutritional risk."[3] A nutritional screen should be done on all patients within the first 24 to 72 hours following admission, although the earlier the screen is performed and acted on, the sooner the patient will, if necessary, receive and benefit from nutritional support. Nutritional screening can be done by any member of the health care team. Because it does not require the high degree of nutrition knowledge and expertise of a registered dietitian, it is best done by a dietetic technician. Box 7-1 outlines the characteristics of the nutritional screening process.[3] The Nutrition Screening Initiative and its outstanding screening forms are discussed later in this chapter.

Screening can be greatly facilitated by using a checklist or form on which pertinent patient information can be entered. Once completed, this form can be placed in the patient's medical record (often referred to as the patient's "chart") for other members of the health care team to refer to. An example of a nutritional screening form is shown in Figure 7-1.[4] Information required to complete the form includes anthropometric, biochemical, clinical, and dietary data. Much of this information can be obtained from the patient's medical record. To use the screening form in Figure 7-1, place a check in every box that applies to the patient and, when appropriate, enter pertinent patient data on the line next to certain items.

Suppose your patient's serum albumin was 2.5 mg/dl. You would check the box following number 1 to indicate that the serum albumin level was ≤ 2.9 mg/dl. Then enter the patient's serum albumin level on the line following that item. Enter the patient's anthropometric data next (Ht = height; Admit Wt = body weight on admission; DBW = desirable body weight). A patient's usual weight is his or her stable weight in the past 6 to 12 months. It can be determined by asking the patient or a significant other or looking in the nurses' notes or in the medical records of previous

BOX 7-1

Characteristics of the Nutritional Screening Process

- It can be completed in any setting, either through personal contact with the patient or by collecting data from the patient's chart.
- It facilitates completion of early intervention.
- It includes the collection of relevant data on risk factors and the interpretation of data for intervention and treatment.
- It determines the need for a more in-depth nutritional assessment.
- It is cost-effective.

Adapted from Posthauer ME, Dorse B, Foiles RA, et al. 1994. ADA's definitions for nutrition screening and nutrition assessment. *Journal of the American Dietetic Association* 94:838–839.

Nutritional Screening Form

Laboratory Values

1. ☐ Albumin $\leq$ 2.9 mg/dl ________

6. ☐ Albumin < 3.5 mg/dl ________

Anthropometrics

Ht ______ Admit Wt ______ Usual Wt ______ DBW ______

BMI ______ % DBW ______ % Wt Lost ______

2. ☐ <80% DBW

3. ☐ >10% Wt Lost

7. ☐ 80%-90% of Usual Wt

8. ☐ 5%-10% Wt Lost

Feeding

4. ☐ TPN/PPN or Tube Feeding

9. ☐ Loss of appetite (<1/2 trays)

10. ☐ Chewing or swallowing difficulty

11. ☐ >3 days of NPO, dextrose, and/or clear liquids only

Nutrition-Related Problems/Diagnoses

5. ☐ Malnutrition ☐ Sepsis

   ☐ Decubitus ulcers ☐ AIDS

   ☐ Dysphagia/renal/hepatic diet restrictions

12. ☐ Nutrition-related diagnosis/ problems ____________________

13. ☐ Serum cholesterol $\geq$ 200 mg/dL

14. ☐ Random glucose $\geq$ 200 mg/dL

15. ☐ BMI $\geq$ 27 kg/m^2 women; $\geq$ 28 kg/m^2 men

☐ No further nutrition evaluation recommended at this time

☐ Patient may benefit from further nutritional evaluation and will be seen by a Registered Dietitian or Dietetic Technician

☐ Care Level I ☐ Care Level II ☐ Care Level III

☐ Diet counseling/education/classes recommended (1 risk in criteria 13-15), which requires a physician order

Patient Information

Current diet order: ____________________

Screened by: ____________________

Date: ____________________

Figure 7-1 An example of a form that can be used to screen patients for nutritional risk. Instructions for using the form are discussed in the text. Adapted from Hedberg AM, Garcia N, Trejus IJ, Weinmann-Winkler S, Gabriel ML, Lutz AL. 1988. Nutritional risk screening: Development of a standardized protocol using dietetic technicians. *Journal of the American Dietetic Association* 88:1553–1556.

BOX 7-2

Diagnoses and Problems That Can Increase Risk of Malnutrition

Trauma
- fracture
- burn
- closed head injury
- gunshot wound
- spinal cord injury
- motor vehicle accident

Dysphagia
Bowel resection
Short bowel syndrome
Small bowel obstruction
Hypoglycemia
Failure to thrive
Congenital heart disease
Chronic obstructive pulmonary disease
Anorexia
Cancer
Diarrhea
Vomiting
Anemia
Stroke or hemiparesis
Gastrointestinal bleeding
Crohn's disease
Dumping syndrome
Decubitus ulcers
Organ transplant
Diabetes mellitus
Coronary artery disease
Pancreatitis

hospitalizations, if these are available. Desirable (or reference) body weight can be obtained from a height-weight chart. The particular height-weight chart used varies among health care facilities. Calculate the percent of desirable weight (or relative weight) and percent of weight lost (these are discussed later in this chapter). Enter the values in the appropriate lines and place checks in the appropriate boxes. Check on the form whether the patient is on total parenteral nutrition (TPN) or peripheral parenteral nutrition (PPN), or receiving tube feedings, has experienced loss of appetite (eating less than one half of the food on meal trays), or has been NPO ("non per os" meaning "nothing by mouth") or received only intravenous fluids (e.g., 5% dextrose in water) or clear liquids for more than 3 days. Certain diagnoses such as decubitus ulcer, sepsis, AIDS, diet restrictions because of dysphagia, renal or hepatic disease, and, of course, a diagnosis of malnutrition place a patient at nutritional risk. Nutritional risk is increased when serum cholesterol, random (or nonfasting) serum glucose, and body mass index are above certain cutpoints. Nutritional risk can also be elevated in certain nutrition-related diagnoses and problems listed in Box 7-2.

A patient receiving one check for items 6 through 12 (found along the right side of the form) falls in Care Level I. Follow-up for these patients can be done by a registered dietitian or a dietetic technician. A patient having one or more checks for items 1 through 5 (found on the left side of the form) or two or more checks for items 6 through 12 falls within Care Level II and should receive further evaluation by a registered dietitian. Patients receiving enteral or parenteral nutrition support are placed in Care Level III and are further evaluated by a registered dietitian. A patient not meeting these criteria requires no further nutrition evaluation unless a change in his or her condition warrants it. If a patient receives a check for items 13 through 15, he or she would likely benefit from diet counseling or education. A check is placed in the appropriate box (Diet Counseling/Education/Classes, and so on) to signal the patient's physician who can then order any necessary intervention.

Levels of Nutritional Assessment

Once nutritional screening has identified a patient to be at nutritional risk, a nutritional assessment should be done to determine the severity and causes of the patient's nutritional impairment, evaluate whether the nutritional impairment might be a factor contributing to the worsening of the patient's medical condition, and monitor the patient's response to nutritional support. If the nutritional impairment is identified and documented as a factor appreciably worsening the patient's health (what is called a comorbidity and complicating condition), it could increase the reimbursement the health care facility receives for that patient's care.[3,5,6] This is an important consideration for dietitians who want to document the revenue-generating ability and cost-effectiveness of nutrition services rather than being a nonreimbursable service and easy target of draconian budget cuts.

The various techniques used in assessing nutritional status can be grouped into three levels according to complexity and cost: primary, secondary, and tertiary.[1,2] The patient's current and past weight and stature, basic evaluation of the patient's dietary habits, information from the physician's history and physical examination, and results of routine laboratory tests (complete blood count and chemistry profile, discussed in Chapter 9) constitute most of the data used in the *primary assessment.* In general, primary assessment allows identification of patients with more obvious nutritional deficits and helps indicate which patients should undergo more detailed evaluation. Because primary assessment involves data that tend to be late indicators of malnutrition and response to therapy, the more sensitive indicators of secondary and tertiary assessment are recommended for assessing critically ill patients.[2]

In addition to data obtained in the primary assessment phase, *secondary assessment* involves more detailed anthropometric and laboratory measures and more in-depth evaluation of the patient's dietary intake. Included among anthropometric measures are skinfold measurements (usually only triceps and subscapular), and measurements of midarm and midcalf circumferences. Additional biochemical measurements may include 24-hour urinary creatinine (for calculating the creatinine-height index), 24-hour urine urea nitrogen (for estimating nitrogen balance), serum proteins (that are more sensitive indicators of protein nutriture and repletion than serum albumin), and testing of delayed cutaneous hypersensitivity. Indirect calorimetry may be used to measure energy expenditure and energy needs. Dietary assessment may include calorie counts, more extensive patient interviewing, and questioning of surrogates having knowledge of the patient's dietary intake.

Tertiary assessment uses such techniques as neutron activation analysis, isotope dilution, whole-body potassium measurement, computed tomography, and magnetic resonance imaging to determine body composition and response to nutritional therapy. Because of high cost, restricted availability, and other drawbacks, these methods are infrequently used in assessing the critically ill. Instead, their use is limited to research applications.

History

Obtaining a patient's history is the first step in clinical assessment of nutritional status.[7] Data on the patient's history can be obtained from the medical record and from interviews with the patient or others knowledgeable about the patient's habits. Parts of the medical record that are particularly helpful include the medical history, entries made by physicians, nurses, social workers and other members of the health care team, and medical records from previous admissions.[8] Other essential components of a patient's history include pertinent facts about past and current health, use of medications, and personal and household information.[1,7,8] Components of the medical history and psychosocial factors to consider in nutritional assessment are discussed in Chapter 10.

Dietary Information

Dietary information includes the patient's food preferences, allergies and intolerances, and usual eating pattern (timing and location of meals and snacks). Data should also be collected about the amount of money available for purchasing food, ability to obtain and prepare food, eligibility for and access to food assistance programs, and use of vitamin, mineral, and other supplements (if not obtained in the history).

A 24-hour recall or simple food frequency questionnaire can provide important data on usual eating patterns and help generate additional questions on dietary intake. Patients sent home to return for later follow-up visits can be asked to complete a food frequency questionnaire or a multiple-day (usually a 3-day) diet record. Food intake of hospitalized patients can be evaluated by a calorie count, in which the caloric and nutrient value of foods eaten from the patient's tray for one or more days are calculated and recorded.

Physical Examination

Two of the most important measurements to obtain are body weight and height (or length in the case of infants and young children unable to stand without assistance). Weight is a gross measure of the body's fluid and tissue mass, and serial weighings indicate changes in those body constituents. Marked weight loss is generally viewed as a manifestation of serious disease.[9] Weight is an important variable in equations predicting energy expenditure and in Quetelet's index.[10] Stature is necessary for determining weight for stature and for calculating Quetelet's index, the creatinine height index, body surface area, and energy expenditure.[11]

Body weight gain can indicate repletion of lean and fat tissues, development of obesity, or abnormal accumulation of body fluids as in edema, ascites, pleural effusion, or fluid overload in a patient receiving excessive intravenous fluid. Loss of body weight can represent the presence, severity, or progress of a disease or nutritional impairment. It can also be seen in patients receiving diuretics. Depletion of lean body mass can be masked by the simultaneous retention of fluid. For these reasons, body weight measurements need to be carefully scrutinized.

One way to evaluate body weight is to compare it to some reference or "desirable" weight. This can be expressed as a percent of desirable body weight. This is the same as relative weight, which was discussed in Chapter 6. The following equation is used for calculating percent of desirable weight (relative weight).

$$\text{Percent desirable body weight} = \frac{\text{current weight}}{\text{"desirable" or reference weight}} \times 100$$

The value for reference or "desirable" weight depends on what a particular health care facility has chosen for its standard. Usually this is a height-weight table similar to the ones shown in Chapter 6. If the patient's percent of desirable body weight (%DBW) is 80%, he or she is 20% below desirable body weight. Many authors regard a %DBW of < 80% as substandard.[7]

Recent changes in body weight are a better indicator of nutritional status than static weight measurements. One way to assess change in body weight is to calculate percent of usual weight. This can be done using the following equation.

$$\text{\% Usual weight} = \frac{\text{current or admit weight}}{\text{usual weight}} \times 100$$

Information about usual weight can be obtained from the patient, a person close to the patient, from the nurses' notes, or from the medical records of previous admissions. An alternate approach to assessing recent changes in body weight is to calculate percent of weight change using the following equation.

$$\text{\% Weight change} = \frac{\text{usual weight} - \text{current weight}}{\text{usual weight}} \times 100$$

A weight loss < 5% is considered small. A 5% to 10% weight loss is considered potentially significant. A weight loss > 10% is considered definitely significant.[12] Rapid changes in body weight should be interpreted with caution. A change in body weight > 1 lb/d (0.5 kg/d) indicates fluid shifts and not a true change in body weight.

The rate of weight loss is as important to consider as the amount lost. A 12% weight loss during the past 6 months is more significant than a similar weight loss during the past 12 months. The pattern of weight loss is also important to consider. Let's imagine two patients, Patient A and Patient B. Patient A lost 12% of her usual weight over a period 6 months to 1 month prior to admission, but regained half that weight in the month just before admission and is continuing to regain. Consequently, she has a net loss of 6% of her body weight. Patient B lost 6% of his usual weight during the 6 months prior to admission and is continuing to lose weight. Some health care professionals would consider the nutritional status of Patient A to be better than that of Patient B.[12]

Because important clinical decisions will be based on the patient's weight and stature, it is important to obtain measurements that are as accurate and precise as possible. This can be done by following the techniques outlined in Chapter 6. Although the patient should be asked about his or her weight history, actual weight and stature should be measured or estimated using the appropriate equation rather than relying on the patient's stated weight and stature. If stated weight and stature are recorded in the patient's chart, they should be labeled as such.

Weighing can be complicated by the patient's condition and the presence of casts, traction devices, and life-support equipment. Nonambulatory patients, for example, can be weighed using bed or wheelchair scales (see Chapter 6), or weight can be estimated from various anthropometric measures, including subscapular skinfold, calf circumference, knee height, and midarm circumference (explained later in this chapter).[13] When patients cannot stand for stature measurements or when stature is likely to be inaccurate because of skeletal deformity, it can be estimated from knee height, as explained in the next section.[11,13] As discussed in Chapter 6, body weight for stature can be compared with height-weight charts, and relative weight and Quetelet's index can be calculated and compared with various standards.

Another valuable indicator of nutritional status is arm muscle area. Arm muscle area is calculated from measures of the triceps skinfold and the midarm circumference.[14] Arm muscle area (discussed later in this chapter) has been shown to be a useful index of total body muscle in young children[8] and in adults.[14]

Besides weight, stature, and other anthropometric measures, the physical examination involves numerous measurements and observations, including measurement of heart and respiratory rate and body temperature; observation of heart, respiratory, and bowel sounds; examination of the head, neck, thorax, abdomen, extremities, integument (skin, hair, and nails), and examination of the nervous and circulatory systems. This information is gathered during the physical examination and initial work-up on admission and is available in the patient's chart.

Knee Height

Knee height is measured with the subject in the supine position (lying facing up) using one of several commercially available large, broad-blade sliding calipers (see Appendix N for sources).[11,13,15,16] Calipers for measuring knee height vary in price from about $50 to $1500. Ross Laboratories has developed an economical knee-height caliper that has been shown to be as accurate and reliable as more expensive calipers (i.e., those manufactured by GPN Anthropological Instruments).[17]

Measurements are made on the *left leg* because this side was used by researchers in developing the equations given in Table 7-1.[11] The knee and ankle of the left leg are positioned at a 90-degree angle, as shown in Figure 7-2. These angles should be verified by a right triangle, square, or other appropriate device. The fixed blade of the caliper is placed under the heel of the left foot, and the moveable blade is placed on the anterior surface of the left thigh. The caliper shaft is positioned parallel to the fibula (the outside bone of the lower leg), over the lateral malleolus (the most prominent bony projection on the outer side of the left ankle), and just posterior to the head of the fibula (Figure 7-3 and Figure 7-4). Pressure is applied to the two blades to compress the soft tissues.[13,15,16] The measurement is recorded to the

TABLE 7-1 Equations for estimating stature from knee height for various groups

Age*	Equation†	Error‡
Black females		
>60	S = 58.72 + (1.96 KH)	8.26 cm
19–60	S = 68.10 + (1.86 KH) − (0.06 A)	7.60 cm
6–18	S = 46.59 + (2.02 KH)	8.78 cm
White females		
>60	S = 75.00 + (1.91 KH) − (0.17 A)	8.82 cm
19–60	S = 70.25 + (1.87 KH) − (0.06 A)	7.20 cm
6–18	S = 43.21 + (2.14 KH)	7.80 cm
Black males		
>60	S = 95.79 + (1.37 KH)	8.44 cm
19–60	S = 73.42 + (1.79 KH)	7.20 cm
6–18	S = 39.60 + (2.18 KH)	9.16 cm
White males		
>60	S = 59.01 + (2.08 KH)	7.84 cm
19–60	S = 71.85 + (1.88 KH)	7.94 cm
6–18	S = 40.54 + (2.22 KH)	8.42 cm

Adapted from Chumlea WC, Guo SS, Steinbaugh ML. 1994. Predication of stature from knee height for black and white adults and children with application to mobility-impaired or handicapped persons. *Journal of the American Dietetic Association*. 94: 1385–88.

*Age in years rounded to the nearest year

†S = stature; KH = knee height; A = age in years

‡Estimated stature will be within this value for 95% of persons within each age, sex, race group.

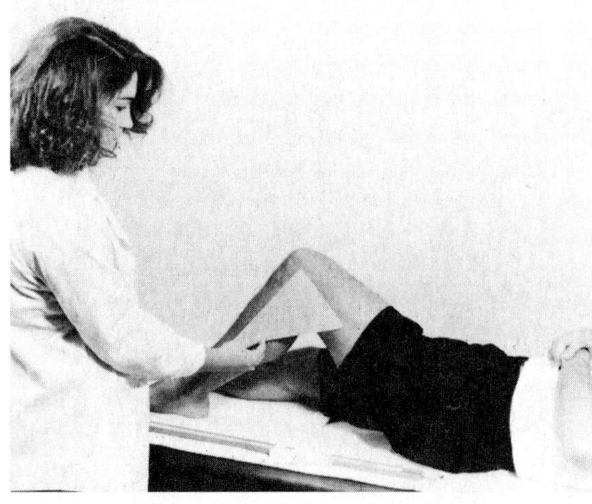

Figure 7-2 When knee height is being measured, the knee and ankle of the left leg should be bent at 90-degree angles.

nearest 0.1 cm. Two measurements made in quick succession should agree to within 0.5 cm.[6]

Estimating Stature

For most patients, stature can be easily obtained. However, for persons who are nonambulatory or who have contractures, severe arthritis, paralysis, amputations, or other conditions limiting their ability to stand erectly, stature may have to be estimated. The most common approach is to estimate stature from knee height because knee height has been shown to correlate highly with stature.[11,17,18] An alternate approach is estimating stature from either upper arm or lower arm length as described by Jarzem.[19]

The sex-, age-, and race-specific equations in Table 7-1 can be used for estimating stature in

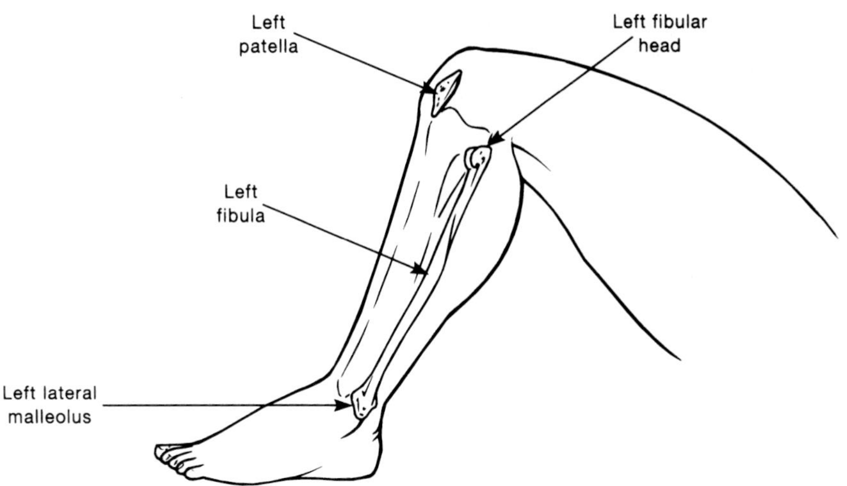

Figure 7-3 Anatomical landmarks for proper placement of the knee height caliper.

children, adults, and older persons. Data from national surveys of healthy, able-bodied persons were used to develop these equations, and they reflect normal patterns of growth and development. The nomogram in Figure 7-5 can be used for estimating stature from age and knee height in persons 60 to 90 years old.

An alternative approach to measuring the stature of a bedridden patient who has no skeletal abnormalities or contractures is to align his or her body so that the lower extremities, trunk, shoulders, and head are in a straight line and mark on the bedsheet the position of the base of the heels and top of the crown, as shown in Figure 7-6. The distance between these two lines can then be measured using a suitable tape measure.

When done carefully, this approach is somewhat more accurate than estimates derived from knee height in patients without skeletal abnormalities or contractures. However, it is always preferable to obtain standing measurements of stature when patients are able to stand and when these measurements are not contraindicated by the patient's condition.

Midarm Circumference

Midarm circumference (MAC), also known as upper midarm circumference, can be used in equations for calculating arm muscle area and estimated body weight.[13,16] As an indicator of muscle and subcutaneous adipose tissue, it is an accepted measure of nutritional status. It and related upper arm anthropometric measurements can be obtained quickly and noninvasively.[20] MAC is the circumference of the upper arm at the triceps skinfold site. In the ambulatory patient, the triceps skinfold site is measured and marked as described in Chapter 6. The arm is relaxed to the side with the palm of the hand facing the thigh. A nonstretchable measuring tape is placed around the arm, perpendicular to the long axis of the arm, and at the level of the triceps skinfold site (see Figure 7-7). The tape should be placed in contact with the arm but without compressing the soft tissues. The measurement should be recorded to the nearest 0.1 cm.[15]

In the nonambulatory patient, MAC is measured while the patient is in the supine position.[11,21] Either the right or left side can be used for this and subsequent recumbent measurements.[15] With the upper arm approximately parallel to the body, the forearm is placed palm down across the middle of the body with the elbow bent 90 degrees. Using a nonstretchable tape measure, the midpoint of the upper arm is located between the tip of the acromion process and the olecranon process and marked, as

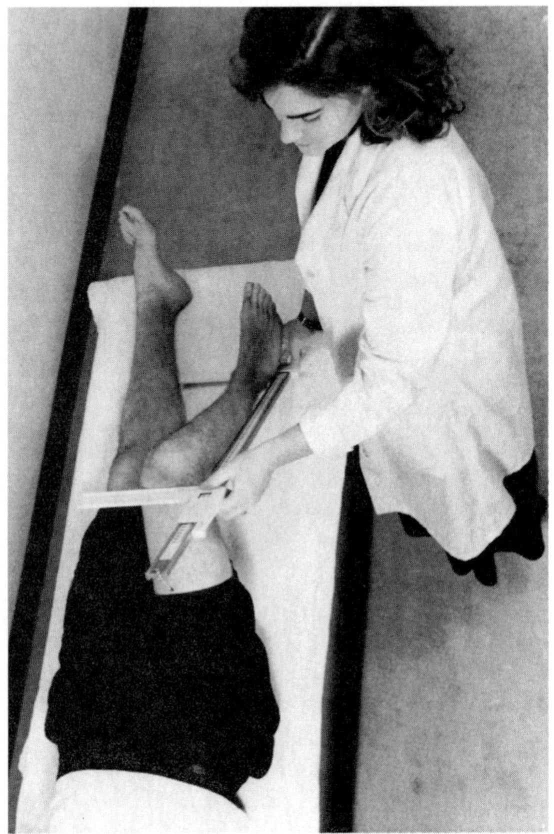

Figure 7-4 The fixed blade of the caliper is placed under the heel, and the moveable shaft is positioned parallel to the fibula, over the lateral malleolus, and just behind the head of the fibula.

shown in Figure 7-8.[13,21] (These are the same anatomical landmarks used for determining the triceps skinfold site described in Chapter 6.)

Once the midpoint of the upper arm is properly marked, the arm is returned to the patient's side with the palm facing upward. The arm is then raised slightly off the surface of the examination table by placing a folded pillow or towel under the patient's elbow. A nonstretchable tape measure is placed around the upper arm at the level of the marked midpoint and perpendicular to the long axis of the arm (Figure 7-9). The tape should come in contact with the skin of the arm but should not be pulled so tight that it indents or compresses the soft tissues. The measurement should be recorded to the nearest 0.1 cm.[13,21]

Calf Circumference

Calf circumference is used in some equations for estimating body weight and is a measure of muscle and subcutaneous adipose tissue. In elderly men, it is significantly correlated with lean body mass.[22] Calf circumference can be measured with the subject either standing, sitting, or in the supine position. If ambulatory, the subject can either sit on an examination table with the right or left leg hanging freely or stand with the feet about 20 cm (8 in) apart with the body weight equally distributed on both feet.[21] A nonstretchable measuring tape should be looped horizontally around the calf and moved up and down until the greatest calf circumference is found. The tape should be tightened around the calf so that it contacts the skin without indenting or compressing the soft tissues. The circumference should be recorded to the nearest 0.1 cm.[21]

If nonambulatory, the subject should be in the supine position with the knee bent at a 90-degree angle. The tape measure should be looped around the calf in a plane perpendicular to the long axis of the lower leg (Figure 7-10) and moved up and down. When the greatest circumference of the lower leg is found, the tape should be tightened around the calf so that it contacts the skin without indenting or compressing the soft tissues. The circumference should be recorded to the nearest 0.1 cm.[13,15]

Recumbent Skinfold Measurements

In the recumbent patient, the triceps and subscapular skinfolds can be measured with the patient lying on the right or left side.[15] Apart from differences in body positioning, the techniques for measuring skinfolds in the recumbent patient are essentially the same as those described in Chapter 6. The reader may want to review the skinfold measuring techniques outlined there.

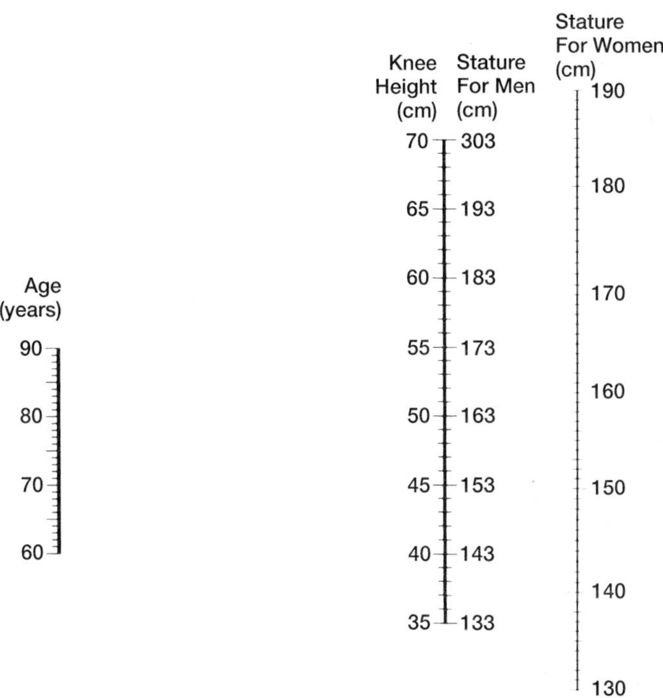

Figure 7-5 Nomogram for estimating stature from knee height in persons ages 60 to 90 years. To use, locate the patient's age and knee height on the appropriate columns and connect these points with a straightedge. The estimated stature can be read where the straightedge crosses the appropriate sex-specific column. Adapted with permission of Ross Laboratories, Columbus, OH 43216, from Chumlea WC, Roche AF, Mukherjee D. 1987. *Nutritional assessment of the elderly through anthropometry*. 1987. Columbus, OH: Ross Laboratories.

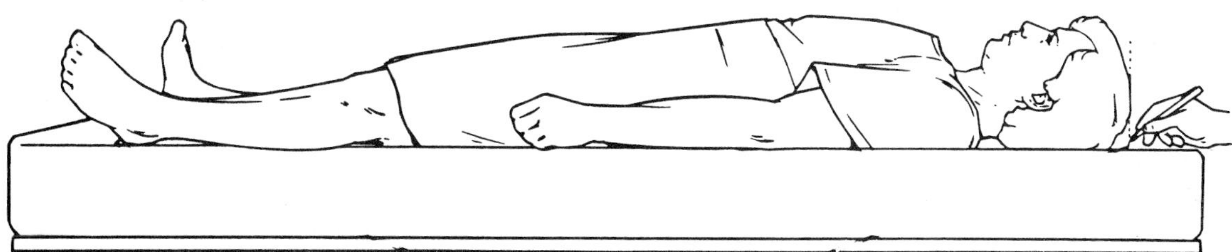

Figure 7-6 An alternative approach to measuring recumbent length in the bedridden patient is to simply place a mark on the bed sheet at the top of the patient's head and at the bottom of his heel. With the patient out of bed or rolled to one side, measure the distance.

The subject is positioned as shown in Figure 7-11. The right arm is in front of the body at a 45-degree angle, the trunk is in a straight line, the shoulders are perpendicular to the spine and examination table, and the arm to be measured is lying on the trunk with the palm down. The legs are slightly flexed at the hips and knees.[13,15]

As in the standing ambulatory patient, the triceps skinfold is measured at the back of the upper arm at the level of the marked midpoint. With the

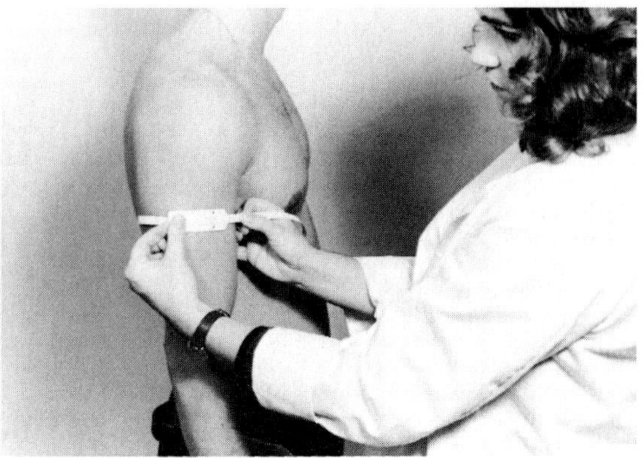

Figure 7-7 Midarm circumference is measured with the subject standing. The tape is placed around the arm, perpendicular to the long axis, and at the level of the triceps skinfold site.

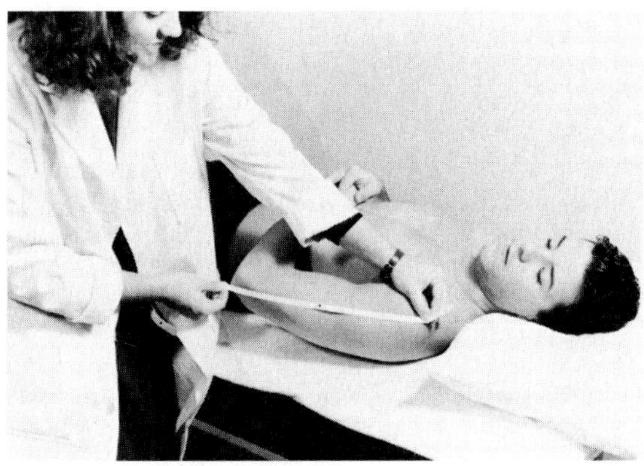

Figure 7-8 When the subject cannot stand, midarm circumference is measured by first locating and marking the midpoint of the upper arm between the tip of the acromion process and the olecranon process.

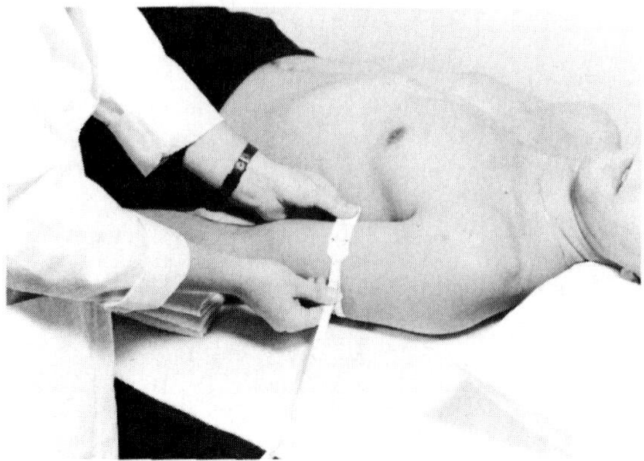

Figure 7-9 Measurement of the midarm circumference of the recumbent subject. A folded towel under the elbow raises the arm off the surface of the table. The tape is perpendicular to the long axis of the arm and touches the arm without compressing soft tissues.

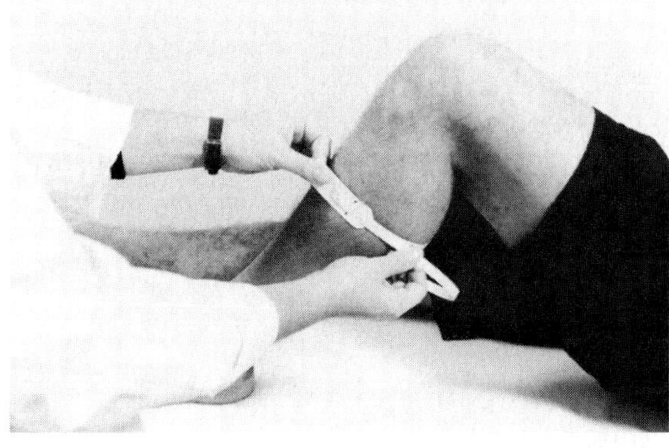

Figure 7-10 Measurement of calf circumference of the recumbent subject. The tape measure is kept in a plane perpendicular to the long axis of the lower leg.

thumb and index finger of the left hand, the measurer grasps a double fold of skin and adipose tissue about 1 cm (½ in) above the marked midpoint of the upper arm. The long axes of the skinfold and arm must be parallel. Holding the skinfold, the measurer places the caliper tips on the skinfold and reads the dial after about 4 seconds (Figure 7-12). The measurer's eyes should be in line with the needle and dial of the caliper to avoid errors caused by parallax.[13,15]

For measuring the subscapular skinfold, the body is positioned as shown in Figure 7-11. The same site is used as when the subject is standing, and the skinfold is grasped and measured along the same axis. (The reader may want to refer to Chapter 6.) Because the subject is lying on the right side, however, the measurement technique is somewhat different. The subscapular skinfold site is just distal to the inferior angle of the left scapula. As shown in Figure 7-13, the measurer

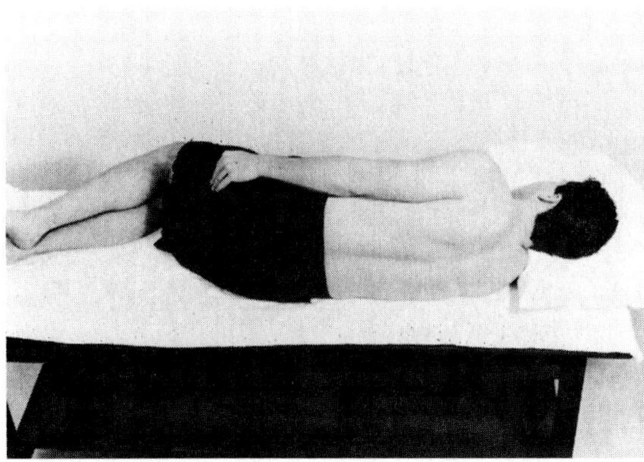

Figure 7-11 Body position for measurement of triceps and subscapular skinfolds of the recumbent subject.

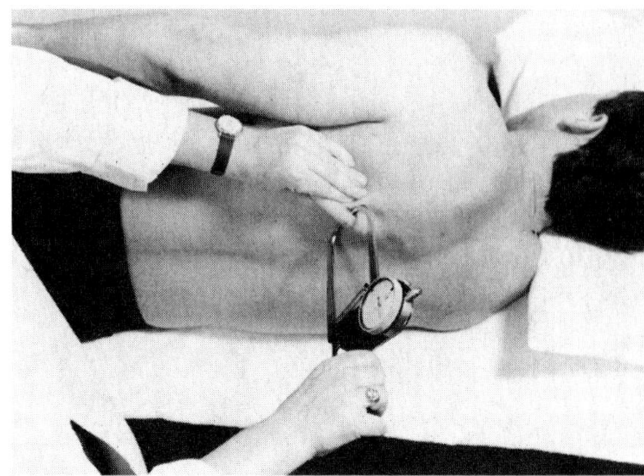

Figure 7-13 Measurement of subscapular skinfold of the recumbent subject.

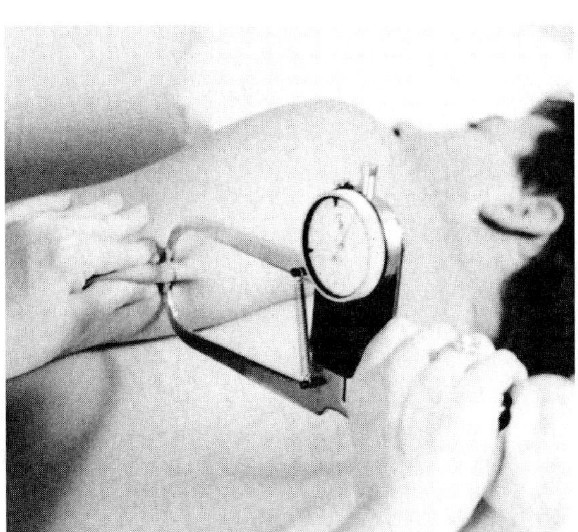

Figure 7-12 Measurement of triceps skinfold of the recumbent subject.

grasps the double layer of skin and adipose tissue along the axis of the skinfold so that the thumb and index finger of the left hand are about 1 cm (½ in) from the actual measurement site. Note that the left hand is distal and lateral to the skinfold site. Holding the skinfold, the measurer places the caliper tips at the site and reads the dial after about 4 seconds. The measurer should look directly at the dial of the caliper to avoid errors caused by parallax.[13,15] A minimum of two measurements should be taken at each site. Successive measurements should be at least 15 seconds apart from each other to allow the skinfold site to return to normal. If consecutive measurements vary by more than 1 mm, additional measurements should be taken until the readings are consistent.

The sum of the triceps and subscapular skinfold thicknesses can be used as an indicator of the body's energy reserves. Appendix Q provides percentiles for the sum of triceps and subscapular skinfold thicknesses for males and females age 1 to 74 years. Although researchers disagree about which standards are the most appropriate, the guidelines in Table 7-2 can be used for interpreting these age-, sex-, and race-specific percentile values.[1] The cutoff point for excess fat was chosen as greater than the 85th percentile because it has been observed that persons above this point are at significantly greater risk of hypertension and hypercholesterolemia than persons at or below the 85th percentile.[23]

Estimating Body Weight

Most patients can be weighed on scales, but sometimes it is difficult or impossible to obtain a patient's weight. This may be because of the patient's medical condition, equipment attached to the patient (for example, life support devices, traction equipment, casts, or braces), or lack of a suitable bed or wheelchair scale.[10] Despite the

TABLE 7-2 Guidelines for interpreting the age-, sex-, and race-specific percentile values for the sum of triceps and subscapular skinfold thicknesses for males and females given in Appendix Q

Percentile	Category
≤5th percentile	Lean
>5th percentile but ≤15th percentile	Below average
>15th percentile but ≤75th percentile	Average
>75th percentile but ≤85th percentile	Above average
>85th percentile	Excess fat

From Frisancho AR. 1990. *Anthropometric standards for the assessment of growth and nutritional status.* Ann Arbor: University of Michigan Press.

critical importance of body weight in delivering nutritional therapy, it is estimated that about 22% of hospitalized adults receiving nutritional support have no record of body weight.[24]

When it is difficult or impossible to obtain a patient's body weight directly, it can be estimated from various anthropometric measures (that is, knee height, midarm circumference, calf circumference, and subscapular skinfold thickness) using equations given in Tables 7-3 and 7-4. The decision of which equation to use will depend on the patient's age and the anthropometric measures that can be obtained or are available.

From Tables 7-3 and 7-4 it can be noted that a certain amount of error is inherent in the process of estimating body weight from anthropometric measures. This error can be minimized by using an equation requiring a larger number of variables (four as opposed to two) and by paying strict attention to measurement technique. Although estimates of body weight may be as much as 14 kg greater than or less than actual body weight, an estimate of body weight recorded on a patient's chart is better than no weight recorded. The use of estimated weights should be reserved for patients who cannot be weighed or for whom weights would be inaccurate, and every reasonable effort should be made to obtain direct measurements of body weights on patients.

If a patient has had an amputation, the patient's current body weight can be adjusted to account for the weight of the amputated body part. Table 7-5 shows the percent of total body weight contributed by individual body parts that are frequently amputated. These values are then used in the following equation to calculate adjusted body weight.[8,25]

$$\text{Adjusted wt} = \frac{\text{current weight}}{100 - \%\text{ of amputation}} \times 100$$

Suppose you had a patient whose current weight was 157 lb and whose leg was amputated at the right knee (right lower leg and foot removed). From Table 7-5 it can be seen that the lower leg and foot contribute approximately 7.1% of total body weight. Given this information and the equation, adjusted body weight can be calculated as shown below.

$$\text{Adjusted wt} = \frac{157\text{ lb}}{100 - 7.1} \times 100$$

$$\text{Adjusted wt} = 169\text{ lb}$$

Thus this patient's adjusted body weight (approximately what it would be without the amputation) is 169 lb.

Arm Muscle Area

Arm muscle area (AMA) is used as an index of lean tissue or muscle in the body.[13,26] This is based on the observation that an organism facing nutritional deprivation draws upon its nutritional reserves in the form of adipose tissue, visceral protein, and skeletal protein. In the case of upper arm anthropometry, thickness of the triceps skinfold is used as an index of fat stores, and arm muscle size is used to represent muscle protein reserves.[26]

As the size of arm muscle changes in response to growth, development, and nutritional status,

TABLE 7-3 Equations for estimating body weight in persons 65 years of age and older from anthropometric measures

Equation	SEE†
Females*	
Weight = (MAC × 1.63) + (CC × 1.43) − 37.46	±4.96 kg
Weight = (MAC × 0.92) + (CC × 1.50) + (SSF × 0.42) − 26.19	±4.21 kg
Weight = (MAC × 0.98) + (CC × 1.27) + (SSF × 0.40) + (KH × 0.87) − 62.35	±3.80 kg
Males*	
Weight = (MAC × 2.31) + (CC × 1.50) − 50.10	±5.37 kg
Weight = (MAC × 1.92) + (CC × 1.44) + (SSF × 0.26) − 39.97	±5.34 kg
Weight = (MAC × 1.73) + (CC × 0.98) + (SSF × 0.37) + (KH × 1.16) − 81.69	±4.48 kg

From Chumlea WC, Guo S, Roche AF, Steinbaugh ML. 1988. Prediction of body weight for the nonambulatory elderly from anthropometry. *Journal of the American Dietetic Association* 88:564–568.

*Weight is in kg; MAC = midarm circumference in cm; CC = calf circumference in cm; SSF = subscapular skinfold thickness in mm; KH = knee height in cm.

†SEE = standard error of the estimate.

TABLE 7-4 Equations for estimating body weight from knee height (KH) and midarm circumference (MAC) for various groups

Age*	Race	Equation†	Accuracy‡
Females			
6–18	Black	Weight = (KH × 0.71) + (MAC × 2.59) − 50.43	±7.65 kg
6–18	White	Weight = (KH × 0.77) + (MAC × 2.47) − 50.16	±7.20 kg
19–59	Black	Weight = (KH × 1.24) + (MAC × 2.97) − 82.48	±11.98 kg
19–59	White	Weight = (KH × 1.01) + (MAC × 2.81) − 66.04	±10.60 kg
60–80	Black	Weight = (KH × 1.50) + (MAC × 2.58) − 84.22	±14.52 kg
60–80	White	Weight = (KH × 1.09) + (MAC × 2.68) − 65.51	±11.42 kg
Males			
6–18	Black	Weight = (KH × 0.59) + (MAC × 2.73) − 48.32	±7.50 kg
6–18	White	Weight = (KH × 0.68) + (MAC × 2.64) − 50.08	±7.82 kg
19–59	Black	Weight = (KH × 1.09) + (MAC × 3.14) − 83.72	±11.30 kg
19–59	White	Weight = (KH × 1.19) + (MAC × 3.21) − 86.82	±11.42 kg
60–80	Black	Weight = (KH × 0.44) + (MAC × 2.86) − 39.21	±7.04 kg
60–80	White	Weight = (KH × 1.10) + (MAC × 3.07) − 75.81	±11.46 kg

From Ross Laboratories, Columbus, OH 43210.

*Age (in years) is rounded to the nearest year.

†Weight is in kg: lb ÷ 2.2 = kg; kg × 2.2 = lb. Knee height is in cm; in. × 2.54 = cm; cm ÷ 2.54 = in.

‡For persons within each group, estimated body weight should be within the stated value for 95% of the subjects.

TABLE 7-5 Percent of total body weight contributed by individual body parts

Body part	Contribution to body weight (%)
Entire arm	6.5
Upper arm	3.5
Forearm	2.3
Hand	0.8
Entire leg	18.5
Upper leg	11.6
Lower leg	5.3
Foot	1.8

From Brunnstrom S. 1983. *Clinical kinesiology,* 4th ed. Philadelphia: Davis.

the resulting change in arm muscle area is greater than the change in midarm circumference. Consequently, changes in upper arm musculature are not as easily detected by measurement of midarm circumference as by measurement of AMA. Therefore, AMA is the preferred nutritional index.[26]

AMA is correlated with creatinine excretion in children[8] and related to total body muscle mass in adults.[14] It is particularly valuable in assessing persons with edema, whose body weights would be augmented by increased intracellular water, and in assessing persons who have undergone amputation.[1]

AMA is estimated from the triceps skinfold measurement and midarm circumference.[13,14,26] The standard equation for calculating arm muscle area is:[26]

$$\text{AMA} = \frac{[\text{MAC} - (\pi \times \text{TSF})]^2}{4\pi}$$

where AMA = arm muscle area in mm^2; MAC = midarm circumference in mm; and TSF = triceps skinfold thickness in mm. Use of the above formula is based on the following assumptions. In cross-section, both the midarm and midarm muscle compartment are circular; the triceps skinfold thickness is twice the average thickness of the subcutaneous fat layer; bone atrophies in proportion to muscle wasting in protein-energy malnutrition; and the cross-sectional area of bone and the sheath containing the nervous and vascular tissues of the upper arm are small and insignificant.[14] In reality, however, several of these factors are a significant source of error in estimating AMA. When estimates of AMA derived from this equation were compared with AMA measured by computed tomography (see Chapter 6), the equation overestimated AMA by 20% to 25%.[14]

Heymsfield and coworkers[14] have developed the following revised equations, which partially correct for the overestimation of AMA by subtracting a constant that accounts for the presence of bone, nervous, and vascular tissue in the upper arm.

$$\text{cAMA for females} = \frac{[\text{MAC} - (\pi \times \text{TSF})]^2}{4\pi} - 6.5$$

$$\text{cAMA for males} = \frac{[\text{MAC} - (\pi \times \text{TSF})]^2}{4\pi} - 10$$

where cAMA = corrected arm muscle area in cm^2; MAC = midarm circumference in cm; and TSF = triceps skinfold thickness in cm. Note that these equations call for all measurements to be made in *centimeters*. The nomogram in Figure 7-14 facilitates calculation of cAMA. Estimates of cAMA have been shown to be within ±8% of actual AMA based on computed tomography. It should be noted that measurements must be carefully taken by trained observers and that the equations and nomogram for cAMA have not been validated for use with elderly persons.[14] In the obese, all of the equations tend to overestimate AMA when compared with values derived from computed tomography, and the magnitude of overestimation is proportional to the degree of adiposity. Heymsfield[14] recommends that AMA prediction equations not be used for persons having a relative weight of ≥125 percent, but Frisancho[23] suggests they not be used for persons whose triceps skinfold thickness exceeds the 85th age and sex percentile. Despite these limitations, estimates of

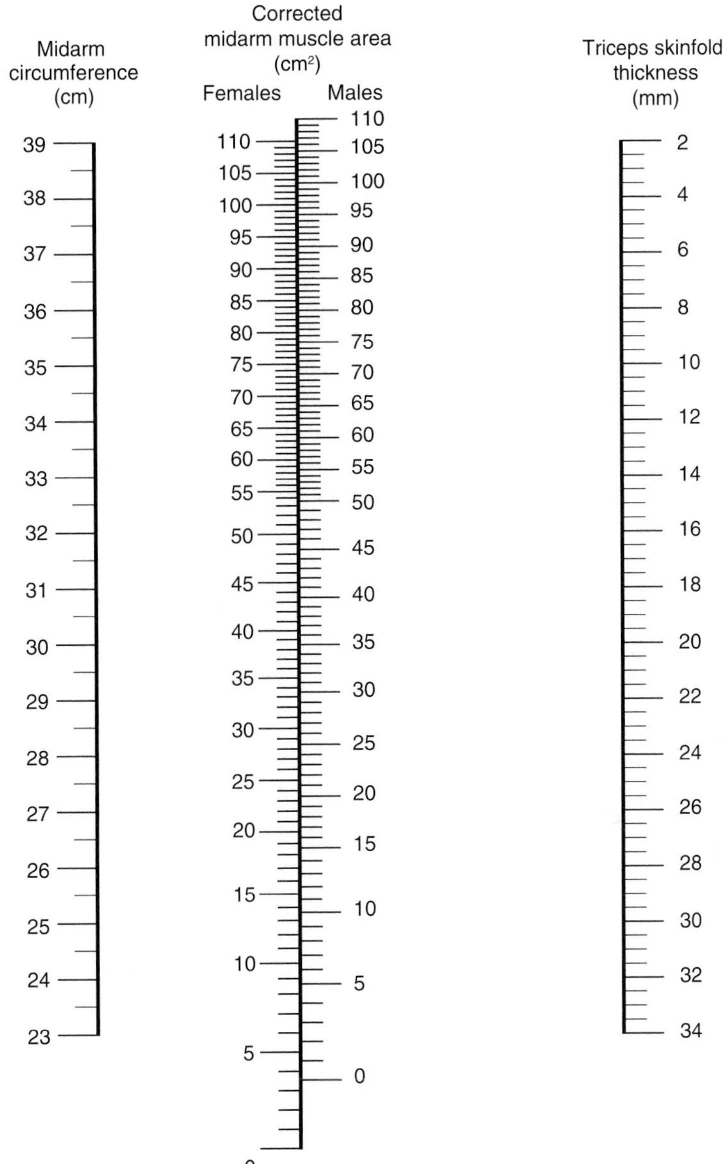

Figure 7-14 Nomogram for estimating corrected arm muscle area. To use, locate the patient's midarm circumference and triceps skinfold in the appropriate columns. Connect these points with a straightedge. The corrected arm muscle area is read where the straightedge crosses the arm muscle area column. Note that there are values for females and males. Adapted with permission of Ross Laboratories, Columbus, OH 43216, from Chumlea WC, Roche AF, Mukherjee D. 1989. *Nutritional assessment of the elderly through anthropometry.*

TABLE 7-6 Guidelines for interpreting the age/sex percentile values for arm muscle area given in Appendix R

Percentile	Category
≤5th percentile	Wasted
>5th percentile but ≤15th percentile	Below average
>15th percentile but ≤85th percentile	Average
>85th percentile but ≤95th percentile	Above average
>95th percentile	High muscle

From Frisancho AR. 1990. *Anthropometric standards for the assessment of growth and nutritional status*. Ann Arbor: University of Michigan Press.

muscle mass derived from anthropometry can be collected inexpensively and easily and are helpful in assessing nutritional status and response to nutritional support.

Appendix R provides means and percentiles of AMA for males and females age 1 to 74 years. For persons age 18 years and older, the values are for corrected AMA. The guidelines in Table 7-6 can be used for interpreting these age/sex percentile values. No single index (for example, AMA) can be used as a reliable indicator of nutritional status. Basic assumptions inferred from anthropometry should be corroborated by data derived from dietary, biochemical, and clinical observations.[23]

DETERMINING ENERGY REQUIREMENTS

Twenty-four-hour energy expenditure is primarily determined by resting energy expenditure, the thermic effect of food, the thermic effect of exercise, and whether disease or injury is present.[27] As Sims and Danforth[27] have pointed out, these "components of energy expenditure are not entirely discrete but are useful divisions when attempting to investigate factors that might regulate or control them."

Twenty-four-hour energy expenditure can be represented by the following equation:

$$24\text{-EE} = \text{REE} + \text{TEF} + \text{TEE} + \text{TED}$$

where 24-EE = 24-hour energy expenditure; REE = resting energy expenditure; TEF = thermic effect of food; TEE = thermic effect of exercise; and TED = thermic effect of disease and injury.

Basal metabolic rate (BMR) is defined as the lowest rate of energy expenditure of an individual. It is calculated from oxygen consumption measured over a 6- to 12-minute period when the subject is in a postabsorptive state (no food consumed during the previous 12 hours) and has rested quietly during the previous 30 minutes in a thermally neutral environment (room temperature is perceived as neither hot nor cold). To be precise, however, the point of lowest energy expenditure—the true BMR—occurs in the early morning hours of deep sleep. Obtaining a truly basal metabolic measurement is impractical in most instances. Therefore, a more appropriate term for metabolic rate or energy expenditure in the awake, resting, postabsorptive subject is resting energy expenditure (REE), also known as resting metabolic rate.

In the clinical setting, achieving optimal conditions for determining REE can be difficult sometimes because of the continuous care patients undergo. In these situations, the term REE is used in the scientific literature to represent energy expenditure measured by indirect calorimetry under conditions that are as controlled as the clinical situation allows.[28,29] As shown in Figure 7-15, REE is the largest component of 24-hour energy expenditure, accounting for roughly 65% to 75% of 24-hour energy expenditure in healthy persons.

The second largest contributor to 24-hour energy expenditure is the energy expended for muscular work or the thermic effect of exercise (TEE).[27] Of all the components of a healthy person's 24-hour energy expenditure, it is the most variable. For most North Americans, it accounts for about 15% to 20% of 24-hour energy expenditure but can increase by a factor of two or more with regular high-intensity, long-duration

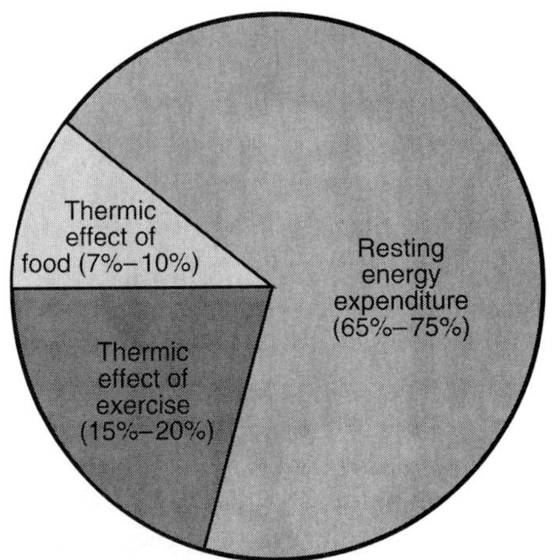

Figure 7-15 The components of 24-hour energy expenditure in healthy persons.

physical activity.[27] Energy expended in exercise generally exceeds the REE in athletes who train several hours daily.

The thermic effect of food (TEF), also known as diet-induced thermogenesis or the specific dynamic action of food, is the increased energy expenditure following food consumption or administration of parenteral or enteral nutrition. The TEF is the energy cost of nutrient absorption, transport, storage, and metabolism. It accounts for about 7% to 10% of 24-hour energy expenditure.[27]

The energy needs of patients can be determined in two ways: measuring energy expenditure or estimating these needs using a variety of guidelines.[2,28,30]

Measuring Energy Expenditure

Calorimetry is the measurement of energy expenditure. Direct calorimetry measures the body's heat output, whereas indirect calorimetry determines energy expenditure by measuring the body's oxygen consumption and carbon dioxide production.

Direct Calorimetry

Although simple in theory, direct calorimetry is cumbersome and expensive in practice.[31,32] It requires a highly sophisticated chamber or specially designed suit, which allows measurement of both the sensible heat given off by the body and the latent heat of vaporized water from the lungs and skin.[28,33,34] Measurements may require a subject to be confined within the chamber or suit for 24 hours or longer. Consequently this approach is not suitable for critically ill patients. The USDA Human Nutrition Research Center in Beltsville, Maryland, has a direct calorimeter that it uses for nutrition research requiring highly accurate measurements of energy expenditure. This is shown in Figure 7-16.

Indirect Calorimetry

Indirect calorimetry is based on the fact that energy metabolism ultimately depends on oxygen utilization (VO_2) and carbon dioxide production (VCO_2).[31,32,35] Thus expired air contains less oxygen and more carbon dioxide than inspired air. When the volume of expired air is known and the differences in oxygen and carbon dioxide concentrations in inspired and expired air are known, the body's energy expenditure can be calculated. Estimations of energy expenditure by indirect calorimetry have been shown to be practically identical to those derived from direct calorimetry.

Several different techniques can be used in indirect calorimetry. In *closed circuit calorimetry,* the subject is connected via a mouthpiece, mask, or endotracheal tube to a spirometer filled with a known amount of 100% oxygen.[29,33,35] The subject rebreathes only the gas within the spirometer—a closed system. Carbon dioxide is removed from the system by a canister of soda lime (potassium hydroxide) placed in the breathing circuit. The subject's VO_2 is determined either from the amount of oxygen consumed from the spirometer or the amount of added oxygen needed to maintain a constant volume within the spirometer.[29] The closed circuit technique is neither portable nor suitable to use on exercising subjects. During exercise, the apparatus offers excessive resistance to gas flow, and the removal of carbon dioxide is inadequate.

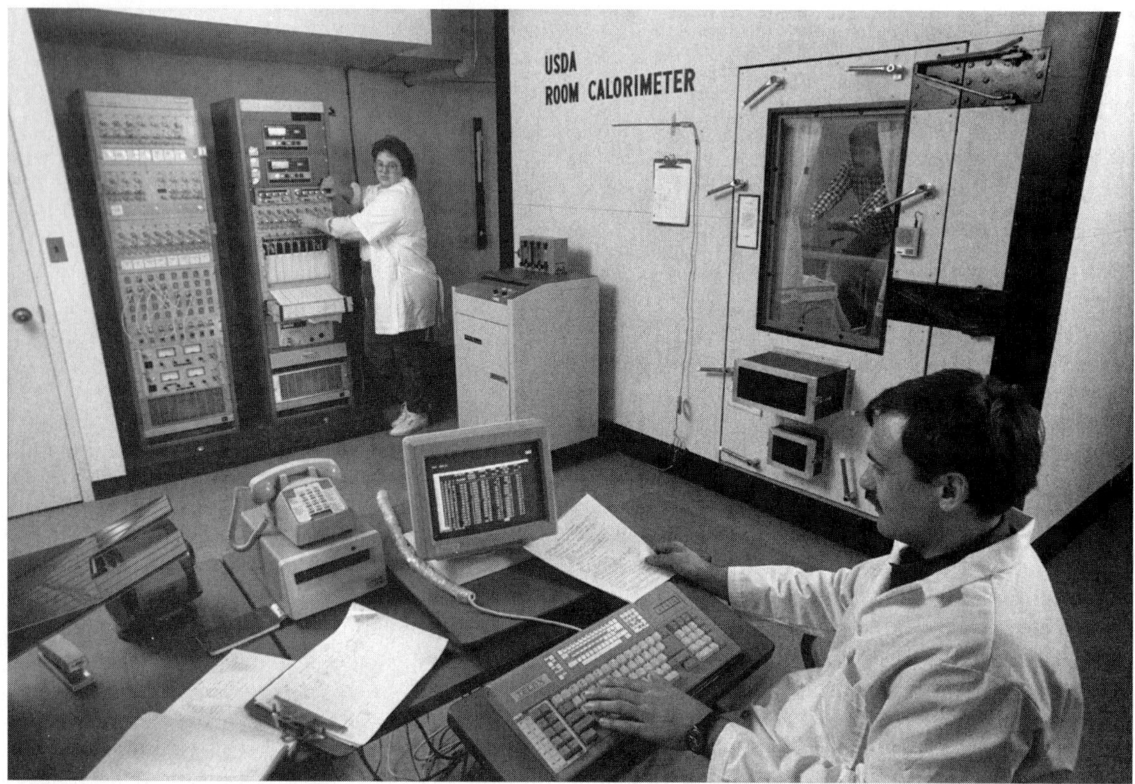

Figure 7-16 The USDA Human Nutrition Research Center's direct calorimeter.

In *open circuit calorimetry,* the subject breathes through a two-way valve in which room air is inspired from one side of the valve, and expired air passes through the opposite side to where it is either analyzed immediately or collected for later analysis. In the *Douglas bag method* of open circuit calorimetry, the expired air is collected in large vinyl bags or latex rubber meteorologic balloons for later analysis. A lightweight, portable apparatus strapped to the subject's back also can be used to measure ventilation and periodically collect samples of expired air for later analysis.[28,33]

A more common approach to open circuit indirect calorimetry in clinical settings is use of a *computerized metabolic cart* or a ventilated hood indirect calorimeter.[28] The metabolic monitor shown in Figure 7-17 can measure the volume of expired air, determine the oxygen and carbon dioxide content of both inspired and expired air, and determine caloric requirements and substrate utilization. Data can be displayed on the unit's video screen, recorded on an optional printer, or downloaded to a computer for storage and/or further analysis. Use of a mouthpiece or face mask often results in discomfort and stress to the patient, which can affect test results. The hood on the monitor in Figure 7-17 avoids this problem and can result in an accurate and representative measurement of metabolic rate in the critically ill patient.[28]

In terms of the accuracy and reproducibility of energy expenditure measurements, computerized metabolic monitors have been shown to compare favorably with more time-consuming approaches. They are relatively easy to operate, and they analyze data quickly. Because of their complexity, however, they are much more expensive to purchase and maintain.

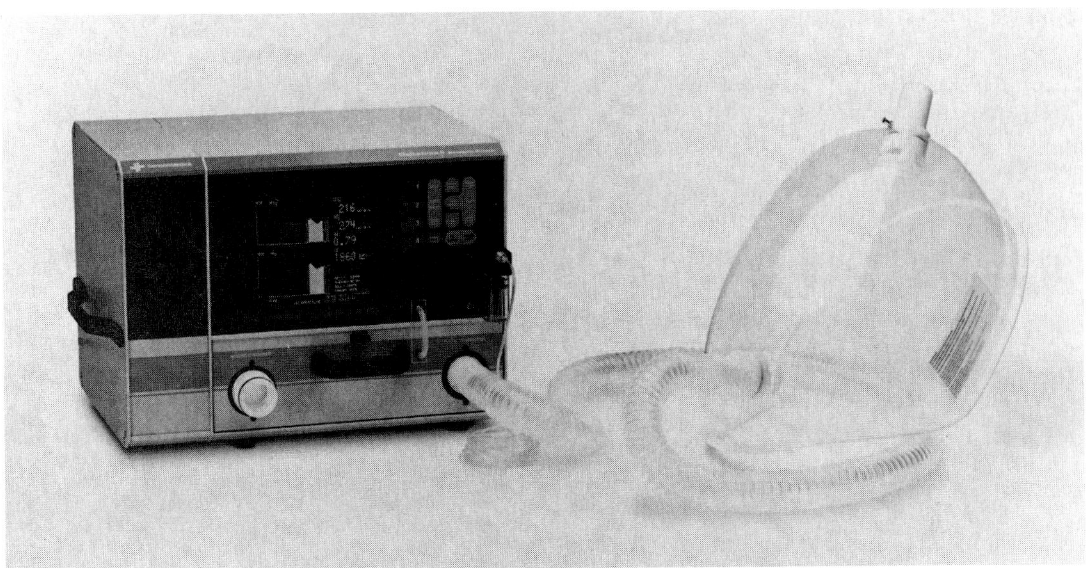

Figure 7-17 This computerized metabolic monitor uses the technique of indirect calorimetry to determine a patient's energy expenditure. The plastic hood allows expired air to be collected without the annoyance of a mask or mouthpiece.

Doubly Labeled Water

Another approach to measuring energy expenditure is the doubly labeled water (DLW) method. Using this approach, a subject drinks a known amount of water ($^2H_2{}^{18}O$) labeled with the stable isotopes deuterium (^2H) and ^{18}O (oxygen 18).[31,32,36] The subject then provides periodic urine and blood samples over the next 1 to 3 weeks, which allow monitoring of the body's elimination of deuterium and ^{18}O. The difference between the rates at which deuterium and ^{18}O are lost from the body is an index of the body's carbon dioxide production. Using standard indirect calorimetric techniques, researchers can calculate energy expenditure with considerable accuracy and precision.

The method has been validated in humans by use of carefully performed energy balance studies and by direct and indirect calorimetry.[37,38] In laboratory testing, DLW has demonstrated an accuracy of 1% and a coefficient of variation of 3% to 6%.[36] Under field conditions, there may be a slight loss of accuracy and precision. Despite this, DLW appears to be the best method of monitoring the energy expenditure of free-living subjects (those outside a controlled setting).[31,39] As mentioned in Chapter 3, comparisons of energy expenditure determined by DLW with reported energy intake from 24-hour recalls and food records have raised serious questions about the accuracy of reported energy intakes in dietary studies.[36,32,40–42]

Estimating Energy Needs

In most clinical settings, energy expenditure usually is not measured. Instead it is estimated using one of numerous available formulas, of which two of the most common are shown in Table 7-7.

Harris-Benedict Equations

There are approximately 190 published guidelines for estimating the nonprotein energy requirements of hospitalized patients.[30] The most widely used equations for predicting REE are those published in 1919 by Harris and Benedict.[43] Indirect calorimetry was used to determine the REE of 239 healthy young adults (136 males and 103 females with a mean age of 27 and 31 years,

TABLE 7-7 Examples of equations for estimating resting energy expenditure in healthy persons*

Harris-Benedict

Females	REE = 655.096 + 9.563 W + 1.850 S − 4.676 A
Males	REE = 66.473 + 13.752 W + 5.003 S − 6.755 A

Harris-Benedict (values rounded for simplicity)

Females	REE = 655.1 + 9.6 W + 1.9 S − 4.7 A
Males	REE = 66.5 + 13.8 W + 5.0 S − 6.8 A

World Health Organization (WHO)

			SD†
Females	3–10 years old	22.5 W + 499	± 63
	10–18 years old	12.2 W + 746	± 117
	18–30 years old	14.7 W + 496	± 121
	30–60 years old	8.7 W + 829	± 108
	>60 years old	10.5 W + 596	± 108
Males	3–10 years old	22.7 W + 495	± 62
	10–18 years old	17.5 W + 651	± 100
	18–30 years old	15.3 W + 679	± 151
	30–60 years old	11.6 W + 879	± 164
	>60 years old	13.5 W + 487	± 148

From Harris JA, Benedict FG. 1919. *A biometric study of basal metabolism in man.* 279. Washington, DC: Carnegie Institution of Washington; World Health Organization. 1985.

Energy and protein requirements. Report of a Joint FAO/WHO/UNU Expert Consultation. Technical Report Series 724. Geneva: World Health Organization.

*REE = resting energy expenditure in kilocalories (kcal); W = body weight in kg; S = stature in cm; A = age;

†SD = standard deviation of the differences between actual and computed values—68% of the time actual REE will be within ± 1 standard deviation of the predicted REE

respectively). From these data, Harris and Benedict derived regression equations (Table 7-7) that best predicted REE using the variables weight, stature, age, and sex.[43,44] Recent research has shown the Harris-Benedict equations' accuracy of prediction among healthy, adequately nourished persons to be within ±14% of REE measured by indirect calorimetry.[44,45] In malnourished, ill patients, however, the Harris-Benedict equations tend to underestimate REE by as much as 22%.[44] Despite these shortcomings, the Harris-Benedict equations are the most widely used in estimating the energy needs of most patients in clinical settings.

World Health Organization Equations

Numerous other equations for predicting REE in healthy populations are available. Some are derived from original research,[33,34,45–47] and others are based on a reanalysis of data published by Harris and Benedict between 1919 and 1935.[44,48] The WHO equations, used for calculating the recommended energy intakes in the tenth edition of the *Recommended Dietary Allowances* (discussed in Chapter 2), were developed by a group of experts and are probably the best equations currently available.[49,50] Because stature was not found to significantly improve the predictive

BOX 7-3

Activity Factors Used to Account for the Thermic Effect of Exercise

Confined to bed	1.2
Ambulatory, low activity	1.3
Average activity	1.5–1.75
Highly active	2.0

From Zeman FJ. 1991. *Clinical nutrition and dietetics.* New York: Macmillan; Long CL. 1984. The energy and protein requirements of the critically ill patient. In Wright RA, Heymsfield SB (eds.) *Nutritional assessment.* Boston: Blackwell Scientific Publications.

ability of the equations, it was omitted from those developed by the WHO.

The Harris-Benedict and WHO equations predict *resting energy expenditure* in kilocalories. To arrive at estimates of 24-hour energy expenditure, the REE must be increased to account for TEE. This is done by multiplying REE by one of the activity factors shown in Box 7-3 to arrive at TEE. Theoretically, REE includes TEF as well as TEE. In most clinical settings, however, no additional allowance is made for TEF. However, use of an additional factor to account for increased metabolism caused by disease, injury, and surgery is often necessary to estimate the 24-hour energy expenditure of patients.

A major decision in developing prediction equations is which variables to include. The major determinant of REE is fat-free mass—what some researchers call the *active protoplasmic tissue* or the *body cell mass.*[34,44,45,47] These are the body's metabolically active, energy consuming cells. Statistical analysis of the data (stepwise multiple regression analysis) has shown that stature and body weight are reasonably well correlated with REE, and because these measures can be easily and accurately performed, one or both are included in most equations.[45,47] Stature was not found to improve the predictability of the WHO equations. Some of the earlier REE equations used body surface area as a variable.

When using these equations, keep in mind that there is a large interindividual variability in REE. Even though a particular equation may be able to predict the *mean* REE for a given *group* of people with a rather high degree of accuracy, the accuracy of that same equation in predicting *one individual's* REE may be quite low. Thus it should be remembered that even the best prediction equation provides only an approximation of REE.

Should actual body weight or desirable body weight be used to predict energy expenditure? This is primarily a concern when working with obese patients. Use of actual body weight has been shown to be better at predicting energy expenditure than use of a patient's desirable body weight.[51] However, if it is the practice of a particular facility to adjust body weight for obese patients, the following equation can be used.[52]

$$\text{Adjusted body weight} = (\text{actual body weight} - \text{DBW}) \times 0.25 + \text{DBW}$$

Energy Expenditure in Disease and Injury

Surgery, trauma, infection, burns, and various diseases can cause 24-hour energy expenditure and urinary nitrogen excretion to markedly increase.[28,29] The effect of various stresses on REE in hospitalized patients is shown in Figure 7-18.[28] The normal range of resting energy expenditure is represented by the light horizontal bar across the middle of the figure. Starvation in the unstressed person results in a hypometabolic state (below average metabolic rate) as the body attempts to conserve its energy reserves. The time when peak energy expenditure occurs in response to stress varies depending on the severity of the illness or injury, and energy needs gradually return to normal during recovery. Figure 7-18 represents average values for both males and females of varying ages and body sizes and

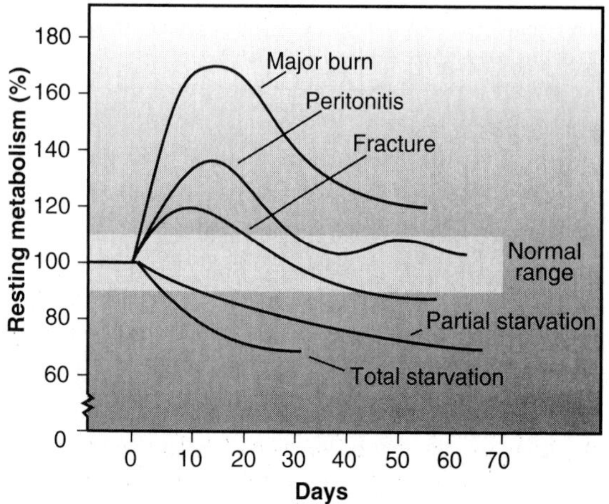

Figure 7-18 Effect of various stresses on resting energy expenditure in hospitalized patients. From Long CL, Schaffel N, et al. 1979. Metabolic response to injury and illness: Estimation of energy and protein needs from indirect calorimetry and nitrogen balance. *Journal of Parenteral and Enteral Nutrition* 3:452–456.

assumes no secondary complications, which can prolong periods of increased energy needs. The clinical course of individual patients can be expected to vary somewhat from these average values.

A common approach to estimating a patient's energy needs is to calculate the 24-hour energy expenditure as outlined in Box 7-4 and then to increase this value by the appropriate injury factors shown in Table 7-8. This second step is necessary because the prediction equations given in Table 7-7 are based on data collected from healthy subjects.

Of all the conditions in Table 7-8, burns have the greatest potential for increasing energy expenditure.[53–56] When caloric intake fails to adequately meet energy expenditure in burn patients, weight loss, delayed wound healing, and poor clinical outcome will result. A number of different equations or approaches have been proposed for

BOX 7-4

Estimating Resting Energy Expenditure (REE) and 24-Hour Energy Expenditure Using the World Health Organization (WHO) Equations

Using the WHO equations (or the Harris-Benedict equations from Table 7-7) is quite easy. As an example, take a 23-year-old female with a body weight of 64 kg (141 lb). Begin by selecting the proper equation for the subject's sex and age. Then calculate the predicted REE using the subject's weight of 64 kg.

$$\text{REE} = 14.7\ \text{W} + 496$$
$$\text{REE} = (14.7 \times 64) + 496$$
$$\text{REE} = 941 + 496$$
$$\text{REE} = 1437\ \text{kcal}$$

To arrive at an estimate of 24-hour energy expenditure the value for REE (1437 kcal) is then multiplied by an activity factor (Table 7-8) that accounts for the thermic effect of exercise—the calories expended during physical activity. Assuming this person has an activity level at the low end of the average activity category, the activity factor of 1.5 will be used.

$$1437\ \text{kcal} \times 1.5 = 2156\ \text{kcal}$$

This gives an estimated 24-hour energy expenditure of 2156 kcal. How do these values compare with those derived from the Harris-Benedict equation in Table 7-7, assuming the subject is 168 cm (66 in.) tall?

TABLE 7-8 Injury factors used to account for the thermic effect of disease and injury

Condition	Injury factor*
Minor surgery	1.0–1.1
Major surgery	1.1–1.3
Mild infection	1.0–1.2
Moderate infection	1.2–1.4
Severe infection	1.4–1.8
Skeletal or blunt trauma	1.2–1.4
Skeletal or head trauma (steroid treated)	1.6–1.8
Burns involving ≤20% BSA†	1.2–1.5
Burns involving 20%–40% BSA	1.5–1.8
Burns involving >40% BSA	1.8–2.0

From Long CL. 1984. The energy and protein requirements of the critically ill patient. In Wright RA, Heymsfield SB (eds.) *Nutritional assessment*. Boston: Blackwell Scientific Publications.

*Multiply the predicted resting energy expenditure adjusted for the thermic effect of food and the thermic effect of exercise by the appropriate injury factor to arrive at an estimate of the patient's 24-hour energy expenditure. The range in values allows adjustment depending on the severity of the disease or injury.

†BSA = body surface area.

estimating the energy and protein needs of burn patients.[53–55,57–60] Several of these are shown in Table 7-9. An approach to estimating the energy requirements of a burn patient is to simply calculate his or her REE using the Harris-Benedict equation and then increase this value by an injury factor (1.6 to 2.2) and possibly an activity factor to account for energy the patient expends while in therapy.[60] A very simple approach shown in Table 7-9 is to merely double the REE derived from the Harris-Benedict equation.[57]

The equations developed by Curreri and coworkers shown in Table 7-9 have been frequently used for calculating the energy needs of burned patients.[53,61] In these equations, energy requirements for patients of different ages are estimated by adding resting energy expenditure (REE) as predicted by the Harris-Benedict equation to the product of the percent of body surface area burned (%BSAB) and an age-dependent constant. In the originally published equation for adults, resting or basal energy requirement was estimated by multiplying the patient's body weight in kilograms by 25.[61] This is based on the observation that REE is approximately 25 kcal/kg of body weight. The Curreri equations have the advantage of linking energy estimates with percent of body surface area burned. However, studies comparing the energy needs of severely burned patients as measured by indirect calorimetry and as estimated by the Curreri equations show that the equations tend to overestimate energy needs, resulting in overfeeding.[55,62,63] One explanation for this may be that recent advances in the management of severe burns result in less of a hypermetabolic response to the thermal injury as when the Curreri formula was originally developed in the early 1970s.[55]

The equation in Table 7-9 developed by Allard and coworkers[58] has been shown to fairly accurately predict the energy requirements of burned patients compared with energy expenditure measured by indirect calorimetry. Referred to as the "Toronto formula," it was derived by multiple regression analysis of data collected from 23 patients with a mean burned body surface area of 39%.[64] Energy requirement is estimated by beginning with a negative value of 4343 kcal and adding or subtracting to this value various products. The equation requires information on the percent body surface area burned (estimated on admission and corrected where amputation was performed), the number of kilocalories the patient received in the previous 24 hours including all dextrose infusions, parenteral and enteral feedings, REE calculated from the Harris-Benedict equation, the average of the hourly rectal temperatures from the previous 24 hours expressed in degrees Celsius, and the number of postburn days as of the previous day. The Toronto formula has been shown to more closely predict the energy requirements of severely burned patients

TABLE 7-9 Equations for estimating the energy requirements of patients with burns*

Age	Equation
Allard[64]	
Adults	kcal = −4343 + (10.5 × %BSAB) + (0.23 CI) + (0.84 REE) + (114 T) − (4.5 PBD)
Cunningham[57]	
0–3 yr	kcal = 2 × REE
Curreri[61]	
0–1 yr	kcal = REE + (15 × %BSAB)
1–3 yr	kcal = REE + (25 × %BSAB)
4–15 yr	kcal = REE + (40 × %BSAB)
16–59 yr	kcal = REE + (40 × %BSAB)
≥60 yr	kcal = REE + (65 × %BSAB)
Hildreth[59]	
Child	kcal = (1800 × m^2 BSA) + (2200 × m^2 BSAB)
Adolescent	kcal = (1500 × m^2 BSA) + (1500 × m^2 BSAB)
Long[60]	
Any age	kcal = REE × injury factor × activity factor

*kcal = estimated daily energy requirement in kilocalories; REE = resting energy expenditure as predicted by the Harris-Benedict equation; BSA = body surface area in m^2; BSAB = body surface area burned in m^2; %BSAB = percent of body surface area burned; CI = the number of kilocalories the patient received in the previous 24 hours; T = average rectal temperature of the previous 24 hours in degrees Celsius; PBD = the number of post-burn days prior to the day the energy requirements are calculated; see Box 7-3 for activity factors and Table 7-8 for injury factors.

than the modified Curreri or the practice of doubling REE derived from the Harris-Benedict equation, both of which tend to overestimate energy requirements.[58] Energy expenditure predictions derived from the Toronto formula have also been shown to compare favorable with measured resting energy expenditure of clinically stable, mechanically ventilated burn patients.[65] The Toronto formula is unique in that it considers the thermic effect of food (which tends to be elevated in critically ill patients), the increased metabolic rate caused by elevations in body temperature, and the gradual fall in metabolic rate with time.

Energy Needs: Estimated or Measured?

Estimates of energy expenditure obtained from any of these and other equations are just that—estimates. They are approximate and should only be used as rough guidelines.[55,66] However, for most hospital patients, estimates of energy expenditure are acceptable in providing the care their conditions demand. For these patients, the time and financial costs of measuring energy needs are not warranted. However, in some instances it may be cost-effective to determine energy expenditure rather than to rely solely on estimates. The use of total parenteral nutrition (TPN) is quite expensive; not only are the solutions themselves costly but their administration requires a considerable time investment by nurses, pharmacists, physicians, and registered dietitians. Basing the administration of TPN solutions on measured energy expenditure may help prevent excessive use of TPN.[30] Not only is undernutrition associated with increased morbidity and mortality, but overnutrition can have negative clinical outcomes, as well.[30]

Measuring energy expenditure will allow administration of TPN solutions to be based on physiologic need and promote patient recovery. Thus the cost of indirect calorimetry may be justified by both improved patient care and savings resulting from more judicious use of costly resources such as TPN solutions and staff time and savings to the hospital because of shorter hospital stays.[30] In the case of burn patients, routine use of indirect calorimetry allows tailoring of nutritional support and is valuable in the early detection of significant undernutrition or overnutrition.[62] Considering the seriousness of thermal injury and the importance of nutrition support in its management, measuring the energy expenditure of severely burned patients should be standard practice.[66]

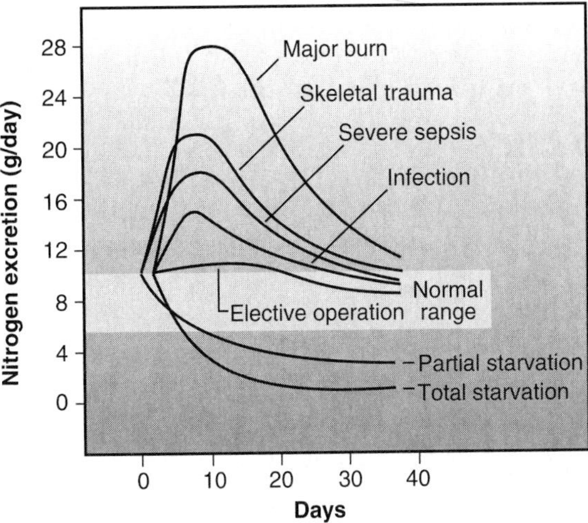

Figure 7-19 Effect of various stresses on urinary nitrogen excretion in hospitalized patients. Used with permission from Long CL, Schaffel N, et al. 1979. Metabolic response to injury and illness: Estimation of energy and protein needs from indirect calorimetry and nitrogen balance. *Journal of Parenteral and Enteral Nutrition* 3:452–456.

DETERMINING PROTEIN REQUIREMENTS

Protein serves as a functional component of body tissues and enzymes and as a fuel source. The protein needs of healthy, nonpregnant, nonlactating adults generally can be met with an intake of 0.8 g/kg body weight per day.[49] In trauma or burn patients, protein catabolism increases markedly, as does protein loss as indicated by urinary nitrogen excretion. Nitrogen makes up about 16% of protein and serves as a convenient way of measuring protein intake and losses.

Protein Losses in Disease and Injury

Figure 7-19 shows how urinary nitrogen losses vary over time among different conditions.[28] The normal range of urinary nitrogen loss is represented by the figure's light horizontal bar. Partial or total starvation in the unstressed person often results in *reduced* nitrogen losses as the body attempts to spare protein. The opposite is true in trauma or burn patients, even though their energy and protein intake often are reduced substantially. Trauma and burns are usually associated with increased protein catabolism and urinary nitrogen losses, although the patient's nutritional status before injury can affect the extent of loss. All other factors being equal, nitrogen losses after trauma and thermal injury are less in depleted persons and the elderly. Under these conditions, the protein reserves may be so depleted that the response is blunted or may not even be observed.

As with changes in REE seen in response to injury and illness (Figure 7-18), urinary nitrogen losses vary in degree and duration with the severity of the injury, may take several days after onset of the disease or trauma to reach their peak, and gradually return to the normal range.

Estimating Protein Needs

In practice, there is no single "best" method for conclusively determining the amount of protein that should be in the diet of patients suffering from trauma, burns, and other injuries. The protein requirements of these patients can only be estimated. Three approaches are commonly used—basing protein intake on body weight, caloric

TABLE 7-10 Suggested ranges of protein intake per kilogram of body weight during peak catabolic response for various injuries and conditions in adults

Stress level	Condition	Protein (g/kg/d)
Normal	Healthy	0.8
Mild	Minor surgery, mild infection	0.8–1.2
Moderate	Major surgery, moderate infection, moderate skeletal trauma	1.2–1.8
Severe	Severe infection, multiple injuries, severe trauma, major burns	1.6–2.2

From Ireton-Jones CS, Hasse JM. 1992. Comprehensive nutritional assessment: The dietitian's contribution to the team effort. *Nutrition* 8:75–81; Long CL. 1984. The energy and protein requirements of the critically ill patient. In Wright RA, Heymsfield SB (eds.) *Nutritional assessment*. Boston: Blackwell Scientific Publications; Waymack JP, Herndon DN. 1992. Nutritional support of the burned patient. *World Journal of Surgery* 16:80–86; Mentegut WJ, Lowry SF. 1993. Nutrition in burn patients. *Seminars in Nephrology* 13:400–408.

intake, or nitrogen balance.[1,2,28] Table 7-10 provides some suggested ranges of protein intake per kilogram of body weight for various injuries and situations. If the energy needs of a patient are reasonably well defined, these can be used to estimate protein requirements. Some authorities consider 1 g of nitrogen (or 6.25 g of protein) for every 150 nonprotein kilocalories to be an adequate daily protein intake for critically ill adults and adults with burns when the percent body surface area burned is ≤10.[28] When injuries are very severe or the burn involves more than 10% body surface area, 1 g of nitrogen is recommended for every 100 nonprotein kilocalories.

Nitrogen balance (discussed in Chapter 9) involves 24-hour measurement of protein intake and an estimate of nitrogen losses where N Bal = nitrogen balance; protein intake = protein intake in g/24 hours; and UUN = urine urea nitrogen in g/24 hours.

$$\text{N Bal} = \frac{\text{Protein intake}}{6.25} - \text{UUN} - 4$$

Protein intake is divided by 6.25 to arrive at an estimate of nitrogen intake. Because protein is 16% nitrogen, dividing grams of protein by 6.25 gives you grams of nitrogen. Nitrogen loss is *estimated* by measuring urine urea nitrogen (which accounts for 85% to 90% of total urinary nitrogen) and subtracting a constant (4 g in the above equation, although this value can vary from 2 to 4 g) to account for dermal, fecal, and nonurea nitrogen losses, which cannot be easily measured.[67,68]

Measuring total urinary nitrogen (TUN) is more difficult, expensive, and time consuming than measuring urinary urea nitrogen (UUN). Consequently, estimating TUN from measurements of UUN is standard practice. However, some researchers question the appropriateness of this practice, suggesting that in trauma and burn patients UUN represents only about 65% of TUN as opposed to 80% to 90% in healthy persons.[69,70] They suggest that TUN should be measured directly rather than estimated from UUN. Other researchers report that estimates of TUN based on UUN are significantly different than direct measures of TUN, but that the differences are small and clinically insignificant to justify the added expense and trouble of directly measuring TUN.[71]

Despite the problems associated with measuring protein intake and nitrogen excretion, nitrogen balance is generally accepted as an appropriate and cost-effective way of monitoring the protein status of burn and other critically ill patients.[28,55,69,71] Although not an exact indicator of nutritional adequacy, nitrogen balance studies serve as an excellent guide to nutrition support when used in conjunction with changes in body weight and energy expenditure measured by indirect calorimetry.[71] However, even if more protein is provided a patient than is calculated from losses in the urine, nitrogen balance is difficult to achieve in the early stage of severe trauma and thermal injury. The catabolism associated with the stress of trauma and thermal injury, as well as the atrophy of muscle caused by immobilization and disuse, result in considerable urinary nitrogen losses. Given time and the provision of adequate energy and protein, the patient gradually will begin to retain more protein than is excreted and replace lost body protein.[28,55]

NUTRITION SCREENING INITIATIVE

The Nutrition Screening Initiative (NSI) was a 5-year endeavor begun in 1991 to encourage routine nutrition screening and better nutrition care in America's health and medical care settings.[72,73] It was a joint project of the American Dietetic Association, the American Academy of Family Physicians, and the National Council on the Aging. Also playing a pivotal role in guiding the NSI was a Blue Ribbon Advisory Committee composed of more than 30 organizations and professionals from the fields of nutrition, medicine, and aging.[73]

The focus of the NSI was older Americans—the most rapidly growing segment of the U.S. population and a group at disproportionate risk of poor nutritional status.[74] Among the major goals of the NSI was determining the best way to identify potential risk factors and major indicators of poor nutritional status among older adults and raising public and professional awareness of poor nutritional status.[74] The NSI defined a risk factor as "a characteristic or occurrence that increases the likelihood that an individual has or will have problems with nutritional status."[73] Risk factors associated with poor nutritional status (Box 7-5) include inappropriate food intake, poverty, social isolation, dependency and disability, acute or chronic diseases or conditions, chronic medication use, and advanced age.[73]

BOX 7-5

Risk Factors for Poor Nutritional Status

- Inappropriate food intake
- Poverty
- Social isolation
- Dependency/disability
- Acute/chronic diseases or conditions
- Chronic medication use
- Advanced age (≥80 years)

From the Nutrition Screening Initiative, a project of the American Academy of Family Physicians, the American Dietetic Association, and the National Council on Aging, and funded in part by a grant from Ross Laboratories, a division of Abbott Laboratories.

The NSI defined an indicator as "an observable, recordable phenomenon such as a physical sign, specific symptom, syndrome, or measurable parameter that indicates that poor nutritional status is already present in the individual and is causing some effect."[73] Major and minor indicators of poor nutritional status are shown in Box 7-6. These can be identified through interviews, observation, physical examination, anthropometric measurements, and laboratory tests.

Public Awareness Checklist

Before people will seek screening for nutritional status, they must be aware that a potential problem exists. This requires increased public awareness that poor nutritional status is a common problem. The NSI developed a public awareness checklist (Figure 7-20) to help identify individuals at greater-than-average risk of poor nutritional status. The checklist is intended to serve two purposes. The first is to provide people with basic nutrition information regarding the characteristics that may increase the likelihood of poor nutritional status. The second is to encourage the public to talk with health and social service providers about their nutritional concerns.[75]

BOX 7-6

Major and Minor Indicators of Poor Nutritional Status in Older Americans

Major Indicators

- Weight loss $\leq$ 10 lb
- Underweight or overweight
- Serum albumin $<$ 3.5 g/dl
- Change in functional status
- Inappropriate food intake
- Midarm muscle circumference $<$ 10th percentile
- Triceps skinfold $<$ 10th percentile or $>$ 95th percentile
- Obesity
- Nutrition-related disorders
- Osteoporosis
- Osteomalacia
- Folate deficiency
- Vitamin B_{12} deficiency

Minor Indicators

- Alcoholism
- Cognitive impairment
- Chronic renal insufficiency
- Multiple concurrent medications
- Malabsorption syndromes
- Anorexia, nausea, dysphagia
- Change in bowel habits
- Fatigue, apathy, memory loss
- Poor oral/dental status
- Dehydration
- Poorly healing wounds
- Loss of subcutaneous fat or muscle mass
- Fluid retention
- Reduced iron, ascorbic acid, zinc

From the Nutrition Screening Initiative, a project of the American Academy of Family Physicians, the American Dietetic Association, and the National Council on Aging, and funded in part by a grant from Ross Laboratories, a division of Abbott Laboratories.

The checklist uses the mnemonic "DETERMINE" to convey basic nutrition information and help users recall the major risk factors and indicators of poor nutritional status. The checklist is not intended to be used as a diagnostic device.

A nutrition score of 0 to 2 is considered good, and a recheck in 6 months is recommended. A recheck in 3 months and a self-help approach to improving nutritional status is encouraged for persons scoring between 3 and 5 points, which is considered moderate nutritional risk. Persons with a nutrition score of 6 or more are regarded at high nutritional risk and are encouraged to take the checklist with them the next time they visit their physician, dietitian, or other health or social service provider.

Screening Tools

A practical approach to nutritional screening recommended by the NSI is outlined in Figure 7-21. The first step is completing the checklist. Persons at increased risk of poor nutritional status then can be screened at one of two screening levels. The Level I Screen (Figure 7-22) is a basic nutrition evaluation instrument that can be administered in a community setting by a social service or health care professional or other trained person. It is designed to distinguish between persons at high risk and those at moderate risk of poor nutritional status. High-risk individuals are those with a documented, significant change in body weight. They should be referred to a physician for

The Warning Signs of poor nutritional health are often overlooked. Use this checklist to find out if you or someone you know is at nutritional risk.

DETERMINE YOUR NUTRITIONAL HEALTH

Read the statements below. Circle the number in the yes column for those that apply to you or someone you know. For each yes answer, score the number in the box. Total the nutritional score.

	YES
I have an illness or condition that made me change the kind and/or amount of food I eat.	2
I eat fewer than 2 meals per day.	3
I eat few fruits or vegetables, or milk products.	2
I have 3 or more drinks of beer, liquor, or wine almost every day.	2
I have tooth or mouth problems that make it hard for me to eat.	2
I don't always have enough money to buy the food I need.	4
I eat alone most of the time.	1
I take 3 or more different prescribed or over-the-counter drugs a day.	1
Without wanting to, I have lost or gained 10 pounds in the past 6 months.	2
I am not always physically able to shop, cook and/or feed myself.	2
TOTAL	

Total Your Nutritional Score. If it's –

0-2 **Good!** Recheck your nutritional score in 6 months.

3-5 **You are at moderate nutritional risk.** See what can be done to improve your eating habits and lifestyle. Your office on aging, senior nutrition program, senior citizens center or health department can help. Recheck your nutritional score in 3 months.

6 or more **You are at high nutritional risk.** Bring this checklist the next time you see your doctor, dietitian, or other qualified health or social service professional. Talk with them about any problems you may have. Ask for help to improve your nutritional health.

Remember that warning signs suggest risk, but do not represent diagnosis of any condition.

These materials developed and distributed by the Nutrition Screening Initiative, a project of: American Academy of Family Physicians, The American Dietetic Association, and National Council on the Aging, Inc.

The Nutrition Checklist is based on the Warning Signs described below. Use the word DETERMINE to remind you of the Warning Signs.

Disease. Any disease, illness, or chronic condition that caused you to change the way you eat, or makes it hard for you to eat, puts your nutritional health at risk. Four out of five adults have chronic diseases that are affected by diet. Confusion or memory loss that keeps getting worse is estimated to affect one out of five or more of older adults. This can make it hard to remember what, when or if you've eaten. Feeling sad or depressed, which happens to about one in eight older adults, can cause big changes in appetite, digestion, energy level, weight, and well-being.

Eating Poorly. Eating too little and eating too much both lead to poor health. Eating the same foods day after day or not eating fruit, vegetables, and milk products daily will also cause poor nutritional health. One in five adults skip meals daily. Only 13% of adults eat the minimum amount of fruit and vegetables needed. One in four older adults drink too much alcohol. Many health problems become worse if you drink more than one or two alcoholic beverages per day.

Tooth Loss/Mouth Pain. A healthy mouth, teeth and gums are needed to eat. Missing, loose or rotten teeth or dentures which don't fit well or cause mouth sores make it hard to eat.

Economic Hardship. As many as 40% of older Americans have incomes of less than $6,000 per year. Having less -- or choosing to spend less -- than $25-$30 per week for food makes it very hard to get the foods you need to stay healthy.

Reduced Social Contact. One third of all older people live alone. Being with people daily has a positive effect on morale, well-being and eating.

Multiple Medicines. Many older Americans must take medicines for health problems. Almost half of older Americans take multiple medicines daily. Growing old may change the way we respond to drugs. The more medicines you take, the greater the chance for side effects such as increased or decreased appetite, change in taste, constipation, weakness, drowsiness, diarrhea, nausea, and others. Vitamins or minerals when taken in large doses act like drugs and can cause harm. Alert your doctor to everything you take.

Involuntary Weight Loss/Gain. Losing or gaining a lot of weight when you are not trying to do so is an important warning sign that must not be ignored. Being overweight or underweight also increases your chance of poor health.

Needs Assistance in Self Care. Although most older people are able to eat, one of every five have trouble walking, shopping, buying, and cooking food, especially as they get older.

Elder Years Above Age 80. Most older people lead full and productive lives. But as age increases, risk of frailty and health problems increase. Checking your nutritional health regularly makes good sense.

The Nutrition Screening Initiative, 2626 Pennsylvania Avenue, NW, Suite 301, Washington, DC 20037

Figure 7-20 The "Determine Your Nutritional Health" checklist developed by the Nutrition Screening Initiative to identify persons at increased risk of poor nutrition status. From the Nutrition Screening Initiative, a project of the American Academy of Family Physicians, the American Dietetic Association, and the National Council on Aging, and funded in part by a grant from Ross Laboratories, a division of Abbott Laboratories.

SCHEMATIC—A PRACTICAL APPPROACH TO NUTRITIONAL SCREENING

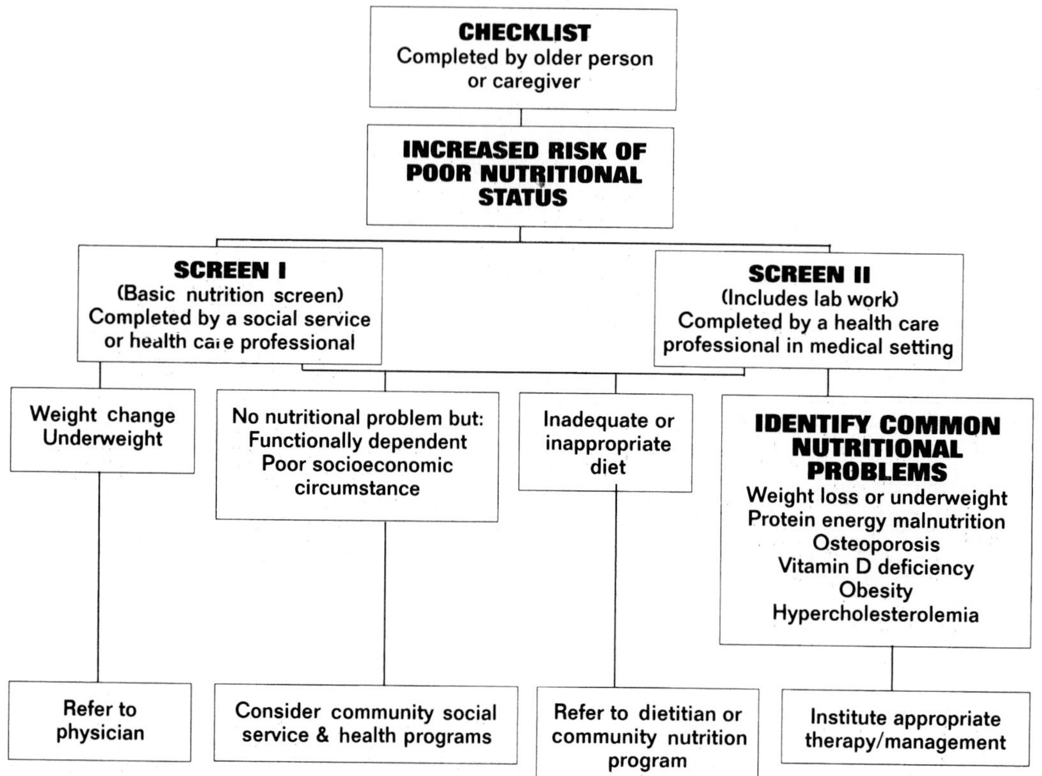

Figure 7-21 Outline of a practical approach to nutritional screening recommended by the Nutrition Screening Initiative. Reprinted with permission by the Nutrition Screening Initiative, a project of the American Academy of Family Physicians, the American Dietetic Association, and the National Council on Aging, and funded in part by a grant from Ross Laboratories, a division of Abbott Laboratories.

more in-depth assessment. Persons at moderate risk may benefit from dietary counseling, dental evaluation, food stamps, home-delivered or congregate meals, economic assistance programs, shopping or transportation assistance, increased socialization, and increased physical activity.[75] The Level I Screen should be repeated annually or if a major change in status occurs.

The Level II Screen (Figure 7-23) is administered by a health professional and requires the input of a physician and dietitian. In addition to the items covered by the Level I Screen, the Level II Screen requires data from laboratory tests, anthropometric measures, physical examination, and tests of mental and cognitive status.[75] Potential problems that may be identified by this screen include unintentional weight loss, protein-energy malnutrition, osteoporosis, vitamin or mineral deficiency, obesity, and elevated serum cholesterol. If potential problems are identified, the person should be referred to the appropriate health care professional.

LEVEL I SCREEN Name: Date:

Level 1 Screen

Body Weight

Measure height to the nearest inch and weight to the nearest pound. Record the values below and mark them on the Body Mass Index (BMI) scale to the right. Then use a straight edge (ruler) to connect the two points and circle the spot where this straight line crosses the center line (body mass index). Record the number below.

Healthy older adults should have a BMI between 24 and 27.

Height (in):_______________

Weight (lbs):_______________

Body Mass Index:_____________

(number from center column)

NOMOGRAM FOR BODY MASS INDEX

WEIGHT

KG LB

150 140 130 120 110 100 95 90 85 80 75 70 65 60 55 50 45 40 35 30 25

340 320 300 280 260 240 220 200 190 180 170 160 150 140 130 120 110 100 95 90 85 80 75 70 65 60 55 50

BODY MASS INDEX [WT/(HT)²]

70 60 50 40 30 20 10

WOMEN: OBESE / OVERWEIGHT / ACCEPTABLE

MEN: OBESE / OVERWEIGHT / ACCEPTABLE

HEIGHT

CM IN

125 130 135 140 145 150 155 160 165 170 175 180 185 190 195 200 205 210

50 55 60 65 70 75 80 85

© George A Bray 1978

Check any boxes that are true for the individual:

- ❑ Has lost or gained 10 pounds (or more) in the past 6 months.
- ❑ Body mass index <24
- ❑ Body mass index >27

For the remaining sections, please ask the individual which of the statements (if any) is true for him or her and place a check by each that applies.

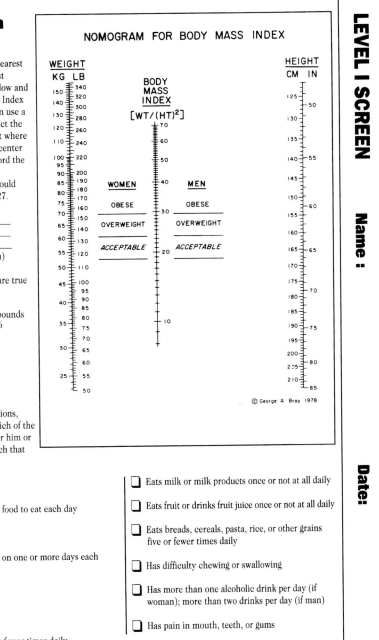

Eating Habits

- ❑ Does not have enough food to eat each day
- ❑ Usually eats alone
- ❑ Does not eat anything on one or more days each month
- ❑ Has poor appetite
- ❑ Is on a special diet
- ❑ Eats vegetables two or fewer times daily
- ❑ Eats milk or milk products once or not at all daily
- ❑ Eats fruit or drinks fruit juice once or not at all daily
- ❑ Eats breads, cereals, pasta, rice, or other grains five or fewer times daily
- ❑ Has difficulty chewing or swallowing
- ❑ Has more than one alcoholic drink per day (if woman); more than two drinks per day (if man)
- ❑ Has pain in mouth, teeth, or gums

Figure 7-22A The Level I Screen developed by the Nutrition Screening Initiative. It is designed to distinguish between persons at high and moderate risk of poor nutritional status and to be administered by a social service or health care professional. From the Nutrition Screening Initiative, a project of the American Academy of Family Physicians, the American Dietetic Association, and the National Council on Aging, and funded in part by a grant from Ross Laboratories, a division of Abbott Laboratories.

A physician should be contacted if the individual has gained or lost 10 pounds unexpectedly or without intending to during the past 6 months. A physician should also be notified if the individual's body mass index is above 27 or below 24.

Living Environment

- ❑ Lives on an income of less than $6000 per year (per individual in the household)
- ❑ Lives alone
- ❑ Is housebound
- ❑ Is concerned about home security
- ❑ Lives in a home with inadequate heating or cooling
- ❑ Does not have a stove and/or refrigerator
- ❑ Is unable or prefers not to spend money on food (<$25-$30 per person spent on food each week)

Functional Status

Usually or always needs assistance with (check each that apply):

- ❑ Bathing
- ❑ Dressing
- ❑ Grooming
- ❑ Toileting
- ❑ Eating
- ❑ Walking or moving about
- ❑ Traveling (outside the home)
- ❑ Preparing food
- ❑ Shopping for food or other necessities

If you have checked one or more statements on this screen, the individual you have interviewed may be at risk for poor nutritional status. Please refer this individual to the appropriate health care or social service professional in your area. For example, a dietitian should be contacted for problems with selecting, preparing, or eating a healthy diet, or a dentist if the individual experiences pain or difficulty when chewing or swallowing. Those individuals whose income, lifestyle, or functional status may endanger their nutritional and overall health should be referred to available community services: home-delivered meals, congregate meal programs, transportation services, counseling services (alcohol abuse, depression, bereavement, etc.), home health care agencies, day care programs, etc.

Please repeat this screen at least once each year--sooner if the individual has a major change in his or her health, income, immediate family (e.g., spouse dies), or functional status.

These materials developed by the Nutrition Screening Initiative.

Figure 7-22B

LEVEL II SCREEN Name: Date:

Level II Screen

Complete the following screen by interviewing the patient directly and/or by referring to the patient chart. If you do not routinely perform all of the described tests or ask all of the listed questions, please consider including them but do not be concerned if the entire screen is not completed. Please try to conduct a minimal screen on as many older patients as possible, and please try to collect serial measurements, which are extremely valuable in monitoring nutritional status. Please refer to the manual for additional information.

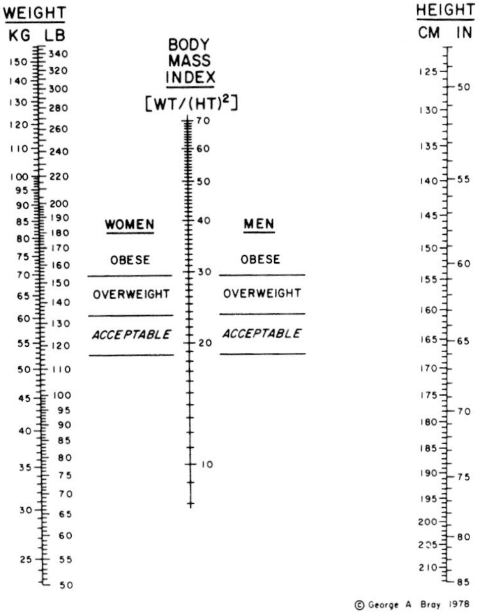

Anthropometrics

Measure height to the nearest inch and weight to the nearest pound. Record the values below and mark them on the Body Mass Index (BMI) scale to the right. Then use a straight edge (paper, ruler) to connect the two points and circle the spot where this straight line crosses the center line (body mass index). Record the number below; healthy older adults should have a BMI between 24 and 27; check the appropriate box to flag an abnormally high or low value.

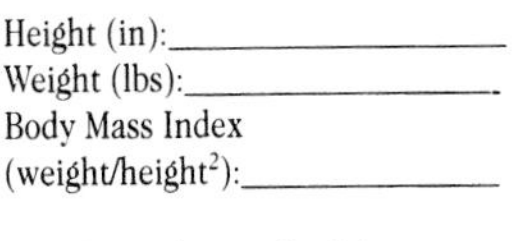

Height (in):________
Weight (lbs):________
Body Mass Index (weight/height^2):________

Please place a check by any statement regarding BMI and recent weight loss that is true for the patient.

- ☐ Body mass index < 24
- ☐ Body mass index > 27
- ☐ Has lost or gained 10 pounds (or more) of body weight in the past 6 months

Record the measurement of mid-arm circumference to the nearest 0.1 centimeter and of triceps skinfold to the nearest 2 millimeters.

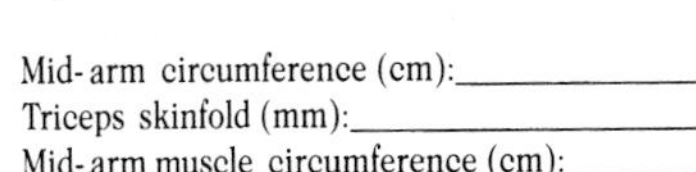

Mid-arm circumference (cm):________
Triceps skinfold (mm):________
Mid-arm muscle circumference (cm):________

Refer to the table and check any abnormal values:

- ☐ Mid-arm muscle circumference <10th percentile

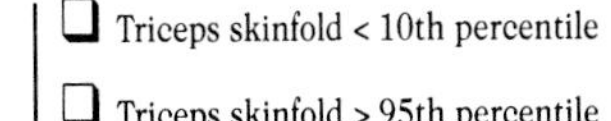

- ☐ Triceps skinfold < 10th percentile
- ☐ Triceps skinfold > 95th percentile

Note: mid-arm circumference (cm) - {0.314 x triceps skinfold (mm)}= mid-arm *muscle* circumference (cm)

For the remaining sections, please place a check by any statements that are true for the patient.

Laboratory Data

- ☐ Serum albumin below 3.5 g/dl
- ☐ Serum cholesterol below 160 mg/dl
- ☐ Serum cholesterol above 240 mg/dl

Drug Use

- ☐ Three or more prescription drugs, OTC medications, and/or vitamin/mineral supplements daily

Figure 7-23A The Level II Screen developed by the Nutrition Screening Initiative. It is designed to identify common problems such as protein-energy malnutrition, obesity, elevated serum cholesterol levels, and osteoporosis. From the Nutrition Screening Initiative, a project of the American Academy of Family Physicians, the American Dietetic Association, and the National Council on Aging, and funded in part by a grant from Ross Laboratories, a division of Abbott Laboratories.

Clinical Features

Presence of (check each that apply):

- ❑ Problems with mouth, teeth, or gums
- ❑ Difficulty chewing
- ❑ Difficulty swallowing
- ❑ Angular stomatitis
- ❑ Glossitis
- ❑ History of bone pain
- ❑ History of bone fractures
- ❑ Skin changes (dry, loose, nonspecific lesions, edema)

Percentile	Men 55-65 y	Men 65-75 y	Women 55-65 y	Women 65-75 y
Arm circumference (cm)				
10th	27.3	26.3	25.7	25.2
50th	31.7	30.7	30.3	29.9
95th	36.9	35.5	38.5	37.3
Arm muscle circumference (cm)				
10th	24.5	23.5	19.6	19.5
50th	27.8	26.8	22.5	22.5
95th	32.0	30.6	28.0	27.9
Triceps skinfold (mm)				
10th	6	6	16	14
50th	11	11	25	24
95th	22	22	38	36

From Frisancho AR. 1981 New norms of upper limb fat and muscle areas for assessment of nutritional status. Am J Clin Nutr: 34:2540-2545. *American Society for Clinical Nutrition.*

Eating Habits

- ❑ Does not have enough food to eat each day
- ❑ Usually eats alone
- ❑ Does not eat anything on one or more days each month
- ❑ Has poor appetite
- ❑ Is on a special diet
- ❑ Eats vegetables two or fewer times daily
- ❑ Eats milk or milk products once or not at all daily
- ❑ Eats fruit or drinks fruit juice once or not at all daily
- ❑ Eats breads, cereals, pasta, rice, or other grains five or fewer times daily
- ❑ Has more than one alcoholic drink per day (if woman); more than two drinks per day (if man)

Living Environment

- ❑ Lives on an income of less than $6000 per year (per individual in the household)
- ❑ Lives alone
- ❑ Is housebound
- ❑ Is concerned about home security
- ❑ Lives in a home with inadequate heating or cooling
- ❑ Does not have a stove and/or refrigerator
- ❑ Is unable or prefers not to spend money on food (<$25-$30 per person spent on food each week)

Functional Status

Usually or always needs assistance with (check each that apply):

- ❑ Bathing
- ❑ Dressing
- ❑ Grooming
- ❑ Toileting
- ❑ Eating
- ❑ Walking or moving about
- ❑ Traveling (outside the home)
- ❑ Preparing food
- ❑ Shopping for food or other necessities

Mental/Cognitive Status

- ❑ Clinical evidence of impairment, e.g., Folstein < 26
- ❑ Clinical evidence of depressive illness, e.g., Beck Depression Inventory > 15, Geriatric Depression Scale > 5

Patients in whom you have identified one or more major indicator of poor nutritional status require immediate medical attention; if minor indicators are found, ensure that they are known to a health professional or to the patient's own physician. Patients who display risk factors of poor nutritional status should be referred to the appropriate health care or social service professional (dietitian, nurse, dentist, case manager, etc.).

These materials developed by the Nutrition Screening Initiative.

Figure 7-23B

SUMMARY

1. Assessing the nutritional status of hospitalized patients involves at least four goals: identifying those at nutritional risk, determining the severity and causes of nutritional impairment, determining the patient's risk of dying from the undernutrition or developing a related disease condition, and monitoring to evaluate response to nutritional therapy.
2. The purpose of nutritional screening is to identify potentially malnourished individuals at nutritional risk. Screening should be done on all patients within the first 24 to 72 hours following admission. It is best done by a dietetic technician.
3. Nutritional assessment techniques can be grouped into three levels: primary, secondary, and tertiary. Primary assessment employs such basic methods as the medical history, dietary evaluation, certain laboratory tests, and physical examination. Secondary assessment involves more detailed anthropometric and laboratory measures and evaluation of the patient's dietary intake in greater depth. Tertiary assessment methods generally are reserved for research applications.
4. The history includes facts about past and current health, use of medications, and personal and household information as it pertains to nutritional status. Dietary information relates to food intake, food preferences, intolerances and allergies, usual eating pattern, use of supplements, and resources for purchasing and preparing food. Physical examination includes anthropometric data as well as findings from the physical examination available from the patient's chart.
5. Stature and body weight are important measures to be obtained from hospitalized patients. Under certain conditions they may have to be calculated from such variables as the patient's knee height, calf circumference, age, and sex, or they may be obtained by measuring body length while the patient is lying in bed. When calculations are performed, care should be exercised in selecting the proper equation.
6. Midarm circumference is the circumference of the upper arm at the triceps skinfold site. It is an indicator of muscle and subcutaneous adipose tissue and can be obtained quickly and noninvasively in both ambulatory and nonambulatory patients. Arm muscle area, calculated from the triceps skinfold measurement and midarm circumference, is used as an index of lean tissue or muscle in the body.
7. Calf circumference is used in estimating body weight and as an indicator of muscle and subcutaneous adipose tissue. Obtaining calf circumference and measures of skinfold thickness in bedridden patients is somewhat different than in ambulatory persons, and the standardized protocol outlined in this chapter should be strictly followed.
8. Energy needs are based on an individual's 24-hour energy expenditure, which is determined by resting energy expenditure, the thermic effect of food, energy expended in physical activity, and whether disease or injury are present. Resting energy expenditure is the largest component of 24-hour energy expenditure.
9. Twenty-four-hour energy expenditure can be determined through indirect calorimetry or roughly approximated from a variety of equations. Indirect calorimetry involves measurement of the body's oxygen consumption and carbon dioxide production and often uses a computerized metabolic cart. The energy expenditure of patients usually is estimated. In critically ill persons or those receiving parenteral or enteral feedings, indirect calorimetry may be preferable to estimating energy expenditure.
10. Surgery, trauma, infection, burns, and various diseases can cause 24-hour energy expenditure and urinary excretion of nitrogen to markedly increase. Energy expenditure in patients can be obtained through indirect

calorimetry or estimates using a variety of equations.

11. The degree and duration of increased protein catabolism following injury vary with the trauma's severity. Protein catabolism may take several days to peak before gradually returning to normal. Recommended protein intake can be based on nitrogen balance, body weight, or energy intake.
12. The Nutrition Screening Initiative (NSI) was a 5-year endeavor begun in 1991 to encourage routine nutrition screening and better nutrition care in America's health and medical care settings. The goals of the NSI included raising public and professional awareness of poor nutritional status and developing assessment tools to identify potential risk factors and major indicators of poor nutritional status, especially among older adults. Assessment tools developed include a public awareness checklist and screening instruments for assessing nutritional status at two different levels.

REFERENCES

1. Bistrian BR. 1984. Nutritional assessment of the hospitalized patient: A practical approach. In Wright RA, Heymsfield SB (eds.) *Nutritional assessment.* Boston: Blackwell Scientific Publications.
2. Grossman GD. 1985. Nutritional assessment of critically ill patients. *Respiratory Care* 30:463–469.
3. Posthauer ME, Dorse B, Foiles RA, et al. 1994. ADA's definitions for nutrition screening and nutrition assessment. *Journal of the American Dietetic Association* 94:838–839.
4. Hedberg AM, Garcia N, Trejus IJ, Weinmann-Winkler S, Gabriel ML, Lutz AL. 1988. Nutritional risk screening: Development of a standardized protocol using dietetic technicians. *Journal of the American Dietetic Association* 88:1553–1556.
5. Trimble JM. 1992. Reimbursement enhancement in a New Jersey hospital: Coding for malnutrition in prospective payment systems. *Journal of the American Dietetic Association* 92:737–734.
6. Sayarath VG. 1993. Nutrition screening for malnutrition: Potential economic impact at a community hospital. *Journal of the American Dietetic Association* 93:1440–1442.
7. Ireton-Jones CS, Hasse JM. 1992. Comprehensive nutritional assessment: The dietitian's contribution to the team effort. *Nutrition* 8:75–81.
8. Hopkins B. 1993. Assessment of Nutritional Status. In Gottschlich MM, Matarese LE, Shronts EP (eds.) *Nutrition support dietetics core curriculum,* 2nd ed. Silver Spring, Md: American Society for Parenteral and Enteral Nutrition.
9. Marton KI, Sox HC, Krupp JR. 1981. Involuntary weight loss: Diagnostic and prognostic significance. *Annals of Internal Medicine* 95: 568–574.
10. Chumlea WC, Guo S, Roche AF, Steinbaugh ML. 1988. Prediction of body weight for the nonambulatory elderly from anthropometry. *Journal of the American Dietetic Association* 88:564–568.
11. Chumlea WC, Guo SS, Steinbaugh ML. 1994. Prediction of stature from knee height for black and white adults and children with application to mobility-impaired or handicapped persons. *Journal of the American Dietetic Association* 94:1385–88.
12. Detsky AS, Smalley PS, Change J. 1994. Is this patient malnourished? *Journal of the American Medical Association* 271:54–58.
13. Chumlea WC, Roche AF, Mukherjee D. 1987. *Nutritional assessment of the elderly through anthropometry.* Columbus, Oh: Ross Laboratories.
14. Heymsfield SB, McManus C, Smith J, Stevens V, Nixon DW. 1982. Anthropometric measurement of muscle mass: Revised equations for calculating bone-free arm muscle area. *American Journal of Clinical Nutrition* 36:680–690.
15. Chumlea WC. 1988. Methods of nutritional anthropometric assessment for special groups. In Lohman TG, Roche AF, Martorell R (eds.) *Anthropometric standardization reference manual.* Champaign, Ill: Human Kinetics Books.
16. Chumlea WC, Roche AF. 1988. Assessment of the nutritional status of healthy and handicapped adults. In Lohman TG, Roche AF, Martorell R (eds.) *Anthropometric standardization reference manual.* Champaign, Ill: Human Kinetics Books.

17. Cockram DB, Baumgartner RN. 1990. Evaluation of accuracy and reliability of calipers for measuring recumbent knee height in elderly people. *American Journal of Clinical Nutrition* 52:397–400.
18. Muncie HL, Sobal J, Hoopes JM, Tenney JH, Warren JW. 1987. A practical method of estimating stature of bedridden female nursing home patients. *Journal of the American Geriatrics Society* 35:285–289.
19. Jarzem PF, Gledhill RB. 1993. Predicting height from arm measurements. *Journal of Pediatric Orthopaedics* 13:761–765.
20. Falciglia G, O'Conner J, Gedling E. 1988. Upper arm anthropometric norms in elderly white subjects. *Journal of the American Dietetic Association* 88:569–574.
21. Callaway CW, Chumlea WC, Bouchard C, Himes JH, Lohman TG, Martin AD, Mitchell CD, Mueller WH, Roche AF, Seefeldt VD. 1988. Circumferences. In Lohman TG, Roche AF, Martorell R (eds.) *Anthropometric standardization reference manual.* Champaign, Ill: Human Kinetics Books.
22. Chumlea WC, Roche AF, Webb P. 1984. Body size, subcutaneous fatness and total body fat in older adults. *International Journal of Obesity* 8:311–317.
23. Frisancho AR. 1990. *Anthropometric standards for the assessment of growth and nutritional status.* Ann Arbor: University of Michigan Press.
24. Guenter PA, Moore K, Crosby LO, Buzby GP, Mullen JL. 1982. Body weight measurement of patients receiving nutritional support. *Journal of Parenteral and Enteral Nutrition* 6:441–443.
25. Brunnstrom S. 1983. *Clinical kinesiology,* 4th ed. Philadelphia: Davis.
26. Frisancho AR. 1981. New norms of upper limb fat and muscle areas for assessment of nutritional status. *American Journal of Clinical Nutrition* 34:2540–2545.
27. Sims AH, Danforth E. 1987. Expenditure and storage of energy in man. *Journal of Clinical Investigation* 79:1019–1025.
28. Long CL. 1984. The energy and protein requirements of the critically ill patient. In Wright RA, Heymsfield SB (eds.) *Nutritional assessment.* Boston: Blackwell Scientific Publications.
29. Damask MC, Schwarz Y, Weissman C. 1987. Energy measurements and requirements of critically ill patients. *Critical Care Clinics* 3:71–96.
30. Foster GD, Knox LS, Dempsey DT, Mullen JL. 1987. Caloric requirements in total parenteral nutrition. *Journal of the American College of Nutrition* 6:231–253.
31. Schutz Y, Jéquier E. 1994. Energy needs: Assessment and requirements. In Shils ME, Olson JA, Shike (eds.) *Modern nutrition in health and disease,* 8th ed. Philadelphia: Lea & Febiger.
32. Murgatroyd PR, Shetty PS, Prentice AM. 1993. Techniques for the measurement of human energy expenditure: A practical guide. *International Journal of Obesity* 17:549–568.
33. Ravussin E, Burnand B, Schutz Y, Jéquier E. 1982. Twenty-four-hour energy expenditure and resting metabolic rate in obese, moderately obese, and control subjects. *American Journal of Clinical Nutrition* 35:566–573.
34. Ravussin E, Lillioja S, Anderson TE, Christin L, Bogardus C. 1986. Determinants of 24-hour energy expenditure in man. *Journal of Clinical Investigation* 78:1568–1578.
35. McClave SA, Snider HL. 1992. Use of indirect calorimetry in clinical nutrition. *Nutrition in Clinical Practice* 7:207–221.
36. Schoeller DA. 1990. How accurate is self-reported dietary energy intake? *Nutrition Reviews* 48: 373–379.
37. Klein PD, James WPT, Wong WW, Irving CS, Murgatroyd PR, Cabrera M, Dallosso HM, Klein ER, Nichols BL. 1984. Calorimetric validation of the doubly labeled water method for determination of energy expenditure in man. *Human Nutrition Clinical Nutrition* 38C:95–106.
38. Seale JL, Rumpler WV, Conway JM, Miles CW. 1990. Comparison of doubly labeled water, intake-balance, and direct- and indirect-calorimetry methods for measuring energy expenditure in adult men. *American Journal of Clinical Nutrition* 52:66–71.
39. Livingstone MBE, Prentice AM, Coward AW, Ceesay SM, Strain JJ, McKenna PG, Nevin GB, Barker ME, Hickey RJ. 1990. Simultaneous measurement of free-living energy expenditure by the doubly labeled water method and heart-rate monitoring. *American Journal of Clinical Nutrition* 52:59–65.

40. Bandini LG, Schoeller DA, Dietz WH. 1990. Energy expenditure in obese and nonobese adolescents. *Pediatric Research* 27:198–202.
41. Prentice AM, Black AE, Coward WA, Davies HL, Goldberg GR, Murgatroyd PR, Ashford J, Sawyer M, Whitehead RG. 1986. High levels of energy expenditure in obese women. *British Medical Journal* 292:983–987.
42. Johnson RK, Goran MI, Poehlman ET. 1994. Correlates of over- and underreporting of energy intake in healthy older men and women. *American Journal of Clinical Nutrition* 59:1286–1290.
43. Harris JA, Benedict FG. 1919. *A biometric study of basal metabolism in man*. Publication 279. Washington, DC: Carnegie Institution of Washington.
44. Roza AM, Shizgal HM. 1984. The Harris Benedict equation reevaluated: Resting energy requirements and the body cell mass. *American Journal of Clinical Nutrition* 40:168–182.
45. Owen OE, Holup JL, D'Alessio DA, Craig ES, Polansky M, Smalley KJ, Karle EC, Bushman MC, Owen LR, Mozzoli MA, Kedrick ZV, Boden GH. 1987. A reappraisal of the caloric requirement of men. *American Journal of Clinical Nutrition* 46:875–885.
46. de Boer JO, van Es AJH, van Raaij JMA, Hautvast JGAJ. 1987. Energy requirements and energy expenditure of lean and overweight women, measured by indirect calorimetry. *American Journal of Clinical Nutrition* 46:13–21.
47. Mifflin MD, St Jeor ST, Hill LA, Scott BJ, Daugherty SA, Koh YO. 1990. A new predictive equation for resting energy expenditure in healthy individuals. *American Journal of Clinical Nutrition* 51:241–247.
48. Cunningham JJ. 1980. A reanalysis of the factors influencing basal metabolic rate in normal adults. *American Journal of Clinical Nutrition* 33: 2372–2374.
49. Food and Nutrition Board, National Research Council. 1989. *Recommended Dietary Allowances,* 10th ed. Washington, DC: National Academy Press.
50. World Health Organization. 1985. *Energy and protein requirements. Report of a joint FAO/WHO/UNU expert consultation*. Technical Report Series 724. Geneva: World Health Organization.
51. Ireton-Jones CS, Turner WW. 1991. Actual or ideal body weight: Which should be used to predict energy expenditure? *Journal of the American Dietetic Association* 91:193–195.
52. Parenteral and Enteral Nutrition Team. 1994. *Parenteral and enteral nutrition manual,* 7th ed. University of Michigan Medical Center, p. 14.
53. Curreri PW. 1990. Assessing nutritional needs for the burned patient. *Journal of Trauma* 30(12 suppl):S20–S23.
54. Bell SJ, Wyatt J. 1986. Nutrition guidelines for burned patients. *Journal of the American Dietetic Association* 86:648–653.
55. Waymack JP, Herndon DN. 1992. Nutritional support of the burned patient. *World Journal of Surgery* 16:80–86.
56. Montegut WJ, Lowry SF. 1993. Nutrition in burn patients. *Seminars in Nephrology* 13:400–408.
57. Cunningham JJ, Lydon MK, Russell WE. 1990. Calorie and protein provision for recovery from severe burns in infants and young children. *American Journal of Clinical Nutrition* 51: 533–537.
58. Allard JP, Pichard C, Hoshino E, Stechison S, Fareholm L, Peters WJ, Jeejeebhoy KN. 1990. Validation of a new formula for calculating the energy requirements of burn patients. *Journal of Parenteral and Enteral Nutrition* 14:115–118.
59. Hildreth MA, Herndon DN, Parks KH. 1987. Evaluation of a caloric requirement formula in burned children treated with early excision. *Journal of Trauma* 27:188–000.
60. Long CL, Schaffel N, Geiger JW, Schiller WR, Blackmore WS. 1979. Metabolic response to injury and illness: Estimation of energy and protein needs from indirect calorimetry and nitrogen balance. *Journal of Parenteral and Enteral Nutrition* 3:452–456.
61. Curreri PW, Richmond D, Marvin J, Baxter CR. 1974. Dietary requirements of patients with major burns. *Journal of the American Dietetic Association* 65:415–417.
62. Saffle JR, Medina E, Raymond J, Westenskow D. 1985. Use of indirect calorimetry in the nutritional management of burned patients. *Journal of Trauma* 25:32–39.
63. Turner WW, Ireton CS, Hunt JL, Baster CR. 1985. Predicting energy expenditure in burned patients. *Journal of Trauma* 25:11–16.

64. Allard JP, Jeejeebhoy KN, Whitwell J, Pashutinski L, Peters WJ. 1988. Factors influencing energy expenditure in patients with burns. *Journal of Trauma* 28:199–202.
65. Royall D, Fairholm L, Peters WJ, Jeejeebhoy KJ, Allard JP. 1994. Continuous measurement of energy expenditure in ventilated burn patients: An analysis. *Critical Care Medicine* 22:399–406.
66. Mancusi-Ungaro HR, Van Way CW, McCool C. 1992. Caloric and nitrogen balance as predictors of nutritional outcome in patients with Burns. *Journal of Burn Care and Rehabilitation* 13:695–702.
67. Benjamin DR. 1989. Laboratory tests and nutritional assessment: Protein-energy status. *Pediatric Clinics of North America* 36:139–161.
68. Heymsfield SB, Tighe A, Zi-Mian W. 1994. Nutritional assessment by anthropometric and biochemical methods. In Shils ME, Olson JA, Shike M (eds.) *Modern nutrition in health and disease,* 8th ed. Philadelphia: Lea & Febiger.
69. Konstantinides FN, Radmer WJ, Becker WK, Herman VK, Warren WE, Solem LD, Williams JB, Cerra FB. 1992. Inaccuracy of nitrogen balance determinations in thermal injury with calculated total urinary nitrogen. *Journal of Burn Care and Rehabilitation* 13:254–260.
70. Loder PB, Kee AJ, Horsburgh R, Jones M, Smith RC. 1989. Validity of urinary urea nitrogen as a measure of total urinary nitrogen in adult patients requiring parenteral nutrition. *Critical Care Medicine* 17:309–312.
71. Milner EA, Cioffi WG, Mason AD, McManus WF, Pruitt BA. 1993. Accuracy of urinary urea nitrogen for predicting total urinary nitrogen in thermally injured patients. *Journal of Parenteral and Enteral Nutrition* 17:414–416.
72. White JV, Ham RJ, Lipschitz DA, Dwyer JT, Wellman NS. 1991. Consensus of the Nutrition Screening Initiative: Risk factors and indicators of poor nutritional status in older Americans. *Journal of the American Dietetic Association* 91:783–787.
73. White JV, Ham RJ, Lipschitz DA. 1991. *Report of nutrition screening 1: Toward a common goal.* Washington, DC: Nutrition Screening Initiative.
74. Dwyer JT. 1991. *Screening older Americans' nutritional health: Current practices and future possibilities.* Washington, DC: Nutrition Screening Initiative.
75. White JV, Dwyer JT, Possner BM, Ham RJ, Lipschitz DA, Wellman NS. 1992. Nutrition Screening Initiative: Development and implementation of the public awareness checklist and screening tools. *Journal of the American Dietetic Association* 92:163–167.

Assessment Activity 7-1

ESTIMATING STATURE AND BODY WEIGHT

Although stature and body weight usually can be easily obtained by direct measurement, there are times when they may have to be estimated. Stature can be estimated from knee height, age, sex, and race using the equations in Table 7-1. Body weight can be estimated from knee height, age, sex, race, and midarm circumference using the equations in Tables 7-3 and 7-4. In this Assessment Activity, you will have an opportunity to practice measuring knee height, midarm circumference, stature, and body weight. You will use the appropriate formulas in Tables 7-1, 7-3, and 7-4 for calculating estimates of stature and body weight and then compare these estimates with values obtained by direct measurement.

Students can divide into groups of two or three and measure each other's knee height and midarm circumference as outlined in this chapter. Two consecutive measurements of knee height should agree with each other to within 0.5 cm and be recorded. Measurements of midarm circumference should be recorded to within 0.1 cm. Be sure to mark the triceps skinfold site (where the midarm circumference is measured) if you plan to measure the triceps skinfold site in Assessment Activity 7-2. These values then can be substituted into the appropriate equations to obtain estimates of stature and body weight. Stature and body weight then can be measured directly following the guidelines in Chapter 6.

Once all students have completed their measurements and calculations, these can be listed on the board or on a sheet of paper distributed to all students. The means and standard deviations of all estimates and measures can be quickly calculated using a pocket calculator with statistical functions. In addition, the differences between estimated and measured values for stature and body weight can be calculated, and the mean and standard deviations of these can be calculated as well.

What was the difference between the estimated and measured values? Although it is clearly better to directly measure stature and body weight, estimates are generally better than no values at all.

Assessment Activity 7-2

ARM MUSCLE AREA

Arm muscle area is used as an index of lean tissue or muscle in the body and represents muscle protein reserves. This Assessment Activity will help familiarize you with the anthropometric measurements and calculations required in arriving at estimates of arm muscle area.

In addition to midarm circumference (already obtained in Assessment Activity 7-1), the formula for arm muscle area requires measurement of the triceps skinfold. If you marked the triceps skinfold site in Assessment Activity 7-1, it will be easy to make this measurement. Review the section on triceps skinfold measurement in Chapter 6 if necessary. A pocket calculator and the following equations can be used for calculating corrected arm muscle area:

$$\text{cAMA for females} = \frac{[\text{MAC} - (\pi \times \text{TSF})]^2}{4\pi} - 6.5$$

$$\text{cAMA for males} = \frac{[\text{MAC} - (\pi \times \text{TSF})]^2}{4\pi} - 10$$

where cAMA = corrected arm muscle area in cm^2; MAC = midarm circumference in cm; and TSF = triceps skinfold thickness in cm. Note that these equations call for all measurements to be made in *centimeters*. The nomogram in Figure 7-14 also can be used to calculate corrected arm muscle area.

Appendix R provides means, standard deviations, and percentiles of arm muscle area for males and females age 1 to 74 years. For persons age 18 years and older, the values are for corrected arm muscle area. Table 7-6 can be used for interpreting these age/sex percentile values. No single index (for example, arm muscle area) is a reliable indicator of nutritional status. Basic assumptions inferred from anthropometry should be corroborated by data derived from dietary, biochemical, and clinical observations.

EIGHT

NUTRITIONAL ASSESSMENT IN DISEASE PREVENTION

OUTLINE

INTRODUCTION

The prominent role of diet and nutritional status in several leading causes of death for Americans gives nutritional assessment an important role to play in disease prevention. This chapter addresses nutritional assessment as it relates to three major causes of death and disability: coronary heart disease, osteoporosis, and diabetes.

Several risk factors of coronary heart disease, the leading cause of death for Americans, are related to diet. Among these are elevated serum total and low-density-lipoprotein cholesterol (LDL-C), low levels of high-density-lipoprotein cholesterol (HDL-C), obesity, hypertension, and diabetes. This chapter also discusses issues in measuring lipid and lipoprotein levels, which apply to practically all measurements in nutritional assessment.

Osteoporosis, a loss of mineral from bones that leave them weakened and more likely to fracture, is a major cause of disability and death among older persons. Available methods for assessing bone mineral content are discussed. We conclude the chapter with a discussion of criteria for diagnosing diabetes.

Reducing the individual and societal burden imposed by these and other diseases lies in our ability to prevent their premature onset through early diagnosis and research into more effective preventive measures. Nutritional assessment plays a prominent role in each of these.

CORONARY HEART DISEASE

Coronary heart disease, also referred to as coronary artery disease, is one of more than 20 different diseases affecting the heart and blood vessels, which collectively are known as cardiovascular diseases. Coronary heart disease results when the coronary arteries supplying the heart with vital oxygen and nutrients become narrowed and inelastic because of atherosclerosis. Evidence supports the view that atherosclerosis begins in childhood with the formation of a fatty streak as lipids (primarily cholesterol and its esters) become deposited in macrophages (large phagocytic cells located within connective tissue) and smooth muscle cells within the inner lining of large elastic and muscular arteries.[1,2,3] These early lesions do not disturb blood flow in the affected artery. As more lipid collects within the artery wall during adolescence and early adulthood, a fibrous plaque develops that projects into the channel or lumen of the artery, resulting in ischemia, or impaired blood flow. Ischemia within the heart muscle or myocardium can result in angina pectoris, which is chest pain caused by insufficient blood flow to the heart. If the impaired blood flow is severe enough, the tissues fed by the obstructed artery may die. This is known as an infarct. When this process affects the coronary arteries, a heart attack or myocardial infarction occurs. When the cerebral arteries are affected (known as cerebrovascular disease), a stroke results. Atherosclerotic changes within the aorta and iliac and femoral arteries can result in peripheral vascular disease.[1,2]

Coronary heart disease (CHD) is the single largest cause of death of American males and females.[4] More than 6 million Americans alive today have CHD. According to American Heart Association estimates, about 1.5 million Americans have heart attacks each year. Each year 500,000 people die of heart attack. Half of these deaths occur before the victims reach the hospital. This is due in part to the unfortunate fact that about half of all heart attack victims wait more than 2 hours before seeking help. Everyone should be familiar with the warning signs of heart attack (outlined in Box 8-1) and promptly seek medical care if they occur. Coronary heart disease costs the United States more than $56 billion per year in direct and indirect costs. Despite a more than 50% decline in the death rate from CHD since 1950, it remains the leading cause of death in the United States and many Western nations.[4]

BOX 8-1

Warning Signals of a Heart Attack

- Uncomfortable pressure, fullness, squeezing, or pain in the center of the chest that lasts more than a few minutes or goes away and comes back.
- Pain spreading to the shoulders, neck, or arms.
- Chest discomfort with lightheadedness, fainting, sweating, nausea, or shortness of breath.

Not all of these warning signs occur in every heart attack. If some start to occur, however, don't wait. Get help immediately. Adapted from *Heart Stroke and Facts*. 1992. Dallas, Tex: American Heart Association.

Coronary Heart Disease Risk Factors

Several factors or traits influence a person's risk of developing CHD and how rapidly atherosclerosis progresses.[2,4,5] The risk factors other than LDL-C levels are shown in Box 8-2. The "positive" risk factors are those that increase CHD risk. An HDL-C level ≥ 60 mg/dl is considered a "negative" risk factor because it decreases risk of CHD, as discussed later in this chapter. Some of these risk factors are modifiable (e.g., cigarette smoking, physical activity, and to a somewhat lesser degree hypertension, obesity, and diabetes mellitus) while others are obviously not modifiable (e.g., age, male sex, and family history of premature CHD). The risk factors most directly associated with CHD are elevated serum cholesterol, high blood pressure, cigarette smoking, and diabetes mellitus.

BOX 8-2

Risk Status Based on Presence of CHD Risk Factors other than LDL-C

Positive Risk Factors

- Age:
  Male: ≥45 years
  Female: ≥55 years or premature menopause without estrogen replacement therapy
- Family history of premature CHD (definite myocardial infarction or sudden death before 55 years of age in father or other male first-degree relative, or before 65 years of age in mother or other female first-degree relative)
- Current cigarette smoking
- Hypertension (>140/90 mm Hg* or taking antihypertensive medication)
- Low HDL-C (<35 mg/dl*)
- Diabetes mellitus

Negative Risk Factors†

- High HDL-C (≥60 mg/dl)

From National Cholesterol Education Program. 1993. *Second report of the expert panel on detection, evaluation, and treatment of high blood cholesterol in adults*. Bethesda, Md: US Department of Health and Human Services, Public Health Service; National Institutes of Health; National Heart, Lung, Blood Institute.

High risk, defined as a net of two or more CHD risk factors, leads to more vigorous intervention. Age (defined differently for men and for women) is treated as a risk factor because rates of CHD are higher in the elderly than in the young, and in men than in women of the same age. Obesity is not listed as a risk factor because it operates through other risk factors that are included (hypertension, hyperlipidemia, decreased HDL-C, and diabetes mellitus), but it should be considered a target for intervention. Physical inactivity is similarly not listed as a risk factor, but it too should be considered a target for intervention, and physical activity is recommended as desirable for everyone.

*Confirmed by measurements on several occasions.

†If the HDL-C level is ≥ 60 mg/dl, subtract one risk factor (because high HDL-C levels decrease CHD risk).

Serum Lipids and Lipoproteins

Cholesterol is a lipid or fatlike substance present only in foods of animal origin and synthesized by the body. It serves as a structural component of cell membranes and a precursor for steroid hormones and vitamin D and is used by the liver to form bile acids, which facilitate fat digestion and absorption. About 93% of the body's cholesterol is present in cell membranes, whereas only about 7% circulates in the blood.[6] Triglyceride, a compound consisting of three fatty acids esterified to a molecule of glycerol, is the usual storage form of lipid in humans and animals.

There is a strong positive relationship between elevated levels of total blood cholesterol and incidence of and mortality from CHD.[2,5,7–9] In 1984, the National Institutes of Health Consensus Development Conference on Lowering Blood Cholesterol conducted an exhaustive review of the evidence relating cholesterol levels and CHD. The panel unanimously concluded that "elevated blood cholesterol is a major cause of coronary artery disease. It has been established beyond a reasonable doubt that lowering definitely elevated blood cholesterol levels (specifically blood levels of low-density lipoprotein cholesterol) will reduce the risk of heart attacks caused by coronary heart disease."[8]

Because lipids such as cholesterol and triglycerides are fat soluble, they must be transported within the bloodstream from sites of absorption or synthesis to sites of storage or metabolism by lipoproteins. The major lipid-transporting lipoproteins are chylomicrons, very-low-density lipoproteins (VLDL), low-density lipoproteins (LDL), and high-density lipoproteins (HDL).[5,9–11] Lipoproteins are spherical macromolecular complexes of lipids (triglycerides, cholesterol, cholesterol esters, and phospholipids) and special proteins known as apoproteins. Apoproteins control the interaction and metabolic fate of lipoproteins. They activate enzymes that modify the composition and structure of lipoproteins, are involved in the binding and ingestion of lipoproteins by cells, and participate in the exchange of lipids between lipoproteins of different classes.[6] Figure 8-1 shows the relative size and the lipid composition of the three major lipoprotein particles.

Chylomicrons are the largest lipoproteins, containing about 90% triglycerides by weight. They are synthesized in the intestine and transport dietary triglycerides from the small intestine to adipose tissue, muscle, and the liver. The dietary cholesterol they carry is taken up by the liver for production of bile acids or later incorporation into VLDL. Chylomicrons are not found in fasting serum, except in certain disease states.[6]

VLDL are 60% triglyceride by weight and contain 10% to 15% of the serum's total cholesterol. They are synthesized in the liver and primarily carry triglyceride to the cells for storage and metabolism. Removal of triglycerides from VLDL results in smaller, denser particles known as intermediate-density lipoproteins (IDL). The density of IDL falls between that of VLDL and LDL. About half the IDL is catabolized by the liver, and the remaining IDL undergoes additional changes (for example, uptake of cholesterol) that transform it into LDL. Thus LDL levels are linked to hepatic VLDL production and IDL catabolism.[6]

The primary role of LDL is to transport cholesterol to the various cells of the body. LDL contains approximately 70% of the serum's total cholesterol, is considered the most atherogenic (atherosclerosis-producing) lipoprotein, and *is the prime target of attempts to lower serum cholesterol.* Clinical trials have shown, for example, that for every 1% decrease in serum total cholesterol (most of which is found in the LDL particle), CHD risk falls roughly 2%.[5,12] About 70% to 80% of LDL is removed from the serum by LDL receptors located on the plasma membranes of hepatic and peripheral cells. The remaining 20% to 30% are degraded by macrophages.[6,13]

Most clinical laboratories do not measure LDL-C directly. Instead, they calculate it based on measurements of total cholesterol, HDL-C, and triglycerides. In this procedure, VLDL-cholesterol (VLDL-C) is estimated by dividing triglycerides

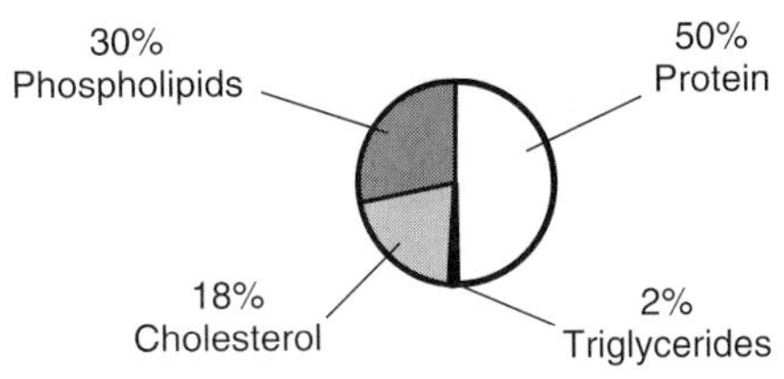

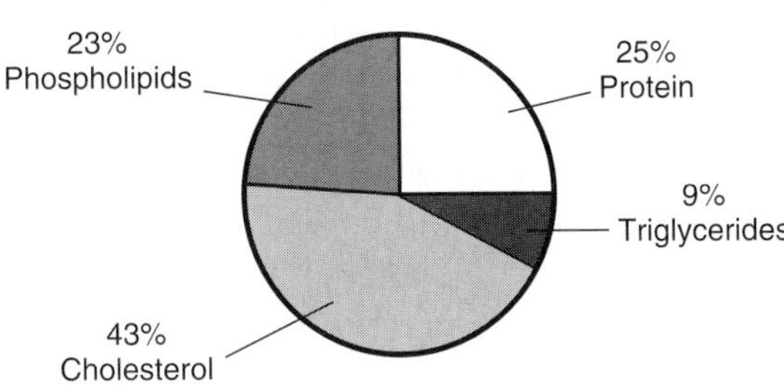

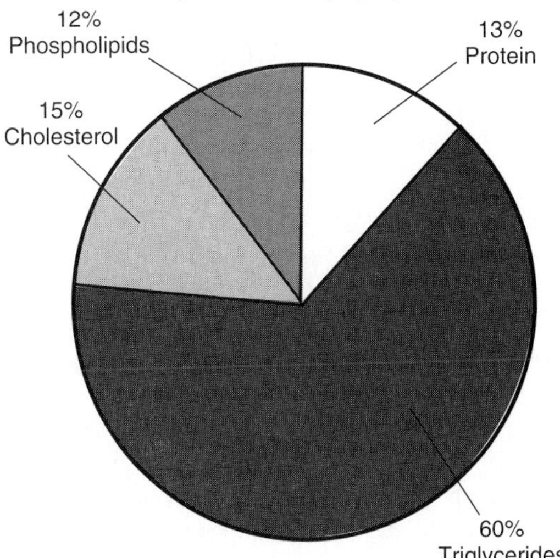

Figure 8-1 The relative size and the lipid composition of the three major lipoprotein particles found in fasting serum. From Haskell WL. 1994. The influence of exercise on the concentrations of triglyceride and cholesterol in human plasma. *Exercise and Sports Science Review,* 12:205–244.

by 5. The following equation is recommended by the National Cholesterol Education Program:[5]

$$\text{LDL-C} = \text{TC} - \text{HDL-C} - (\text{TG} \div 5)$$

where TC = total cholesterol and TG triglycerides. This formula cannot be used when the triglyceride level is > 400 mg/dl.

HDL is the smallest and densest of the lipoproteins. Secreted by the liver and small intestine in a disc-shaped form, HDL eventually assumes a spherical shape as it takes up phospholipids and cholesterol from other lipoproteins and body cells.[13,14] As serum HDL levels *rise,* risk of CHD *decreases.* In other words, higher serum levels of HDL are protective against risk of CHD.[15–17]

Data from several studies have shown that a 1% increase in serum HDL cholesterol (the cholesterol carried by the HDL particle) translates into a 1.5% to 2% reduction in CHD risk.[18]

HDL is involved in the reverse transport of cholesterol.[14,15,19] It is currently thought that HDL picks up cholesterol from the blood stream and various cells of the body and transports it to the liver and other lipoproteins where it is excreted in the bile, converted to bile acids, or reprocessed into VLDL.[14,19] It is hypothesized that this reverse transport process is responsible, at least in part, for the strong inverse relationship between serum HDL-C and CHD risk, although it is likely that other mechanisms are involved as well.[6,14,15]

A more recently discovered lipoprotein, and one in which there is currently considerable interest, is lipoprotein(a) [Lp(a)] or "lipoprotein small a." Lp(a) is a low-density lipoprotein-like particle that shares many characteristics with plasminogen.[20–22] Some research suggests that Lp(a) may promote blood coagulation by interfering with the action of plasminogen and plasmin, which are involved in the lysis or dissolution of blood clots and inhibition of blood clotting. This could potentially lead to thrombus formation in atherosclerotic arteries and increased risk of heart attack or stroke. However, the role of Lp(a) in blood coagulation is not clear. Studies investigating the relationship of Lp(a) to CHD risk have yielded conflicting results.[22–25] In those studies

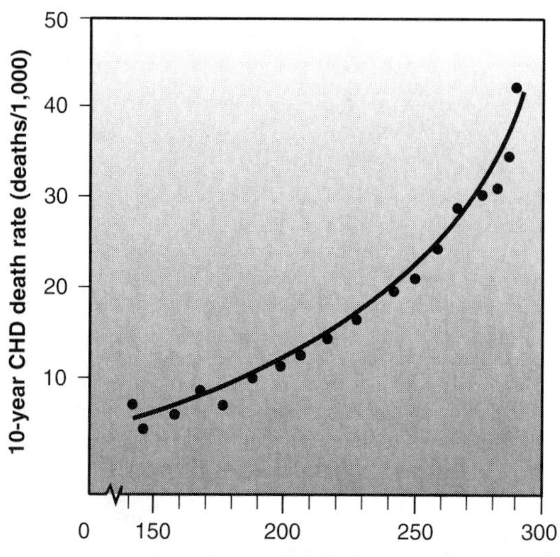

Figure 8-2 The relationship between serum total cholesterol and coronary heart disease (CHD) mortality in men. From National Cholesterol Education Program. 1993. *Second report of the expert panel on detection, evaluation, and treatment of high blood cholesterol in adults.* Bethesda, Md: US Department of Health and Human Services, Public Health Service; National Institutes of Health; National Heart, Lung, and Blood Institute.

TABLE 8-1 Initial classification based on total cholesterol and HDL-C

Total cholesterol	mg/dl	mmol/L
Desirable	<200	<5.17
Borderline high	200–239	5.17–6.19
High	≥240	≥6.20
HDL-C		
Low HDL-C	<35	<0.9

From National Cholesterol Education Program. 1993. *Second report of the expert panel on detection, evaluation, and treatment of high blood cholesterol in adults.* Bethesda, Md: US Department of Health and Human Services, Public Health Service; National Institutes of Health; National Heart, Lung, Blood Institute.

suggesting that Lp(a) is an independent risk factor for CHD, the mechanism underlying its association with CHD has not been defined.[22,24] Simple and accurate methods for measuring Lp(a) have yet to be developed, and its potential use as a marker of increased risk for CHD is still in the research stage. In addition, there is no effective therapy for lowering elevated Lp(a) levels.

Lipoproteins, Cholesterol, and Coronary Heart Disease

The relationship between serum total cholesterol and CHD mortality is shown in Figure 8-2.[26] It can be noted that CHD risk steadily increases as serum cholesterol rises. The increase in CHD risk is particularly steep after serum cholesterol rises above 200 mg/dl (5.17 mmol/L). For example, men whose cholesterol levels are at or above the 90th percentile have four times the risk of CHD compared with men whose cholesterol levels are at or below the 10th percentile.[6,26]

Guidelines developed by the National Cholesterol Education Program (NCEP) for classifying total cholesterol and HDL-C levels in adults are shown in Table 8-1. The cutoff point that defines "high blood cholesterol" (total cholesterol of 240 mg/dl) is the value above which risk of CHD rises steeply and corresponds to approximately the 80th percentile for the adult U.S. population based on data from the third National Health and Nutrition Examination Survey (NHANES III).[5] Reference values for serum levels of total cholesterol, LDL cholesterol, and HDL cholesterol and the ratio of total cholesterol to HDL cholesterol (TC/HDL-C) are given in Appendix S.

The atherosclerotic process begins in childhood and progresses slowly into adulthood.[2,3,27] There is also evidence that children and adolescents with elevated serum cholesterol frequently come from families whose adult members have a high incidence of CHD or elevated serum cholesterol levels.[3,27] For these reasons, the NCEP has established guidelines for classifying total cholesterol and LDL-C levels in children and adolescents from families with elevated serum cholesterol levels or premature CHD. These are

TABLE 8-2 The National Cholesterol Education Program's classification of total cholesterol and LDL-C levels in children and adolescents from families with hypercholesterolemia or premature coronary heart disease

	Total cholesterol		Low-density-lipoprotein cholesterol	
	mg/dl	mmol/L	mg/dl	mmol/L
Acceptable	<170	<4.40	<110	<2.84
Borderline	170–199	4.40–5.15	110–129	2.84–3.34
High	≥200	≥5.17	≥130	≥3.36

From NCEP. 1991. *Report of the expert panel on blood cholesterol levels in children and adolescents*. Bethesda, Md: US Department of Health and Human Services, Public Health Service; National Institutes of Health; National Heart, Lung, and Blood Institute.

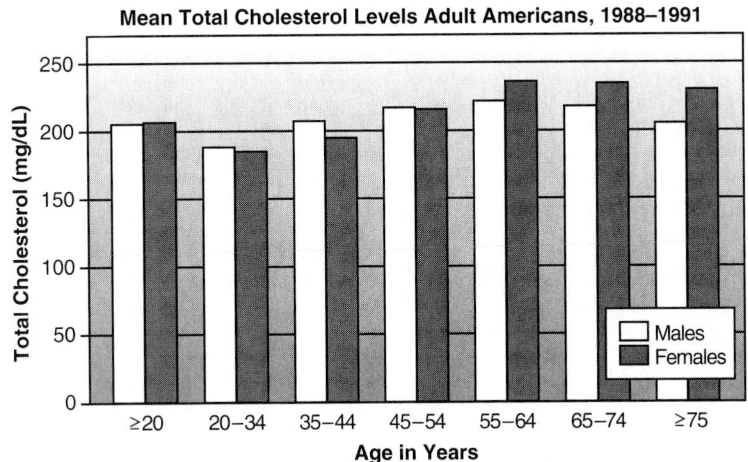

Figure 8-3 As Americans age, their mean serum total cholesterol levels rise. After about age 35, serum total cholesterol levels for most Americans are greater than that recommended by the National Cholesterol Education Program. Data from the National Center for Health Statistics.

shown in Table 8-2. The average total cholesterol and LDL-C levels in persons age 1 to 19 years are approximately 160 mg/dl (4.14 mmol/L) and 100 mg/dl (2.59 mmol/L), respectively. The cutoff points for the "borderline" (170 mg/dl) and "high" (200 mg/dl) values in this age group correspond to the 75th and 95th percentiles, respectively.[27]

How do mean (average) cholesterol levels for adult Americans compare with these standards? According to data from NHANES III shown in Figure 8-3, the mean total cholesterol levels for all U.S. males and females age 20 years and over are 205 mg/dl and 207 mg/dl, respectively. Mean total cholesterol levels for males age 20 to 34 years and for females age 20 to 44 years are within the range considered as "desirable" by the NCEP. For the rest of adult Americans, mean levels are greater than desirable. Thus the majority of Americans could benefit from lower serum cholesterol.

In contrast to total cholesterol and LDL-C levels, CHD risk *falls* as HDL-C levels *rise*.[2,14–16,28] According to data from the Framingham Heart Study, in the presence of high serum HDL-C levels, the risk of CHD is relatively low even in subjects with increased serum total cholesterol or LDL-C. In contrast, persons with low HDL-C levels are at increased CHD risk even if their total cholesterol and LDL-C levels are within the "desirable" range.[16,17,29] Some researchers believe that HDL-C levels are a stronger predictive factor for CHD than serum total or LDL-C levels.[14]

According to the NCEP, an HDL-C level below 35 mg/dl (0.9 mmol/L) is defined as a "low" serum level and is considered a major risk factor.[5] This cutoff point corresponds to the 5th percentile for U.S. women and approximately the 10th percentile for U.S. men.[30] As mentioned earlier, an HDL-C level ≥ 60 mg/dl (≥1.6 mmol/L) is considered a "negative risk factor" that decreases CHD risk.[5]

Lipoprotein Ratios

Another approach to evaluating HDL-C levels that is suggested by some investigators is to calculate the ratio of two lipid values—for example, the LDL-C/HDL-C ratio (LDL-C level divided by HDL-C level) and the TC/HDL-C ratio (total cholesterol level divided by HDL-C level).[16,31–33] Data from the Framingham Heart Study show that the higher a person's TC/HDL-C ratio, the greater is his or her risk of having symptomatic CHD. In other words, as total cholesterol increases in proportion to HDL-C, CHD risk increases as well. According to Framingham data, 50- to 70-year-old men having a TC/HDL-C ratio of 4.4 have an average risk of CHD compared with men their age. This cutoff point roughly corresponds to a total cholesterol of 200 mg/dl (5.17 mmol/L) and an HDL-C of 45 mg/dl (1.16 mmol/L). Those having a TC/HDL-C ratio of 3.0 have half the risk, and those with a ratio of 6.2, 7.7, or 9.5 have two, three, or four times the average risk, respectively.[34] Although not a substitute for measurements of individual lipid and lipoprotein levels, the TC/HDL-C ratio appears, in many instances, to be a valuable adjunct to evaluating CHD risk.

The NCEP, in its *Second Report of the Expert Panel on Detection, Evaluation, and Treatment of High Blood Cholesterol in Adults,* decided not to use the TC/HDL-C ratio as part of its guidelines. Questions exist about the value of the TC/HDL-C ratio in persons with very low or very high LDL-C levels. The report also points out that LDL (the major component of total cholesterol) and HDL are independent risk factors for CHD and that risk assessment and therapy should focus on LDL and HDL separately.[5]

Triglyceride and Coronary Heart Disease

The connection between serum triglyceride levels and CHD risk is controversial.[5,17,34] Most population studies show serum plasma triglyceride levels to be positively associated with increased CHD risk. However, in most of these studies, triglyceride was not shown to act independently to increase CHD risk after statistical adjustments were made for closely associated factors such as total cholesterol, HDL-C, high blood pressure, cigarette smoking, and obesity.[5] Some researchers argue that elevated triglyceride levels reflect certain lipoprotein alterations (elevated VLDL-C and LDL-C and decreased HDL-C) or accompany other disease states known to increase CHD risk such as diabetes mellitus, nephrotic syndrome, and chronic renal disease.[5,34] Elevated triglyceride levels produce increases in several clotting factors and decrease fibrinolytic activity, both of which contribute to the atherosclerotic process.[17] Guidelines for classifying triglyceride levels developed by the NCEP are shown in Table 8-3.

Coronary Heart Disease Risk Prediction Chart

Data from the Framingham Heart Study have been used to compile the CHD risk prediction chart shown in Table 8-4. Professionals or patients can use the chart to obtain a "good approximation" of CHD risk during a 5- or 10-year period.[35] The chart uses the following variables: age, total cholesterol level, HDL-C level, systolic blood pressure, cigarette smoking (yes or no), diabetes (defined as

TABLE 8-3 Guidelines for classifying serum triglyceride levels

Serum triglyceride	mg/dl	mmol/L
Normal triglycerides	<200	<2.3
Borderline high triglycerides	200–399	2.3–4.5
High triglycerides	400–1000	4.5–11.3
Very high triglycerides	>1000	>11.3

From National Cholesterol Education Program. 1993. *Second report of the expert panel on detection, evaluation, and treatment of high blood cholesterol in adults.* Bethesda, Md: US Department of Health and Human Services, Public Health Service; National Institutes of Health; National Heart, Lung, Blood Institute.

treatment with insulin or oral agents or having a fasting glucose ≥ 140 mg/dl), and definite left-ventricular hypertrophy (increased thickness of the walls surrounding the heart's left ventricle) diagnosed by electrocardiogram (ECG). An example of how the chart is used is given in Assessment Activity 8-2.

The chart is not appropriate for use with persons in whom CHD has been diagnosed, those with extremely elevated risk factors such as malignant hypertension or severe diabetes mellitus, or those with extremely elevated total cholesterol and HDL-C levels.[35] The chart may not be applicable to populations with very low CHD incidence rates, and it cannot be used if a value for any of the risk factors is missing.

National Cholesterol Education Program's Guidelines

The NCEP was created by the National Heart, Lung, and Blood Institute in November 1985 with the overall goal of reducing the prevalence of high blood cholesterol in the United States. It has issued reports written by different panels of experts that address elevated cholesterol levels in several populations. These reports recommend the *patient-based approach* and/or the *population-based* or *public health approach*.[5] The former establishes guidelines for the identification and treatment by physicians of individuals with elevated cholesterol levels. The latter approach emphasizes dietary and lifestyle changes that can be made by all people to lower average cholesterol levels in the entire population. The two approaches are complementary, and together represent a coordinated strategy for reducing coronary risk.

Two somewhat related concepts are primary prevention and secondary prevention. Primary prevention involves risk factor reduction (smoking cessation, lowering of elevated total and LDL-cholesterol levels, control of high blood pressure, and so on) in patients with no evidence or diagnosis of CHD. Secondary prevention involves risk factor reduction in patients who have evidence of and in whom CHD or some other atherosclerotic disease has been diagnosed.

In 1988, the NCEP published the *Report of the Expert Panel on Detection, Evaluation, and Treatment of High Blood Cholesterol in Adults.*[36] This report was revised in 1993 when the NCEP published its *Second Report of the Expert Panel on Detection, Evaluation, and Treatment of High Blood Cholesterol in Adults.*[5] These reports took the patient-based approach. In 1990, the *Report of the Expert Panel on Population Strategies for Blood Cholesterol Reduction* was published.[7] As the title states, it took the population-based or public health approach. In 1991, the *Report of the Expert Panel on Blood Cholesterol Levels in Children and Adolescents* was published.[27] These reports make similar dietary recommendations, which are discussed in the following sections.

Blood Cholesterol in Adults

The *Second Report of the Expert Panel on Detection, Evaluation, and Treatment of High Blood Cholesterol in Adults,* (also known as the Adult Treatment Panel II or ATP II), recommends that all persons 20 years of age or older have their total cholesterol and HDL-C measured at least once

TABLE 8-4 Framingham Heart Study Coronary Heart Disease Risk Prediction Chart

1. Find points for each risk factor

Age (if female) (yr)				Age (if male) (yr)				HDL-C*			
Age	Points	Age	Points	Age	Points	Age	Points	HDL	Points	HDL	Points
30	−12	41	1	30	−2	48–49	9	25–26	7	67–73	−4
31	−11	42–43	2	31	−1	50–51	10	27–29	6	74–80	−5
32	−9	44	3	32–33	0	52–54	11	30–32	5	81–87	−6
33	−8	45–46	4	34	1	55–56	12	33–35	4	88–96	−7
34	−6	47–48	5	35–36	2	57–59	13	36–38	3		
35	−5	49–50	6	37–38	3	60–61	14	39–42	2		
36	−4	51–52	7	39	4	62–64	15	43–46	1		
37	−3	53–55	8	40–41	5	65–67	16	47–50	0		
38	−2	56–60	9	42–43	6	68–70	17	51–55	−1		
39	−1	61–67	10	44–45	7	71–73	18	56–60	−2		
40	0	68–74	11	46–47	8	74	19	61–66	−3		

Total cholesterol (mg/dl)				Systolic blood pressure (mm Hg)			
Chol	Points	Chol	Points	SBP	Points	SBP	Points
139–151	−3	220–239	2	98–104	−2	150–160	4
152–166	−2	240–262	3	105–112	−1	161–172	5
167–182	−1	263–288	4	113–120	0	173–185	6
183–199	0	289–315	5	121–129	1		
200–219	1	316–330	6	130–139	2		
				140–149	3		

Other factors	Points: Yes	Points: No
Cigarette smoking	4	0
Diabetes		
Male	3	0
Female	6	0
ECG-LVH	9	0

2. Add points for all risk factors

_____ (Age) + _____ (Total chol) + _____ (HDL) + _____ (SBP) + _____ (Smoking) + _____ (Diabetes) + _____ (ECG-LVH) = _____ (Total)

Note: *Subtract minus points from total.*

TABLE 8-4 Framingham Heart Study Coronary Heart Disease Risk Prediction Chart—cont'd

3. Look up risk corresponding to point total

Points	Probability (%) 5 yr	10 yr	Points	Probability (%) 5 yr	10 yr	Points	Probability (%) 5 yr	10 yr	Points	Probability (%) 5 yr	10 yr
≤1	<1	<2	9	2	5	17	6	13	25	14	27
2	1	2	10	2	6	18	7	14	26	16	29
3	1	2	11	3	6	19	8	16	27	17	31
4	1	2	12	3	7	20	8	18	28	19	33
5	1	3	13	3	8	21	9	19	29	20	36
6	1	3	14	4	9	22	11	21	30	22	38
7	1	4	15	5	10	23	12	23	31	24	40
8	2	4	16	5	12	24	13	25	32	25	42

4. Compare with average 10-yr risk

Age (yr)	Probability (%) Women	Men	Age (yr)	Probability (%) Women	Men	Age (yr)	Probability (%) Women	Men
30–34	<1	3	45–49	5	10	60–64	13	21
35–39	<1	5	50–54	8	14	65–69	9	30
40–44	2	6	55–59	12	16	70–74	12	24

From *An Updated Coronary Risk Profile*. 1991. American Heart Association.

*HDL-C, high density lipoprotein cholesterol; SBP, systolic blood pressure; ECG-LVH, left ventricular hypertrophy by electrocardiography.

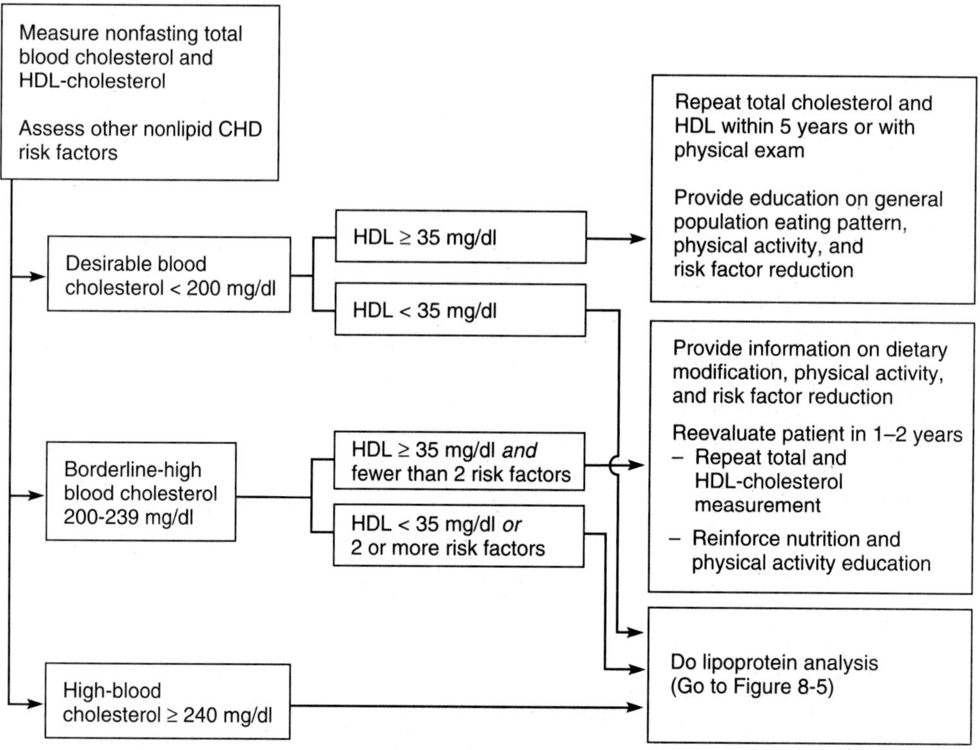

Figure 8-4 Primary prevention in adults without evidence of CHD, initial classification based on total cholesterol and HDL-cholesterol. CHD = coronary heart disease; HDL = high-density lipoprotein. From National Cholesterol Education Program. 1993. *Second report of the expert panel on detection, evaluation, and treatment of high blood cholesterol in adults*. Bethesda, Md: US Department of Health and Human Services, Public Health Service; National Institutes of Health; National Heart, Lung, and Blood Institute.

every 5 years.[5] These measurements can be made in the nonfasting state and should be accompanied by an evaluation of other nonlipid risk factors shown in Box 8-2. For primary prevention in adults without evidence of CHD, initial classification is based on total cholesterol and HDL-C using the criteria shown in Table 8-1. Once these values are known, the steps outlined in Figure 8-4 should be taken as appropriate for the situation. In some instances it may be indicated to perform a lipoprotein analysis, which involves measuring fasting levels of total cholesterol, total triglyceride, and HDL-C. From these values, LDL-C can be calculated using the equation discussed earlier in the chapter.

In the case of primary prevention (Figure 8-4), persons having a total cholesterol < 200 mg/dl and an HDL-C ≥ 35 mg/dl should receive general information on CHD risk factor reduction and be advised to have these tests repeated within 5 years. Persons with a borderline-high total cholesterol, an HDL-C ≥ 35 mg/dl and fewer than two CHD risk factors should receive general information on CHD risk factor reduction and be advised to have these tests repeated in 1 to 2 years. Lipoprotein analysis is indicated for persons with a total cholesterol < 200 mg/dl and an HDL-C < 35 mg/dl; persons with a total cholesterol of 202 to 239 mg/dl and either an HDL-C < 35 mg/dl or two or more CHD risk factors; and

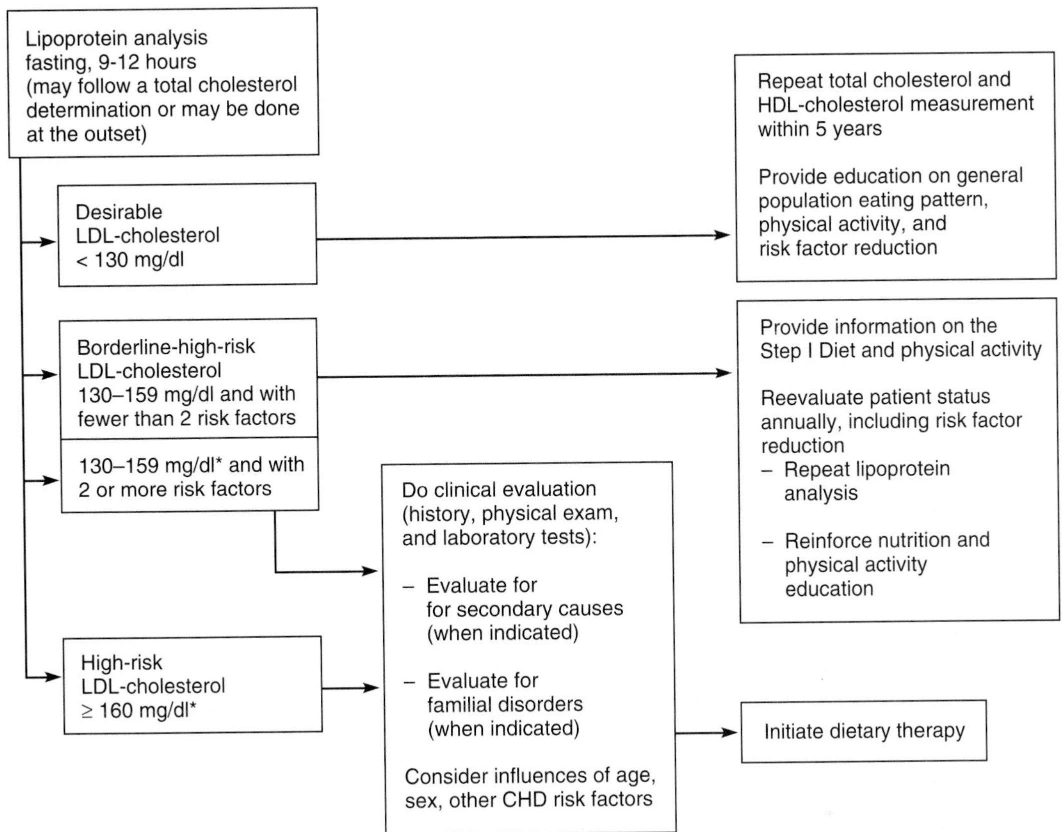
Lipoprotein analysis
fasting, 9-12 hours
(may follow a total cholesterol determination or may be done at the outset)
Desirable
LDL-cholesterol
< 130 mg/dl
Repeat total cholesterol and HDL-cholesterol measurement within 5 years
Provide education on general population eating pattern, physical activity, and risk factor reduction
Borderline-high-risk
LDL-cholesterol
130–159 mg/dl and with fewer than 2 risk factors
Provide information on the Step I Diet and physical activity
Reevaluate patient status annually, including risk factor reduction
– Repeat lipoprotein analysis
– Reinforce nutrition and physical activity education
130–159 mg/dl* and with 2 or more risk factors
Do clinical evaluation (history, physical exam, and laboratory tests):
– Evaluate for for secondary causes (when indicated)
– Evaluate for familial disorders (when indicated)
Consider influences of age, sex, other CHD risk factors
High-risk
LDL-cholesterol
≥ 160 mg/dl*
Initiate dietary therapy
*On the basis of the average of two determinations. If the first two LDL-cholesterol tests differ by more than 30 mg/dl, a third test should be obtained within 1-8 weeks and the average value of three tests used.

Figure 8-5 Primary prevention in adults without evidence of CHD, subsequent classification based on LDL-C. CHD = coronary heart disease; HDL = high-density lipoprotein. From National Cholesterol Education Program. 1993. *Second Report of the expert panel on detection, evaluation, and treatment of high blood cholesterol in adults*. Bethesda, Md: US Department of Health and Human Services, Public Health Service; National Institutes of Health; National Heart, Lung, and Blood Institute.

any person with a total cholesterol ≥ 240 mg/dl. Because of potential errors in the lipoprotein analysis, the test should be done twice within a period of 1 to 8 weeks, with the values for LDL-C averaged. If the two LDL-C values differ by more than 30 mg/dl, a third analysis should be performed and the three values averaged together.

The decision to initiate dietary or drug treatment is based on LDL-C levels, as shown in Figure 8-5. In the case of primary prevention, the desirable LDL-C level is < 130 mg/dl. Persons having an LDL-C level < 130 mg/dl require only general information on CHD risk factor reduction and repeat testing of total cholesterol and HDL-C within 5 years. Persons whose LDL-C is 130 to 159 mg/dl and who have fewer than two CHD risk factors should be given instruction in dietary modification and physical activity and be reevaluated for risk status and lipoprotein profile in 1 year. Persons with an LDL-C of 130 to

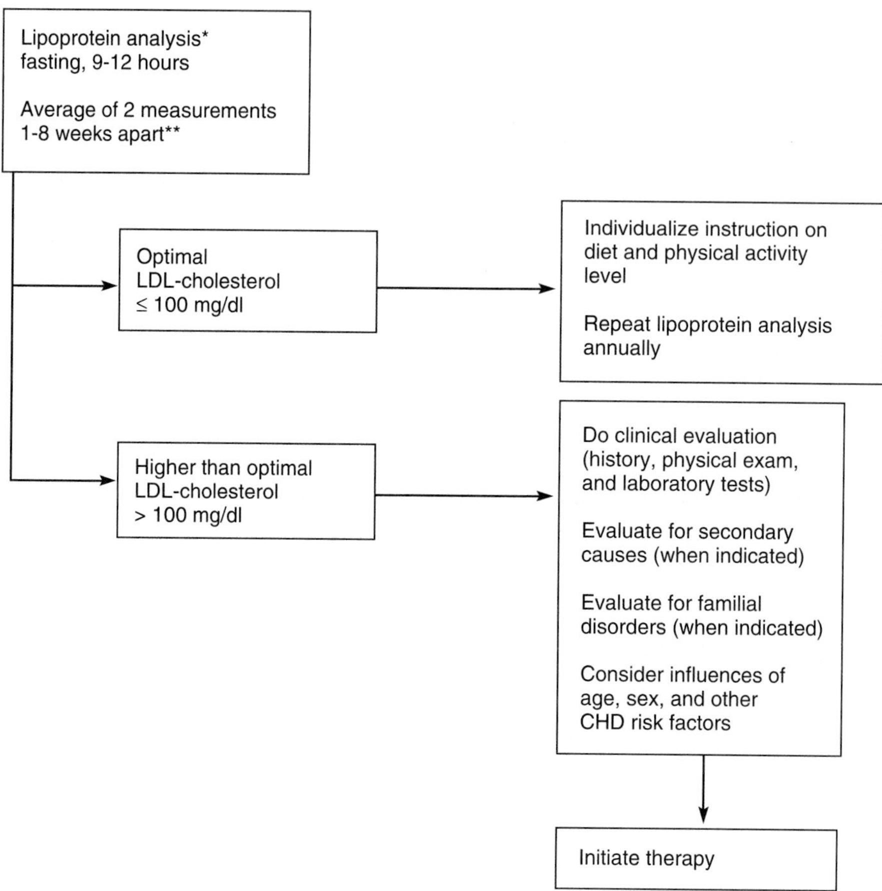
Lipoprotein analysis*
fasting, 9-12 hours
Average of 2 measurements
1-8 weeks apart**
Optimal
LDL-cholesterol
≤ 100 mg/dl
Individualize instruction on
diet and physical activity
level
Repeat lipoprotein analysis
annually
Higher than optimal
LDL-cholesterol
> 100 mg/dl
Do clinical evaluation
(history, physical exam,
and laboratory tests)
Evaluate for secondary
causes (when indicated)
Evaluate for familial
disorders (when indicated)
Consider influences of
age, sex, and other
CHD risk factors
Initiate therapy

*Lipoprotein analysis should be performed when the patient is not in the recovery phase from an acute coronary or other medical event that would lower his or her usual LDL-cholesterol level.

**If the first two LDL-cholesterol tests differ by more than 30 mg/dl, a third test should be obtained within 1-8 weeks and the average value of the three tests used.

Figure 8-6 Secondary prevention in adults with evidence of CHD, classification based on LDL-C. LDL = low-density lipoprotein. From National Cholesterol Education Program, 1993. *Second report of the expert panel on detection, evaluation, and treatment of high blood cholesterol in adults.* Bethesda, Md: US Department of Health and Human Services, Public Health Service; National Institutes of Health; National Heart, Lung, and Blood Institute.

159 mg/dl and who have two or more CHD risk factors and those with an LDL-C ≥ 160 mg/dl should evaluated clinically to determine if their elevated LDL-C levels are due to a genetic disorder or caused by some other condition such as diabetes mellitus, hypothyroidism, nephrotic syndrome, or obstructive liver disease, or use of drugs known to elevate LDL-C such as progestins, anabolic steroids, corticosteroids, and certain antihypertensive drugs. Thereafter, cholesterol-lowering dietary therapy should be started.

Steps to follow in secondary prevention for adults with evidence of CHD or other atherosclerotic disease are outlined in Figure 8-6. Lipoprotein analysis is required when determining which treatment course to pursue. As in the case with primary prevention, lipoprotein analysis should be done twice within 1 to 8 weeks and repeated

BOX 8-3

Treatment Decisions Based on LDL-C. The Initiation Level is the LDL-C Level at which either Dietary or Drug Therapy Should Begin, Given the Various Conditions such as Whether CHD and Risk Factors are Present. The Goal of Therapy is to Bring Levels of LDL within the LDL Goal.

Dietary Therapy	Initiation Level	LDL Goal
Without CHD and with fewer than 2 risk factors	≥160 mg/dl	<160 mg/dl
Without CHD and with 2 or more risk factors	≥130 mg/dl	<130 mg/dl
With CHD	>100 mg/dl	≤100 mg/dl
Drug Treatment	Consideration Level	LDL Goal
Without CHD and with fewer than 2 risk factors	≥190 mg/dl*	<160 mg/dl
Without CHD and with 2 or more risk factors	≥160 mg/dl	<130 mg/dl
With CHD	≥130 mg/dl†	≤100 mg/dl

From: National Cholesterol Education Program. 1993. *Second report of the expert panel on detection, evaluation, and treatment of high blood cholesterol in adults*. Bethesda, Md: US Department of Health and Human Services, Public Health Service; National Institutes of Health; National Heart, Lung, Blood Institute.

*In men under 35 years of age and premenopausal women with LDL-C levels 190–219 mg/dl, drug therapy should be delayed except in high-risk patients such as those with diabetes.

†In patients with CHD whose LDL-C levels are 100–129 mg/dl, the physician should exercise clinical judgment in deciding whether to initiate drug treatment.

a third time if the first two LDL-C values differ by more than 30 mg/dl. As discussed later in this chapter, results of the lipoprotein analysis must be interpreted with caution in persons recovering from a recent heart attack or unstable angina. In the case of secondary prevention, the desirable LDL-C level is ≤100 mg/dl, and persons with this level require only instruction on diet and physical activity and a repeat lipoprotein analysis in one year. When LDL-C is > 100 mg/dl, a clinical evaluation should be done to rule out a genetic disorder or secondary causes. Box 8-3 gives the recommended LDL-C levels at which dietary and drug treatment should be initiated based on whether CHD or risk factors are present. The treatment goals ("LDL Goal") are expressed in terms of LDL-C levels.

Dietary treatment is considered the cornerstone of therapy to reduce blood cholesterol levels. The general aim of dietary therapy is to reduce serum total cholesterol and LDL-cholesterol while providing a nutritionally adequate diet. Dietary therapy occurs in two steps, the Step I and Step II Diets. These are designed to progressively reduce intakes of saturated fatty acids and cholesterol and to promote weight loss in overweight patients. These diets are outlined in Table 8-5. The rationale for these diets is thoroughly discussed in the ATP II and is briefly reviewed later in this chapter. Because the eating pattern recommended by the NCEP for the general public is similar to the Step I Diet, many patients may have already adopted the recommended diet. Consequently it is important to assess the patient's current eating habits before recommending a therapeutic diet. This can be done using the MEDFICTS dietary assessment questionnaire discussed in Chapter 3. If greater accuracy in determining

TABLE 8-5 Dietary therapy of high blood cholesterol using the Step I and Step II Diets

Nutrient*	Recommended Intake†	
	Step I Diet	Step II Diet
Total fat	≤30% of kcal	
SFA	8%–10% of kcal	<7% of kcal
PUFA	up to 10% of kcal	
MUFA	up to 15% of kcal	
Carbohydrates	≥55% of kcal	
Protein	approximately 15% of kcal	
Cholesterol	<300 mg/day	<200 mg/day
Total of kcal	to achieve and maintain desirable weight	

*Kilocalories from alcohol not included; SFA = saturated fatty acids; PUFA = polyunsaturated fatty acids; MUFA = monounsaturated fatty acids

†Kcal = kilocalories

nutrient intake is needed, other methods such as multiple 24-hour recalls, a 3-day food record, or a food frequency questionnaire can be used. If a patient has not adopted a Step I Diet, this should be the first step in dietary therapy. If the patient is already following the Step I Diet at the time of detection, or if the Step I Diet is inadequate to meet the goals of dietary therapy, the patient should proceed to the Step II Diet.

The Step I Diet is the recommended initial approach for most persons. With adequate training, physicians or members of their staffs can assist patients in nutritional education and behavioral change. However, some patients may need counseling from a registered dietitian from the outset. It should be emphasized to patients that the goal is not a temporary "diet," but a permanent change in eating behavior.[5]

Serum cholesterol should be measured at 4 to 6 weeks and again at 3 months after the diet has been started. If the minimal goals of therapy are not achieved after 3 months, the patient may benefit from referral to a registered dietitian for evaluation and counseling. If another trial of the Step I Diet fails to adequately lower cholesterol levels, or if the Step I Diet has been properly adhered to without adequate success, the patient can progress to the Step II Diet. The ATP II suggests that candidates for the Step II Diet be referred to a registered dietitian with expertise in dietary management of cholesterol levels. In case of primary prevention, the attempt to lower serum cholesterol by diet should last for 6 months. However, it may be wise to begin drug therapy sooner in patients with severe elevations of serum cholesterol or those with definite CHD.[5]

Once treatment goals are achieved, monitoring of serum cholesterol levels and reinforcement of behavioral change should continue. If the cholesterol-lowering goal is not achieved, drug treatment should be considered. However, for most patients, at least 6 months of intensive dietary therapy should be carried out before considering drug therapy. For some patients who are not at immediate risk for developing CHD and are continuing to make favorable changes in diet and exercise, a 12-month trial of dietary therapy may be appropriate.

Inadequate lowering of cholesterol levels can result from several factors.[5] Inherited metabolic disorders of lipid metabolism (for example, absent or dysfunctional LDL receptors or hepatic lipoprotein overproduction) can result in severe elevations of serum cholesterol that are resistant to lowering, no matter how strict the diet. Some patients are biologically resistant to LDL lowering by dietary modification and will not achieve the cholesterol-lowering goal despite good adherence to diet.

Some patients refuse to change their eating habits despite the intensive efforts of the physician and counselors. However, a concerted effort by health professionals to promote behavioral change should minimize the size of this patient group. It may take up to a year, or even longer, for some patients to adopt the recommended dietary changes. Thus adequate time should be allowed for patients to attempt to modify their diets to achieve the desired therapeutic goals.[5]

Lowering Cholesterol in the Population

In the *Report of the Expert Panel on Population Strategies for Blood Cholesterol Reduction,* similar CHD risk factors are identified and the same total cholesterol and LDL-C cutoff points are used in classifying persons.[7] The Expert Panel has recommended that all healthy Americans about age 2 years and older adopt the Step I Diet (see Table 8-5). The rationale for the Step I and Step II Diets is outlined later in this chapter in the section entitled "Dietary Treatment in Coronary Heart Disease."

Will population strategies be successful in lowering the average serum cholesterol levels of Americans? Even before government agencies made a concerted effort to promote a heart-healthy diet, the average cholesterol level of Americans was declining, as shown in Figure 8-7. A comparison of data from the first National Health Examination Survey (1960–62) with data collected during Phase I of NHANES III (1988–91) shows that mean serum total cholesterol levels of U.S. males and females age 20 to 74 years have declined 12 mg/dl in males and 17 mg/dl in females, respectively.[37] This fact, along with a decrease in cigarette smoking and a possible

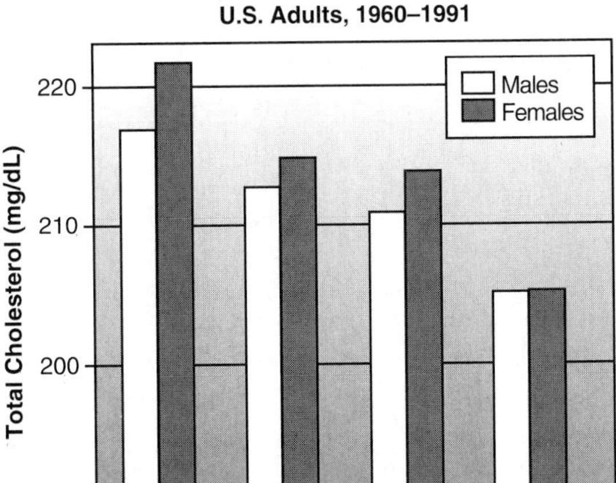

Figure 8-7 Since between 1960 and 1962, mean serum cholesterol levels of U.S. males and females ages 20 through 74 years have declined 12 mg/dl and 17 mg/dl, respectively. Values shown are age-adjusted. From Johnson CL, Rikfind BM, Sempos CT, Carroll MD, Bachorik PS, Briefel RR, Gordon DJ, Burt Vl, Brown CD, Lippel K, Cleeman JI. 1993. Declining serum total cholesterol levels among U.S. adults. *Journal of the American Medical Association*. 269: 3002–3008.

increase in leisure-time physical activity, have no doubt contributed to the 27% decline in heart disease mortality between 1970 and 1991, as shown in Figure 8-8. During the same period, there was 34% reduction in age-adjusted stroke mortality, as shown in Figure 8-9. Despite these reductions, heart disease mortality is nearly 40% greater for black men than it is for white men, and 64% greater for black women than for white women. Stroke mortality is twice as high for black men compared to white men and 80% greater for black women compared to the rate for white women.

Not only is there good evidence that lowering serum cholesterol levels reduces CHD risk, several studies have shown that cholesterol lowering can slow the progression of and even reverse atherosclerotic narrowing.[38–43] According to the NCEP, "the conclusion now seems inescapable that definite regression can be expected in 16% to

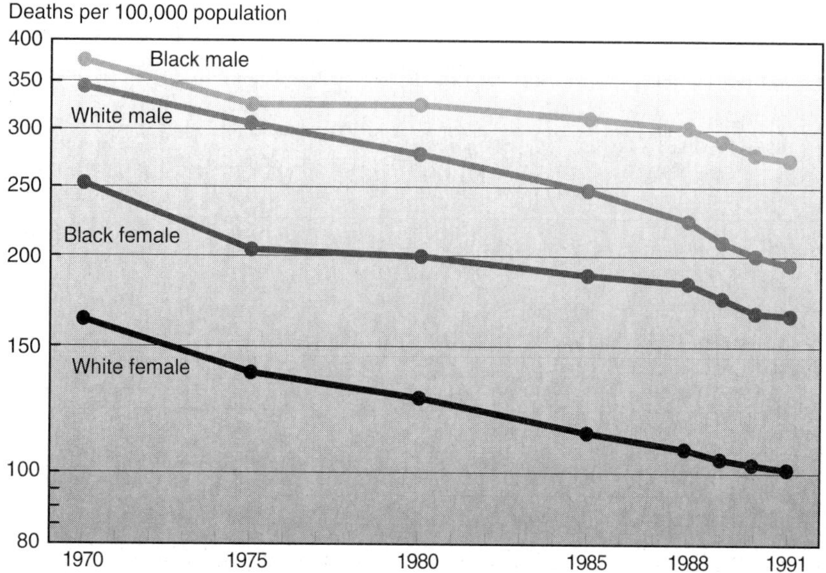

Figure 8-8 Since 1970, the age-adjusted death rate for heart disease, the leading cause of death for U.S. men and women, declined 27%. Data from the National Center for Health Statistics.

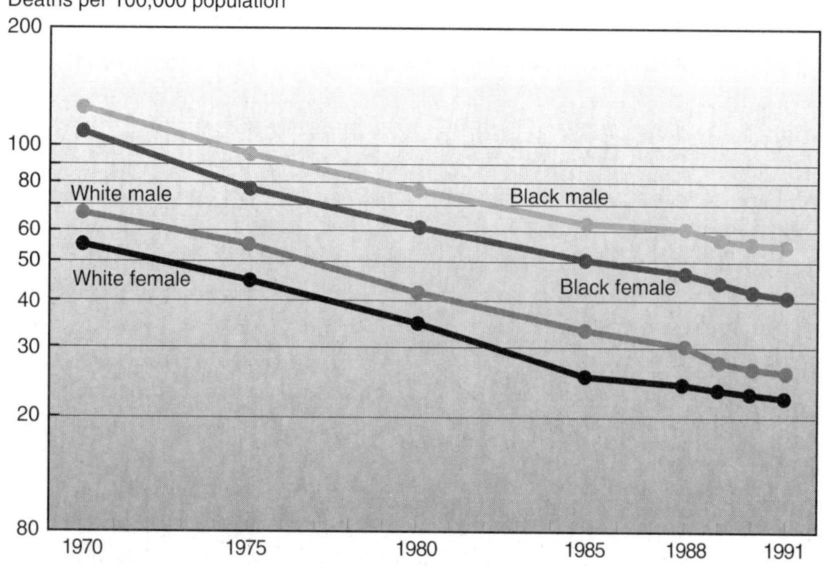

Figure 8-9 Since 1970, the age-adjusted death rate for stroke, the third leading cause of death for U.S. men and women, declined 34%. Data from the National Center for Health Statistics.

TABLE 8-6 Dietary saturated fatty acids and cholesterol intake and serum total cholesterol in boys age 7 to 9 years in six countries

Country	Dietary intake		Serum total cholesterol (mg/dl)
	Saturated fatty acids (% of energy)	Cholesterol (mg/1000 kcal)	
Philippines	9.3	97	147
Italy	10.4	159	159
Ghana	10.5	48	128
United States	13.5	151	167
Netherlands	15.1	142	174
Finland	17.7	157	190

From National Cholesterol Education Program. 1991. *Report of the expert panel on blood cholesterol levels in children and adolescents*. Bethesda, Md: US Department of Health and Human Services, Public Health Service; National Institutes of Health; National Heart, Lung, Blood Institute.

47% of patients, provided that large decreases in LDL-cholesterol (of the order of 34% to 48%) are induced for a period of 2 to 5 years."[27]

Coronary Heart Disease in Children and Adolescents

As mentioned earlier in this chapter, there is considerable scientific evidence that CHD begins in childhood. For example, there are good data indicating that atherosclerosis was present in the coronary arteries of U.S. soldiers killed in the Korean and Vietnam wars.[44,45] These studies showed lesions and narrowing consistent with CHD in 77% of the soldiers whose average age was 22 years. Data from a number of researchers studying the development and progression of coronary artery lesions in infants and children support the view that atherosclerosis begins in childhood and progresses slowly into adulthood.[46–49] Evidence from the Pathobiological Determinants of Atherosclerosis in Youth study, for example, indicates that early atherosclerotic lesions in the coronary arteries of adolescents and young adults are associated with smoking, high serum total cholesterol, LDL-C and VLDL-C levels, and low HDL-C levels. Data from the study have provided strong justification for reducing CHD risk factors in young persons.[50–52]

Other research has shown that children and adolescents in the United States have higher cholesterol levels than their counterparts in many other countries.[53–56] This probably is because children in the United States and children in other countries who have higher total cholesterol levels have a higher intake of saturated fatty acids and dietary cholesterol. In Table 8-6, it can be seen that as the percent of kilocalories from saturated fatty acids increases, serum total cholesterol increases as well. One exception is the case of Ghana, where intake of dietary cholesterol is low.

Reducing Cholesterol Levels in Children and Adolescents

Clearly, prevention of CHD needs to begin in childhood. A convenient and apparently effective starting place is the cholesterol levels of children and adolescents. The *Report of the Expert Panel on Blood Cholesterol Levels in Children and Adolescents* makes both patient-based and population-based recommendations for reducing cholesterol levels in these age groups.[27]

BOX 8-4

Other Risk Factors that may Contribute to Early Onset of CHD

- Family history of premature CHD, cerebrovascular or occlusive peripheral vascular disease (definite onset before age 55 in a sibling, parent, or sibling of a parent)
- Cigarette smoking
- Elevated blood pressure
- Low HDL-C (>35 mg/dl)
- Severe obesity (≥30 percent overweight or ≥95th percentile weight for height by National Center for Health Statistics growth charts)
- Diabetes mellitus
- Physical inactivity

From National Cholesterol Education Program. 1991. *Report of the expert panel on blood cholesterol levels in children and adolescents*. Bethesda, Md: US Department of Health and Human Services, Public Health Service; National Institutes of Health; National Heart, Lung, Blood Institute.

The goal of the population-based recommendations is "to lower average population levels of blood cholesterol in children and adolescents in order to reduce the incidence of adult CHD and generally to improve health."[27] These recommendations are essentially the same as those suggested for adults—adoption of the Step I Diet (see Table 8-5) beginning at about age 2 years. The panel suggested that "nutritional adequacy be achieved by eating a wide variety of foods," that energy "be adequate to support growth and development and to reach or maintain desirable body weight," that dietary cholesterol intake be less than 300 mg/day, and that no more than 10% and 30% of calories be derived from saturated fatty acids and total fat, respectively.[27] The rationale for the Step I Diet is given later in this chapter in the section entitled "Dietary Treatment in Coronary Heart Disease." The reader is referred to the Expert Panel's report for its outstanding suggestions for implementing the population approach.[27]

The goal of the patient-based approach is to identify those children and adolescents with elevated serum cholesterol levels or with other CHD risk factors that are likely to increase their risk of CHD as adults.[27] The Expert Panel did not recommend that all U.S. children and adolescents have their cholesterol levels measured (that is, universal screening). They did recommend that serum cholesterol be measured in a specific subgroup of youth (that is, selective screening)—those at greatest risk of having high blood cholesterol as adults and an increased risk of CHD.[27] Elevated serum cholesterol levels and other CHD risk factors tend to aggregate or cluster in families as a result of both shared environments and genetic factors. Children with high cholesterol levels often have high levels as adults, but not always. There are many instances when an adult's cholesterol level is not as high as would be expected based on childhood levels. The Expert Panel suggested that the following children and adolescents, age 2 years or older, be screened for elevated cholesterol and other risk factors:[27]

- Those whose parents or grandparents, by age 55 years or less, underwent diagnostic coronary arteriography and were found to have coronary atherosclerosis, or had balloon angioplasty or coronary artery bypass surgery.
- Those whose parents or grandparents, by age 55 years or less, suffered documented myocardial infarction, angina pectoris, peripheral vascular disease, cerebrovascular disease, or sudden cardiac death.
- Those with a parent having high serum cholesterol (≥240 mg/dl).
- Those whose parental or grandparental history is unknown, especially if the youth has other CHD risk factors, as outlined in Box 8-4.
- Health care providers may decide to screen youth judged at high risk of CHD—for example, youth who are overweight, are cigarette smokers, have high blood pressure or diabetes, are on certain medications such as isotretinoin (Accutane) or steroids, or who consume excessive amounts of saturated fatty acids, total fat, and cholesterol.

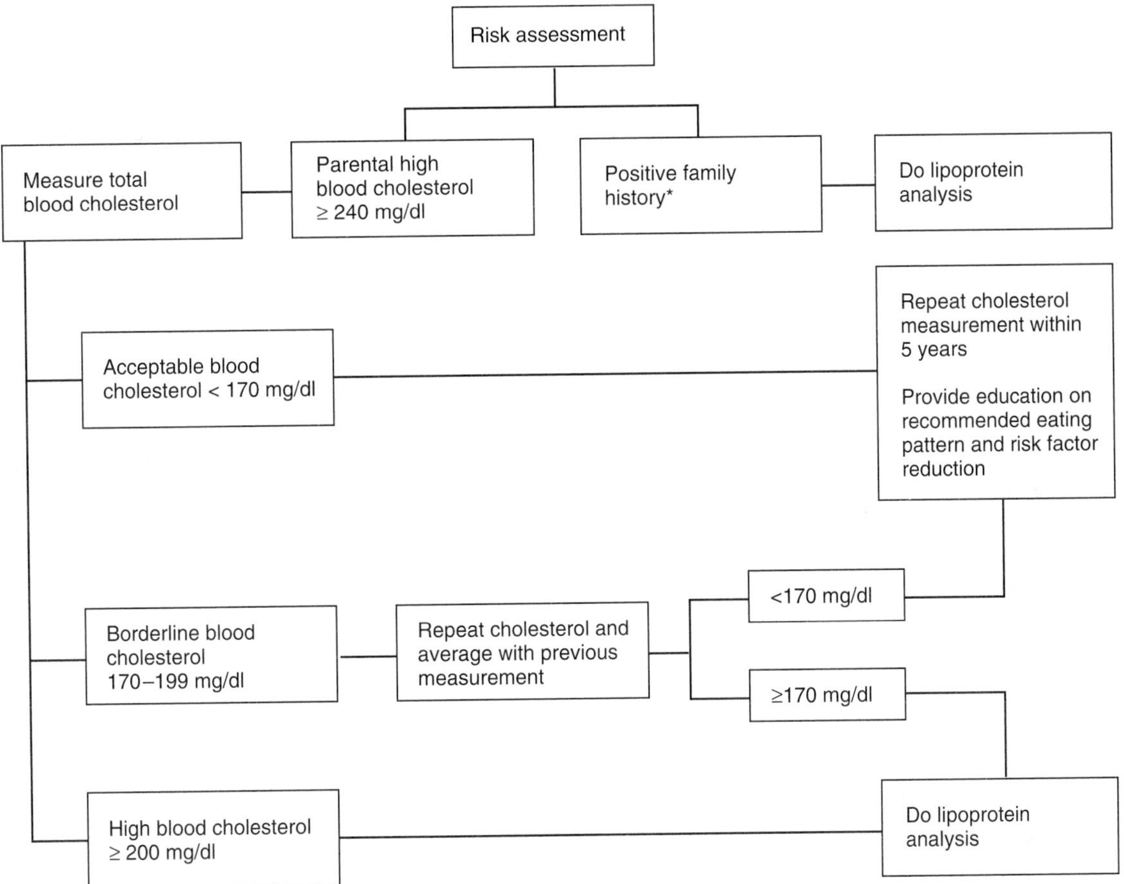

Figure 8-10 Steps in assessing cholesterol and lipoprotein levels in children and adolescents. From National Cholesterol Education Program. 1991. *Report of the expert panel of blood cholesterol levels in children and adolescents.* Bethesda, Md: US Department of Health and Human Services, Public Health Service; National Institutes of Health; National Heart, Lung, and Blood Institute.

Figure 8-10 outlines the steps for risk assessment. The panel recommended that a child's total cholesterol be measured when his or her parent has high blood cholesterol. Once a borderline-high or high blood cholesterol is established (Table 8-2), then lipoprotein analysis is recommended. In youth having a positive family history for CHD (Box 8-4), lipoprotein analysis is recommended at the outset. Classification, education, and follow-up are based on LDL-C levels, as shown in Figure 8-11. As is the case with elevated LDL-C levels in adults, the suggested dietary approach to treating elevated cholesterol levels in children and adolescents is the Step I and Step II Diets, as outlined in Figure 8-12.

DIETARY TREATMENT IN CORONARY HEART DISEASE

In recent years, various U.S. organizations have proposed dietary recommendations for the control of elevated blood cholesterol levels. The

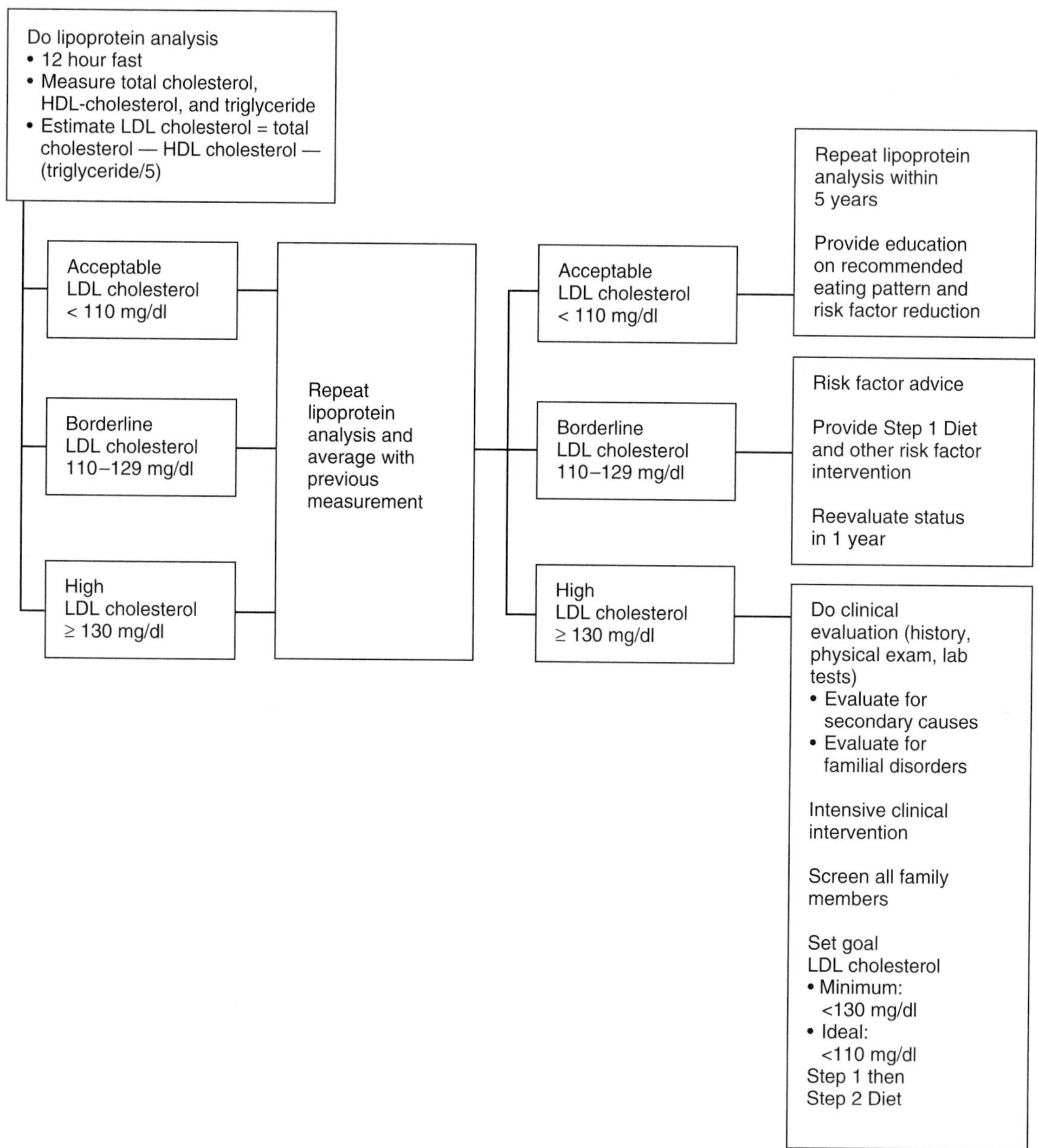

Figure 8-11 Classification, education, and follow-up of children and adolescents based on their low-density lipoprotein (LDL)-cholesterol levels. From National Cholesterol Education Program. 1991. *Report of the expert panel of blood cholesterol levels in children and adolescents*. Bethesda, Md: US Department of Health and Human Services, Public Health Service; National Institutes of Health; National Heart, Lung, and Blood Institute.

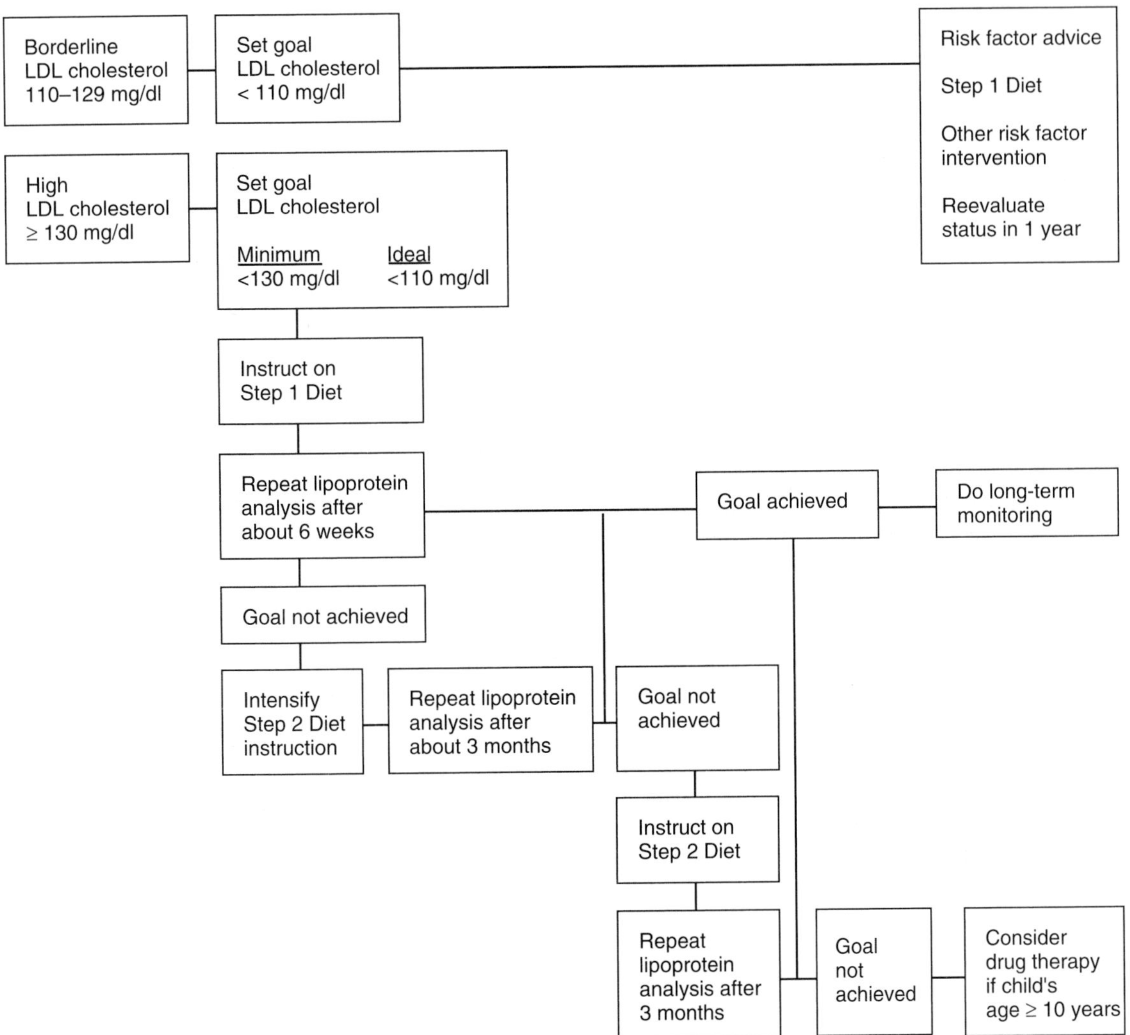

Figure 8-12 Recommended approach to dietary treatment of elevated low-density lipoprotein (LDL)-cholesterol levels in children and adolescents. From National Cholesterol Education Program. 1991. *Report of the expert panel of blood cholesterol levels in children and adolescents*. Bethesda, Md: US Department of Health and Human Services, Public Health Service; National Institutes of Health; National Heart, Lung, and Blood Institute.

Step I and Step II Diets shown in Table 8-5 can be recommended for the entire population of persons about age 2 years and older and, especially, for those whose serum cholesterol is classified as borderline high or high (Tables 8-1 and 8-2). Dietary studies show that adoption of the Step I Diet can reduce serum cholesterol levels by 3% to 4%. Progressing to the Step II Diet should yield another 3% to 7% reduction, depending on the degree to which saturated fat and cholesterol are restricted.[5]

Dietary recommendations from government and private organizations are consistent in giving emphasis to the two most important dietary factors influencing serum total cholesterol and LDL-C levels: intake of saturated fatty acids and dietary cholesterol.

Saturated Fatty Acids

It is well documented that saturated fatty acids (SFA) raise serum total cholesterol and LDL-C levels. One exception to this rule is stearic acid (18:0), an SFA that appears to have a neutral effect on cholesterol and lipoprotein levels.[57] Moderation still should be practiced in the consumption of fats high in stearic acid, such as beef fat and cocoa butter, because these fats contain a substantial amount of the other SFAs that raise serum cholesterol.[57]

According to data from NHANES III, Americans currently consume an average of 12% of total calories from SFA, although intakes in some people can be markedly higher. A reduction in SFA intake from 17% to 6% of total calories will decrease serum total cholesterol by about 24 mg/dl (0.52 mmol/L).[58] Although SFA are provided by both animal and plant foods, in children 1 to 5 years of age and adults, about 55% to 60% of SFA intake comes from meat, fish, poultry, and dairy products, and from mixed dishes containing these animal products as major ingredients.[59] Particular attention should be given to monitoring the intake of these foods when evaluating the diets of persons with elevated serum cholesterol levels.

Dietary Cholesterol

Dietary cholesterol (cholesterol in food) also raises serum total cholesterol and LDL-C levels (especially the latter), although the elevations are not as great as those seen in diets high in SFA.[5,60,61] According to data from NHANES III, mean dietary cholesterol intake for American males and females is 322 mg and 221 mg per day, respectively. However, mean dietary cholesterol intake for males and females age 20 to 49 years is approximately 369 mg and 243 mg per day, respectively.[62]

Several long-term prospective studies have shown that dietary cholesterol intake is positively associated with CHD risk.[63–66] In several studies, researchers have found dietary cholesterol to be an independent predictor of CHD, *apart from its effects on serum cholesterol*.[63,67]

Confusion about dietary cholesterol's influence on serum cholesterol is primarily due to the high variability of response of serum total cholesterol and LDL-C to consumption of dietary cholesterol.[2] A report of an 88-year-old man having a plasma total cholesterol level of 200 mg/dl (5.17 mmol/L) despite eating about 25 eggs per day for more than 15 years is a case in point.[68] Amazingly, he was almost completely free of any clinically important atherosclerosis. He absorbed only 18% of the cholesterol he ate (people normally absorb 45% to 55%), he had twice the normal rate of bile acid synthesis, and his body synthesized less than average amounts of cholesterol. Despite this *one* individual's highly unusual cholesterol metabolism, it remains prudent for the rest of us with more normal cholesterol metabolism to follow a low-cholesterol diet.

Total Calories

Another significant dietary factor is total caloric intake with its implications for obesity. Because obesity is associated with elevated serum LDL-C levels and is an independent risk factor for CHD, the ATP II recommends reduction of calories to achieve weight reduction in overweight persons.[5] In overweight persons, weight reduction has been shown to lower serum LDL-C and triglycerides and raise HDL-C, as discussed later in this chapter.[2,5,29]

Total and Unsaturated Fat

Data from NHANES III show that total fat currently contributes about 34% of calories in the American diet.[62] The ATP II recommends that total fat not exceed 30% of calories to help reduce saturated fat intake and to promote weight reduction. Some authorities recommend a reduction in fat calories in the range of 20% to 25% of calories (or even less) to maximize reduction of saturated fat and weight reduction. The ATP II recommends that when these diets are used, care should be taken to ensure adequate calcium and iron intake. Advocates of the Mediterranean diet, on the other hand, recommend a more liberal fat intake as long as saturated fat intake is kept very low and the majority of fats come from monounsaturates such as olive oil.

When monounsaturated fatty acids (having one double bond) and polyunsaturated fatty acids (having more than one double bond) replace saturated fatty acids in the diet, serum total cholesterol and LDL-C tend to decrease. Data from NHANES III show that the American diet provides approximately 7% and 13% polyunsaturated and monounsaturated fatty acids, respectively.[62]

Protein and Carbohydrate

The ATP II recommends that protein compose about 15% of total calories. Although the ATP II makes no recommendations regarding protein type, there are definite advantages to obtaining protein from plant sources. Plant foods contain no cholesterol (unless prepared with some type of animal product) and tend to be low in both total and saturated fat. Mortality from CHD is higher in nonvegetarians than in vegetarians, who generally rely heavily on plant foods for protein, energy, and other nutrient needs.[69,70] Most of the decreased CHD mortality rate in vegetarians is likely due to the differences in the types and amounts of fat found in plants compared with foods of animal origin; however, several nondietary factors no doubt play a role as well. There is some evidence, however, that dietary substitution of certain plant proteins (for example, soy protein) for animal proteins can lower serum total cholesterol and LDL-C.[71] Plants also contain phytochemicals, some of which have antioxidant and other beneficial properties that confer protection against heart disease, stroke, and cancer.

An intake of carbohydrates at 55% or more of total calories is recommended. This includes simple sugars (monosaccharides and disaccharides), complex digestible carbohydrates (starches), and complex indigestible carbohydrates (fiber). To ensure that adequate vitamins, minerals, and fiber are consumed, consumption of complex digestible carbohydrates should be kept high and that of simple sugars relatively low. In most people, when digestible carbohydrates are substituted for saturated fatty acids, serum LDL-C generally falls to about the same extent as when oleic and linoleic acids are substituted in this manner.[5]

Fiber can be defined as plant materials in the diet that are resistant to digestion by enzymes produced by the human intestinal tract.[72] Fiber can be divided into the soluble and insoluble fractions. The soluble fibers (gums, pectins, mucilages, and some hemicelluloses) are effective in lowering serum total cholesterol and LDL-C levels, although these effects are not as pronounced in persons with lower serum total cholesterol as in those having higher levels.[72–74]

Probable mechanisms for this effect include soluble fiber's ability to bind bile acids and promote their excretion in the feces and reduction of cholesterol absorption by fiber's interference with micelle formation.[75–76] The release of short-chain fatty acids (especially propionate) from the bacterial fermentation of dietary fiber may act to decrease hepatic cholesterol synthesis, thus lowering serum cholesterol levels and providing several other beneficial effects.[77,78] Concerns that carbohydrate intakes as high as 60% of total calories may result in elevated serum triglycerides and reduced HDL-C levels are not supported by the scientific literature. On the contrary, a high-carbohydrate diet is consistent with good health and is recommended.[79]

General Principles

The goal of dietary treatment of elevated cholesterol levels is not a temporary "diet" but rather a permanent change in eating behavior that is consistent with good overall nutrition.[5] Consumption of a variety of foods is important because no single food item provides all the essential nutrients in the amounts needed. One of the best ways to ensure an adequate diet is to include in one's meals a variety of foods from all food groups.[27]

Although preventing obesity by controlling energy consumption is a major concern of many people, supplying the nutrient and energy needs of growing and developing children and adolescents must not be overlooked. For example, the energy needs of 2- to 3-year-old children per unit of body weight are particularly high. In addition, the capacity of a child's gastrointestinal tract for food at any one time is limited. Consequently, children's diets should include foods that are good sources of energy and nutrients and yet low in SFA and cholesterol.[27] In some instances, young children may need snacks to help them meet their energy and nutrient needs, and suitable selections are available that will keep children's diets within the Step I and Step II guidelines.

ISSUES IN MEASURING LIPID AND LIPOPROTEIN LEVELS

Two particularly important aspects of any measurement, whether a clinical laboratory test (such as a blood test) or a measurement of weight or stature, are *precision* and *accuracy*.[80,81] Although these concepts apply to any measurement, they are discussed in this section as they relate to measurement of lipid and lipoprotein levels. *Precision* or reproducibility relates to the difference in results when the same measurement is repeatedly performed. The difference or variability in results from repeated or replicate measurements should be within acceptable limits. *Accuracy* relates to the difference between the measured value as reported by the clinical laboratory and the "true" or "real" value that has been previously established by comparison with a known standard (reference material) and/or a definitive measurement method.[80,81]

Precision

Because consistent accuracy is not possible if measurements are imprecise, the Laboratory Standardization Panel (LSP) of the NCEP in its report

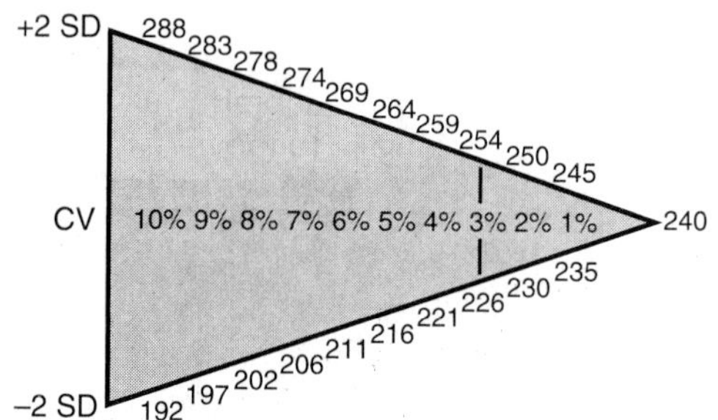

Figure 8-13 Effect of differing degrees of imprecision in analysis of a blood specimen with a "true" cholesterol value of 240 mg/dl. An analytic method having a precision consistent with a coefficient of variation (CV) of 3% would yield, on repeat measurements of the same sample, values ranging from 226 to 254 mg/dl. SD = standard deviation. From National Cholesterol Education Program. 1988. *Current status of blood cholesterol measurement in clinical laboratories in the United States: A report from the Laboratory Standardization Panel of the National Cholesterol Education Program*. Bethesda, Md: US Department of Health and Human Service, Public Health Service; National Institutes of Health; National Heart, Lung, and Blood Institute.

Current Status of Blood Cholesterol Measurement in Clinical Laboratories in the United States recommends that initial efforts be focused on making blood cholesterol measurement in the United States adequately precise.[80] The importance of precision in diagnosing and monitoring persons with high cholesterol levels is illustrated in Figure 8-13. The figure shows the effect of differing degrees of imprecision in cholesterol measurement. If a person's serum sample has a "true" cholesterol value of 240 mg/dl (6.21 mmol/L), values from replicate measurements of that sample could be scattered over a wide range depending on the precision of the measurement as represented by the coefficient of variation (CV). CV is a measure of precision and is calculated by dividing the standard deviation (SD) by the mean and multiplying by 100 (CV = SD ÷ mean × 100).

Figure 8-13 shows, for example, that if the precision of a cholesterol measurement method is such that the CV is 10%, replicate cholesterol measurements of one sample having a true value of 240 mg/dl would yield values ranging from 192 to 288 mg/dl. Obviously, with this degree of imprecision, it would be most difficult to properly identify persons with elevated cholesterol.

In its 1988 report, the LSP recommended that clinical laboratories achieve an overall precision consistent with a CV ≤ 3% by 1992.[73] Given the same blood sample with a true cholesterol value of 240 mg/dl, a measurement method having a CV of 3% would result in values ranging from 226 to 254 mg/dl.

How precise are the total cholesterol measurements of clinical laboratories in the United States? The College of American Pathologists has the world's largest proficiency testing program for clinical laboratories. Data for 1987 indicating precision within single laboratories (*intra*laboratory precision) showed that 75% of the 2000 North American laboratories participating in the College of American Pathologists Quality Assurance Program met the 1992 performance requirement of a CV ≤ 3%. An assessment of precision among 5400 North American laboratories (*inter*laboratory precision) by the College of American Pathologists in 1988 ranged from 5.5% to 7.2% CV, and proficiency testing of 613 laboratories by the U.S. Centers for Disease Control and Prevention in 1985 revealed a CV of approximately 7%.[81]

Accuracy

Accuracy is also necessary to diagnose, treat, and monitor elevated lipid and lipoprotein levels. Inaccurate measurement can lead to clinical misdiagnosis because of reporting of false positive values (measurement results falsely classifying a person as having a condition) or false negative values (measurement results falsely classifying a person as not having a condition).[80]

Bias is a measure of inaccuracy or departure from accuracy. If a laboratory's particular method of measuring serum cholesterol has a *positive bias* of 10% and a subject's true cholesterol value is 200 mg/dl (5.17 mmol/L), the laboratory's reported value would be 220 mg/dl (5.69 mmol/L) or 10% greater than the true value. If a person's true value was 240 mg/dl (6.21 mmol/L), a 10% *negative bias* would result in a reported value of 216 mg/dl (5.59 mmol/L) or 10% less than the true value. If the true value was 240 mg/dl (6.21 mmol/L), a 10% positive bias would yield a reported value of 264 mg/dl (6.83 mmol/L). Thus at a given bias, the higher the true cholesterol value, the greater the magnitude of error.

At the time of its release, the LSP's report recommended that biases in measurement methods not exceed ±5% from the true value and that by 1992 the national goal of ≤ 3% be achieved.[80] In proficiency testing conducted by the American College of Pathologists from 1985 through 1987, only 59% of laboratories tested met the ideal goal of ≤ 3% bias.[81]

Sources of Error in Cholesterol Measurement

It is estimated that approximately one third of within-individual variability in cholesterol analyses is due to laboratory errors. These factors are beyond the scope of this text and will not be addressed. A detailed discussion of them can be found in the LSP's report *Recommendations for Improving Cholesterol Measurement*.[81]

The remaining two thirds of within-individual variability is due to a variety of factors occurring before the sample is actually analyzed. These can be referred to as *preanalytical factors*.[81,82] Preanalytical factors operate before or during blood sampling or during sample storage or shipment to the laboratory. They can be divided into biologic factors contributing to the patient's usual cholesterol level and those factors altering the patient's usual cholesterol level. (Table 8-7).

Factors Altering Usual Cholesterol Level

Because factors that alter usual cholesterol level can be controlled by those workers involved in the drawing, preparation, storage, and shipment of blood specimens, they will be discussed, along with recommendations from the LSP for their control.

TABLE 8-7 Preanalytical factors affecting within-individual variability in cholesterol levels

Biologic factors contributing to a patient's usual cholesterol level	Factors altering a patient's usual cholesterol level
Age and sex	Fasting
Diurnal variation	Posture
Seasonal variation	Venous occlusion
Diet and alcohol	Anticoagulants
Exercise	Recent myocardial infarction and stroke
Primary dyslipoproteinemia*	Trauma and acute infection
Secondary dyslipoproteinemia†	Pregnancy
Drugs	

From National Cholesterol Education Program. 1990. *Recommendations for improving cholesterol measurement: A report from the Laboratory Standardization Panel of the National Cholesterol Education Program*. Bethesda, Md: US Department of Health and Human Services, Public Health Service; National Institutes of Health; National Heart, Lung, Blood Institute.

*Primary dyslipoproteinemias: a defect in lipoprotein clearance or excessive body synthesis of lipoproteins stemming from a genetic disorder.

†Secondary dyslipoproteinemias: a defect in lipoprotein clearance or excessive body synthesis of lipoproteins resulting from another disease or some cause that is not apparently genetic in nature. Secondary causes can be corrected by treating the underlying disease.

Fasting

Total cholesterol and HDL-C levels can be measured in nonfasting persons. Recent food intake affects plasma total cholesterol levels by only about 1.5% or less.[81] The LSP recommended that plasma triglyceride concentrations should be measured only after a fast of at least 12 hours because absorption of fat after a meal will elevate blood triglyceride levels. When a patient's LDL-C value is desired, a fast of at least 12 hours also is necessary because LDL-C typically is calculated from measurements of triglyceride, cholesterol, and HDL-C. If the triglyceride concentration is > 400 mg/dl (>4.52 mmol/L), the LDL-C should be measured directly instead of being calculated.[81]

Posture

When a person sits or lies down after standing for several minutes, his or her plasma volume increases, and the concentration of cholesterol (and other nondiffusible plasma components) decreases. Compared with values in blood drawn while a person is standing, cholesterol levels can be significantly lower in blood drawn from the same person after he or she has been lying down for 5 minutes and may be as much as 10% to 15% lower in blood drawn after the person has been lying down for 20 minutes. Cholesterol levels in blood drawn after a person has been sitting for 10 to 15 minutes have been shown to be 6% lower than those in blood drawn from the same person while standing. The LSP recommended that blood sampling conditions be standardized to the sitting position. The patient should sit quietly for about 5 minutes before the sample is drawn.[81]

Venous Occlusion

If a tourniquet is applied to a vein for a prolonged period, the concentration of cholesterol (and other nondiffusible plasma components) will increase. The cholesterol concentration of blood drawn from a vein following a 2-minute tourniquet application can be 2% to 5% higher than that of venous blood drawn after a 30- to 60-second tourniquet application. A 10% to 15% average increase can result from a 5-minute tourniquet application. The LSP recommended that venipuncture should be completed as rapidly as possible, preferably within 1 minute.[81]

Anticoagulants

Plasma is derived from whole blood that is treated with an anticoagulant. The anticoagulants heparin and ethylenediamine tetraacetic acid are preferred. Fluoride, citrate, and oxalate anticoagulants should not be used because they cause plasma components to be diluted (cholesterol concentration is lower when these are used).[81]

Recent Heart Attack and Stroke

The LSP recommended that when a person has suffered a heart attack or stroke, his or her total cholesterol and LDL-C should not be measured for 8 weeks following the attack. These levels fall considerably in a heart attack or stroke victim and remain low for several weeks.

Trauma and Acute Infections

Cholesterol levels can fall by as much as 40% in a person who has suffered severe trauma and can fall temporarily in response to severe pain, surgery, and short-term physical strain. The LSP recommended that cholesterol measurements be performed no sooner than 8 weeks after the above conditions have occurred.

Pregnancy

Increases in LDL and VLDL during pregnancy can lead to increases in cholesterol levels by as much as 20% to 35%. The LSP recommended that lipid measurements should not be made until 3 to 4 months after delivery.

HYPERTENSION

Hypertension (high blood pressure) is one of the most common risk factors for cardiovascular and renal diseases. It is associated with increased risk of developing CHD, stroke, congestive heart failure, renal insufficiency, and peripheral vascular disease.[83,84] Figure 8-14 shows that as systolic blood pressure (SBP) increases above 120 mm Hg and as diastolic blood pressure (DBP) increases above 80 mm Hg, there is an increased risk of death from cardiovascular disease.

According to NHANES III, approximately 50 million Americans have hypertension or are taking antihypertensive medication; that is one in every four U.S. adults.[85] The prevalence of hypertension, based on NHANES III data, for different age and sex groups is shown in Figure 8-15. Because of the cross-sectional nature of NHANES III, these estimates are based on reported use of antihypertensive medication or on blood pressure measurements obtained at a single visit to the Mobile Examination Center (see Chapter 4). More conservative estimates based on two or more evaluations of blood pressure or use of antihypertensive medication place the prevalence of hypertension at 30 to 40 million Americans. Regardless of which estimate is used, hypertension is a very common problem. Hypertension is more common in black males and females than in white males and females, as shown in Figure 8-16. The figure also shows that the percentage of black and white males and females with hypertension has decreased since the 1970s.

Arterial blood pressure is measured using a device called a sphygmomanometer ("blood pressure cuff") and is expressed in millimeters of mercury (mm Hg). Systolic blood pressure is the blood pressure following systole, the phase of cardiac contraction. Diastolic blood pressure is that following diastole, the phase of cardiac relaxation. Blood pressure is expressed as two numbers, as in 120/80. The first number (120 mm Hg) is systolic blood pressure, and the second is diastolic blood pressure (80 mm Hg). From the standpoint of cardiovascular disease, an "optimal" blood pressure is one that is less than 120/80, although unusually low blood pressure readings should be evaluated for clinical significance. Guidelines developed by the National High Blood Pressure Education Program for classifying blood pressure are shown in Figure 8-17. For blood pressure to be considered within the

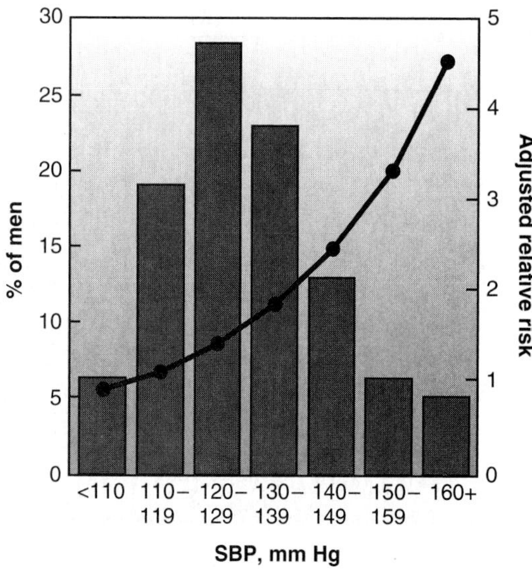

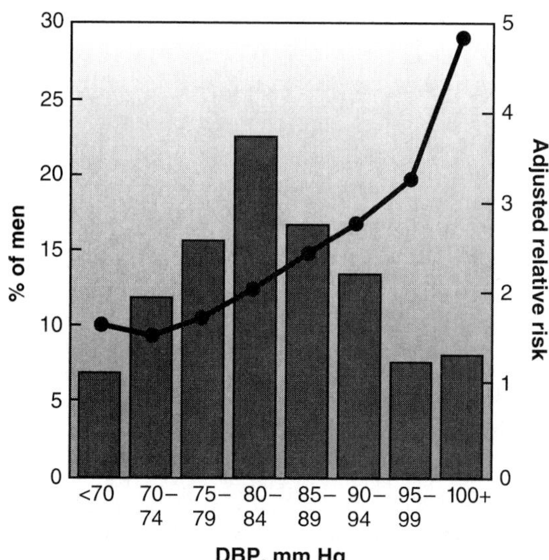

Figure 8-14 The bars in this figure represent the distribution of systolic blood pressure (chart on the left) and diastolic blood pressure (chart on the right) for males ages 35 to 57 years participating in the Multiple Risk Factor Intervention Trial (*N* = 347,978). The curved lines represent the 12-year rate of cardiovascular mortality for each level of systolic blood pressure (SBP) and diastolic blood pressure (DBP). As either SBP or DBP increase, risk of death from cardiovascular disease increases. Adapted from National High Blood Pressure Education Program Working Group. 1993. National High Blood Pressure Education Program Working Group report on primary prevention of hypertension. *Archives of Internal Medicine*. 153:186–208.

"normal" range, systolic blood pressure must be 120 to 129 mm Hg with diastolic pressure being no more than 84 mm Hg, or the diastolic must be within the 80 to 84 mm Hg range with a systolic pressure of no more than 129 mm Hg.

Most of the effort expended to reduce morbidity and mortality related to hypertension has revolved around detecting and treating hypertension, what we call the patient-based approach. This has resulted in a considerable measure of success, as demonstrated by the recent declining death rates from stroke shown in Figure 8-9. However, the patient-based approach has definite limitations. About 35% of NHANES III survey participants with a SBP ≥ 140 mm Hg or a DBP ≥ 90 mm Hg were unaware that they might have hypertension. Only 49% of the survey's participants with hypertension were receiving antihypertensive medications, and only 21% of those being treated with antihypertensive medications had a blood pressure < 140/90 mm Hg. Thus large numbers of hypertensive patients are unaware of their condition, and many being treated for hypertension have suboptimal blood pressure control. This lack of awareness and inadequate control can result in significant vascular damage to the eyes, heart, kidneys, and brain. In addition, antihypertensive therapy is expensive and poses the possibility of adverse reactions from drug treatment. Even with optimal blood pressure control, persons with hypertension still have a higher morbidity and mortality than persons with normal or optimal blood pressure.[83]

Primary Prevention of Hypertension

In recent years, however, there has been increasing attention given to the primary prevention of hypertension (also known as the population-based approach) through modification of risk

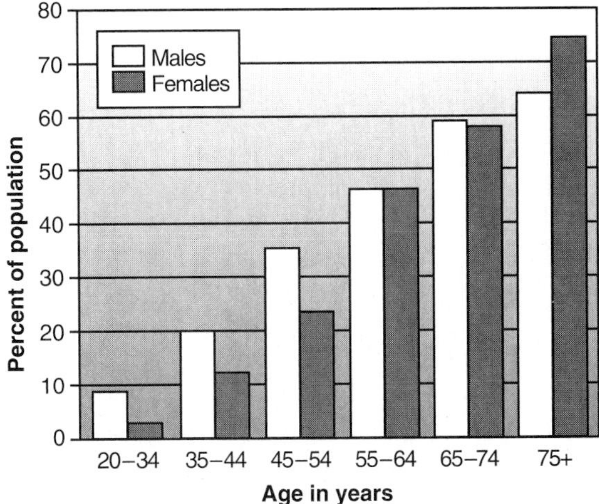

Figure 8-15 Data from NHANES III show that the prevalence of hypertension in the United States varies by age and sex. Between age 20 and 54 years, hypertension is more common in males than in females. Prevalence is roughly equal in both sexes between age 55 and 74 years. After age 75 years, females are more likely to have hypertension than males. Data from the National Center for Health Statistics.

Average DBP mm Hg	Average SBP mm Hg			
	<120	120–129	130–139	≥140
<80	Optimal[a]	Normal	High Normal	High
80–84	Normal	Normal	High Normal	High
85–89	High Normal	High Normal	High Normal	High
≥90	High	High	High	High

Figure 8-17 The National High Blood Pressure Education Program's classifications for blood pressure for persons age 18 years and older. SPB = systolic blood pressure; DBP = diastolic blood pressure. Optimal blood pressure, with regard to cardiovascular risk, is SBP < 120 mm Hg and DBP < 80 mm Hg. However, unusually low readings should be evaluated for clinical significance. From National High Blood Pressure Education Program. 1993. *Fifth Report of the Joint National Committee on Detection, Evaluation, and Treatment of High Blood Pressure.* Bethesda, Md: US Department of Health and Human Services, Public Health Service; National Institutes of Health; National Heart, Lung, and Blood Institute.

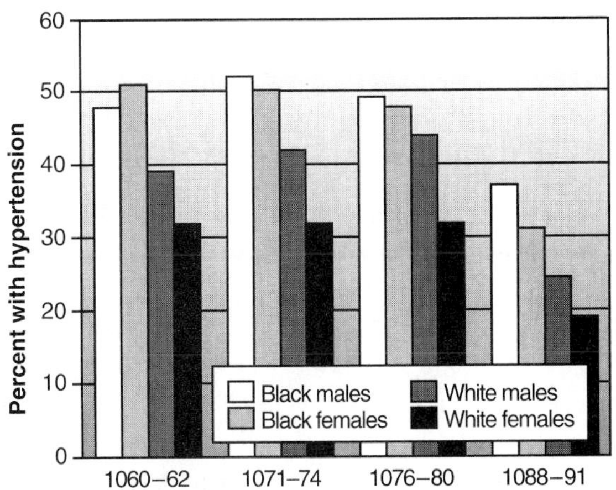

Figure 8-16 Black males and females are more likely to have hypertension than white males and females. However, prevalence rates for black and white males and females have declined since the 1970s. Data from the National Center for Health Statistics.

factors associated with hypertension. The most important of these risk factors are a high sodium intake, excessive consumption of energy, physical inactivity, excessive alcohol consumption, and inadequate potassium intake. Box 8-5 lists factors having proved efficacy in lowering blood pressure and several others with limited or unproved efficacy. Primary prevention can be complemented by special attempts to lower blood pressure in populations most likely to develop hypertension such as black persons, persons with a high-normal blood pressure, those with a family history of hypertension, and those who are overweight, consume excessive amounts of sodium, are physically inactive, or have a high intake of alcohol.[84]

BOX 8-5

Factors Having Proven Efficacy in Lowering Blood Pressure and Those with Limited or Unproven Efficacy

Factors with documented efficacy
- Weight loss
- Reduced sodium intake
- Reduced alcohol consumption
- Exercise

Factors with limited or unproved efficacy
- Stress management
- Potassium (pill supplementation)
- Fish oil (pill supplementation)
- Calcium (pill supplementation)
- Magnesium (pill supplementation)
- Macronutrient alteration
- Fiber supplementation

From National High Blood Pressure Education Program. 1993. *Fifth Report of the Joint National Committee on Detection, Evaluation, and Treatment of High Blood Pressure.* Bethesda, Md: US Department of Health and Human Services; Public Health Service; National Institutes of Health; National Heart, Lung, Blood Institute.

Body Weight

The evidence linking body weight to blood pressure and overweight to hypertension is strong and consistent. It is estimated that 20% to 30% of hypertension can be attributed to overweight. Several studies have shown that loss of excess body weight reduces both SBP and DBP and that the degree of blood pressure reduction is related to the extent of weight loss. The largest randomized controlled trial to evaluate the impact of weight loss in persons with high-normal blood pressure, the Trials of Hypertension Prevention, showed that an average weight loss of 8.4 lb (3.8 kg) resulted in a 2.9 mm Hg and 2.3 mm Hg reduction in SBP and DBP, respectively.[86] Although this may seem like an insignificant decline in blood pressure, it has been estimated that a 2-mm Hg decline in the population mean SBP might reduce the annual mortality from stroke, CHD, and all causes by 6%, 4%, and 3%, respectively.[83,84] Not only is weight loss an effective means of lowering blood pressure, it also tends to improve the lipid and lipoprotein profile and reduce the risk of development of noninsulin-dependent diabetes mellitus and possibly breast cancer.

Sodium

Research on the association between sodium intake and blood pressure has been hampered by several methodologic challenges. These include difficulty in measuring sodium intake, the large day-to-day intraindividual (within-person) variation in sodium intake, the presence of a wide range of blood pressure values at any level of sodium intake, and the small interindividual (between-person) variation in sodium intakes within a given population group. Despite these challenges, there is compelling evidence of a direct association between sodium intake and risk of hypertension.[83,84]

The mean sodium intake of Americans is estimated at 3.3 g per day.[87] This corresponds to 8.3 g per day of salt (sodium chloride) and is far in excess of our physiologic need. It is also much greater than the amounts typically eaten by less industrialized societies that do not experience North America's age-related increase in blood pressure. Research shows that a reduction in sodium intake of 1.2 g (50 mEq) per day is associated with an average 7 mm Hg reduction in SBP in hypertensive persons and a 5 mm Hg reduction in normotensive persons (those without hypertension). Black persons, older persons, and persons with hypertension will likely be more sensitive to changes in dietary sodium. This modest reduction in sodium intake is sufficient to control mild hypertension in some patients. In most others who still need antihypertensive medication, the requirement for medication will be reduced.[84]

Alcohol

Despite the difficulty of measuring the alcohol intake of study participants, there is consistent evidence of a strong positive relationship between alcohol consumption and blood pressure. It is estimated that as much as 5% to 7% of the overall prevalence of hypertension in the U.S. can be attributed to an alcohol intake of three drinks or more per day.[83] One drink of alcohol (0.5 fluid ounce of ethanol) is equivalent to 12-fluid ounces of beer, 4 fluid ounces of wine, or one ounce of 100 proof spirits. Furthermore, when alcohol intake is reduced, there is a subsequent reduction in blood pressure. A reduction in alcohol intake has been shown to be effective in lowering blood pressure in both hypertensive and normotensive individuals, and may help prevent hypertension. Persons with hypertension should be advised to limit their alcohol intake to no more than two drinks per day.[84]

Physical Activity

Numerous studies have shown an inverse relationship between leisure-time and work-related physical activity and blood pressure. Other studies have shown that blood pressure tends to be lower in physically fit individuals. Although these studies have certain design limitations, they provide consistent evidence that increased physical activity results in an average reduction of approximately 6 to 7 mm Hg for both SBP and DBP. This reduction is not dependent on weight loss. A low-to-moderate exercise intensity (40% to 60% of maximum oxygen consumption) is as effective at lowering blood pressure in patients with mild-to-moderate hypertension as higher-intensity exercise.

Potassium

A number of studies have identified an inverse relationship between blood pressure and measures of serum, urine, total-body, and dietary intake of potassium. For example, SBP was shown to be 2.7 mm Hg lower in persons having a 2.3-gram-per-day greater urinary potassium excretion. However, it appears that the ratio of urinary sodium to potassium is more closely related to blood pressure than to either electrolyte alone. One study showed a 3.4-mm Hg reduction in SBP when the 24-hour urinary sodium-potassium ratio changed from a population median of 3.1 (170 mEq of sodium/55 mEq of potassium) to 1.0 (70 mEq of sodium/70 mEq of potassium). The lower consumption of potassium by U.S. black persons compared with white persons may account for the former group's higher prevalence of hypertension. Although potassium (either as a supplement or in the diet) appears to have a role in the control of blood pressure, it is unlikely to be as important as sodium restriction or weight management. However, increased potassium intake used in conjunction with other nonpharmacologic approaches does show promise. This may be particularly important for groups such as U.S. black persons who have a low dietary potassium intake.

OSTEOPOROSIS

Osteoporosis is a condition in which the mass of bone per unit volume is reduced (see Figure 8-18), resulting in greater susceptibility to bone fracture.[2,88] Osteoporosis is a major public health problem afflicting about 25 million Americans (85% of which are women) and each year causing an estimated 1.5 million fractures of the pelvis, vertebrae, hip, distal forearm, and humerus. It is estimated that 5 million men have osteoporosis.[89] Along with heart disease and breast cancer, it is one of the three most serious diseases affecting women.[89] It is estimated that 50% of females over age 45 years and 90% of females over age 75 years suffer from osteoporosis.[90] For any given age, osteoporotic fractures are twice as common in females than in males, and because they live longer than males, females experience an even higher absolute incidence during their lifetime.[2,91] Twenty percent of persons with hip fractures will

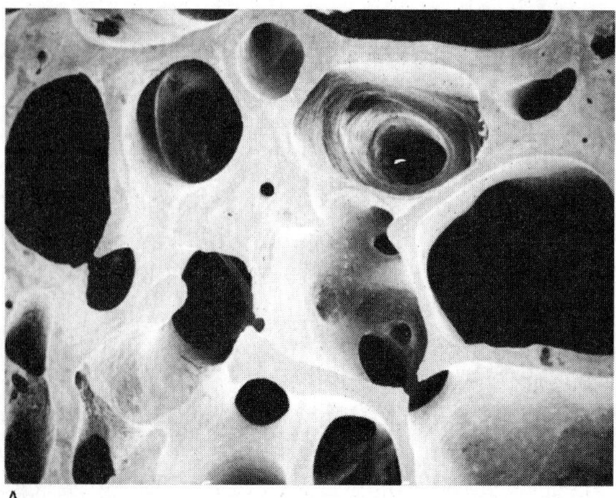

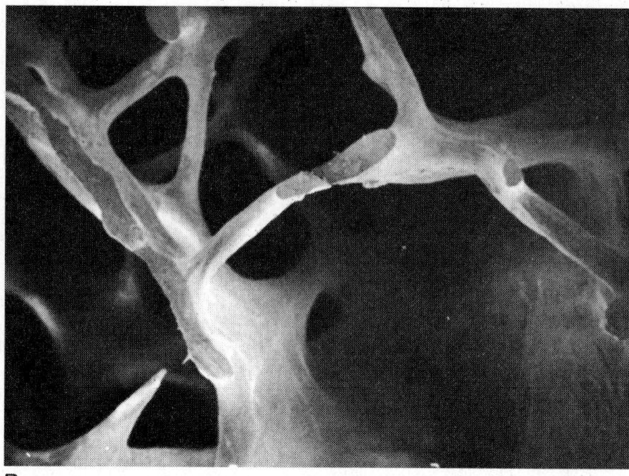

Figure 8-18 Scanning electron micrographs of bone biopsy specimens from the iliac crest: **A** is normal, and **B** is from a person with osteoporosis.

die within a year, and 50% of survivors will require assistance to walk. It is estimated that the annual medical costs of osteoporosis for the U.S. is $10 billion.[89]

By about age 20 or 25 years, the bones of the human skeleton reach 90% to 95% of their *peak bone mass* (the point of maximum bone mineralization). Over the next 10 years, the final 5% to 10% of bone mineral is added, in a process known as *consolidation*.[2,92] There is considerable inter-individual variation in peak bone mass because of such factors as heredity, sex, race, and environmental factors. On average, males have 10% to 15% greater peak bone mass than females, and the bones of black persons are about 10% denser than those of white persons. Black males have the most dense bones, followed by white males, black females, and white females.[89,92]

Once peak mass is reached, bone mineral content begins to decline in both sexes at an annual rate of 0.3% to 0.5%.[93] In males, this gradual decline remains fairly constant, resulting in a lifetime bone mineral loss of 20% to 30%. In females, around the time of menopause (generally occurring at age 45 to 55 years) or following surgical removal of both ovaries, the rate of bone mineral loss temporarily accelerates to as high as 4% to 8% annually. Lifetime losses in females may be 40% to 50% or more of peak bone mass. The major factor in the higher rate of bone demineralization in the years immediately following menopause is apparently due to estrogen deficiency.[88]

Bones: Structure and Remodeling

Bones can be classified as being composed of two different types of structural tissue: *cortical* or *compact* tissue and *trabecular* or *cancellous* tissue. The very dense cortical tissue forms the outer shells of bones, encasing the trabecular tissue, which is composed of a fine, spongelike mesh with numerous small voids. The marrow elements occupy these voids.[88] The total skeleton is composed of 80% cortical bone and 20% trabecular bone. Cortical bone is found primarily in the appendicular skeleton (bones of the limbs), whereas most of the trabecular bone is found in the axial skeleton (the skull and vertebral bones).[94]

Bone is a dynamic tissue and is constantly undergoing change in a process known as *remodeling*. The bone resorption cells or osteoclasts are active at numerous points within bone. They secrete enzymes that dissolve bone before it is reformed and provide a source for blood calcium when dietary intake is inadequate. The bone-forming cells or osteoblasts secrete an organic matrix composed largely of collagen. This matrix then becomes hardened by deposits of calcium and phosphate crystals known as *hydroxyapatite*. The rate of remodeling or turnover rate is approximately eight times faster in trabecular bone than in cortical bone, leading to a faster decline in bone mineral content in trabecular bone.[94] Consequently, symptoms of osteoporosis appear earlier in trabecular bone, for example the spine (vertebral bodies) and wrist (distal radius).[88,94]

Osteoporosis: Classification and Risk Factors

Osteoporosis can be classified as either primary (not related to other disease) or secondary (when an identifiable cause other than age or menopause is present). Osteoporosis can be secondary to such conditions as Cushing's syndrome, malignancies of the bone (myeloma), hyperthyroidism, hyperparathyroidism, male hypogonadism, and amenorrhea. Certain inherited diseases such as osteogenesis imperfecta can also result in osteoporosis as can long-term use of such medications as thiazide diuretics and heparin.[88,93] The most common form is primary osteoporosis, in which no other disease is apparent. This is most frequently seen in middle-aged and older females and older males. In these age groups, Type I and Type II primary osteoporosis are most commonly seen.[88,93]

Type I is seen in postmenopausal females between 51 and 75 years of age and primarily involves loss of trabecular bone. Low estrogen levels accompanying menopause lead to increased bone remodeling and accelerated bone loss. Production of vitamin D_3 and intestinal absorption of calcium often are decreased in postmenopausal women, exacerbating bone loss. This leads to fractures at sites where trabecular bone predominates (for example, vertebral bodies and the distal radius).[88,93]

Type II osteoporosis is seen in both sexes after age 70 years. It is related to several age-related changes such as decreased osteoblast function, decreased calcium absorption, decreased vitamin D_3 synthesis, and decreased levels of calcitonin (calcitonin inhibits bone resorption).[88] In Type II osteoporosis, bone mineral is lost from both trabecular and cortical bone. The most common sites of fractures are the hip and vertebrae. Multiple fractures of the vertebrae can lead to a marked curvature of the thoracic spine known as *thoracic kyphosis* or "dowager's hump." Other sites include the proximal humerus (bone of the upper arm), pelvis, and proximal tibia (large bone of the lower leg).

Various risk factors are associated with development of osteoporosis.[95] These are shown in Table 8-8. Compared with leaner persons, obese persons tend to be a lower risk of osteoporosis because of the greater density of their bones, which must support a greater body weight. Early menopause, either natural or surgically induced by removal of both ovaries (bilateral oophorectomy), shortens the time that a woman experiences estrogen's protective effects and thus increases risk. Risk is also increased by menstrual irregularities (oligomenorrhea or amenorrhea) resulting from an unhealthfully low percent body fat. This may be due to excessive physical activity coupled with caloric restriction (as seen in some long-distance runners, gymnasts, and ballet dancers) or from eating disorders such as anorexia nervosa or bulemia.

Peak bone mass is a major factor determining risk of developing osteoporosis. At any given age, risk of fracture is less in people who have achieved a greater peak bone mass during the period of bone development than in those with a lower peak bone mass. Because they have the greatest average peak bone mass, black males tend to develop osteoporosis least often of any sex/race group. Compared with white females, black females have a higher peak bone mass and consequently less incidence of osteoporosis.[88]

Bone Densitometry

Bone densitometry, the measurement of bone mineral content, is important in the early detection and treatment of osteoporosis and in monitoring its

TABLE 8-8 Risk factors for osteoporosis and their scientific validity

Well-established evidence	Moderate evidence
Obesity (−)	Alcohol (+)
African ancestry (−)	Cigarette smoking (−)
Estrogen use (−)	Thiazide diuretic use (+)
High peak bone mass (−)	Moderate exercise (−)
Heavy exercise (−)	Caffeine use (+)
Female (+)	Fluoridated water use (−)
Caucasian/Asian (+)	
Age (+)	
Early menopause (+)	
Menstrual irregularities (+)	
Family history (+)	
Bilateral oophorectomy (+)	
Low dietary calcium (+)	
Corticosteroid use (+)	
Bed rest (+)	

From McBean LD, Forgac, T, Finn SC. 1994. Osteoporosis: Visions for care and prevention—a conference report. *Journal of the American Dietetic Association* 94:668–671; Peck WA, Riggs BL, Bell NH. 1988. Research directions in osteoporosis. *American Journal of Medicine* 84:275–282; US Dept. of Health and Human Services. 1991. *Osteoporosis research, education, and health promotion*. Bethesda, Md: National Institute of Arthritis and Musculoskeletal and Skin Diseases, National Institute of Health.
(−) = decreased risk; (+) = increased risk.

progression and response to treatment.[94,96] In addition to radiogrammetry, four basic approaches are used to quantify bone density. These include single-photon absorptiometry, dual-photon absorptiometry, dual-energy x-ray absorptiometry, and quantitative computed tomography. Other techniques, such as neutron activation analysis, Compton scattering, ultrasonic transmission velocity or attenuation, and magnetic resonance, are either not widely available or are in the early stages of development.[97]

Single-photon absorptiometry primarily measures content of cortical bone in the peripheral appendicular skeleton (for example, the bones of the forearm, wrist, and hands).[94] Dual-photon absorptiometry and dual-energy x-ray absorptiometry are capable of measuring both cortical and trabecular bone in the spine, hip, and total skeleton. Quantitative computed tomography provides a measure of trabecular bone in the vertebrae and other sites.[94] The various features of each are summarized in Table 8-9.

Radiogrammetry

Radiogrammetry uses standard x-rays of bones from which measurements of cortical bone thickness are obtained using a caliper or other measuring device. It usually is performed on the bones of the hands (metacarpals) and is widely available, easy to perform, reproducible, and backed by a large body of normative data.[94,96] Measurements of bone mineral content within the appendicular skeleton, however, fail to reflect mineral status of the axial skeleton. Therefore, this method is of limited value in assessing early

TABLE 8-9 Comparison of bone densitometry techniques*

	SPA	DPA	QCT	DEXA
Precision (%)	2–3	2–4	2–5	1–2
Accuracy (%)	5	4–10	5–20	3–5
Duration of examination (min)	15	20–45	10–20	5
Absorbed dose (mrem)	10	5	100–1,000	1–3
Radiation source	Iodine-125	Gadolinium-153	x-ray	x-ray
Source renewal (months)	6	12–18	N/A	N/A
Cost	Low	Moderate	High	Low

From National High Blood Pressure Education Program Working Group. 1993. National High Blood Pressure Education Program Working Group Report on Primary Prevention of Hypertension. *Archives of Internal Medicine* 153:186–208; Sartoris DJ, Resnick D. 1990. Current and innovative methods for noninvasive bone densitometry. *Orthopedics* 28:257–278; US Dept. of Health and Human Services. 1991. *Osteoporosis research, education, and health promotion.* Bethesda, Md: National Institute of Arthritis and Musculoskeletal and Skin Diseases, National Institutes of Health.

*SPA = single-photon absorptiometry; DPA = dual-photon absorptiometry; QCT = quantitative computerized tomography; DEXA = dual-energy x-ray absorptiometry; N/A = not applicable.

osteoporosis and fracture and in assessing bones in which improvements in mineral content caused by treatment are likely to be seen.[94,96]

Single-Photon Absorptiometry

In single-photon absorptiometry (SPA), a single-energy beam of photons from a radioisotope (iodine-125) is directed through the bone and overlying soft tissue and received by a detector and counter. The measured transmission rate of the photon beam is inversely proportional to the bone mineral content, which is expressed as bone mineral per square centimeter scanned.[96] The method involves a low radiation dose, and individual examinations are inexpensive. The instruments are portable and thus suited to epidemiologic studies in remote populations.

Usual sites for SPA measurements are those within the appendicular skeleton—the distal third of the radius, the calcaneus (the heel bone), and the distal femur.[94,96] Results from SPA are influenced by the variable thicknesses of soft tissue. Renewal of the radiation source every 6 months requires additional attention and expense. Thus the general consensus is that SPA primarily measures cortical bone and consequently is not well suited for predicting bone strength and fracture risk at typical osteoporotic fracture sites or for monitoring change caused by osteoporosis treatment.[94,96,98] Experts in metabolic bone disease have little or no use today for appendicular bone densitometry, even by sophisticated methods.[99]

Dual-Photon Absorptiometry

Dual-photon absorptiometry (DPA) is similar in concept to SPA except it uses photon beams at two different energy levels derived from a radioisotopic source (gadolinium-153). This allows measurement of bone mineral content that is independent of the thickness or density of soft tissues in the photon path, which is a drawback of SPA.[94,96] However, DPA measurements can be adversely affected by calcification of blood vessels, other soft tissue calcification, and abnormal outgrowths of bones. Bone mineral content is expressed in grams per centimeter,[2] which is an expression based on area rather than density.[94]

Usual sites for measurement with DPA are the spine, hip, upper femur, and total body. Measurements express both cortical and trabecular bone. The main advantages of DPA are low radiation dose, sufficient accuracy for making clinical judgments, a large number of accessible anatomic sites, and independence from the effects of soft tissues. Limiting factors include DPA's long scanning time (20 to 45 minutes), the expense involved in replacing the radiation source every 12 to 18 months, and low short-term precision that is insufficient for detecting bone mineral changes over follow-up periods typically used in clinical studies of treatments for osteoporosis.[94,96] DPA is a significant improvement over SPA, but overall it appears that measurements by quantitative CT and dual-energy x-ray absorptiometry are better at assessing mineral content of trabecular bone and more predictive of vertebral fracture than DPA.[94,96]

Quantitative Computed Tomography

Quantitative computed tomography (QCT) uses a device consisting of an array of x-ray sources and radiation detectors aligned opposite each other. As the x-ray beams pass through the subject, they are weakened or attenuated by the body's tissues and eventually picked up by the detectors. Data from the detectors then are transmitted to a computer, which reconstructs the subject's cross-sectional anatomy using mathematic equations adapted for computer processing.[100]

QCT can provide a quantitative measure of mineral content in cortical and/or trabecular bone within either the appendicular or axial skeleton.[94,96] In measurements of the axial skeleton, it has several advantages over dual-photon absorptiometry. It distinguishes between cortical and trabecular bone and is unaffected by mineral deposits outside the skeleton. Dual-energy QCT has been shown to measure changes in trabecular mineral content in the spine, radius, and tibia with considerable precision. However, it requires sophisticated calibration and positioning and careful technical monitoring.[94] The accuracy of single-energy QCT is more variable, depending on the amount of fat in the bone marrow.[98] The potential for using QCT in assessing bone mineral content is limited by problems of high radiation exposure, high cost, and limited availability of the method.[98,101] However, technical advances are resulting in lower radiation doses, lower costs, and greater availability, thus making QCT increasingly important in evaluating bone diseases.[96,97]

Dual-Energy X-Ray Absorptiometry

Dual-energy x-ray absorptiometry (DEXA) is a more recently developed approach to measuring bone mineral content in the appendicular skeleton, axial skeleton, or whole body. It is similar in concept to dual-photon absorptiometry but has several advantages. In DEXA the energy source is an x-ray tube, which provides an energy beam of greater intensity than the radioisotope used with DPA.[94,96] DEXA has a much shorter scanning time (5 minutes versus 20 minutes), which reduces errors from patient movement, allows better use of instruments, reduces patient costs, and shortens the duration of discomfort in patients with osteoporosis who are experiencing back pain.[94,98] Radiation exposure from DEXA is substantially less than in QCT.[99] A major advantage over DPA is the improved precision, which allows changes in bone mineral content to be detected over short periods.[96,98,99] Development of new software has permitted measurement of total and regional body calcium and body composition.[97,102]

Of all the methods compared, DEXA has the lowest precision error and is the most sensitive method for detecting changes in bone mineral density in the axial skeleton, where the earliest losses of bone mineral and their consequences occur. This, coupled with its speed, ease of use, and low radiation dose, has made DEXA the clinical method of choice for studying bone changes associated with metabolic diseases.[99,102]

Prevention and Treatment

Preventing and treating osteoporosis involves attaining the greatest genetically possible bone mineral density and then minimizing its loss. The three major interacting factors influencing bone health are diet, exercise, and estrogen.[89,97] Calcium, phosphorus, and vitamins D and C are particularly important in achieving optimal bone mineral density. Protein, sodium, caffeine play interactive roles, while more research is needed on the roles of vitamin K, manganese, copper, and zinc.[103] Primary prevention of osteoporosis begins in childhood and continues throughout adolescence and into the mid-30s, when the skeleton is acquiring its genetically programmed peak mineral mass. Secondary prevention is also critical to reducing morbidity and mortality. Although lost bone mineral cannot be replaced, the rate at which losses occur can be reduced by diet, exercise, and estrogen replacement therapy. It is estimated that adequate nutrition can reduce the impact of osteoporosis by as much as one half or more. Exercise by older adults can also help maintain muscular strength, stability, and balance, which will help reduce falls and risk of osteoporotic-related injury.[89]

Studies show that adequate calcium intake during childhood and adolescence is associated with improved bone mineral density, thus contributing to peak bone mineral density.[104,105] In adult women at least 5 years following menopause, adequate calcium intake has been shown to slow the rate of bone demineralization.[103,106] In an 18-month study of 1765 women age 69 years and over, women increased their calcium intake from 500 mg to 1700 mg per day and consumed 20 μmg of vitamin D (cholecalciferol). Nonvertebral fractures were reduced by 32% and hip fractures were reduced by 43%.[107] Finnish researchers studied the influence of supplemental vitamin D given to males and females age 75 years and older who had a vitamin D deficiency but had adequate calcium intake. Participants received annual injections of 3750 μmg or 7500 μmg of vitamin D (ergocalciferol) over a period of 2 to 5 years. For females receiving supplemental vitamin D, fractures of the upper limb and ribs were approximately half of that seen for females in the control group. There was no significant difference in the rate of fractures of the lower limbs in females. Among males, the fracture rate in those receiving vitamin D did not differ significantly from that of the control group.[108] Thus the benefits of increased calcium and vitamin D intake can be seen in younger persons as well as in older persons. Although there is not uniform agreement among studies, the weight of evidence clearly shows the efficacy of increased calcium intake in slowing the rate of bone mineral loss and markedly reducing the risk of fracture in older adults.[106–108] The lack of agreement stems from the difficulty of measuring dietary calcium intake and the fact that diet and exercise appear to have little, if any, effect on slowing the rate of bone demineralization during the first 5 years following menopause.[103]

In the light of these studies, some are asking if the RDAs for calcium and vitamin D are adequate to prevent osteoporosis. It has been suggested that the RDAs for calcium be increased to 1600 mg/d for adolescents (currently 1200 mg/d), 1000 mg/d for mature adults (currently 800 mg/d), and 1500 mg/d for postmenopausal women (currently 800 mg/d). Some have suggested that the RDA for vitamin D (currently set at 5 μmg/d) be increased to 20 μmg/d.[109]

Because osteoporosis is a multifactorial disease, measures such as estrogen replacement therapy for postmenopausal women, weight-bearing exercise, and smoking cessation should be included along with dietary attempts to delay the rate of bone demineralization.

DIABETES MELLITUS

Diabetes mellitus is a group of diseases characterized by a lack of insulin secretion and/or increased cellular resistance to insulin resulting in elevated plasma (or serum) glucose levels, abnormalities of carbohydrate and lipid metabolism, characteristic pathologic changes in the nerves and small blood vessels, and aggravation of atherosclerosis.[110,111] Since 1932, diabetes mellitus has been among the top 10 leading causes of death in America.[112,113] It is a major cause of blindness, renal failure, congenital malformation, and lower extremity amputation. The prevalence of coronary artery disease and peripheral vascular disease is twice as common among persons with

BOX 8-6

Major Risk Factors for Noninsulin–Dependent Diabetes Mellitus

- History of diabetes in parent or sibling
- >20% desirable body weight
- American Indian, Hispanic, or African American race
- Age > 40 years, plus any of the above factors
- Previously identified impaired glucose tolerance
- Hypertension or significant hyperlipidemia (i.e., serum cholesterol ≥ 240 mg/dl or triglycerides ≥ 250 mg/dl)
- History of gestational diabetes or delivery of a baby having birth weight > 9 lbs

From American Diabetes Association. 1989. Screening for diabetes. *Diabetes Care* 12:588–590.

diabetes compared with those without diabetes.[112] It afflicts nearly 14 million Americans, or approximately 6% of the population.[111]

Types of Diabetes

Among the diseases classified as diabetes are insulin-dependent diabetes mellitus, noninsulin-dependent diabetes mellitus, gestational diabetes, and impaired glucose tolerance.[110,111] Insulin-dependent diabetes mellitus (IDDM), also known as Type I diabetes, is generally (but not always) diagnosed in persons less than 30 years of age. Of all people diagnosed with IDDM and noninsulin-dependent diabetes mellitus, 5% to 10% have IDDM. Because the onset of symptoms is relatively abrupt and the disease requires immediate medical care, it rarely goes undiagnosed for long.[114]

Noninsulin-dependent diabetes mellitus (NIDDM), also known as Type II diabetes, generally is found in persons more than 30 years of age. NIDDM accounts for about 90% to 95% of all persons diagnosed with IDDM and NIDDM. Risk factors for NIDDM are outlined in Box 8-6.[112,114,115] Sixty percent to 90% of people with NIDDM are overweight. NIDDM develops slowly and is often symptom-free. It is estimated that as many as 50% of people with NIDDM are not diagnosed.[114]

The onset or first recognition of gestational diabetes mellitus (GDM) occurs during pregnancy. About 2% to 4% of all pregnant women develop GDM, making it the most common medical disorder affecting pregnancy. It typically is diagnosed during the third trimester of pregnancy and generally reverses after delivery. NIDDM may develop within 15 to 20 years in 40% to 60% of women who had GDM during pregnancy, although weight management and regular physical activity decreases this risk. The symptoms of GDM are mild and not threatening to the life of the mother but do increase the risk of fetal morbidity and mortality.[111,114,116]

Impaired glucose tolerance (IGT) occurs when blood glucose levels are elevated (but not enough to be diagnostic of diabetes) and symptoms of diabetes are absent.[111,114] Data from the second National Health and Nutrition Examination Survey (NHANES II) indicated that 4.8% of Americans age 20 to 74 years have IGT. Both overweight and family history of diabetes are associated with higher rates of IGT.[117] Because persons with IGT are at increased risk for CHD and peripheral vascular disease, treatment is now being encouraged for persons with IGT.[111,118]

Diagnosis of Diabetes

Despite the public health significance of diabetes, data from NHANES II show that only about 50% of people with diabetes are identified as having the disease. Diabetes has been diagnosed in about 3.4% of the U.S. population, and another 3.2% meet criteria for the disease. It is estimated that an additional 11.2% of the U.S. population has impaired glucose tolerance.[112]

Blood Glucose

Diagnosis of diabetes mellitus is not difficult when a person has the classic signs and symptoms of diabetes (discussed below) and a markedly elevated blood glucose level. It is also

BOX 8-7

Diagnosis of Diabetes

In nonpregnant adults, a diagnosis of diabetes can be made if any of the following is present:

- random plasma glucose (nonfasting) ≥ 200 mg/dl *and* classic signs and symptoms of diabetes (excessive thirst, excessive consumption of food, frequent urination, weight loss, blurred vision, and recurrent infections)
- FPG ≥ 140 mg/dl on two occasions
- FPG < 140 mg/dl with a plasma glucose during an OGTT of > 200 mg/dl at 2 hours and one other plasma glucose level > 200 mg/dl during the OGTT

From American Diabetes Association. 1994. *Maximizing the role of nutrition in diabetes management.* Alexandria, Va: American Diabetes Association.

FPG = fasting plasma glucose, OGTT = oral glucose tolerance test

relatively easy when a patient with no symptoms has persistently elevated fasting blood glucose levels. In other instances, the diagnosis of diabetes may rest on use of the oral glucose tolerance test (OGTT) or the oral glucose challenge.

A normal fasting glucose level is considered approximately 60 to 115 mg/dl (3.3 to 6.4 mmol/L). For the purpose of some glucose measurements, fasting can be defined as no consumption of food or beverage other than water for at least 3 hours before testing.[114] The diagnostic criteria for diabetes are shown in Box 8-7. A definitive diagnosis of diabetes can be made when the fasting plasma glucose (FPG) is ≥ 200 mg/dl (11.1 mmol/L) and the classic signs and symptoms of diabetes are present. These include excessive thirst (polydipsia), excessive consumption of food (polyphagia), excessive urination (polyuria), weight loss, blurred vision, and recurrent infections.[114] In the absence of these symptoms (as would be expected in someone with NIDDM), a diagnosis of diabetes can be made when the FPG is ≥ 140 mg/dl (≥ 7.8 mmol/L) on two occasions. If the FPG is > 115 mg/dl but < 140 mg/dl on two occasions, an oral glucose tolerance test may be recommended.

Oral Glucose Tolerance Test

The oral glucose tolerance test (OGTT) involves having the patient drink a beverage containing a known amount of glucose, usually 75 grams for adults or 1.75 g/kg for children.[119] Venous blood is drawn immediately before the glucose beverage is consumed and then at set intervals following consumption to monitor changes in blood sugar level. In preparing for the OGTT, it is best for the patient to consume more than 150 g of carbohydrate per day, abstain from alcohol, and have unrestricted activity for 3 days before the test.[119] On the morning of the test, the fasting subject consumes the glucose beverage within a 5- to 10-minute period. Plasma glucose is measured while fasting and usually at 1-hour intervals for 2 or 3 hours.

Plasma glucose levels ≥ 200 mg/dl (≥ 11.1 mmol/L) at 1 and 2 hours are diagnostic of diabetes. Figure 8-19 shows examples of how plasma glucose might respond to an OGTT in a person with diabetes and in one without diabetes. In the curve representing the person with diabetes, the plasma glucose exceeds 200 mg/dl at 1 hour and 2 hours after consuming the glucose load.

The 1 hour, 50 g oral glucose challenge is used as a screening test for GDM. The American Diabetes Association recommends that all pregnant women undergo this test at 24 to 28 weeks of gestation.[116] According to the American Diabetes Association, this test can be administered at any time of day and without regard to when the last meal was eaten. If the plasma glucose is > 140 mg/dl (> 7.8 mmol/L) at 1 hour following consumption of the glucose beverage, an OGTT should be performed.

Self-Monitoring of Blood Glucose

In self-monitoring of blood glucose (SMBG), persons with diabetes periodically measure the amount of glucose in a small sample of their

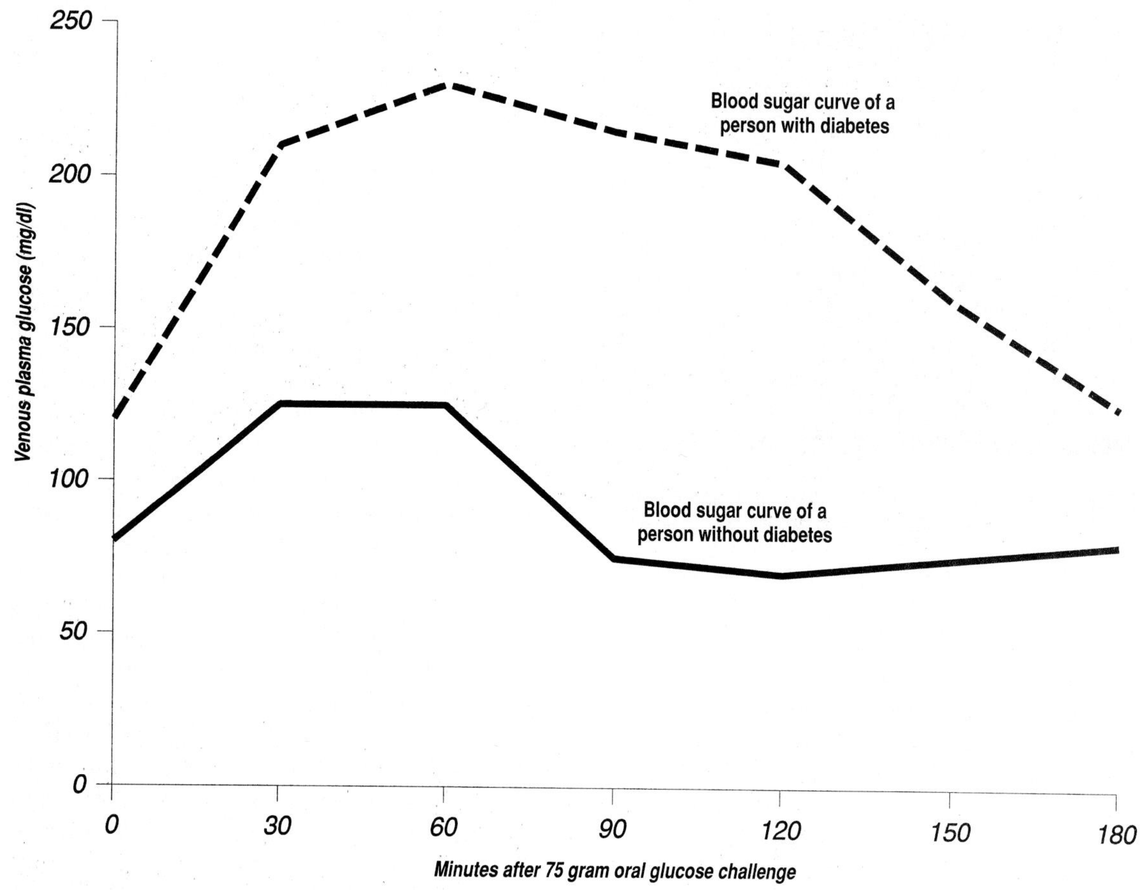

Figure 8-19 Examples of oral glucose tolerance test (OGTT) curves in a patient without diabetes and one with diabetes.

blood. This process is critical to glycemic control—maintaining blood glucose levels within an acceptable range. Self-monitoring of blood glucose allows a person with diabetes to evaluate how various combinations of diet, exercise, and medication affect blood glucose levels and determine the best combinations for optimal blood glucose control.

Self-monitoring of blood glucose can be accurately and precisely done using specially designed reagent strips. The reagent strip is a small piece of plastic with a test pad affixed to one end. The test pad is impregnated with an enzyme and chemicals that react to the glucose in a drop of blood applied to the test pad. The finger is first pricked using a lancet. A drop of blood from the finger is applied to the test pad of the reagent strip and then wiped away after a certain number of seconds. The enzymatic and chemical reaction results in the test pad changing color. The change in color is proportional to the amount of glucose in the blood. To determine blood glucose level, the color change can be compared with a color chart included with the reagent strips or the reagent strip can be inserted in a small, battery-operated meter that optically "reads" the color on the test pad and indicates the blood glucose level on the meter's electronic display (see Figure 8-20).

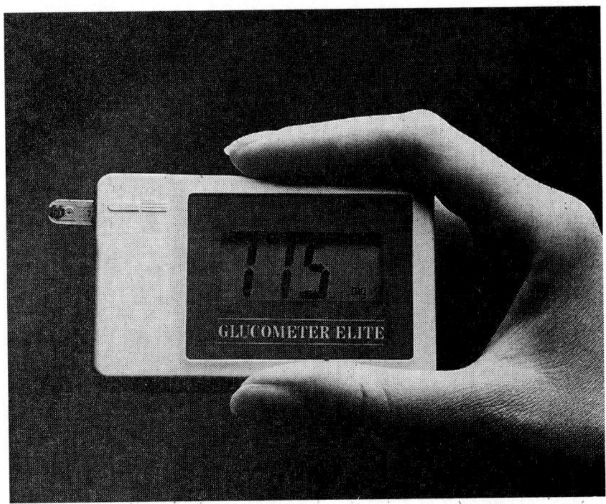

Figure 8-20 Example of a portable, battery-operated glucose meter for performing self-monitoring of blood glucose.

The frequency of SMBG depends primarily on the type of diabetes and a person's overall therapy. In some instances, monitoring as often as seven times a day may be appropriate. For persons with IDDM, it is recommended that SMBG be done before each meal and at bedtime. In some instances it may be appropriate to do additional testing 1 to 2 hours after meals and occasionally in the middle of the night to monitor glycemic control. Recommendations for NIDDM depend on the type of therapy. For NIDDM controlled by diet and exercise alone, SMBG can be done one to two times per week. For persons using diet and exercise along with oral hypoglycemic agents (medications taken orally to help control blood glucose levels), SMBG should be done daily at different times during the day. If glycemic control is good, these individuals can reduce the frequency of SMBG to one to two times per week. For those with NIDDM who also take insulin, it is recommended that SMBG be done at least twice a day at different times. Testing should be more frequent when there are changes in a person's schedule, exercise habits, medications, diet, and body weight, and when illness occurs.[111]

Glycosylated Hemoglobin

One drawback of blood glucose measurements is that they are only an index of glycemic control at the time the testing is done. For example, a person with diabetes who ordinarily runs a high blood glucose might be extra careful about maintaining glycemic control just before his or her visit with a physician. To assess mean glucose levels for the past 6 to 12 weeks, a physician can use a test measuring the amount of hemoglobin that is glycosylated. During the life span of a red blood cell, glucose in the blood binds to the major form of hemoglobin (Hb) in the red blood cell, hemoblogin A (HbA). When this occurs, the hemoglobin is said to be glycosylated. There are several forms of HbA in the red blood cell. The form of glycosylated HbA that most closely correlates to mean blood glucose levels is referred to as hemoglobin A_{1C} (HbA_{1C}). This binding of glucose to HbA is almost irreversible during the life span of the red blood cell. Consequently, HbA_{1C} reflects average blood glucose levels during the past 6 to 12 weeks. The proportion of HbA_{1C} does not decline with a temporary fall in blood glucose. It only decreases when glycemic control has been consistent over a period of several weeks, and older red blood cells with a high proportion of HbA_{1C} gradually die and are replaced by new red blood cells with a low proportion of HbA_{1C}. Consequently, the test is a good way to assess a patient's adherence to his or her program of blood glucose control.

In persons without diabetes, HbA_{1C} accounts for about 4% to 8% of the total hemoglobin. In persons with diabetes, blood glucose levels are usually elevated, more of the Hb becomes glycosylated, and the proportion of HbA_{1C} is greater. In persons with diabetes, an HbA_{1C} of 7% indicates good glycemic control. An HbA_{1C} of 10% indicates fair glycemic control, and a value of 13% to 20% indicates poor glycemic control.[119] It is important to note that values will vary with different measurement methods and even between different laboratories using the same methods. It is recommended to use only those laboratories participating in a recognized proficiency testing program. When evaluating values for HbA_{1C}, use the reference values provided by the laboratory performing the test.

The importance of glycemic control was shown by the Diabetes Control and Complications Trial (DCCT), a prospective clinical study investigating the effects of glycemic control on the incidence of microvascular complications such as neuropathy (nerve damage), retinopathy (damage to the retina that can lead to blindness), and nephropathy (damage to the nephron of the kidney). In the DCCT, 1441 persons age 13 to 39 years who had IDDM were randomly assigned to either a standard treatment group or an experimental treatment group.[120] The standard treatment group received conventional treatment for their IDDM—one or two insulin injections per day, periodic self-monitoring of urine or blood glucose, clinic appointments every 3 months, and nutrition education as requested by the participant. Those in the experimental treatment group received intensive therapy that involved continuous subcutaneous insulin infusion with an insulin pump or multiple insulin injections and monthly clinic appointments. Insulin adjustments were guided by self-monitoring of blood glucose done at least four times per day and at 3 AM once per week.

Persons in the standard treatment group had a mean glucose level of 231 mg/dl and a mean HbA_{1C} of 9%. Those in the experimental treatment group had a mean glucose level of 155 mg/dl and a mean HbA_{1C} of 7%. Compared with those in the standard treatment group, persons in the experimental group receiving intensive therapy had a dramatic reduction in the incidence of microvascular complications related to diabetes. There was a 76% reduction in retinopathy, a 60% reduction in neuropathy, and a 39% reduction in microalbuminuria (a sign of kidney disease).[111] Thus frequent SMBG and periodic monitoring of HbA_{1C} are useful for persons with diabetes who wish to maintain glycemic control.

Medical Nutrition Therapy

In 1994, the American Diabetes Association issued new nutrition recommendations and principles for people with diabetes.[121] These recommendations presented two major philosophical changes in the nutritional management of diabetes. One was that the focus of therapy for persons with NIDDM should include reasonable goals for the control of blood glucose and lipid levels, in addition to weight loss, if necessary. The other philosophical change was that a client's diet should be individually tailored according to his or her lifestyle and nutritional and metabolic needs. Rather than clients merely receiving and following a generic set of instructions from health professionals through the process of "diabetes patient education," they are encouraged to become more fully informed of and involved in the management of their condition through the process of "self-management training." Instead of "diet therapy" for persons with diabetes, the new recommendations employ "medical nutrition therapy."[122]

Medical nutrition therapy is a four-part approach that involves assessing an individual's nutritional, metabolic, and lifestyle needs; identifying nutrition and lifestyle goals; designing an intervention to achieve these goals; and evaluating therapeutic outcomes.[122] This four-step model is outlined in Figure 8-21. The goals of medical nutrition therapy are to achieve goals for blood glucose, blood lipids, and blood pressure; to provide adequate calories for reasonable weight, normal growth and development, and pregnancy and lactation; to prevent, delay, or treat nutrition-related complications of diabetes; and to improve health through optimal nutrition.[111,118]

Medical nutrition therapy is assessment based; goal setting, intervention, and evaluation depend in large part on data collected through nutritional assessment. Assessment begins with establishing rapport with the client and then proceeds with

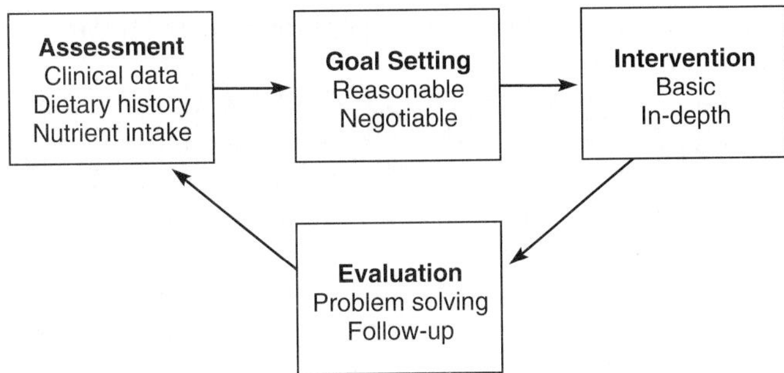

Figure 8-21 The four-step model for medical nutrition therapy for diabetes. From Tinker LF, Heins JM, Holler HJ. 1994. Commentary and translation: 1994 nutrition recommendations for diabetes. *Journal of the American Dietetic Association* 94:507–511.

BOX 8-8

Components of Nutritional Assessment for People with Diabetes

Clinical Data

Obtain height and weight
Determine body frame size
Determine desirable or healthy weight
Measure blood pressure
Assess laboratory values:
- blood glucose levels
- blood lipid levels
- glycosylated hemoglobin
- protein in urine

Identify diabetes medication:
- insulin
- oral hypoglycemic agents

Dietary History

Determine usual food intake
Assess nutrition and health attitudes
Assess previous dietary education and outcomes

Nutritional Intake

Assess overall nutritional adequacy
Assess energy intake
Assess nutrient distribution
Assess type of carbohydrate, protein, and fat
Determine appropriate nutrition intervention

Adapted from American Diabetes Association. 1994. Nutrition recommendations and principles for people with diabetes mellitus. *Diabetes Care* 17:519–522; Tinker LF, Heins JM, Holler HJ. 1994. Commentary and translation: 1994 nutrition recommendations for diabetes. *Journal of the American Dietetic Association* 94:507–511.

collecting pertinent clinical data, obtaining a diet history, and assessing current nutrient intake. The types of information included in these three components are shown in Box 8-8. Nutritional assessment shows what the client is currently doing, suggests what he or she is able and willing to do, and how likely he or she will be to adhere to nutritional recommendations. Once data from the assessment is discussed with the client, the process of goal setting can begin. Goal setting allows the client to set his or her own goals that are reasonable, specific, and measurable. Although goal setting is the responsibility of the client, the dietitian can negotiate with the client so that goals promote positive changes in eating and other lifestyle habits, resulting in improvements in blood

TABLE 8-10 Changes in dietary recommendations for persons with diabetes during the 20th century

Year	Carbohydrate (% kcal)	Distribution of Energy Fat (% kcal)	Protein (% kcal)
Pre-1921		Starvation diets	
1921	20	70	10
1950	40	40	20
1971	45	35	20
1986	50–60	30	12–20
1994	Based on assessment	<10% SFA* Up to 10% PUFA Based on assessment	10–20

Adapted from American Diabetes Association. 1994. *Maximizing the role of nutrition in diabetes management.* Alexandria, Va: American Diabetes Association; Franz MJ, Horton ES, Bantle JP, Beebe CA, Brunzell JD, Coulston AM, Henry RR, Hoogwerf BJ, Stagpoole PW. 1994. Nutrition principles for the management of diabetes and related complications. *Diabetes Care* 17:490–518; Tinker LF, Heins JM, Holler JH. 1994. Commentary and translation: 1994 nutrition recommendations for diabetes. *Journal of the American Dietetic Association* 94:507–511.

*SFA = saturated fatty acids; PUFA = polyunsaturated fatty acids

glucose and lipid levels and nutrient intake. Remember that as a client's metabolic control changes over time (e.g., glucose and lipid levels improve), goals will also change.

Rather than prescribing a set energy level and percentage of energy from carbohydrates, protein, and fat, the nutrition intervention should be individually tailored to address any metabolic abnormality. Through a process known as self-management training, the intervention should help the client acquire the knowledge and meal planning skills necessary to adapt diet and lifestyle to achieve his or her goals despite the various situations demanded by modern life.

Nutritional Recommendations

Over the course of the twentieth century nutritional recommendations for diabetes have changed markedly, as shown by Table 8-10. The goals for carbohydrate now address the total amount of carbohydrate consumed rather than the source of the carbohydrate. Use of sucrose as part of the meal plan does not impair blood sugar control, as long as it is substituted for other carbohydrates and foods and not merely added to the meal plan. However, the overall nutrient content of the sucrose-containing foods should be considered, as well as the presence of other nutrients frequently ingested with sucrose, such as fat and cholesterol. There now appears to be no advantage to using fructose and sugar alcohols (polyols) in place of other nutritive sweeteners. Fiber is recognized as beneficial in treating or preventing several gastrointestinal disorders including constipation and colon cancer, and soluble fiber has a beneficial effect on elevated serum lipids. The effect of dietary fiber on glycemic control, however, appears insignificant. The dietary recommendations for dietary fiber are now the same as for the general population: 20 to 35 g per day from a wide variety of food sources.

It is recommended that saturated fatty acids provide less than 10% of kilocalories and that intake of polyunsaturated fatty acids not exceed 10% of kilocalories. Apart from these restrictions, the amount of energy derived from fat should be based on the nutritional assessment and treatment goals. Persons with hypertriglyceridemia may be sensitive to carbohydrate and want to lower their carbohydrate and saturated fat intake and modestly increase their intake of monounsaturated fat. Evidence is mounting that a high-fat diet may contribute to obesity and that a low-fat diet, independent of energy reduction, may be beneficial in weight loss.[123] Therefore it may be prudent for obese persons with diabetes to reduce fat and increase carbohydrate intake. Dietary cholesterol should be limited to 300 mg/d per day or less; however, persons with elevated levels of LDL-C may want to adopt the more stringent recommendations for both dietary cholesterol and saturated fat of the National Cholesterol Education Program's Step II diet.

When diabetes is well controlled, blood glucose levels are not generally affected by an alcohol intake of no more than two drinks per day ingested with and in addition to the usual meal plan. Because alcohol consumption may increase the risk of hypoglycemia in persons treated with insulin and oral hypoglycemic agents, if consumed, it should be consumed with meals. Abstention is advised during pregnancy and for persons with a history of alcohol abuse. Abstention or reduced intake may be advisable for individuals with pancreatitis, dyslipidemia, or nephropathy.

Energy supplied by protein can range between 10% and 20%, although with the onset of nephropathy, a protein intake approaching the RDA (0.8 g/kg of body weight per day or about 10% of energy) should be considered. Sodium recommendations are no different than those for the general population, ranging between 2400 and 3000 mg/d. However, for persons with mild-to-moderate hypertension, 2400 mg/d is recommended. Potassium supplementation may be required in some persons taking diuretics. Vitamin and mineral supplementation is not necessary for most people with diabetes when dietary intake is adequate. There appears to be no benefit of taking chromium and magnesium supplements unless a documented deficiency of these nutrients exits.

SUMMARY

1. Coronary heart disease (CHD) remains the leading cause of death in the United States despite a more than 50% decline in CHD death rates since 1950. CHD is causally associated with several risk factors, especially elevated blood cholesterol levels, high blood pressure, and cigarette smoking.
2. Because cholesterol, triglycerides, and other lipids are fat soluble, they are transported in the blood by lipoproteins. CHD risk is directly related to serum levels of total cholesterol and low-density-lipoprotein cholesterol (LDL-C) and inversely related to levels of high-density-lipoprotein cholesterol (HDL-C). The National Cholesterol Education Program (NCEP) has set desirable levels of total cholesterol and LDL-C in adults at <200 mg/dl and <130 mg/dl, respectively.
3. Atherosclerosis begins in childhood and progresses slowly into adulthood. Children and adolescents with elevated serum cholesterol frequently come from families whose adult members have a high incidence of CHD or elevated serum cholesterol levels. According to the NCEP, acceptable levels of total cholesterol and LDL-C in children and adolescents are <170 mg/dl and <110 mg/dl, respectively.
4. Two ways of addressing the problem of high serum cholesterol levels are the population-based and the patient-based approaches. The former emphasizes dietary and lifestyle changes for all people to lower average cholesterol levels in the entire population. The latter promotes identification and treatment of individuals with elevated cholesterol levels by physicians.
5. A two-step dietary approach is recommended for lowering cholesterol levels. The Step I diet recommends <10% of total calories from saturated fat and <300 mg/day of dietary cholesterol. The Step II diet recommends <7% of total calories from saturated fat and <200 mg/day of dietary cholesterol. Both diets recommend <30% of calories from total fat, up to

10% of calories from polyunsaturated fat, 10% to 15% of calories from monounsaturated fat, 50% to 60% and 10% to 20% of calories from carbohydrates and protein, respectively, and a reduction in total calories to achieve and maintain desirable weight.

6. After about age 2 years, children can safely follow the Step I or Step II diets. Although the NCEP discourages cholesterol screening for all children, it advises cholesterol testing for children whose parents or grandparents have elevated cholesterol and lipoprotein levels or who have definite CHD or other cardiovascular disease by age 55 years, as well as cholesterol testing for children at high risk of CHD because of overweight, cigarette smoking, high blood pressure, diabetes, and so on.
7. A number of dietary factors can influence serum cholesterol and lipoprotein levels. Saturated fatty acids tend to raise total cholesterol and LDL-C levels, whereas substitution of saturated fats with polyunsaturated and monounsaturated fats tends to lower total cholesterol and LDL-C. Dietary cholesterol tends to raise serum cholesterol, but it is not as potent an elevator as saturated fats. Obesity elevates total cholesterol and LDL-C levels and depresses HDL-C levels. Consumption of soluble dietary fiber tends to lower elevated total cholesterol and LDL-C levels.
8. Precision or reproducibility relates to the difference in results when the same blood sample is repeatedly measured. The coefficient of variation (CV) is a measure of precision and is calculated by dividing the standard deviation (SD) by the mean and multiplying by 100 (CV = SD ÷ mean × 100). The NCEP recommends that laboratories achieve a CV ≤ 3%.
9. Accuracy relates to the difference between the measured value reported by the clinical laboratory and the "true" or "real" value that has been previously established by comparison with a known standard (reference material) and/or a definitive measurement method. Bias is a measure of inaccuracy or departure from accuracy. Inaccurate measurement leads to clinical misdiagnosis caused by reporting of false positive or false negative values.
10. Hypertension is one of the most common risk factors for cardiovascular and renal diseases. One of every four Americans has hypertension or is taking antihypertensive medication. As systolic blood pressure increases above 120 mm Hg and diastolic blood pressure increases above 80 mm Hg, risk of death from cardiovascular disease increases.
11. The most important risk factors for hypertension are high sodium intake, excessive energy consumption and physical inactivity (both promoting obesity), excessive alcohol consumption, and inadequate potassium intake.
12. Osteoporosis is a condition in which bone mineral content is decreased, resulting in greater susceptibility to fracture. Common fracture sites include the pelvis, vertebrae, hip, distal forearm, and humerus. Osteoporotic fractures are twice as common in females than in males, and because they live longer than males, females experience an even higher absolute incidence during their lifetimes.
13. Peak bone mass, a major factor determining risk of osteoporosis development, varies considerably among individuals because of heredity, sex, race, and environmental factors. On average, males have 20% to 30% greater peak bone mass than females, and the bones of black males and females are about 10% denser than those of white males and females.
14. Bone densitometry, the measurement of bone mineral content, is important in early detection and treatment of osteoporosis and in monitoring its progression and response to treatment. Approaches to bone densitometry include radiogrammetry, single-photon absorptiometry, dual-photon absorptiometry, quantitative computed tomography, and dual-energy x-ray absorptiometry.

15. In children and adolescents, optimal calcium intake increases bone mineral density. In postmenopausal women, calcium and vitamin D supplementation and estrogen replacement therapy decreases the rate of bone deminerization and reduces fracture risk.
16. Diabetes is a group of diseases characterized by lack of insulin secretion and/or increased insulin resistance, elevated plasma glucose levels, abnormal carbohydrate and lipid metabolism, pathologic changes in the nerves and small blood vessels, and aggravation of atherosclerosis. Among the diseases classified as diabetes are insulin-dependent diabetes mellitus, noninsulin-dependent diabetes mellitus, gestational diabetes, and impaired glucose tolerance.
17. Despite its public health significance, diabetes is undiagnosed in about 50% of people who have the disease. Diagnostic criteria for diabetes include the presence of symptoms of diabetes and fasting glucose measurements of >140 mg/dl (>7.8 mmol/L) on two occasions. The oral glucose tolerance test also can be used to diagnose diabetes.
18. Glycosylated hemoglobin (HbA_{1C}) is a useful test for assessing a person's mean glucose levels during the past 6 to 12 weeks. Self-monitoring blood glucose is an accurate and precise way to monitor how changes in diet, exercise, and medications affect glycemic control. Glycemic control has been shown to be effective in reducing the risk of microvascular complications in persons with IDDM.
19. The American Diabetes Association's new nutrition recommendations for people with diabetes represent a philosophical shift toward encouraging people with diabetes to become better informed about diabetes and its nutritional management rather than simply follow a standard "diabetic diet."
20. Medical nutrition therapy is an approach involving nutritional assessment, goal setting, intervention, and evaluation. Its goals are to control blood glucose, blood lipids, and blood pressure; provide adequate calories normal growth and development, pregnancy, and lactation; prevent delay, or treat nutrition-related complications of diabetes; and improve health through optimal nutrition.

REFERENCES

1. Bierman EL. 1994. Atherosclerosis and other forms of arteriosclerosis. In Isselbacher KJ, Braunwald E, Wilson JD, Martin JB, Fauci AS, Kasper DL, eds. *Harrison's principles of internal medicine,* 13th ed. New York: McGraw-Hill.
2. National Research Council. 1989. *Diet and health: Implications for reducing chronic disease risk.* Washington, DC: National Academy Press.
3. Kwiterovich PO. 1990. Diagnosis and management of familial dyslipoproteinemia in children and adolescents. *Pediatric Clinics of North America* 37:1489–1523.
4. American Heart Association. 1993. *Heart and stroke facts statistics.* Dallas, Tex: American Heart Association.
5. National Cholesterol Education Program. 1993. *Second report of the expert panel on detection, evaluation, and treatment of high blood cholesterol in adults.* Bethesda, Md: US Department of Health and Human Services, Public Health Service; National Institutes of Health; National Heart, Lung, and Blood Institute.
6. Merck, Sharp, & Dohme. 1989. *The hypercholesterolemia handbook.* West Point, Pa: Merck Sharp & Dohme.
7. National Cholesterol Education Program. 1990. *Report of the expert panel on population strategies for blood cholesterol reduction.* Bethesda, Md: US Department of Health and Human Services, Public Health Service; National Institutes of Health; National Heart, Lung, and Blood Institute.
8. National Institutes of Health Consensus Development Conference Statement. 1985. Lowering blood cholesterol levels to prevent heart disease. *Journal of the American Medical Association* 253:2080–2086.
9. LaRosa JC, Hunninghake D, Bush D, et al. 1990. The cholesterol facts. A summary of the evidence relating to dietary fats, serum cholesterol, and coronary heart disease. A joint statement by the

American Heart Association and the National Heart, Lung, and Blood Institute. *Circulation* 8:1721–1733.

10. Schaefer EJ, Levy RI. 1985. Pathogenesis and management of lipoprotein disorders. *New England Journal of Medicine* 312:1300–1310.
11. Haskell WL. 1984. The influence of exercise on the concentrations of triglyceride and cholesterol in human plasma. *Exercise and Sports Science Review* 12:205–244.
12. Lipid Research Clinics Program. 1984. The Lipid Research Clinics Coronary Primary Prevention Trial results II. The relationship of reduction in incidence of coronary heart disease to cholesterol lowering. *Journal of the American Medical Association* 251:365–374.
13. Gotto AM. 1990. Interrelationships of triglycerides with lipoproteins and high-density lipoproteins. *American Journal of Cardiology* 66:20A–23A.
14. Frohlich JJ, Pritchard PH. 1989. The clinical significance of serum high density lipoproteins. *Clinical Biochemistry* 22:417–423.
15. Tall AR. 1990. Plasma high density lipoproteins. *Journal of Clinical Investigation* 86:379–384.
16. Atherosclerosis Study Group. 1984. Optimal resources for primary prevention of atherosclerotic diseases. *Circulation* 70:157A–205A.
17. National Institutes of Health Consensus Development Panel on Triglyceride, High-Density Lipoprotein, and Coronary Heart Disease. 1993. Triglyceride, high-density lipoprotein, and coronary heart disease. *Journal of the American Medical Association* 269:505–510.
18. Gordon DJ, Probstfield JL, Garrison RJ, Neaton JD, Castelli WP, Knoke JD, Jacobs DR, Bangdiwala S, Tyroler A. 1989. High-density lipoprotein cholesterol and cardiovascular disease. Four prospective American studies. *Circulation* 79:8–15.
19. Miller NE. 1990. HDL metabolism and its role in lipid transport. *European Heart Journal* 11(suppl):H1–H3.
20. Scanu AM. 1988. Lipoprotein(a). *Archives of Pathology and Laboratory Medicine* 112:1045–1047.
21. Scanu AM. 1991. Lipoprotein(a) and atherosclerosis. *Annals of Internal Medicine* 115:209–218.
22. Schaefer EJ, Lamon-Fava S, Jenner JL, McNamara JR, Ordovas JM, Davis E, Abolafia JM, Lippel K, Levy RI. 1994. Lipoprotein(a) levels and risk of coronary heart disease in men. *Journal of the American Medical Association* 271:999–1003.
23. Ridker PM, Hennekens CH, Stampfer MJ. 1993. A prospective study of lipoprotein(a) and the risk of myocardial infarction. *Journal of the American Medical Association* 270:2195–2199.
24. Rosengren A, Wilhelmsen L, Eriksson E, Risberg B, Wedel H. 1990. Lipoprotein(a) and coronary heart disease: A prospective case-control study in the general population sample of middle aged men. *British Medical Journal* 301:1248–1251.
25. Jauhiainen M, Koskinen P, Ehnholm C, Frick MH. 1991. Lipoprotein(a) and coronary heart disease risk: A nested case-control study of the Helsinki Heart Study participants. *Atherosclerosis* 89:59–67.
26. Martin MJ, Hulley SB, Browner WS, Kuller LH, Wentworth D. 1986. Serum cholesterol, blood pressure, and mortality: Implications from a cohort of 361,622 men. *Lancet* 2:933–936.
27. National Cholesterol Education Program. 1991. *Report of the expert panel on blood cholesterol levels in children and adolescents.* Bethesda, Md: US Department of Health and Human Services, Public Health Service; National Institutes of Health; National Heart, Lung, and Blood Institute.
28. Rifkind BM. 1990. High-density lipoprotein cholesterol and coronary artery disease: Survey of the evidence. *American Journal of Cardiology* 66:3A–6A.
29. Wilson PWF. 1990. High-density lipoprotein, low-density lipoprotein and coronary artery disease. *American Journal of Cardiology* 66:7A–10A.
30. US Department of Health and Human Services. 1980. *The Lipid Research Clinics population studies data book. Volume I (The Prevalence Study).* Washington, DC: US Department of Health and Human Services.
31. Linn S, Fulwood R, Carroll M, Brook JG, Johnson C, Kalsbeek WD, Rifkind BM. 1991. Serum total cholesterol: HDL cholesterol ratios in US white and black adults by selected demographic and socioeconomic variables (HANES II). *American Journal of Public Health* 81:1038–1043.

32. Kinosian B, Glick H, Garland G. 1994. Cholesterol and coronary heart disease: Predicting risk by levels and ratios. *Annals of Internal Medicine* 121:641–647.
33. Castelli WP, Anderson K, Wilson PW, Levy D. 1992. Lipids and risk of coronary heart disease: The Framingham Study. *Annals of Epidemiology* 2:23–28.
34. Grundy SM, Greenland P, Herd A, Huebsch JA, Jones RJ, Mitchell JH, Schlant RC. 1987. Cardiovascular and risk factor evaluation of healthy American adults. *Circulation* 75:1339A–1362A.
35. Anderson KM, Wilson PWF, Odell PM, Kannel WB. 1991. An updated coronary risk profile. *Circulation* 83:356–362.
36. National Cholesterol Education Program. 1988. *Report of the expert panel on detection, evaluation, and treatment of high blood cholesterol in adults*. Bethesda, Md: US Department of Health and Human Services, Public Health Service; National Institutes of Health; National Heart, Lung, and Blood Institute.
37. Johnson CL, Rikfind BM, Sempos CT, Carroll MD, Bachorik PS, Briefel RR, Gordon DJ, Burt VL, Brown CD, Lippel K, Cleeman JI. 1993. Declining serum total cholesterol levels among US adults. *Journal of the American Medical Association* 269:3002–3008.
38. Brensike JF, Levy RI, Kelsey SF, Passamani ER, Richardson JM, Loh IK, et al. 1984. Effects of therapy with cholestyramine on progression of coronary arteriosclerosis: Results of the NHLBI Type II Coronary Intervention Study. *Circulation* 69:313–324.
39. Blankenhorn DH, Nessim SA, Johnson RL, Sanmarco ME, Azen SP, Cashin-Hemphill L. 1987. Beneficial effects of combined colestipol-niacin therapy on coronary atherosclerosis and coronary venous bypass grafts. *Journal of the American Medical Association* 257:3233–3240.
40. Blankenhorn DH, Johnson RL, Mack WJ, El Zein HA, Vailas LI. 1990. The influence of diet on the appearance of new lesions in human coronary arteries. *Journal of the American Medical Association* 263:1646–1652.
41. Buchwald H, Varco RL, Matts JP, Long JM, Fitch LL, Campbell GS, and the POSCH Group. 1990. Effect of partial ileal bypass surgery on mortality and morbidity from coronary heart disease on patients with hypercholesterolemia: Report of the Program on the Surgical Control of Hyperlipidemias (POSCH). *New England Journal of Medicine* 323:946–955.
42. Kane JP, Mallory MJ, Ports TA, Phillips R, Diehl JC, Havel RJ. 1990. Regression of coronary atherosclerosis during treatment of familial hypercholesterolemia with combined drug regimens. *Journal of the American Medical Association* 264:3007–3012.
43. Ornish D, Brown SE, Scherwitz LW, Billings JH, Armstrong WT, Ports TA, McLanahan SM, Kirkeeide RL, Brand RJ, Gould KL. 1990. Can lifestyle changes reverse coronary heart disease? *Lancet* 336:129–133.
44. Enos WF, Beyer JC, Holmes RH. 1955. Pathogenesis of coronary disease in American soldiers killed in Korea. *Journal of the American Medical Association* 158:912–914.
45. McNamara JJ, Molot MA, Stremple JF, Cutting RT. 1971. Coronary artery disease in combat casualties in Vietnam. *Journal of the American Medical Association* 216:1185–1187.
46. Stary HC. 1989. Evolution and progression of atherosclerotic lesions in coronary arteries of children and young adults. *Arteriosclerosis* 9 (Suppl):I19–I32.
47. Stary HC. 1990. The sequence of cell and matrix changes in atherosclerotic lesions of coronary arteries in the first forty years of life. *European Heart Journal* 11(Suppl):E3–E19.
48. Strong JP, McGill HC. 1969. The pediatric aspects of atherosclerosis. *Journal of Atherosclerosis Research* 9:251–265.
49. McGill HC, Arias-Stella J, Carbonell LM, Correa P, DeVeyra EA, Donoso S, et al. 1968. General findings of the International Atherosclerosis Project. *Laboratory Investigation* 18:498–502.
50. PDAY Research Group. 1990. Relationship of atherosclerosis in young men to serum lipoprotein cholesterol concentrations and smoking. A preliminary report from the Pathobiological Determinants of Atherosclerosis in Youth (PDAY) Research Group. *Journal of the American Medical Association* 264:3018–3024.
51. Strong JP. 1995. Natural history and risk factors for early human atherogenesis. Pathobiological Determinants of Atherosclerosis in Youth (PDAY). *Clinical Chemistry* 41:134–138.

52. Wissler RW. 1994. New insights into the pathogenesis of atherosclerosis as revealed by PDAY. Pathobiological Determinants of Atherosclerosis in Youth. *Atherosclerosis* 108(suppl):S3–S20.
53. National Center for Health Statistics. 1983. Dietary intake source data: United States 1976–80. *Vital and Health Statistics,* Series 11, No. 231. Hyattsville, Md: US Department of Health and Human Services, Public Health Service; National Center for Health Statistics.
54. National Center for Health Statistics. 1978. *Total serum cholesterol levels in children 4–17 years: United States, 1971–74.* Hyattsville, Md: US Department of Health and Human Services, Public Health Service; National Center for Health Statistics.
55. Knuiman JT, Hermus RJ, Hautvast JG. 1980. Serum total and high density lipoprotein (HDL) cholesterol concentrations in rural and urban boys from 16 countries. *Atherosclerosis* 36:529–537.
56. Knuiman JT, Westenbrink S, van der Heyden L, West CE, Burema J, DeBoer J, et al. 1983. Determinants of total and high density lipoprotein cholesterol in boys from Finland, the Netherlands, Italy, the Philippines and Ghana with special reference to diet. *Human Nutrition: Clinical Nutrition* 37C:237–254.
57. Rosenberg IH, Schaefer EJ. 1988. Dietary saturated fatty acids and blood cholesterol. *New England Journal of Medicine* 318:1270–1271.
58. Hegsted DM. 1986. Serum-cholesterol response to dietary cholesterol: A re-evaluation. *American Journal of Clinical Nutrition* 44:299–305.
59. Park YK, Yetley EA. 1990. Trend changes in use and current intakes of tropical oils in the United States. *American Journal of Clinical Nutrition* 51:738–748.
60. Beynen AC, Katan MB. 1985. Effect of egg yolk feeding on the concentration and composition of serum lipoprotein in man. *Atherosclerosis* 54: 157–166.
61. Schonfeld G, Patsch W, Rudel LL, Nelson C, Epstein M, Olson RE. 1982. Effects of dietary cholesterol and fatty acids on plasma lipoproteins. *Journal of Clinical Investigation* 69:1072–1080.
62. McDowell MA, Briefel RR, Alaimo K, Bischof AM, Caughman CR, Carroll MD, Loria CM, Johnson CL. 1994. Energy and macronutrient intakes of persons ages 2 months and over in the United States: Third National Health and Nutrition Examination Survey, Phase 1, 1988–91. *Advance Data from Vital and Health Statistics.* No. 255. Hyattsville, Md: National Center for Health Statistics.
63. Shekelle RB, Shryock AM, Paul O, Lepper M, Stamler J, Liu S, Raynor WJ. 1981. Diet, serum cholesterol, and death from coronary heart disease. The Western Electric Study. *New England Journal of Medicine* 304:65–70.
64. McGee DL, Reed DM, Yano K, Kagan A, Tillotson J. 1984. Ten-year incidence of coronary heart disease in the Honolulu Heart Program. Relationship to nutrient intake. *American Journal of Epidemiology* 119:667–676.
65. Kromhout D, de Lezenne Coulander C. 1984. Diet, prevalence and 10-year mortality from coronary heart disease in 871 middle-aged men. The Zutphen Study. *American Journal of Epidemiology* 119:733–741.
66. Kushi LH, Lew RA, Stare FJ, Ellison CR, Lozy M, Bourke G, Daly L, Graham I, Hickey N, Mulcahy R, Kevaney J. 1985. Diet and 20-year mortality from coronary heart disease. The Ireland-Boston Diet-Heart Study. *New England Journal of Medicine* 312:811–818.
67. Gotto AM. 1991. Cholesterol intake and serum cholesterol level. *New England Journal of Medicine* 324:912–913.
68. Kern F. 1991. Normal plasma cholesterol in an 88-year-old man who eats 25 eggs a day. *New England Journal of Medicine* 312:896–899.
69. Burr ML, Sweetnam PM. 1982. Vegetarianism, dietary fiber, and mortality. *American Journal of Clinical Nutrition* 36:873–877.
70. Phillips RL, Kuzma JW, Beeson WL, Lotz T. 1980. Influence of selection versus lifestyle on risk of fatal cancer and cardiovascular disease among Seventh-day Adventists. *American Journal of Epidemiology* 112:296–314.
71. Carroll KK. 1991. Review of clinical studies on cholesterol-lowering response to soy protein. *Journal of the American Dietetic Association* 91:820–827.
72. Life Sciences Research Office. 1987. *Physiological effects and health consequences of dietary fiber.* Bethesda, Md: Life Sciences Research Office, Federation of American Societies for Experimental Biology.

73. Jenkins DJA, Reynolds D, Slavin B, Leeds AR, Jenkins AL, Jepson EM. 1980. Dietary fiber and blood lipids: Treatment of hypercholesterolemia with guar crispbreads. *American Journal of Clinical Nutrition* 33:575–581.
74. Jenkins DJA, Leeds AR, Slavin B, Mann J, Jepson EM. 1979. Dietary fiber and blood lipids: Reduction of serum cholesterol in type II hyperlipidemia by guar gum. *American Journal of Clinical Nutrition* 32:16–18.
75. Story JA, Kritchevsky D. 1976. Comparison of the binding of various bile acids and bile salts in vitro by several types of fiber. *Journal of Nutrition* 106:1292–1294.
76. Story JA. 1985. Dietary fiber and lipid metabolism. *Proceedings of the Society for Experimental Biology and Medicine* 180:447–452.
77. Chen WJL, Anderson JW, Jennings D. 1984. Propionate may mediate the hypocholesterolemic effects of certain soluble plant fibers in cholesterol-fed rats. *Proceedings of the Society for Experimental Biology and Medicine* 175:215–218.
78. Cummings JH, Englyst HN. 1987. Fermentation in the human large intestine and the available substrates. *American Journal of Clinical Nutrition* 45:1243–1255.
79. Mann J. 1987. Complex carbohydrates: Replacement energy for fat or useful in their own right? *American Journal of Clinical Nutrition* 45:1202–1206.
80. National Cholesterol Education Program. 1988. *Current status of blood cholesterol measurement in clinical laboratories in the United States: A report from the Laboratory Standardization Panel of the National Cholesterol Education Program.* Bethesda, Md: US Department of Health and Human Services, Public Health Service; National Institutes of Health; National Heart, Lung, and Blood Institute.
81. National Cholesterol Education Program. 1990. *Recommendations for improving cholesterol measurement: A report from the Laboratory Standardization Panel of the National Cholesterol Education Program.* Bethesda, Md: US Department of Health and Human Services, Public Health Service; National Institutes of Health; National Heart, Lung, and Blood Institute.
82. Cooper GR, Myers GL, Smith SJ, Schlant RC. 1992. Blood lipid measurements: Variations and practical utility. *Journal of the American Medical Association* 267:1652–1660.
83. National High Blood Pressure Education Program. 1993. *Fifth report of the Joint National Committee on Detection, Evaluation, and Treatment of High Blood Pressure.* US Department of Health and Human Services, Public Health Service; National Institutes of Health; National Heart, Lung, and Blood Institute.
84. National High Blood Pressure Education Program Working Group. 1993. National High Blood Pressure Education Program Working Group report on primary prevention of hypertension. *Archives of Internal Medicine* 153:186–208.
85. National Center for Health Statistics. 1994. Health, United States, 1993. Hyattsville, Md: US Public Health Service.
86. The Trials of Hypertension Prevention Collaborative Research Group. 1992. The effects of nonpharmacologic interventions on blood pressure of persons with high normal levels: Results of the Trials of Hypertension Prevention. Phase I. *Journal of the American Medical Association* 267:1213–1220.
87. Alaimo K, McDowell MA, Briefel RR, Bischof AM, Caughman CR, Loria CM, Johnson CL. 1994. Dietary intake of vitamins, minerals, and fiber of persons ages 2 months and over in the United States: Third National Health and Nutrition Examination Survey, Phase 1, 1988–91. *Advance Data from Vital and Health Statistics.* No. 258. Hyattsville, Md: US Center for Health Statistics.
88. Gillespy T, Gillespy MP. 1991. Osteoporosis. *Radiologic Clinics of North America* 29:77–84.
89. McBean LD, Forgac T, Finn SC. 1994. Osteoporosis: Visions for care and prevention—a conference report. *Journal of the American Dietetic Association* 94:668–671.
90. National Institute of Arthritis and Musculoskeletal and Skin Diseases. 1988. *Arthritis, rheumatic diseases, and related disorders: Moyer report.* Bethesda, Md: US Department of Health and Human Services, Public Health Service; National Institutes of Health.
91. US Department of Health and Human Services. 1991. *Healthy people 2000: National health promotion and disease prevention objectives.* Washington, DC: US Government Printing Office.
92. Department of Health. 1991. *Dietary reference values for food energy and nutrients for the United Kingdom. Report of the Panel on Dietary Reference Values of the Committee on medical*

aspects of food policy. Report on Health and Social Subjects No. 41. London: Her Majesty's Stationery Office.

93. Krane SM, Holick MF. 1994. Metabolic bone disease. In Isselbacher KJ, Braunwald E, Wilson JD, Martin JB, Fauci JB, Kasper DL, eds. *Harrison's principles of internal medicine,* 13th ed. New York: McGraw-Hill.
94. Lang P, Steiger P, Faulkner K, Glüer C, Genant HK. 1991. Osteoporosis: Current techniques and recent developments in quantitative bone densitometry. *Radiologic Clinics of North America* 29:49–76.
95. Peck WA, Riggs BL, Bell NH. 1988. Research directions in osteoporosis. *American Journal of Medicine* 84:275–282.
96. Sartoris DJ, Resnick D. 1990. Current and innovative methods for noninvasive bone densitometry. *Orthopedics* 28:257–278.
97. US Department of Health and Human Services. 1991. *Osteoporosis research, education, and health promotion.* Bethesda, Md: National Institute of Arthritis and Musculoskeletal and Skin Diseases, National Institutes of Health.
98. Sartoris DJ, Moscona A, Reskick D. 1990. Progress in radiology: Dual-energy radiographic absorptiometry for bone density. *Annals New York Academy of Sciences* 592:307–325.
99. Mazess RB, Barden HS, Bisek JP, Hanson J. 1990. Dual-energy x-ray absorptiometry for total-body and regional bone-mineral and soft-tissue composition. *American Journal of Clinical Nutrition* 51:1106–1112.
100. Bushong SC. 1993. *Radiologic science for technologists: Physics, biology, and protection,* 5th ed. St. Louis: Mosby.
101. Lukaski HC. 1987. Methods for the assessment of human body composition: Traditional and new. *American Journal of Clinical Nutrition* 46:537–556.
102. Roubenoff R, Kehayias JJ, Dawson-Hughes B, Heymsfield SB. 1993. Use of dual-energy x-ray absorptiometry in body composition studies: Not yet a "gold standard." *American Journal of Clinical Nutrition* 58:589–591.
103. Heaney RP. 1993. Nutritional factors in osteoporosis. *Annual Review of Nutrition* 13:287–316.
104. Johnston CC, Miller JZ, Slemenda CW, Reister TK, Hui S, Christian JC, Peacock M. 1992. Calcium supplementation and increases in bone mineral density in children. *New England Journal of Medicine* 327:82–87.
105. Lloyd T, Andon MB, Rollings N, Martel JK, Landis JR, Demers LM, Eggli DF, Kieselhorst K, Kulin HE. 1993. Calcium supplementation and bone mineral density in adolescent girls. *Journal of the American Medical Association* 270:841–844.
106. Dawson-Hughes B, Sallal GE, Krall EA, Sadowski L, Sahyoun N, Tannenbaum S. 1990. A controlled trial of the effect of calcium supplementation on bone density in postmenopausal women. *New England Journal of Medicine* 323:878–883.
107. Chapuy MC, Arlot ME, Duboeuf F, Brun J, Crouzet B, Arnaud S, Delmas PD, Meunier PJ. 1992. Vitamin D3 and calcium to prevent hip fractures in elderly women. *New England Journal of Medicine* 327:1637–1642.
108. Heikinheimo RJ, Inkovaara JA, Harju EJ, Haavisto MV, Kaarela RH, Kataja JM, Kokko AM, Kolho LA, Rajala SA. 1992. Annual injection of vitamin D and fractures of aged bones. *Calcified Tissue International* 51:105–110.
109. Matkovic V, Heaney RP. 1992. Calcium balance during human growth: Evidence for threshold behavior. *American Journal of Clinical Nutrition* 55:992–996.
110. Foster DW. 1994. Diabetes mellitus. In Isselbacher KJ, Braunwald E, Wilson JD, Martin JB, Fauci AS, Kasper DL, eds. *Harrison's principles of internal medicine,* 13th ed. New York: McGraw-Hill.
111. American Diabetes Association. 1994. *Maximizing the role of nutrition in diabetes management.* Alexandria, Va: American Diabetes Association.
112. Kovar MG, Harris MI, Hadden WG. 1987. The scope of diabetes in the United States population. *American Journal of Public Health* 77:1549–1550.
113. National Center for Health Statistics. 1994. Annual summary of births, marriages, divorces, and deaths: United States 1993. *Monthly Vital Statistics Report,* Vol. 42, No. 13. Hyattsville, Md: US Department of Health and Human Services, Public Health Service; Centers for Disease Control.
114. American Diabetic Association. 1989. Screening for diabetes. *Diabetes Care* 12:588–590.

115. Morris RD, Rimm DL, Hartz AJ, Kalkhoff RK, Rimm AA. 1989. Obesity and heredity in the etiology of non-insulin-dependent diabetes mellitus in 32,662 adult white women. *American Journal of Epidemiology* 130:112–121.
116. American Diabetes Association. 1993. *Medical management of pregnancy complicated by diabetes*. Alexandria, Va: American Diabetes Association.
117. Harris MJ. 1989. Impaired glucose tolerance in the US population. *Diabetes Care* 12:464–474.
118. Franz MJ, Horton ES, Bantle JP, Beebe CA, Brunzell JD, Coulston AM, Henry RR, Hoogwerf BJ, Stagpoole PW. 1994. Nutrition principles for the management of diabetes and related complications. *Diabetes Care*. 17:490–518.
119. Wallach J. 1992. *Interpretation of diagnostic tests,* 5th ed. Boston: Little, Brown.
120. DCCT Research Group. 1993. Expanded role of the dietitian in the Diabetes Control and Complications Trial: Implications for clinical practice. *Journal of the American Dietetic Association* 93:758–767.
121. American Diabetes Association. 1994. Nutrition recommendations and principles for people with diabetes mellitus. *Diabetes Care* 17:519–522.
122. Tinker LF, Heins JM, Holler HJ. 1994. Commentary and translation: 1994 nutrition recommendations for diabetes. *Journal of the American Dietetic Association* 94:507–511.
123. Astrup A, Buemann B, Western P, Toubro S, Raben A, Christensen NJ. 1994. Obesity as an adaptation to a high-fat diet: Evidence from a cross-sectional study. *American Journal of Clinical Nutrition* 59:350–355.

Assessment Activity 8-1

LIPID AND LIPOPROTEIN LEVELS AND CORONARY HEART DISEASE RISK

The National Cholesterol Education Program recommends that all adults 20 years of age or older know their serum total cholesterol. Values < 200 mg/dl (5.17 mmol/L) can be repeated at least every 5 years. Values of 200 mg/dl (5.17 mmol/L) or greater should be verified by a repeat measurement within 1 to 8 weeks. If the second value is within 30 mg/dl (0.8 mmol/L) of the first, the average of the two can be used as a guide for subsequent decisions. Otherwise, a third test should be obtained in another 1 to 8 weeks and the average of the three values used.

You are encouraged to have your blood lipid and lipoprotein levels measured and to know these values. There are several ways you can do this. Your professor may be able to arrange with student health services or a local hospital or clinical laboratory to have cholesterol and lipoprotein measurements performed on all interested students in your class. If measurements are done on several members of your class, they may be done at a reduced price; for example, triglycerides, total cholesterol, low-density-lipoprotein cholesterol, and high-density-lipoprotein cholesterol may be measured for $20 or less.

As an alternative or in addition to the above, your professor may be able to arrange to have a desktop blood analyzer brought to class so that each member who desires can have his or her total cholesterol measured. A variety of desktop analyzers are available including the Abbott Vision, the Boehringer-Mannheim Reflotron, and the Kodak Ektachem DT60 Analyzer. If this is not possible, you may want to have your cholesterol or lipid and lipoprotein levels measured on your own. Some hospitals offer low-priced testing as a community service.

When you receive your results, answer the following questions:

1. What are the highest, lowest, mean, and median values for each of the lipids and lipoproteins measured?
2. How do these compare with the population norms given in Appendix S?
3. What are the highest, lowest, mean, and median values for the ratio of total cholesterol to high-density-lipoprotein cholesterol?
4. How do these compare with the values shown in Appendix S?
5. Is there anyone in your class needing follow-up testing according to the National Cholesterol Education Program's guidelines given in this chapter?

Assessment Activity 8-2

CORONARY HEART DISEASE RISK PREDICTION CHART

The Framingham Heart Study Coronary Heart Disease Risk Prediction Chart is shown in Box 8-4. This chart can be used to approximate risk of coronary heart disease (CHD) during a 5- or 10-year period in persons who are currently free of CHD. As an example, take a 45-year-old male who has a total cholesterol of 223 mg/dl (5.77 mmol/L), a high-density-lipoprotein cholesterol (HDL-C) level of 43 mg/dl (1.11 mmol/L), and a systolic blood pressure of 127 mm Hg; is a non-smoker; has no diabetes; and has no left ventricular hypertrophy.

Using the Risk Prediction Chart, find the points for each risk factor. These are seven points for age, two points for total cholesterol, one point for HDL-C level, and one point for systolic blood pressure. A person smoking any amount of cigarettes is considered to be a smoker. According to the chart, a person has diabetes if he or she receives insulin or oral agents or has a fasting plasma glucose $\geq$ 140 mg/dl ($\geq$ 7.8 mmol/L); otherwise respond "no" for diabetes. A person has left ventricular hypertrophy (LVH) only if this has been definitely diagnosed by electrocardiogram (ECG); otherwise respond "no" for ECG-LVH. Subtract any minus points from the total. The total for this subject should be 11 points.

Determine the 5-year and 10-year CHD risk by looking up the risk corresponding to the subject's point total. With a total of 11 points, this subject has a 3% and 6% probability of CHD in the next 5 and 10 years, respectively. The average 10-year risk for males age 45 to 49 years is 10%. Thus this subject's 10-year risk of CHD is approximately 60% of average. Notice how predicted risk changes dramatically when one or two risk factors such as smoking or diabetes are altered. If you know your risk factor values, complete the chart for yourself.

NINE

BIOCHEMICAL ASSESSMENT OF NUTRITIONAL STATUS

OUTLINE

INTRODUCTION

Compared with the other methods of nutritional assessment (anthropometric, clinical methods, and dietary), biochemical tests provide the most objective and quantitative data on nutritional status. Biochemical tests often can detect nutrient deficits long before anthropometric measures are altered and clinical signs and symptoms appear. Some of these tests are useful indicators of recent nutrient intake and can be used in conjunction with dietary methods to assess food and nutrient consumption.

This chapter discusses the topic of biochemical methods in nutritional assessment, reviews the more commonly encountered tests for those nutrients of public health importance, and provides examples of various biochemical techniques in nutritional assessment.

Nutritional science is a relatively young discipline, and use of biochemical methods as indicators of nutritional status is still in its early development. This, along with all that yet remains unknown about the human body, makes the use of these measures in nutritional assessment a rapidly developing field and one with many research opportunities.

USE OF BIOCHEMICAL MEASURES

Biochemical tests available for assessing nutritional status can be grouped into two general and somewhat arbitrary categories: *static tests* and *functional tests*. These are sometimes referred to as *direct* and *indirect tests,* respectively.[1] Other, more detailed classification schemes also may be encountered.[2]

Static tests are based on measurement of a nutrient or its metabolite in the blood, urine, or body tissue—for example, serum measurements of albumin, calcium, or vitamin A. These are among the most readily available tests, but they have certain limitations. Although they indicate nutrient levels in the particular tissue or fluid sampled, they often fail to reflect the overall nutrient status of an individual or whether the body as a whole is in a state of nutrient excess or depletion.[3] For example, the amount of calcium in serum can be easily determined, but that single static measurement is a poor indicator of the body's overall calcium status or of bone mineral content.

Functional tests of nutritional status are based on the idea that "the final outcome of a nutrient deficiency and its biologic importance are not merely a measured level in a tissue or blood, but the failure of one or more physiologic processes that rely on that nutrient for optimal performance."[2] Included among these functional tests are measurement of dark adaptation (assesses vitamin A status), urinary excretion of xanthurenic acid in response to consumption of tryptophan (assesses vitamin B_6 status), and impairment of immune status resulting from protein-energy malnutrition and other nutrient deficits. Although many functional tests remain in the experimental stage, this is an area of active research and one that is likely to be fruitful.[2] One drawback of some functional tests, however, is a tendency to be nonspecific; they may indicate general nutritional status but not allow identification of specific nutrient deficiencies.[2]

Biochemical tests can also be used to examine the validity of various methods of measuring dietary intake or to determine if respondents are underreporting or overreporting what they eat. The ability of a food frequency questionnaire to accurately measure protein intake, for example, can be assessed by 24-hour urine nitrogen excretion. When properly used, this method is sufficiently accurate to use as a validation method in dietary surveys. As with any test requiring a 24-hour urine sample, however, each collection must be complete (i.e., respondents must collect all urine during an exact 24-hour period). Urinary nitrogen is best estimated using multiple 24-hour urine samples, and any extrarenal nitrogen losses must be accounted for.[4] The doubly labeled water technique, as mentioned in Chapters 3 and 7, is another biochemical test useful for determining validity and accuracy of reporting. It can be an accurate way of measuring energy expenditure without interfering with a respondent's everyday life.[5] If reported energy and protein consumption fail to match estimates of energy and protein intake derived from these properly performed biochemical tests, then the dietary assessment method may be faulty or the respondent did not accurately report food intake.

Biochemical tests are a valuable adjunct in assessing and managing nutritional status; however, their use is not without problems. Most notable among these is the influence that nonnutritional factors can have on test results. A variety of pathologic conditions, use of certain medications, and technical problems in a sample collection or assay can affect test results in ways that make them unusable. Another problem with some biochemical tests is their nonspecificity. A certain test may indicate that a patient's general nutritional status is impaired yet lack the specificity to indicate which particular nutrient is deficient. Additionally, no single test, index, or group of tests by itself is sufficient for monitoring nutritional status. Biochemical tests must be used in conjunction with measures of dietary intake, anthropometric measures, and clinical methods.

PROTEIN STATUS

The importance of assessing protein status has been well summarized by Phinney:[6]

> Protein is the principal compound upon which body structure and function is based. Unlike the major fuels, fat and carbohydrate, it is not stored to any degree in a non-functional form awaiting use. In this context, a gain or loss of protein represents an equivalent gain or loss of function, and thus evaluation of a patient's protein nutriture can be very important.

Assessing protein status can be approached by use of anthropometric (Chapters 6 and 7), biochemical, clinical (Chapter 10), and dietary data (Chapters 3 and 4). Although each of these approaches has its strengths and limitations, biochemical methods have the potential of being the most objective and quantitative.[7]

Biochemical assessment of protein status has typically been approached from the perspective of the "two-compartment" model: evaluation of somatic protein and visceral protein status. The body's somatic protein is found within skeletal muscle. Visceral protein can be regarded as consisting of protein within the organs or viscera of the body (liver, kidneys, pancreas, heart, and so on), the erythrocytes (red blood cells), and the granulocytes and lymphocytes (white blood cells), as well as the serum proteins.[8] The somatic and visceral pools contain the metabolically available protein (known as body cell mass), which can be drawn upon, when necessary, to meet various bodily needs. The somatic and visceral protein pools comprise about 75% and 25% of the body cell mass, respectively.[6] Together, they comprise about 30% to 50% of total body protein.[8] The remaining body protein is found primarily in the skin and connective tissue (bone matrix, cartilage, tendons, and ligaments) and is not readily exchangeable with the somatic and visceral protein pools.[6] Division of the body's protein into these two "compartments" is somewhat arbitrary and artificial. Although the somatic compartment is homogeneous, the visceral protein pool is composed of hundreds of different proteins serving many different structural and functional roles.

Although protein is not considered a public health issue among the general population of developed nations, protein-energy malnutrition (PEM), also known as protein-calorie malnutrition, can be a result of certain diseases and is clearly a pressing concern in many developing nations. Protein-energy malnutrition can be seen in persons with cancer and acquired immunodeficiency syndrome (AIDS), children who fail to thrive, and homeless persons.

Because of its high prevalence and relationship to infant mortality and impaired physical growth, PEM is considered the most important nutritional disease in developing countries.[9] It is also of concern in developed nations. According to some reports, PEM has been observed in nearly half of the patients hospitalized in medical and surgical wards in the United States. In more recent studies, the prevalence of PEM ranged from 30% to 40% among patients with hip fractures, patients undergoing thoracic surgery for lung cancer, patients receiving ambulatory peritoneal dialysis, and children and adolescents with juvenile rheumatoid arthritis.[10–13]

Assessment of protein status is central to the prevention, diagnosis, and treatment of PEM. The causes of PEM can either be primary (inadequate food intake) or secondary (other diseases leading to insufficient food intake, inadequate nutrient absorption or utilization, increased nutritional requirement, and increased nutrient losses).[7,9] The protein and energy needs of hospitalized patients can be two or more times those of healthy persons as a result of hypermetabolism accompanying trauma, infection, burns, and surgical recovery.[14] PEM can result in kwashiorkor (principally a protein deficiency), marasmus (predominantly an energy deficiency), or marasmic kwashiorkor (a combination of chronic energy deficit and chronic or acute protein deficiency).[9] Clinical findings pertinent to kwashiorkor and marasmus are discussed in Chapter 10.

As Young and coworkers[7] have written, "no single test or group of tests can be recommended at this time as a routine and reliable indicator of protein status." Each of the approaches discussed in this and other sections of this text has certain limitations.

Densitometry, total body potassium, and total body nitrogen (discussed in Chapter 6) stand out as relatively precise and accurate methods of assessing protein status but have limited clinical application because of their expense, limited availability, and problems with patient tolerance. Total body nitrogen as measured by neutron activation analysis and total body potassium as measured by either potassium-40 counting or neutron activation analysis are limited by the expense of the procedures and the availability of equipment. Body weight is a readily obtained indicator of energy and protein reserves. However, it must be carefully interpreted because it fails to distinguish between fat mass and fat-free mass, and losses of skeletal muscle and adipose tissue can be masked by water retention resulting from edema and ascites. The creatinine-height index is also well suited to the clinical setting but has limited precision and accuracy. Use of midarm muscle circumference and midarm muscle area are two other approaches to assessing somatic protein status. These are discussed in Chapter 7.

Rather than relying on any single indicator, a combination of measures can produce a more complete picture of protein status. The choice of approaches depends on methods available to the particular facility. Biochemical data on nutritional status constitute only part of the necessary information to properly quantitate nutritional depletion and PEM. Data relating to dietary intake, pertinent anthropometric measures, and clinical findings are necessary, as well.

Creatinine Excretion and Creatinine-Height Index

A biochemical test sometimes used for estimating body muscle mass is 24-hour urinary creatinine excretion. Creatinine, a product of skeletal muscle, is excreted in a relatively constant proportion to the mass of muscle in the body. It is

TABLE 9-1 Expected 24-hour urinary creatinine values for height for adult males and females

Adult males*		Adult females†	
Height (cm)	Creatinine (mg)	Height (cm)	Creatinine (mg)
157.5	1288	147.3	830
160.0	1325	149.9	851
162.6	1359	152.4	875
165.1	1386	154.9	900
167.6	1426	157.5	925
170.2	1467	160.0	949
172.7	1513	162.6	977
175.3	1555	165.1	1006
177.8	1596	167.6	1044
180.3	1642	170.2	1076
182.9	1691	172.7	1109
185.4	1739	175.3	1141
188.0	1785	177.8	1174
190.5	1831	180.3	1206
193.0	1891	182.9	1240

Adapted from Blackburn GL, Bistrian BR, Maini BS, Schlamm HT, Smith MR. 1977. Nutritional and metabolic assessment of the hospitalized patient. *Journal of Parenteral and Enteral Nutrition* 1:11–12.

*Creatinine coefficient for males = 23 mg/kg of "ideal" body weight.

†Creatinine coefficient for females = 18 mg/kg of "ideal" body weight.

readily measured by any clinical laboratory. Lean body mass can be estimated by comparing 24-hour urine creatinine excretion with a standard based on stature (Table 9-1) or from reference values of 23 and 18 mg/kg of recommended body weight for males and females, respectively. Another approach is using the creatinine-height index (CHI), a ratio of a patient's measured 24-hour urinary creatinine excretion and the expected excretion of a reference adult of the same sex and stature. The CHI is expressed by the following formula:

$$\text{CHI} = \frac{\text{24-hr urine creatinine (mg)} \times 100}{\text{expected 24-hr urine creatinine (mg)}}$$

Expected 24-hour urine creatinine values are shown in Table 9-1. These should be matched to the subject's sex and height.

The CHI is expressed as a percent of expected value. A CHI of 60% to 80% is considered indicative of mild protein depletion; 40% to 60% reflects moderate protein depletion; and a value under 40% represents severe depletion.[2]

As mentioned earlier in this chapter, a major concern when using any test requiring a 24-hour urine sample is obtaining a complete urine sample collected during an exact 24-hour period. The value of protein status measurements based on urinary creatinine measurements can also be compromised by the effect of diet on urine creatinine levels, variability in creatinine excretion, and use of height-weight tables for determining expected creatinine excretion based on sex and stature.[6] These limitations are discussed in Chapter 6.

3-Methylhistidine

Measurement of urinary excretion of 3-methylhistidine is another potential approach for assessing muscle mass. It is subject to many of the same problems as assessment of urinary creatinine excretion (see Chapter 6), and values can be affected by a variety of factors such as age, sex, maturity, hormonal status, degree of physical fitness, recent intense exercise, injury, and disease.[2,7] There also appears to be a significant pool of 3-methylhistidine outside of skeletal muscle, further complicating its use as an index of skeletal muscle protein breakdown.[15] Additional research into this approach is needed. However, it is doubtful that this method will become a routine biochemical assessment technique.

Nitrogen Balance

A person is said to be in nitrogen balance when the amount of nitrogen (consumed as protein) equals the amount excreted by the body. Nitrogen balance is the expected state of the healthy adult. It occurs when the rate of protein synthesis or anabolism equals the rate of protein degradation or catabolism. Positive nitrogen balance occurs when nitrogen intake exceeds nitrogen loss and is seen in periods of anabolism such as childhood or recovery from trauma, surgery, or illness. Negative nitrogen balance occurs when nitrogen losses exceed nitrogen intake and can result from insufficient protein intake, catabolic states (for example, sepsis, trauma, surgery, and cancer), or during periods of excessive protein loss (as a result of burns or certain gastrointestinal and renal diseases characterized by unusual protein loss). Nutritional support can help return a patient to positive nitrogen balance or at least prevent severe losses of energy stores and body protein.[2,14]

Nitrogen balance studies involve 24-hour measurement of protein intake and an estimate of nitrogen losses from the body. The following formula is used:

$$N_2 \text{ Balance} = \frac{\text{PRO}}{6.25} - \text{UUN} - 4$$

where N_2 Balance = nitrogen balance; PRO = protein intake (g/24 hr); and UUN = urine urea nitrogen (g/24 hr).

Protein intake, measured by dietary assessment methods, is divided by 6.25 to arrive at an estimate of nitrogen intake. Nitrogen loss is generally estimated by measuring urine urea nitrogen (which accounts for 85% to 90% of nitrogen in the urine) and adding a constant (for example, 4 g) to account for nitrogen losses from the skin, stool, wound drainage, nonurea nitrogen, and so on, which cannot be easily measured.[2,14]

Problems associated with measuring protein intake and nitrogen excretion limit the usefulness of this approach. For example, it is difficult to account for the unusually high nonurine nitrogen losses seen in some patients with burns, diarrhea, vomiting, or fistula drainage. In such cases, this approach to calculating nitrogen balance may not yield accurate results.

Serum Proteins

Serum proteins concentrations can be useful in assessing protein status, determining whether a patient is at risk of experiencing medical complications, and for evaluating a patient's response to nutritional support. The serum proteins of primary interest in nutritional assessment are shown in Table 9-2.[14] In most instances, their measurement is simple and accurate. Use of serum protein measurements is based on the assumption that decreases in serum concentrations are due to decreased liver production (the primary site of synthesis). This is considered a consequence of a limited supply of amino acids from which the serum proteins are synthesized or a decrease in the liver's capacity to synthesize serum proteins. The extent to which nutritional status or liver function affects serum protein concentrations cannot always be determined. A number of factors other than inadequate protein intake affect serum protein concentrations. These are noted in the following sections or in Table 9-2.

TABLE 9-2 Serum proteins used in nutritional assessment

Serum protein	Normal value, Mean ± SD or (Range)*	Half-life	Function	Comments†
Albumin	45 (35–50)	18–20 days	Maintains plasma oncotic pressure; carrier for small molecules.	In addition to protein status, other factors affect serum concentrations as discussed in text.
Transferrin	2.3 (2.6–4.3)	8–9 days	Binds iron in plasma and transports to bone marrow.	Iron deficiency increases hepatic synthesis and plasma levels; increases during pregnancy, during estrogen therapy, and acute hepatitis; reduced in protein-losing enteropathy and nephropathy, chronic infections, uremia, and acute catabolic states; often measured indirectly by total iron-binding capacity; equations for indirect prediction should be developed locally
Prealbumin	0.30 (0.2–0.4)	2–3 days	Binds T_3 and, to a lesser extent, T_4; carrier for retinol-binding protein	Increased in patients with chronic renal failure on dialysis due to decreased renal catabolism; reduced in acute catabolic states, after surgery, in hyperthyroidism, in protein-losing enteropathy; increased in some cases of nephrotic syndrome; serum level determined by overall energy balance as well as nitrogen balance

Continued

TABLE 9-2 Serum proteins used in nutritional assessment—cont'd

Serum protein	Normal value, Mean ± SD or (Range)*	Half-life	Function	Comments†
Retinol-binding protein (RBP)	0.372 ± 0.0073‡	12 hr	Transports vitamin A in plasma; binds noncovalently to prealbumin	Catabolized in renal proximal tubular cell; with renal disease, RBP increases and half-life is prolonged; low in vitamin A deficiency, acute catabolic states, after surgery, and in hyperthyroidism
Insulin-like growth factor-1 (IGF-1)	0.83 IU/ml (0.55–1.4)	2–6 hr	One of a family of insulin-like peptides that have anabolic actions on fat, muscle, cartilage, and cultured cells	Referred to earlier as somatomedin-C; levels fall rapidly with fasting and quickly recover during refeeding; low values in hypothyroid patients, with estrogen administration, and possibly in obesity; may be a valid nutritional marker during acute-phase response
Fibronectin	Plasma: 2.92 ± 0.2 Serum: 1.82 ± 0.16	4–24 hr	A glycoprotein found in many tissues; a soluble form appears in blood and behaves as an opsonic glycoprotein; may exert chemotactic activity and be involved in wound healing	Plasma fibronectin deficiency may contribute to host defense suppression with malnutrition; may be a sensitive marker during nutritional depletion and repletion; levels may be influenced by acute-phase response; more clinical studies needed; reference ranges not well studied

Adapted from Heymsfield SB, Tighe A, Wang ZM. 1994. Nutritional assessment by anthropometric and biochemical methods. In Shils ME, Olson JA, Shike M (eds.). *Modern nutrition in health and disease,* 8th ed. Philadelphia: Lea & Febiger.

*Units are g/l. Normal range varies among centers; check local values.

†All the listed proteins are influenced by hydration and the presence of hepatocellular dysfunction.

‡Normal values are age and sex dependent. Table value is for pooled subjects.

TABLE 9-3 Factors determining serum albumin levels

Rate of synthesis	Biosynthesis is decreased by lack of dietary protein, physiologic stress, liver disease, hypothyroidism, and the presence of excessive levels of serum cortisol.
Distribution in body	Normally, 30% to 40% of the body's albumin is found in the blood and lymphatic vessels (the intravascular space) with the remainder in lean tissues outside the blood and lymphatic vessels (the extravascular space), especially the skin. Following surgery or thermal injury, albumin shifts from the intravascular space to the extravascular space, with a concomitant fall in serum albumin levels. In semistarvation, albumin shifts from the extravascular space to the intravascular space.
Rate of catabolism	The catabolic rate is decreased in semistarvation and hypometabolism and increased by physiologic stress, hypermetabolism, Cushing's syndrome, and some malignant tumors.
Abnormal losses from the body	Causes of abnormal losses include thermal burns, nephrotic syndrome, and protein-losing enteropathies.
Altered fluid status	Levels decline when blood volume increases from such causes as congestive heart failure, fluid overload, and renal failure. Dehydration decreases blood volume and results in increased albumin levels.

Albumin

The most familiar and abundant of the serum proteins, as well as the most readily available clinically, is albumin. Serum albumin level has been shown to be an indicator of depleted protein status and decreased dietary protein intake. Measured over the course of several weeks, it has been shown to correlate with other measures of protein status (for example, measures of immunocompetence) and to respond to protein repletion. Low concentrations of serum albumin are associated with increased morbidity and mortality in hospitalized patients.[7,16,17] Despite these correlations, the value of albumin as a protein status indicator is limited by several factors. Its relatively long half-life (14 to 20 days) and large body pool (4 to 5 g/kg of body weight) cause serum levels to respond slowly to nutritional change, making it a poor indicator of early protein depletion and repletion.[2,7,14]

Serum albumin level is determined by several factors: the rate of synthesis, its distribution in the body, the rate at which it is catabolized, abnormal losses from the body, and altered fluid status.[14] These are summarized in Table 9-3. About 60% of the body's albumin is found outside the bloodstream. When serum concentrations begin falling during early PEM, this extravascular albumin moves into the bloodstream, helping to maintain normal serum concentrations despite protein and energy deficit.[2,7,14] During the acute catabolic phase of an injury, infection, or surgery, there is increased synthesis of substances known as acute-phase reactants. Included among these are C-reactive protein, fibrinogen, haptoglobin, and $Á_1$-glycoprotein. Acute-phase reactants decrease synthesis of albumin, prealbumin, and transferrin. Consequently, levels of these serum proteins may remain low during this catabolic phase despite the provision of adequate nutritional support.[14] The practice of administrating albumin to severely ill patients also can interfere with its use as an indicator of protein status.[4]

Transferrin

Serum transferrin is a β-globulin synthesized in the liver that binds and transports iron in the plasma. Because of its smaller body pool and shorter half-life, it has been considered a better index of changes in protein status compared to albumin.[2] Although serum transferrin has been shown to be associated with clinical outcome in children with kwashiorkor and marasmus, its use to predict morbidity and mortality outcomes in hospitalized patients has produced conflicting results.[8]

Serum transferrin can be measured directly (by radial immunodiffusion and nephelometry), but it is frequently estimated indirectly from total iron-binding capacity (TIBC) using a prediction formula suited to the particular facility's method for measuring TIBC.[8]

The use of transferrin as an index of nutritional status and repletion is limited by several factors other than protein status that affect its serum concentration. As outlined in Table 9-2, transferrin levels decrease in chronic infections, protein-losing enteropathies, chronically draining wounds, nephropathy, acute catabolic states (e.g., surgery and trauma), and uremia. Serum levels can be increased during pregnancy, estrogen therapy, and acute hepatitis.[14,18]

Prealbumin

Prealbumin, also known as transthyretin and thyroxine-binding prealbumin, is synthesized in the liver and serves as a transport protein for thyroxine (T_4) and as a carrier protein for retinol-binding protein. Because of its short half-life (2 to 3 days) and small body pool (0.01 g/kg body weight), it is considered a more sensitive indicator of protein nutriture and one that responds more rapidly to changes in protein status than albumin or transferrin.

Prealbumin decreases rapidly in response to deficits of either protein or energy and is sensitive to the early stages of malnutrition. Because serum concentration quickly returns to expected levels once adequate nutritional therapy begins, it is not recommended as an endpoint for terminating nutritional support. It may prove to be better suited as an indicator of recent dietary intake than as a means of assessing nutritional status.[2] Serum concentration also will return to expected levels in response to adequate energy in the absence of sufficient protein intake. Its use as an indicator of protein status appears to be preferable to the use of albumin or transferrin. However, like the other serum proteins outlined in Table 9-2, several factors other than protein status affect its concentration in serum. Levels are reduced in liver disease, sepsis, protein-losing enteropathies, hyperthyroidism, and acute catabolic states (e.g., following surgery or trauma). Serum prealbumin can be increased in patients with chronic renal failure who are on dialysis due to decreased renal catabolism.[14,18]

Retinol-Binding Protein

Retinol-binding protein, a liver protein, acts as a carrier for retinol (vitamin A alcohol) when complexed with prealbumin. It circulates in the blood as a 1:1:1 trimolecular complex with retinol and prealbumin.[19] Retinol-binding protein shares several features with prealbumin. It responds quickly to protein-energy deprivation and adequate nutritional therapy, as well as to ample energy in the absence of sufficient protein. Like prealbumin, it may be a better indicator of recent dietary intake than of overall nutritional status. It has a much shorter half-life (about 12 hours) than prealbumin. Its smaller body pool (0.002 g/kg body weight), however, complicates its precise measurement. There is no convincing evidence that its use in nutritional assessment is preferred over prealbumin. Because it is catabolized in the renal proximal tubule cell, serum levels are increased in renal disease and its half-life is prolonged. Serum levels can be decreased in vitamin A deficiency, acute catabolic states, and hyperthyroidism.[14]

Insulin-like Growth Factor-1

Also referred to as somatomedin C, insulin-like growth factor-1 (IGF-1) is a growth-promoting peptide produced by the liver in response to growth hormone stimulation. Although technically not a serum protein, it is included in this section for the sake of convenience. Decreased serum concentration of IGF-1 is seen in PEM.[7] Unlike prealbumin, its concentration in serum is restored by adequate administration of protein, but not when ample energy is present in the absence of protein deficit. Low serum concentrations of IGF-1 in patients with PEM were shown to return to expected levels after 3 to 16 days of nutritional therapy. During the same period, no significant changes were seen in serum albumin, transferrin, prealbumin, and retinol-binding protein, suggesting that IGF-1 is a more sensitive indicator of protein status.[22] IGF-1 may be a valid indicator of nutritional status during the acute phase response.[14]

The combination of low serum concentration of IGF-1 and normal or elevated concentration of growth hormone indicates the presence of PEM. Although this pattern of IGF-1 and growth hormone can result from several other conditions as well (for example, hypothyroidism, renal failure, cirrhosis of the liver, and peripheral growth hormone resistance), most of these conditions can be ruled out by other biochemical tests or physical examination.[2,14]

IGF-1 shows promise as an indicator of protein status, but additional research is required before it becomes a routine test in the clinical setting.[7]

Fibronectin

Fibronectin is a glycoprotein synthesized by many cell types, including liver cells, endothelial cells, and fibroblasts. In contrast to the previously discussed serum proteins, the nonliver sources appear to be most important. Fibronectin functions in cell adhesion, wound healing, hemostasis, and macrophage function.[2] Nutritional deprivation results in decreased serum concentrations, which return to expected levels upon nutritional therapy.[21–25] In malnourished children, low serum concentrations of fibronectin respond to nutritional therapy more readily than other signs.[21] Children with PEM who receive intravenous administration of fibronectin as an adjunct to nutritional therapy have decreased mortality and faster normalization of albumin, transferrin, and prealbumin serum concentrations compared with children in a control group.[24]

Other factors affecting serum concentrations of fibronectin include trauma, burns, shock, and sepsis. Fibronectin holds promise as a useful indicator of nutritional status, but additional research is required before it becomes a routine part of clinical care.[2]

Immunocompetence

A close and complex relationship exists between nutrition and immunity. Nutritional deficits can lead to impaired immunocompetence, infection, and inflammation, which in turn can have profound effects on nutrition and nutrient metabolism.[2,25] Tests of immunocompetence can be useful functional indicators of nutritional status. Because changes in immune response can occur early in nutritional deficiency, immunocompetence can be used as an early functional indicator of nutritional status and as an index of response to nutritional support.[25,26]

Anergy and other immunological changes can be used as prognostic indicators for complications, duration of hospitalization, and mortality in medical and surgical patients.[26] Immune responses may be useful in determining safe upper and lower limits of nutrient intake. Although sensitive to impaired nutritional status, they often lack specificity: they are good indicators of general nutritional deficit but can rarely identify the specific nutritional deficiency.[2,7,25] A variety of factors other than nutritional status also can affect immunocompetence.

Specific and Nonspecific Immunity

The immune system's defense mechanisms can be divided into two broad categories: nonspecific and antigen specific.[26] The nonspecific defenses include the skin, mucous membranes, phagocytic cells, mucus, cilia, complement, lysozyme, and interferon. These are naturally present defenses that act as the first line of protection against infection and are not influenced by prior contact with infectious agents. The antigen-specific defenses act in response to exposure to specific infectious agents and antigens (molecules that stimulate antibody production) and involve the B-lymphocytes and T-lymphocytes. B-lymphocytes, responsible for humoral immunity, secrete antibodies. T-lymphocytes, responsible for cell-mediated immunity, attack host cells that have become infected with viruses or fungi, transplanted human cells, and cancerous cells.[27] Compared with other parts of the immune system, the effects of malnutrition on cell-mediated immunity are more frequent, develop earlier, and are more clinically significant.[2] A variety of responses to nutrient deficiency, especially PEM, have been identified and used as indicators of nutritional status.

Total Lymphocyte Count

The total number of lymphocytes can be derived from a routine complete blood count that includes a *differential count.* The differential gives the percentage of different white blood cells in the sample examined. The percentage of lymphocytes in the sample is multiplied by the number of white blood cells (WBCs) and divided by 100:

$$\text{TLC} = \frac{\%\text{ of lymphocytes} \times \text{WBC count}}{100}$$

where TLC = total lymphocyte count; % lymphocytes = percentage of lymphocytes from the differential count; and WBC count = white blood cell count (cells/mm^3).

According to Grant and coworkers, mild nutritional depletion would be represented by a total lymphocyte count within the range of 1200 to 1800 lymphocytes/mm^3, moderate depletion would be in the range of 800 to 1199 lymphocytes/mm^3, and less than 800 lymphocytes/mm^3 would represent severe depletion.

Factors affecting total lymphocyte count besides nutritional status include cancer, inflammation, infection, stress, sepsis, and certain drugs, such as steroids, chemotherapeutic agents, and immunosuppressive agents.

Delayed Cutaneous Hypersensitivity

Delayed cutaneous hypersensitivity (DCH) involves the injection of a small amount of antigen within the skin (intradermally) to determine the subject's reaction. Because the degree of reactivity to the antigen is a function of the subject's cell-mediated immunity (the T-lymphocytes),[28] the test is sometimes referred to as cell-mediated hypersensitivity.[29] Under normal conditions, the injection site should become inflamed, with a characteristic hardening (induration) and redness (erythema) noted between 24 and 72 hours after injection. In persons with compromised cell-mediated immunity, the response would be less than expected or absent (known as *anergy*). Antigens used include streptokinase-streptodornase, candidin, trichophyton, tuberculin (purified protein derivative), and mumps.[29]

DCH is reported to be decreased in PEM and deficiencies of vitamins B_6 and A, zinc, and iron. As summarized by Twomey and coworkers,[30] a subject's reactivity also is affected by a variety of technical factors (including antigen source and batch, method of administration, and reader variability), patient factors (such as age, prior exposure to antigen, and psychologic state), several drugs, and a number of diseases (including infection, inflammation, immune alterations, and cancers).

IRON STATUS

Iron deficiency is the most common single nutrient deficiency in the United States and the most

TABLE 9-4 Stages of iron depletion and the laboratory tests used to identify them

Stage	Descriptive term	Biochemical test
First	Depleted iron stores	Serum ferritin level
Second	Iron deficiency (without anemia)	Transferrin saturation Erythrocyte protoporphyrin
Third	Iron-deficiency anemia	Hemoglobin Mean corpuscular

From Life Sciences Research Office, Federation of American Societies of Experimental Biology. 1989. *Nutrition monitoring in the United States: An update report on nutrition monitoring*. Washington, DC: U.S. Department of Health and Human Services, Public Health Services.

common cause of anemia. Although the prevalence of iron deficiency appears to have declined in recent years, it remains relatively high in vulnerable groups such as women of childbearing age.[31]

Iron deficiency results when ingestion or absorption of dietary iron is inadequate to meet iron losses or iron requirements imposed by growth or pregnancy. Considerable iron can be lost from heavy menstruation, frequent blood donations, early feeding of cow's milk to infants, frequent aspirin use, or disorders characterized by gastrointestinal bleeding. Risk of iron deficiency increases during periods of rapid growth, notably in infancy (especially in premature infants), adolescence, and pregnancy. The consequences of iron deficiency include reduced work capacity, impaired body temperature regulation, impairments in behavior and intellectual performance, increased susceptibility to lead poisoning, and decreased resistance to infections.[31]

Anemia is a hemoglobin level below the normal reference range for individuals of the same sex and age. Descriptive terms such as *microcytic, macrocytic,* and *hypochromic* are sometimes used to describe anemias. Microcytic refers to abnormally small red blood cells defined by a mean corpuscular volume (MCV) < 80 femtoliters (fL), whereas macrocytic describes unusually large red blood cells defined as an MCV > 100 fL. Hypochromic cells are those with abnormally low levels of hemoglobin as defined by a mean corpuscular hemoglobin concentration < 320 g of hemoglobin/L or by a mean corpuscular hemoglobin < 27 picograms (pg, 10^{-12} grams).

Although the most common cause of anemia is iron deficiency, it also may result from infection, chronic disease, and deficiencies of folate and vitamin B_{12}. Of particular concern to physicians working with individual patients and nutritional epidemiologists attempting to estimate the prevalence of iron deficiency in populations is differentiating iron-deficiency anemia from anemia caused by inflammatory disease, infection, chronic diseases, and thalassemia traits.[32]

Stages of Iron Depletion

The risk of iron deficiency increases as the body's iron stores are depleted. Iron depletion can be divided into three stages. These stages and the biochemical tests used in identifying them are shown in Table 9-4. Figure 9-1 illustrates how values for these different tests change throughout the different stages of iron deficiency.

The first stage of iron depletion, depleted iron stores, is not associated with any adverse physiologic effects, but it does represent a state of vulnerability.[31,33] Low stores occur in healthy persons and appear to be the usual physiologic condition for growing children and menstruating women.[31,34] As shown in Figure 9-1, during this

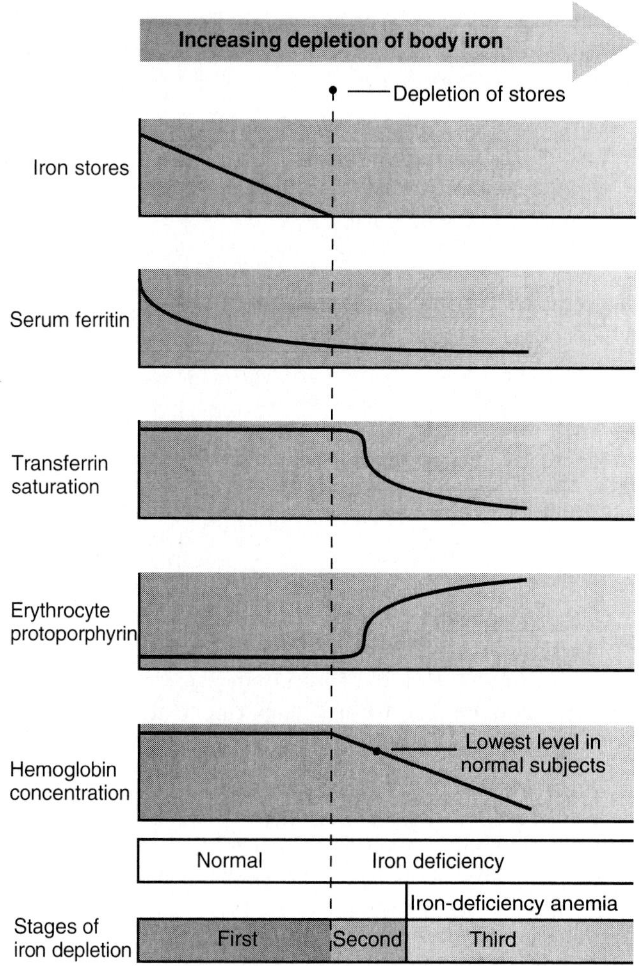

Figure 9-1 Changes in body iron compartments and laboratory assessments of iron status during the stages of iron depletion. From Life Sciences Research Office, Federation of American Societies for Experimental Biology. 1989. *Nutrition monitoring in the United States: An update report on nutrition monitoring*. Washington, DC: U.S. Government Printing Office.

first stage, low iron stores are reflected by decreased serum ferritin levels, but values for the other biochemical tests remain within normal limits.

The second stage of iron depletion, iron deficiency without anemia, can be considered representative of early or mild iron deficiency because, at this point, adverse physiologic consequences can begin to occur. This stage is characterized by changes indicating insufficient iron for normal production of hemoglobin and other essential iron compounds (for example, myoglobin and iron-containing enzymes).[31,33] As shown in Figure 9-1, this stage is assessed by decreased transferrin saturation and increased erythrocyte protoporphyrin levels. A precursor of hemoglobin, erythrocyte protoporphyrin increases when too little iron is available for optimal hemoglobin synthesis. Although hemoglobin may be decreased at this stage, it may not fall below the lowest levels seen in normal subjects. Consequently, hemoglobin is not a useful indicator of either stage one or stage two iron depletion.[31]

The third stage of iron depletion, iron-fjdeficiency anemia, is characterized by decreased serum ferritin, transferrin saturation, hemoglobin, and MCV and increased erythrocyte protoporphyrin.[31,33]

No single biochemical test is diagnostic of impaired iron status. Several different static tests used together provide a much better measure of iron status.[31] These indicators are discussed in the following sections.

Serum Ferritin

When the protein apoferritin combines with iron, ferritin is formed. Ferritin, the primary storage form for iron in the body, is found primarily in the liver, spleen, and bone marrow. In healthy persons, approximately 30% of all iron in the body is in the storage form, most of this as ferritin but some as hemosiderin. As iron stores become depleted, tissue ferritin levels decrease. This is accompanied by a fall in serum ferritin concentration.[35] Measurement of serum ferritin concentration is the most sensitive test available for detecting iron deficiency, and decreases occur before morphologic changes are seen in red blood cells, in the other indicators shown in Figure 9-1, or before anemia occurs.[35] From Figures 9-1 and 9-2 it can also be noted that once serum stores are depleted, serum ferritin levels no longer reflect the severity of iron deficiency. Cutoff values for serum ferritin and other tests used to indicate the presence of iron deficiency in the second National Health and Nutrition Examination Survey (NHANES II) are shown in Table 9-5.[31]

Serum ferritin levels can be increased by the presence of inflammation, infection, trauma, certain chronic diseases, iron overload (excessive iron stores), viral hepatitis, and certain cancers (for example, Hodgkin's disease).[35]

Transferrin, Serum Iron, and Total Iron-binding Capacity

Iron is transported in the blood bound to transferrin, a β-globulin protein molecule synthesized in the liver. Transferrin accepts iron from sites of hemoglobin destruction (the primary source for iron bound to transferrin) and from storage sites and iron absorbed through the intestinal tract. It then delivers the iron to sites where it is utilized—primarily the bone marrow for hemoglobin synthesis, as well as storage sites, the placenta for fetal needs, and to all cells for incorporation into iron-containing enzymes. Each molecule of transferrin has the capacity to transport two atoms of iron, but under most circumstances only about 30% of the available iron-binding sites are occupied or saturated.[34]

Because iron is carried in the blood by transferrin, serum iron level is a measure of the amount of iron bound to transferrin. Levels fall sometime between depletion of tissue iron stores and development of anemia, although they may actually be normal in persons with iron deficiency.[34,35]

Total iron-binding capacity measures the amount of iron capable of being bound to serum proteins and provides an estimate of serum transferrin. It is usually measured by adding an excess of iron to serum (thus saturating iron-binding proteins in serum), removing all iron not bound to protein in the serum, and then measuring serum iron. Because it is assumed that most serum iron is bound to transferrin, TIBC is an indirect measure of serum transferrin. Because other serum proteins can bind iron, TIBC is not an exact measure of transferrin, especially in cases of iron overload and certain other conditions. In about 30% to 40% of persons with iron-deficiency anemia, TIBC is not elevated.[35]

Transferrin saturation is the ratio of serum iron to TIBC and is calculated using the following formula:

$$TS = \frac{\text{Serum iron } (\mu \text{ mol/L})}{\text{TIBC } (\mu \text{ mol/L})} \times 100$$

where TS = percent transferrin saturation, and TIBC = total iron-binding capacity.

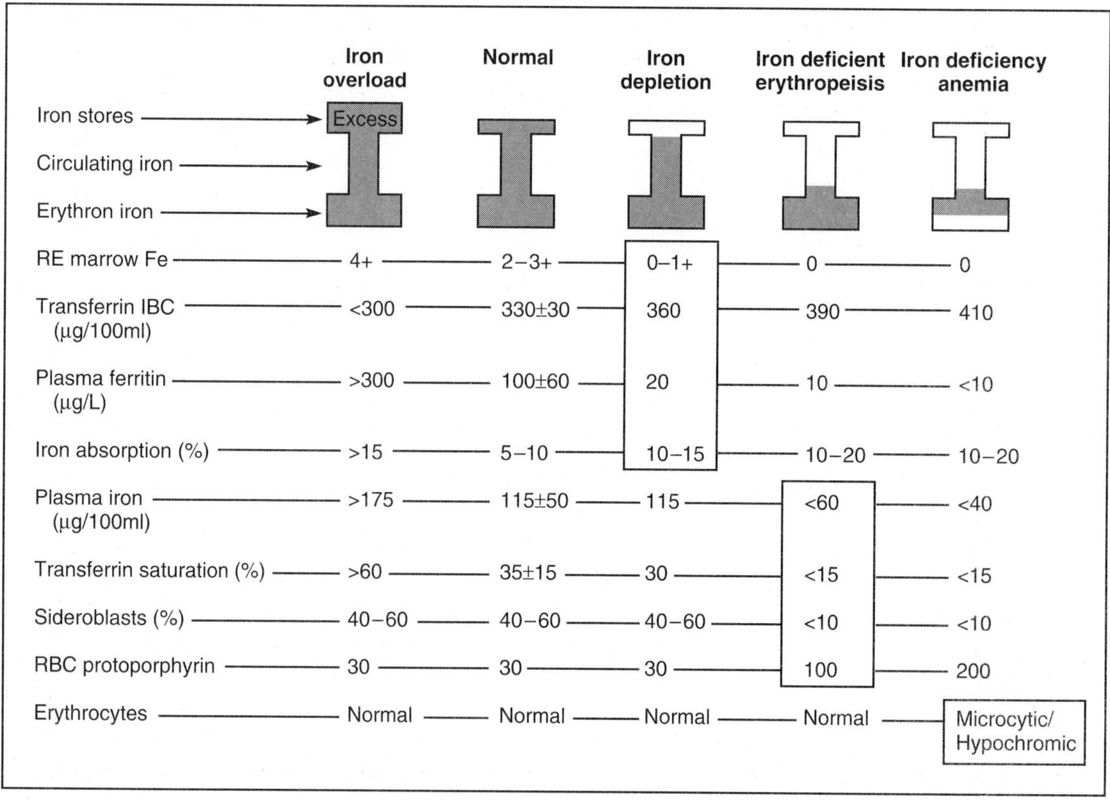

Figure 9-2 Sequence of events in developing iron deficiency and overload. The shaded areas indicate the relative quantities of iron in each compartment (e.g., in stores, circulating, and in the erythrocytes). The sequence of increasingly unshaded areas shows its proportional disappearance during successive stages of iron deficiency. RE = reticuloendothelial; IBC = iron-binding capacity; RBC = red blood cell. To convert µg to SI units (nmol), multiply by 17.9. From Herbert V. 1987. The 1986 Herman Award Lecture. Nutrition science as a continually unfolding story: The folate and vitamin B_{12} paradigm. *American Journal of Clinical Nutrition* 46:387–402.

Transferrin saturation is the percent of transferrin that is saturated with iron. In uncomplicated iron-deficiency anemia, serum iron levels decrease and TIBC increases, resulting in a decreased transferrin saturation. Cutoff values for transferrin saturation that are indicative of the presence of iron deficiency are shown in Table 9-5.

Measures of serum iron, TIBC, transferrin saturation, and serum ferritin concentration are useful in distinguishing iron deficiency from other disorders capable of causing microcytic anemias (anemias in which the erythrocytes are smaller than normal).[34] Transferrin saturation, however, is considered to be a more sensitive indicator of iron deficiency than either serum iron or TIBC.[35]

A variety of factors can affect these measures.[34,35] There is a considerable diurnal (cyclic changes within a 24-hour period) and day-to-day variation in serum iron concentrations. Serum iron can be as much as 50% greater in the morning than in the evening, and values taken at the same time of day can vary as much as 30% from one day to the next. The primary factor affecting TIBC is the status of body iron stores. TIBC is increased with depletion of iron stores and decreased in

TABLE 9-5 Cutoff values indicative of iron deficiency developed for use with data from the second National Health and Nutrition Examination Survey*

Age (yr)	Serum ferritin (μg/l)	Transferrin saturation (%)	Erythrocyte protoporphyrin (μmol/L RBC)	MCV (fl)
1–2	—	<12	>1.42	<73
3–4	<10	<14	>1.33	<75
5–10	<10	<15	>1.24	<76
11–14	<10	<16	>1.24	<78
15–74	<12	<16	>1.24	<80

From Life Sciences Research Office, Federation of American Societies for Experimental Biology. 1989. *Nutrition monitoring in the United States: An update report on nutrition monitoring*. Washington, DC: U.S. Department of Health and Human Services, Public Health Services.

*RBC = red blood cell; MCV = mean corpuscular volume; fL = femtoliter, 10^{-15} liter.

iron overload and in response to inflammation. There is no diurnal variation in TIBC.

Erythrocyte Protoporphyrin

Protoporphyrin is a precursor of heme and accumulates in red blood cells (erythrocytes) when the amount of heme that can be produced is limited by iron deficiency. Protoporphyrin concentration is generally reported in the range of 0.622 ± 0.27 μmol/L of red blood cells, although the value can vary depending on the analytic method. As can be seen from Table 9-5, iron deficiency can lead to a more than twofold increase over normal values. Erythrocyte protoporphyrin increases as iron depletion worsens, as can be seen in Figures 9-1 and 9-2. Lead poisoning also can result in increased erythrocyte protoporphyrin levels.

Hemoglobin

Hemoglobin is an iron-containing molecule capable of carrying oxygen and is found in red blood cells. Grams of hemoglobin per liter (or deciliter) of blood is an index of the blood's oxygen-carrying capacity. Measurement of hemoglobin in whole blood is the most widely used screening test for iron-deficiency anemia.

The amount of hemoglobin in blood primarily depends on the number of red blood cells and to a lesser extent on the amount of hemoglobin in each red blood cell.[35] Reference values are 14 to 180 g/l (14 to 18 g/dl) for men and 120 to 160 g/l (12 to 16 g/dl) for women. Hemoglobin levels for black men and women average 5 to 10 g/l less than levels for white men and women at most ages.[35] Hemoglobin and hematocrit values useful for defining anemia and iron-deficiency anemia are shown in Table 9-6. These were developed by the U.S. Centers for Disease Control and Prevention and are based on the 5th percentile values for a reference population from NHANES II. During pregnancy, the plasma volume increases, leading to a condition known as hemodilution, resulting in lower hemoglobin levels.[35] Depending on the trimester of pregnancy, hemoglobin levels as low as 105 g/l (10.5 g/dl) are considered within normal limits. As can be seen in Table 9-6, boys and girls have similar hemoglobin levels up until about age 11 years, after which values for males tend to be 5 to 15 g/l higher than for females, depending on the age.[35]

Although hemoglobin and hematocrit values are useful in diagnosing anemia, they tend not to become abnormal until the late stages of iron

TABLE 9-6 Hemoglobin and hematocrit values for determining anemia and iron-deficiency anemia

Age (yr)	Hemoglobin (g/l)	Hematocrit (%)
1.0–1.9	110	33
2.0–4.9	112	34
5.0–7.9	114	35
8.0–11.9	116	36
12.0–14.9 (females)	118	36
12.0–14.9 (males)	123	37
15.0–17.9 (females)	120	36
15.0–17.9 (males)	126	38
18+ (females)	120	36
18+ (males)	135	40
Pregnancy		
1st trimester	110	33
2nd trimester	105	32
3rd trimester	110	33

From Life Sciences Research Office, Federation of American Societies for Experimental Biology. 1989. *Nutrition monitoring in the United States: An update report on nutrition monitoring*. Washington, DC: U.S. Department of Health and Human Services, Public Health Services.

deficiency and are not good indicators of early iron deficiency.

The use of cutoff points (as in Table 9-6) to classify laboratory values inevitably results in some degree of misclassification. No matter where the cutoff value is placed in Figure 9-3, there will be some individuals with adequate iron status whose hemoglobin levels fall below the cutoff value. These are the false positives. There will be some, on the other hand, with an inadequate iron status whose hemoglobin levels fall above the cutoff value. These are the false negatives.

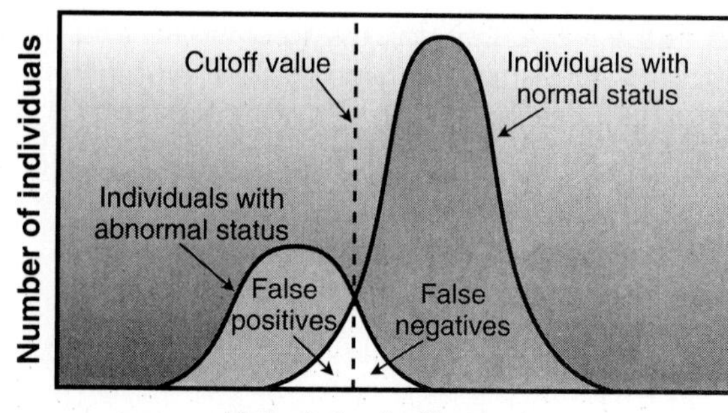

Figure 9-3 Effect of applying a cutoff value for an indicator of nutritional status to the distributions of values for individuals with adequate status and individuals with inadequate status. From Life Sciences Research Office, Federation of American Societies for Experimental Biology. 1989. *Nutrition monitoring in the United States: An update report on nutrition monitoring*. Washington, DC: U.S. Government Printing Office.

Hematocrit

Hematocrit (also known as the *packed cell volume*) is defined as the percentage of red blood cells making up the entire volume of whole blood. It can be measured manually by comparing the height of whole blood in a capillary tube with the height of the RBC column after the tube is centrifuged. In automated counters, it is calculated from the RBC count (number of RBCs per liter of blood) and the mean corpuscular volume (discussed below). Hematocrit depends largely on the number of red blood cells and to a lesser extent on their average size. Normal ranges for hematocrit are 40% to 54% and 37% to 47% for males and females, respectively.[35]

Mean Corpuscular Hemoglobin

The mean corpuscular hemoglobin (MCH) is the amount of hemoglobin in red blood cells. It is calculated by dividing hemoglobin level by the red blood cell count. Reference values are approximately 26 to 34 pg. MCH is influenced by the size of the red blood cell and the amount of hemoglobin in relation to the size of the cell.[35]

TABLE 9-7 Reference blood cell values for adults

	Males		Females
Hemoglobin (g/l of blood)	140–180		120–160
Hematocrit (%)	40–54		37–47
Red cell count (× 10^{12}/l blood)	4.5–6.0		4.0–5.5
Mean corpuscular hemoglobin (pg)		26–34	
Mean corpuscular hemoglobin concentration (g/l of blood)		320–360	
Mean corpuscular volume (fl)		80–100	

From Ravel R. 1994. *Clinical laboratory medicine: Clinical application of laboratory data,* 6th ed. St Louis: Mosby.

A similar measure, mean corpuscular hemoglobin concentration (MCHC) is the average concentration of hemoglobin in the average red blood cell. It is calculated by dividing the hemoglobin value by the value for hematocrit. Normal values lie in the range of 320 to 360 g/l (32 to 36 g/dl).[35]

Mean Corpuscular Volume

Mean corpuscular volume (MCV) is the volume of the average red blood cell. It is calculated by dividing the hematocrit value by the RBC count. Values for MCV are normally in the range of 80 to 100 fL for both males and females.

Factors increasing MCV (resulting in macrocytosis) include deficiencies of folate or vitamin B_{12}, chronic liver disease, alcoholism, and cytotoxic chemotherapy. Among factors decreasing MCV (resulting in microcytosis) are chronic iron deficiency, thalassemia, anemia of chronic diseases, and lead poisoning.[35] Reference blood cell values for adults are shown in Table 9-7.

Models Assessing Impaired Iron Status

Because no single biochemical test exists for reliably assessing impaired iron status, several different indicators should be used together.[19,31,33] Different models using multiple biochemical values have been developed for evaluating iron status (Table 9-8).[31–33] The *ferritin model* uses three indicators: serum ferritin, transferrin saturation, and erythrocyte protoporphyrin. The *MCV model* employs MCV, transferrin saturation, and erythrocyte protoporphyrin as indicators. Both models require that at least two of the three indicators be abnormal. The ferritin model tends to overestimate the presence of iron deficiency because it includes ferritin, which reflects stores in the first stage of iron depletion. The MCV model, on the other hand, includes three biochemical tests, all of which reflect altered red blood cell formation.[31] Both models are capable of identifying persons in the second and third stages of iron depletion.

A concern about these models is that iron status indicators sometime fail to distinguish iron-deficiency anemia from the other common causes of anemia. When data from all four indicators (serum ferritin, erythrocyte protoporphyrin, transferrin saturation, and MCV) are combined in what is called the *four-variable model,* anemias caused by inflammatory conditions are better distinguished from iron-deficiency anemia. The model is considered diagnostic for iron-deficiency anemia when either the value for serum ferritin or for MCV plus one additional value are abnormal according to the values in Table 9-5.[31]

When estimating the prevalence of iron-deficiency anemia in populations from data derived from such studies as NHANES, two other approaches are helpful in discriminating between

TABLE 9-8 Laboratory measurements used in four models for assessing iron deficiency

Model	Measurements used
Ferritin model*	Serum ferritin Transferrin saturation Erythrocyte protoporphyrin
Mean corpuscular volume (MCV) model*	MCV Transferrin saturation Erythrocyte protoporphyrin
Four-variable model†	MCV or serum ferritin Transferrin saturation Erythrocyte protoporphyrin
Hemoglobin-percentile shift model‡	Hemoglobin Transferrin saturation Erythrocyte protoporphyrin

From Life Sciences Research Office, Federation of American Societies for Experimental Biology. 1989. *Nutrition monitoring in the United States: An update report on nutrition monitoring*. Washington, DC: U.S. Department of Health and Human Services, Public Health Services; Johnson MA. 1990. Iron: Nutrition monitoring and nutrition status assessment. *Journal of Nutrition* 120:1486–1491.

*Two of three values must be abnormal.

†Values for either MCV or serum ferritin (or both) must be abnormal, in addition to at least one other abnormal value.

‡The hemoglobin percentile shift model estimates the median change in hemoglobin of a population after excluding individuals with low transferrin saturation and/or high erythrocyte protoporphyrin.

anemias related to inflammatory conditions and those caused by iron deficiency. One is the hemoglobin percentile shift, which estimates the median change in hemoglobin of a population after excluding individuals with low transferrin saturation (<16%) and/or high concentrations of erythrocyte protoporphyrin (>1.2 μmol/L of red blood cells).[32,33]

Another approach is to consider values from one of several nonspecific indicators of infection, inflammatory disease, and malignancy when evaluating indicators of iron status. These include erythrocyte sedimentation rate (ESR), zeta-sedimentation rate (ZSR), and C-reactive protein (CRP).

ESR and ZSR measure the rate at which red blood cells sediment in anticoagulated blood under a given set of conditions.[32,35] CRP is a glycoprotein found in only trace amounts in healthy people but elevated during acute inflammation or tissue destruction. It is not influenced by anemia or plasma protein changes and begins to rise about 4 to 6 hours after the onset of inflammation. CRP is considered by many to be the best indicator for acute inflammation, whereas ESR is the preferred indicator for chronic inflammation. These indicators are of value both in clinical practice and in population studies to help distinguish iron-deficiency anemia from anemia resulting from chronic disease.[32]

CALCIUM STATUS

Calcium is essential for bone and tooth formation, muscle contraction, blood clotting, and cell membrane integrity.[31] Of the 1200 g of calcium in the adult body, approximately 99% is contained in the bones. The remaining 1% is found in extracellular fluids, intracellular structures, and cell membranes.[19]

Osteoporosis, a calcium-related health condition of concern, is discussed in Chapter 8. Interest in osteoporosis prevention and treatment, coupled with data showing low calcium intakes in certain groups, especially women, has made calcium a current public health issue. This has sparked interest in assessing the body's calcium status.

At the current time, there are no appropriate biochemical indicators for assessing calcium status. This is due in large part to the biologic mechanisms that tightly control serum calcium levels despite wide variations in dietary intake.[31,36] Potential approaches to assessing calcium status can be categorized in three areas: bone mineral content measurement, biochemical markers, and measures of calcium metabolism.[36] Of these three approaches, measurement of bone mineral content by such methods as quantitative computed tomography, single- and dual-photon absorptiometry, and dual-energy x-ray absorptiometry is currently the most feasible approach to assessing calcium status. These techniques are discussed in Chapter 8. However, fewer biochemical markers and measures of calcium metabolism are available. Attempts to identify a calcium status indicator in blood have been unsuccessful.[36]

TABLE 9-9 Normal values for calcium in body fluids

	Mean	Normal range
Plasma		
Total calcium (mmol/L)	2.5	2.3–2.75
Ionized (mmol/L)	1.18	1.1–1.28
Complexed (mmol/L)		0.15–0.30
Protein bound (mmol/L)		0.93–1.08
Urine		
24-hour calcium (mmol/L)		
Women	4.55	1.25–10
Men	6.22	1.25–12.5
Fasting calcium:creatinine ratio (molar)		
Postmenopausal women	0.341 ± 0.183*	
Men	0.169 ± 0.099*	

From Weaver CM. 1990. Assessing calcium status and metabolism. *Journal of Nutrition* 120:1470–1473.

*mean ± SD.

Serum Calcium Fractions

Serum calcium exists in three fractions: protein bound, ionized, and complexed.[37] These and other values for calcium in body fluids are shown in Table 9-9. The protein-bound calcium is considered physiologically inactive, whereas the ionized fraction is considered physiologically active and functions as an intracellular regulator.[36–38] Complexed calcium is complexed with small negative ions such as citrate, phosphate, and lactate. Its biologic role is uncertain. Because the ionized and complexed calcium are diffusible across semipermeable membranes, these two fractions can be collectively referred to as *ultrafilterable calcium*. Serum levels of calcium are so tightly controlled by the body that there is little, if any, association between dietary calcium intake and serum levels.[38] Altered serum calcium levels are rare and indicate serious metabolic problems rather than low or high dietary intakes. Low serum calcium or hypocalcemia (serum calcium concentration < 2.3 mmol/L) can result from a variety of conditions including hypoparathyroidism (deficient or absent levels of parathyroid hormone), renal disease, and acute pancreatitis. High serum calcium concentrations or hypercalcemia (serum calcium > 2.75 mmol/L) can be due to increased intestinal absorption, bone resorption, or renal tubular reabsorption resulting from such conditions as hyperparathyroidism, hyperthyroidism, and hypervitaminosis D (excessive intake of vitamin D).[36]

The association between total serum calcium and blood pressure has been investigated, although results have been somewhat conflicting. Several studies[39,40] have found ultrafilterable calcium to be negatively correlated with hypertension but found no significant correlation between total serum calcium and the presence of hypertension. Other investigators,[41,42] however, have reported positive associations between total serum calcium and blood pressure. Clearly, more research is needed to sort out these apparent discrepancies.

Increased levels of complexed calcium and ionized calcium in postmenopausal women have been reported, suggesting that these have potential as markers of low bone mass.[38,43]

Urinary Calcium

Urinary calcium levels are more responsive to changes in dietary calcium intake than are serum levels.[36] However, urinary calcium is affected by a number of other factors, including those factors leading to hypercalcemia. When serum levels are high, more calcium is available to be excreted through the urine. There is a diurnal variation in urinary calcium, with concentrations higher during the day and lower in the evening.[37] Calcium output tends to be increased when the diet is rich in dietary protein and is low in phosphate and decreased by high-protein diets rich in phosphate.[37] Urinary calcium losses are increased when the volume of urine output is higher and when the ability of the kidney to reabsorb calcium is impaired.[36,37] Hypocalciuria can result from those factors leading to hypocalcemia as well as from renal failure.[36,37]

Use of the ratio of calcium to creatinine calculated from 2-hour fasting urine samples has been suggested as a possible indicator of calcium status but requires further research. The calcium level in an overnight urine sample shows potential as an indicator of compliance with calcium supplementation.[36]

Zinc Status

Zinc's most important physiologic function is as a component of numerous enzymes.[55] Consequently, zinc is involved in many metabolic processes, including protein synthesis, wound healing, immune function, and tissue growth and maintenance. Severe zinc deficiency characterized by hypogonadism and dwarfism has been observed in the Middle East. Evidence of milder forms of zinc deficiency (detected by biochemical and clinical measurements) has been found in several population groups in the United States. In humans and laboratory animals, a reduction or cessation of growth is an early response to zinc deficiency, and supplementation in growth-retarded infants and children who are mildly zinc deficient can result in a growth response.[45–47]

Because there is concern about the adequacy of zinc intake among certain groups, especially females, zinc is considered a potential public health issue for which further study is needed. Nutrient intake data and other scientific findings suggest that several U.S. population groups may have marginal zinc intakes. According to NHANES III data, the average intake of zinc among females age 20 to 49 years (approximately 9.6 mg/d) is roughly 80% of the RDA. Biochemical and clinical data derived from U.S. government nutritional monitoring activities, however, show no impairment of zinc status.

Serum Zinc Concentrations

There is currently no specific sensitive biochemical or functional indicator of zinc status.[45] Static measurements of serum zinc are available, but their use is complicated by the body's homeostatic control of zinc levels and by factors influencing serum zinc levels that are unrelated to nutritional status.[44,45]

There is little, if any, functional reserve of zinc in the body, as there is of some other nutrients (for example, iron, calcium, and vitamin A). The body's zinc levels are maintained by both conservation and redistribution of tissue zinc. In mild zinc deficiency, conservation is manifested by reduction or cessation of growth in growing organisms and by decreased excretion in nongrowing organisms. In most instances of mild deficiency, this appears to be the extent of clinical and biochemical changes. If the deficiency is severe, however, additional clinical signs soon appear.[45]

Mature animals and humans have a remarkable capacity to conserve zinc when intakes are low. As a result, inducing zinc deficiency in full-grown animals can be difficult.[45] Several mechanisms are responsible for this. Fecal zinc excretion, for example, can be cut by as much as 60% when dietary intake is low. Not only is the efficiency of intestinal absorption of zinc increased, but losses via the gastrointestinal tract, urine, and sweat are diminished.[45,48,49]

In laboratory animals, deficiency can lead to selective redistribution of zinc from certain tissues to support other higher-priority tissues. In mild zinc deficiency, plasma zinc levels apparently can be maintained at the expense of zinc from other tissues.[48,50] Some evidence suggests that redistribution of total body zinc also occurs in humans.

The result of the body's conservation of and ability to redistribute zinc is that measurements of serum zinc are not a reliable indicator of dietary zinc intake or changes in whole-body zinc status.[31,45] This is especially the case in mild zinc deficiency. For example, serum zinc concentrations in growth-retarded children whose growth responded to zinc supplementation were not significantly different from normally developed children either before or after supplementation.[61] Despite these limitations, measurement of serum zinc concentration may be a useful, albeit late, indicator of the size of the body's exchangeable zinc pool. Less-than-expected values may signal a loss of zinc from bone and liver and increased risk for clinical and metabolic signs of zinc deficiency.[45]

Several factors unrelated to nutritional status can influence serum zinc levels. Decreased levels can result from stress, infection or inflammation, and use of estrogens, oral contraceptives, and corticosteroids.[44,45] Serum zinc can fall by 15% to 20% following a meal.[45] Increased serum zinc concentrations can result from fasting and red blood cell hemolysis.

Metallothionen and Zinc Status

Metallothionen holds promise as a potential indicator of zinc status, particularly when used in conjunction with serum zinc levels.[45] Metallothionen is a protein found in most tissues but primarily in the liver, pancreas, kidney, and intestinal mucosa. Measurable amounts are found in serum and in red blood cells. Metallothionen has the capacity of binding zinc and copper, and tissue metallothionen concentrations often are proportional to zinc status. In animals, levels are almost undetectable in zinc deficiency and are responsive to zinc supplementation. Whereas serum zinc levels fall in response to acute stimuli (for example, stress, infection, and inflammation), hepatic and serum metallothionen levels are increased in response to these stimuli. Thus when serum levels of zinc fall and metallothionen rise, it is likely that tissue zinc has been redistributed in response to acute stimuli and that a zinc deficiency is not present because metallothionen is not responsive to acute stimuli in zinc-deficient animals. If serum zinc and metallothionen are both below expected levels, it is likely that zinc deficiency is present. Erythrocyte metallothionen (which is not affected by stress) also can be used as an indicator of zinc status.[45]

Hair Zinc

Several researchers have investigated the use of zinc in hair as an indicator of body zinc status.[67,68] Decreased concentration of zinc in hair has been reported in zinc-deficient dwarfs, marginally deficient children and adolescents, and in conditions related to zinc deficiency such as celiac disease, acrodermatitis enteropathica, and sickle cell disease.[53] Because hair grows slowly (about 1 cm per month), levels of zinc and other trace elements in hair reflect nutritional status over many months and thus are not affected by diurnal variations or short-term fluctuations in nutritional status. Because of this, hair zinc levels may not be correlated with measurements of zinc in serum or erythrocytes, which reflect shorter-term zinc status.[53] Obtaining a sample is noninvasive, and analyzing hair for zinc and other trace elements is relatively easy.

It is important to note that trace elements in hair can come from endogenous sources (those that are ingested or inhaled by the subject and then enter the hair through the hair follicle) and exogenous sources (contamination from trace elements in dust, water, cosmetics, and so on).[51–53] A major drawback in using hair as an indicator of trace element status is its susceptibility to contamination from these exogenous sources. Some exogenous contaminants can be removed by carefully washing the hair sample before analysis, and several standardized washing procedures have been suggested.[53] However, some contaminants may be difficult or impossible to remove. Selenium, an ingredient in some antidandruff shampoos, is known to increase the selenium content of hair and cannot be removed by the recommended washing procedures.[54]

A variety of other nonnutritional factors may affect the trace element content of hair. Included among these are certain diseases, rate of hair growth, hair color, sex, pregnancy, and age.[49,51,53] It has been reported, for example, that higher concentrations of zinc, iron, nickel, and copper can be found in red hair compared with brown hair and that iron and manganese are found in higher concentrations in brown hair than in blonde hair.[55] These factors limit the usefulness of hair as an index of zinc and other trace element status.

Urinary Zinc

Lower-than-expected concentrations of zinc have been reported in the urine of zinc-depleted persons.[53] However, factors other than nutritional status can influence urine zinc levels, such as liver cirrhosis, viral hepatitis, sickle cell anemia, surgery, and total parenteral nutrition. Problems associated with obtaining 24-hour urine collections can also complicate use of this indicator. Consequently, urine measurements of zinc are not the preferred approach to assessing zinc status.

TABLE 9-10 Functional tests that may be indicative of zinc status

Experimental wound healing	Growth response to zinc supplementation
Nitrogen retention	Collagen accumulation in implant sponge
Lymphocyte (T-cell) blastogenesis	Delayed cutaneous hypersensitivity
Zinc uptake by erythrocyte	Platelet aggregation
Sperm count	Dark adaptometry
Olfactory acuity	Taste acuity

From King JC, Keen CL. 1994. Zinc. In Shils ME, Olson JA, Shike M., eds. *Modern nutrition in health and disease,* 8th ed. Philadelphia: Lea & Febiger; King JC. 1990. Assessment of zinc status. *Journal of Nutrition* 120:1474–1479.

Functional Indicators

Several functional indicators have been proposed for assessing zinc status. These are listed in Table 9-10. Although some of these indicators are sensitive to nutritional status in general and zinc status in particular, a positive response when applied could be indicative of a lack of one of several nutrients, protein, and/or energy. Some of the tests are cumbersome to use and are limited by inter- and intraobserver error and a lack of standardized protocols for their administration and interpretation.

VITAMIN A STATUS

Vitamin A status can be grouped into five categories: deficient, marginal, adequate, excessive, and toxic. In the deficient and toxic states, clinical signs are evident, while biochemical or static tests of vitamin A status must be relied upon in the marginal, adequate, and excessive states.[56] Biochemical assessment of vitamin A status generally involves static measurements of vitamin levels in serum, breast milk, and liver tissue and functional tests such as dose-response tests, examination of epithelial cells of the conjunctiva, and assessment of dark adaptation.[56–58]

Serum Levels

Measurement of serum vitamin A is the most common biochemical measure of vitamin A status.[57] Under normal conditions, about 95% of serum vitamin A is in the form of retinol and bound to retinol-binding protein, and about 5% is unbound and in the form of retinyl esters.[58] Serum measurements are predictive of vitamin A status only when the body's reserves are either critically depleted or overfilled. Because serum vitamin A may be within the expected range despite low vitamin A concentrations within the liver, some investigators do not recommend serum measurements as a screening test for vitamin A status.[59] However, data from serum measurements can be of some value in drawing conclusions about the relationship of serum measurements to clinical signs of deficiency, dietary intake data, and various socioeconomic factors. Serum concentrations < 10 μg/dl (0.35 μmol/L) have generally been considered deficient, and values < 20 μg/dl (0.70 μmol/L) have been considered low.[56,57] Serum values > 30 μg/dl (> 1.05 μmol/L) are indicative of adequate status, while serum levels > 100 μg/dl are diagnostic of hypervitaminosis A, particularly when 50% or more of the vitamin is found in the form of retinyl ester.[56] Guidelines based on data from NHANES suggest that some persons within the population surveyed, particularly postadolescents, are likely vitamin A deficient even when their serum concentrations are in the range of 20 to 29 μg/dl (0.70 to 1.05 μmol/L), as shown in Table 9-11.[60]

Vitamin A levels in breast milk can also be used as an index of vitamin A status. Levels < 10 μg/dl (0.35 μmol/L) suggest the nursing child is at risk for vitamin A deficiency. Adequate vitamin A for growth and development will be provided when levels in breast milk are > 20 μg/dl (0.70 μmol/L). The nursing child's body reserves will increase when breast milk levels are > 40 μg/dl (1.40 μmol/L).[56]

Relative Dose Response

The relative dose-response test (RDR) and modified relative dose-response test (MRDR) are based on the principle that "when stores of retinol are high, plasma retinol concentration is little affected by oral administration of vitamin A. But when reserves are low, the plasma retinol concentration increases markedly, reaching a peak 5 h after an oral dose."[59] As hepatic vitamin A stores become depleted, retinol-binding protein (RBP) accumulates in the liver in an unbound state known as *apo-RBP*. When vitamin A is given to a subject whose stores are depleted, the vitamin A is absorbed from the intestinal tract, taken up by the liver where it binds to the apo-RBP, and then is released from the liver in the form of *holo-RBP* (the complex of RBP and vitamin A). In the RDR, a fasting blood sample is taken, followed by oral administration of vitamin A as retinyl palmitate. Another blood sample is drawn 5 hours later. Comparison of the fasting and postdosing holo-RBP measurements represents the extent of apo-RBP accumulation, which is directly related to the shortage of vitamin A.[3,61]

The RDR is calculated using the following formula:[57]

$$\text{RDR} = \frac{\text{vit A}_5 - \text{vit A}_0}{\text{vit A}_5} \times 100$$

where vit A_5 = serum vitamin A level 5 hours after receiving the dose of vitamin A, and vit A_0 = fasting serum vitamin A level.

An RDR $> 50\%$ is considered indicative of acute deficiency, values between 20% and 50% indicate marginal status, and values $< 20\%$ suggest adequate intake.[56]

Limitations of the RDR include the 5-hour waiting period and the need to draw two blood samples.[3]

TABLE 9-11 Guidelines for interpretation of serum total vitamin A levels in selected low ranges in populations

Serum vitamin A levels (μg/dl)	3–11 years	12–17 years	18–74 years
<10	Vitamin A status* is very likely to improve with increased consumption of vitamin A; impairment of function† is likely.		
<20	Vitamin A status is likely to improve with increased consumption of vitamin A.	Vitamin A status is likely to improve with increased consumption of vitamin A; some individuals may exhibit impairment of function.	Vitamin A status is very likely to improve with increased consumption of vitamin A; impairment of function is likely.
20–29	Vitamin A status of some individuals may improve with increased consumption of vitamin A; improvement is most likely in those with values 20–24 μg/dl.	Vitamin A status may improve with increased consumption of vitamin A; improvement is more likely in those with values 20–24 μg/dl.	Vitamin A status may improve with increased consumption of vitamin A; some individuals may exhibit impairment of function.

From Pilch SM. 1987. Analysis of vitamin A data from the Health and Nutrition Examination Surveys. *Journal of Nutrition* 117:636–640.

*Vitamin A status refers to serum vitamin A levels and tissue levels of the nutrient.

†Impairment of function may include impaired dark adaptation, night blindness, ocular lesions, and possibly impaired immune function.

The MRDR is based on the same principle but uses only one blood sample 5 hours after administration of the test dose of dehydroretinol, a naturally occurring form of vitamin A but one rarely present in most diets.[3] The measured response is the molar ratio of dehydroretinol to retinol in the serum sample. A ratio > 0.06 indicates marginal or poorer vitamin A status. A ratio < 0.03 indicates adequate vitamin A status.[56]

The assay is limited by the fact that there currently is no commercial source for dehydroretinol, and the assay requires the use of high-pressure liquid chromatography to distinguish the two forms of vitamin A. The assay is still under development but does have the advantage of requiring only one blood sample.[3]

Conjunctival Impression Cytology

Vitamin A deficiency can result in morphologic changes in epithelial cells covering the body and lining its cavities. It can result in a decline in the number of mucus-producing goblet cells in the epithelium of the conjunctiva of the eye. The epithelial cells also may take on a more squamous appearance—flatter cells, smaller nuclei, and with the cytoplasm making up a greater proportion of the total cell.[57] The conjunctival impression cytology test involves the microscopic examination of the conjunctival epithelial cells to determine morphologic changes indicative of vitamin A deficiency.[57,62]

A minute sample of epithelial cells can be obtained by touching a strip of cellulose ester filter paper to the outer portion of the conjunctiva for 3 to 5 seconds and then gently removing it. The filter paper with the adherent epithelial cells is placed in a fixative solution, where it can be stored until being stained and examined by ordinary light microscopy.[57,63]

The test is limited by several factors. It is difficult to get tissue samples from children under 3 years of age, and the cytologists must follow standardized criteria in evaluating samples. The sensitivity of the test is limited by conjunctival and systemic infections and possibly by severe malnutrition.[57] Theoretically, test results allow the vitamin A status of persons to be categorized in one of four groups: normal, marginal (+), marginal (−), and deficient. Because of difficulty in interpreting the two intermediate categories, conjunctival impression cytology is primarily used to detect populations at risk of deficiency. A population would be considered at risk of vitamin A deficiency if more than 50% of persons in a sample selected from the population had results that were not in the normal category.[56]

Dark Adaptation

The best-defined function of vitamin A is its role in the visual process. The visual pigment rhodopsin is generated when the protein opsin in the rods of the retina combines with a *cis*-isomer of retinol. When light strikes the eye, rhodopsin is split into opsin and a *trans*-isomer of retinol, generating the visual-response signal. The *trans*-isomer is then converted back to the *cis*-isomer, which then combines with opsin to reform rhodopsin. During this process, some of the retinol isomer is lost and must be replaced by vitamin A present in the retina. Under normal conditions, sufficient retinol is present, and rhodopsin is readily formed. When vitamin A is in short supply, less rhodopsin is formed, and the eye fails to adapt as readily to low light levels after exposure to bright light levels.[56,57]

Tests are available to directly measure the level of rhodopsin and its rate of regeneration. Field tests measuring visual acuity in dim light after exposure to bright light also can be used.[57] However, the relative dose response, when available, is a more specific and objective test of vitamin A status and is preferred over functional tests of dark adaptation.

Direct Measurement of Liver Stores

Direct measurement of hepatic vitamin A stores in liver tissue can be used as an indicator of vitamin

A status.[56] In many countries, the median vitamin A concentration in liver tissue of well-nourished persons is approximately 100 μg of retinol/g of liver tissue. A concentration > 20 μg of retinol/g of liver tissue is considered adequate for both children and adults of all ages.[56] Concentrations < 5 μg of retinol/g of liver tissue are associated with vitamin A deficiency.

The assay can be done on a very small amount of liver tissue obtained by inserting a biopsy needle through the abdominal wall. Because of the invasiveness of the biopsy procedure, assaying liver tissue for vitamin A is limited to situations when a liver biopsy is necessary for diagnostic purposes or when liver tissue can be obtained from postmortem examinations.[57]

VITAMIN C

Vitamin C is a generic term for compounds exhibiting the biologic activity of ascorbic acid. The reduced form of vitamin C is known as *ascorbic acid,* and the oxidized form is known as *dehydroascorbic acid.* The sum of ascorbic acid and dehydroascorbic acid constitutes all the naturally occurring biologically active vitamin C.[64] When used in this chapter, the term "vitamin C" refers to total vitamin C—the sum of ascorbic acid and dehydroascorbic acid.

Vitamin C is necessary for the formation of collagen, the maintenance of capillaries, bone, and teeth, the promotion of iron absorption, and the protection of vitamins and minerals from oxidation. Some evidence suggests a protective effect against certain cancers. Deficiency of vitamin C results in scurvy, a condition characterized by weakness, hemorrhages in the skin and gums, and defects in bone development in children.

Data from NHANES III show that mean vitamin C intakes in the United States are well above the RDA.[65] However, intakes among certain groups (women and children of lower socioeconomic status) may be inadequate, causing vitamin C to be a potential public health issue for which more study is needed.[31]

Assessing vitamin C status is limited primarily to measuring levels in serum (or plasma) and in leukocytes (white blood cells).[64,66] Several functional tests of vitamin C status have been suggested, but these do not appear to be reliable or suitable for field use.[64,67,68]

Serum and Leukocyte Vitamin C

Measurement of serum (or plasma) vitamin C is the most commonly used biochemical procedure for assessing vitamin C status.[66,68] However, in recent years there has been increasing interest in using the level of vitamin C in polymorphonuclear leukocytes (the granular leukocytes: neutrophils, eosinophils, and basophils) and the mononuclear leukocytes (the agranular leukocytes: lymphocytes and monocytes) as indicators of vitamin C status.[69–71] Serum levels of ascorbic acid have been shown to correlate with dietary vitamin C intake and with vitamin C levels in leukocytes (white blood cells).[72,73] However, research suggests that vitamin C concentration in serum is a better indicator of recent dietary intake of vitamin C than leukocyte levels and that leukocyte vitamin C levels better represent cellular stores and the total body pool of the vitamin.[72–74]

An obvious deficient state with biochemical and/or clinical symptoms exists when serum ascorbic acid values are < 11 μmol/L. Marginal vitamin C status with moderate risk of developing clinical signs of deficiency exists when serum ascorbic acid values are between 11 and 23 μmol/L. The lower limit of normal serum ascorbic acid is considered 28 μmol/L.[64]

Factors affecting vitamin C levels in tissues and fluids include cigarette smoking and sex.[64] Compared with nonsmokers, cigarette smokers tend to have lower vitamin C levels in serum and leukocytes even after correcting for vitamin C intake.[64,71,75] The metabolic turnover of vitamin C in smokers has been estimated to be 40% higher than that of nonsmokers. This finding led the Subcommittee on the 10th Edition of the RDAs to recommend that cigarette smokers ingest at least 100 mg of vitamin C daily, as opposed to the RDA for adults of 60 mg of vitamin C daily.[19] However, evidence suggests that smokers may need to ingest > 200 mg of vitamin C daily to achieve serum ascorbic acid levels typically seen in nonsmokers meeting the RDA.[76]

After correcting for vitamin C intakes, females consistently show higher vitamin C levels in tissues and fluids than males.[64,71,75] Age does not appear to influence vitamin C levels in adults.[64,69]

Other Approaches

The requirement of vitamin C for a number of biochemical reactions within the body has resulted in a search for functional tests of the vitamin's status. The capillary fragility test was proposed as a functional test of vitamin C status during the early 1930s, but its results lack specificity for vitamin C because a number of factors other than vitamin C status affect capillary fragility.[67] The ascorbic acid saturation test can be a reliable index of vitamin C depletion.[64,66] The required 24-hour urine sample limits it usefulness to highly cooperative subjects in a clinical or research setting. At this time no reliable functional indicator of vitamin C status exists, but as our understanding of the role of vitamin C in human physiology unfolds, one or more may be developed.[64] Functional measures currently under investigation include markers of collagen metabolism, the urinary carnitine-to-creatinine ratio, and in vitro measurement of ascorbate-free radicals.[64]

Measurement of urinary vitamin C does not discriminate well between adequate and deficient vitamin C intakes.[73] This approach also is limited by difficulty in collecting urine samples and by the increase in urinary excretion of vitamin C in response to several drugs (aminopyrine, aspirin, barbiturates, and paraldehyde).[66] The ease with which saliva samples can be obtained has made measurement of salivary vitamin C a desirable assessment approach. Unfortunately, salivary vitamin C levels do not consistently reflect vitamin C intake, and therefore this does not appear to be a useful indicator of vitamin C status.[73]

In general, serum and leukocyte measurements are preferred over those in erythrocytes, urine, and saliva.[64,66,73] Serum levels appear more indicative of dietary intake, but leukocyte levels of vitamin C are a better index of cellular stores and the body's total vitamin C pool.[64,72,73]

VITAMIN B_6

The vitamin B_6 group is composed of three naturally occurring compounds related chemically, metabolically, and functionally: pyridoxine (PN), pyridoxal (PL), and pyridoxamine (PM). Within the liver, erythrocytes, and other tissues of the body, these forms are phosphorylated into pyridoxal 5′-phosphate (PLP) and pyridoxamine phosphate (PMP). PLP and PMP primarily serve as coenzymes in a large variety of reactions.[19,77] Especially important among these are the transamination reactions in protein metabolism. PLP also is involved in other metabolic transformations of amino acids and in the metabolism of carbohydrates, lipids, and nucleic acids.[19,78,79] Because of its role in protein metabolism, the requirement for vitamin B_6 is directly proportional to protein intake.[19]

Data from NHANES III show that mean vitamin B_6 intakes for infants and children of both sexes and for adolescent and adult males (except those 80 years or older) are greater than the RDA. Mean intakes for adolescent and middle-aged females fall below the RDA.[65] The 1985–86 CSFII showed that vitamin B_6 intakes for about 75% of all American women were below the 1989 RDA. However, after adjusting for lower-than-expected protein intakes, many more women met the protein-based vitamin B_6 allowance than the RDA.[31] Another factor complicating the interpretation of vitamin B_6 intakes is the incomplete nutrient composition data; analytical values for vitamin B_6 were available for only 70% of the foods in CSFII 1985–86.[31]

Although frank vitamin B_6 deficiency resulting in clinical manifestations is not considered widespread in the general U.S. population, there is evidence of impaired status among certain groups, most notably the elderly and alcoholic individuals. There is also concern about excessive vitamin B_6 intake and the possibility of peripheral nervous system damage that may result.[80] Because of these concerns, vitamin B_6 is being considered a potential public health issue for which further study is needed.[31]

Vitamin B_6 status can be assessed by several methods. Static measurements can be made of vitamin B_6 concentrations in blood or urine, and functional tests can measure the activity of several enzymes dependent on vitamin B_6.[1,19]

TABLE 9-12 Factors affecting plasma PLP* concentrations

Factors	Effect
Increased vitamin B_6 intake	Increases
Increased protein intake	Decreases
Increased glucose	Decreases (a)†
Increased plasma volume	Decreases
Increased physical activity	Increases (a)
Decreased uptake into nonhepatic tissues	Increases
Increased age	Decreases

From Leklem JE. 1990. Vitamin B_6: A status report. *Journal of Nutrition* 120:1503–1507.

*PLP = pyridoxal 5′-phosphate.

†(a) indicates that the effect is an acute effect.

Plasma and Erythrocyte Pyridoxal 5′-Phosphate

The most frequently used biochemical indicator of vitamin B_6 status is plasma PLP.[1,78,79] PLP accounts for approximately 70% to 90% of the total vitamin B_6 present in plasma.[1] PL is the next most abundant form in plasma, followed by lower levels of PN and PM.[79]

Fasting measurements of plasma PLP are considered the single most informative indicator of vitamin B_6 status for healthy persons.[79] In rats, plasma PLP has been shown to be significantly correlated with muscle PLP.[1] In humans, muscle PLP accounts for more than 80% of the body's vitamin B_6 stores.[81] In response to changes in dietary intake of vitamin B_6, plasma PLP levels have been shown to plateau within 7 to 10 days when intake is in the range of 0.5 to 1.0 mg/day.[79]

Use of this single measure is limited by the fact that abnormally low concentrations of plasma PLP may result from asthma, coronary heart disease, and pregnancy and may not reflect a true vitamin B_6 deficiency.[79] Dietary intake of vitamin B_6 and protein can affect plasma PLP concentrations as well. As shown in Table 9-12, increases in dietary vitamin B_6 intake raises plasma PLP, and plasma levels fall in response to increased protein consumption.[1] Thus although plasma PLP is a valuable measure, the assessment of vitamin B_6 status is best accomplished by using several indicators in conjunction with each other—for example, measures of other vitamin B_6 forms and/or functional tests.[1,82] Table 9-13 lists expected biochemical values for adults with adequate vitamin B_6 status for various measures of the vitamin.

Measurement of PLP in erythrocytes has been suggested as another approach to assessing vitamin B_6 status.[1,82] Certain characteristics of the erythrocyte may make it unrepresentative of other body tissues. The ability of hemoglobin to bind tightly to PLP and PL, along with the relatively long life of red blood cells (about 120 days), may make red blood cells a significant reservoir for vitamin B_6 and complicate the use of erythrocyte PLP levels as a useful indicator of vitamin B_6 status.[1,79,82]

Plasma Pyridoxal

Measurement of plasma PL has been suggested as an additional indicator of B_6 status to use with plasma PLP.[1,82] PL is the major dietary form of the vitamin, crosses all membranes upon absorption

TABLE 9-13 Indices for evaluating vitamin B_6 status and suggested values for adequate status in adults

Indices	Suggested value for adequate status*
Direct	
Blood	
Plasma pyridoxal 5′-phosphate (PLP)	>30 nmol/L
Plasma pyridoxal	NV†
Plasma total vitamin B_6	>40 nmol/L
Erythrocyte PLP	NV
Urine	
4-Pyridoxic acid	>3.0 µmol/day
Total vitamin B_6	>0.5 µmol/day
Indirect	
Blood	
Erythrocyte alanine transaminase index	<1.25‡
Erythrocyte aspartic transaminase index	<1.80
Urine	
2-g tryptophan load; xanthurenic acid	<65 µmol/day
3-g methionine load; cystathionine	<350 µmol/day
Oxalate excretion	NV
Diet intake	
Vitamin B_6 intake, weekly average	>1.2–1.5 mg/day
Vitamin B_6:protein ratio	>0.020
Other	
Electroencephalogram pattern	NV

From Leklem JE. 1990. Vitamin B_6: A status report. *Journal of Nutrition* 120:1503–1507.

*These values are dependent on sex, age, and, for most, protein intake.

†NV = no value established; limited data are available.

‡The index value for each transaminase represents the ratio of the enzyme activity with added PLP to the activity without PLP added.

from the gastrointestinal tract, and comprises about 8% to 30% of the total plasma vitamin B_6. There are questions about how well plasma PL represents vitamin B_6 status, and further research is needed on this indicator. Despite these questions, plasma PL is recommended in the assessment of B_6 status.[1]

Total Vitamin B_6

Total vitamin B_6 in plasma and urine can be measured by microbiological assay using *Saccharomyces uvarum* as the test organism.[1,82] Plasma levels of PL can be estimated from plasma measures of total vitamin B_6 and PLP because PL and

PLP constitute about 90% of total vitamin B_6 in plasma.[1] Because plasma concentrations of total vitamin B_6 have not been frequently measured, the values given in Table 9-13 were derived by multiplying plasma PLP values by 1.25.[1]

Total vitamin B_6 in urine also can be measured by the same microbiological assay used for plasma.[1] However, urinary levels of vitamin B_6 are not considered a useful indicator for assessing B_6 status.[1] Urinary vitamin B_6 has been shown to correlate closely with intake levels in adults, making it a potentially useful indicator of recent dietary intake. Excretions below 0.5 μmol/day are considered indicative of deficiency.[1] Use of urinary levels, however, is complicated by limitations associated with urine collections. Leklem[78] recommends that vitamin B_6 assays be performed on several 24-hour urine samples collected over 1 to 3 weeks. Use of urinary vitamin B_6 measures are not valid in persons receiving vitamin B_6 antagonists such as the drugs isoniazid, penicillamine, or cycloserine. The ingestion of oral contraceptives does not appear to affect urinary excretion of vitamin B_6.

Urinary 4-Pyridoxic Acid

4-Pyridoxic acid (4-PA) is the major urinary metabolite of vitamin B_6. Urinary excretion of 4-PA has been shown to change rapidly in response to alterations in vitamin B_6 intake[1] and to be indicative of immediate dietary intake. Thus it is considered useful as a short-term index of vitamin B_6 status. In studies of subjects whose usual dietary intake of vitamin B_6 was known, males had a 4-PA excretion of 3.5 μmol/day and females had a 4-PA excretion of > 3.2 μmol/day. Urinary excretions of 4-PA of ≥ 3.0 μmol/day appear to be indicative of acceptable vitamin B_6 status.[1] 4-PA is likely to be absent from urine of persons with a marked vitamin B_6 deficiency.

Tryptophan Load Test

Historically, the most widely used indicator of vitamin B_6 status has been the tryptophan load test.[1] This test is based on the requirement for PLP in the metabolism of the amino acid tryptophan (for example, conversion of the tryptophan to nicotinic acid). In the absence of PLP, tryptophan metabolism is altered, resulting in the production and eventual urinary excretion of several metabolites. Of these, xanthurenic acid is the easiest and most commonly measured. Usually a test load of 2 g of L-tryptophan is administered to a subject whose urine is then collected over a 24-hour period.[99] Urinary levels of xanthurenic acid in subjects with adequate vitamin B_6 status usually range from 30 to 40 μmol/day in response to the 2 g of tryptophan. Urinary xanthurenic acid < 65 μmol/day is considered indicative of adequate vitamin B_6 status.[1]

Factors other than vitamin B_6 status can affect urinary excretion of xanthurenic acid. These include protein intake, exercise, lean body mass, individual variations, the amount of tryptophan used in the test dose, use of estrogen and oral contraceptives, and pregnancy. For this reason, use of the tryptophan loading test has been questioned as an appropriate index of vitamin B_6 status. With the more recent development of direct measures for assessing B_6 status, the tryptophan loading test is used less often. However, when conditions that can adversely affect test outcome are absent, the procedure is regarded as a valid, although somewhat outdated, indicator of hepatic vitamin B_6 status.[1]

Methionine Load Test

The principle of the methionine load test is similar to that of the tryptophan load test. PLP is required in the metabolism of the amino acid methionine. Compared with persons with adequate vitamin B_6 status, those with impaired vitamin B_6 status have higher urine levels of the metabolites cystathionine and cysteine sulfonic acid following consumption of 3 g of methionine.[1]

Use of this test is limited by the required 24-hour urine sample and factors other than vitamin B_6 status that can affect test results (for example, protein intake). Because this test has been used in a limited number of studies, no definitive values for urinary cystathionine are available. The value of < 350 μmol/day given in Table 9-13 is based on three studies.[1]

Erythrocyte Transaminases

Another commonly used functional indicator of vitamin B_6 status is measurement of the activity of two enzymes known to be sensitive to B_6 status: erythrocyte alanine transaminase (EALT or EGPT) and erythrocyte aspartic acid transaminase (EAST or EGOT).[1] In persons whose vitamin B_6 reserves have been depleted, activity of these two enzymes is decreased and activity is increased after the in vitro addition of excess PLP. Consequently, measurements of the activity of EALT and EAST appear to be of value in assessing vitamin B_6 status.

The test employs two measurements: the activity of the enzymes at the unstimulated or basal level (as removed from the subject), and the stimulated level of enzyme activity (after the in vitro addition of excess PLP). From these data, two additional values are calculated. One is the stimulation index, which is the ratio of stimulated activity to unstimulated activity. The other is the percent stimulation, which is calculated from the following formula:[78]

$$\text{Percent stimulation} = \frac{(SA - UA) \times 100}{UA}$$

where SA = stimulated activity and UA = unstimulated activity.

Of the two measures, EALT appears to be the more responsive to changes in vitamin B_6 status and is considered a better indicator.[78]

The approach is limited by the considerable interindividual variation seen in the erythrocyte transaminase activities of persons with apparently adequate vitamin B_6 status, with or without stimulation by added PLP. This has been shown to vary by as much as 25% and 50% for EALT and EAST, respectively. Test results also may be adversely affected by a concomitant riboflavin deficiency. There are also limited data on the degree of stimulation and percent stimulation in response to varying levels of vitamin B_6 depletion and repletion over time. Because a uniform method of reporting data has not been followed, it is difficult to interpret data and compare results of studies using this method. A standardized approach to reporting results from this assay is needed.[1]

FOLATE

Folate or folacin is a group of compounds with properties and chemical structures similar to folic acid or pteroylglutamic acid.[31,83] Folate functions as a coenzyme transporting single carbon groups from one compound to another in amino acid metabolism and nucleic acid synthesis. One of the most significant of folate's functions appears to be purine and pyrimidine synthesis. Folate deficiency can lead to inhibition of DNA synthesis, impaired cell division, and alterations in protein synthesis. These effects are especially seen in rapidly dividing cells (such as erythrocytes and leukocytes).[19,84]

Data from NHANES III show that the mean intake of folate is above the RDA for all groups except for pregnant and lactating females.[65] Data from the 1985–86 CSFII showed that mean folate consumption was below the 1989 RDA for about 50% of women whose income was less than 130% of the Federal Poverty Income guidelines. About 25% of all women had folate intakes less than the 1989 RDA. Serum and RBC folate levels measured in subgroups of NHANES II indicated that women age 20 to 44 years were at greatest risk for folate deficiency. Other groups known to be at risk include premature infants and women during the last half of pregnancy. Because oral contraceptives may depress folate absorption, women taking them are also considered at risk for folate deficiency. However, NHANES II showed no significant difference between blood folate levels of oral contraceptive users and those of nonusers. Folate is considered to be a potential public health issue requiring further study.[31] A primary concern is extensive evidence showing that females with a marginal folate status have an increased risk of giving birth to infants with neural

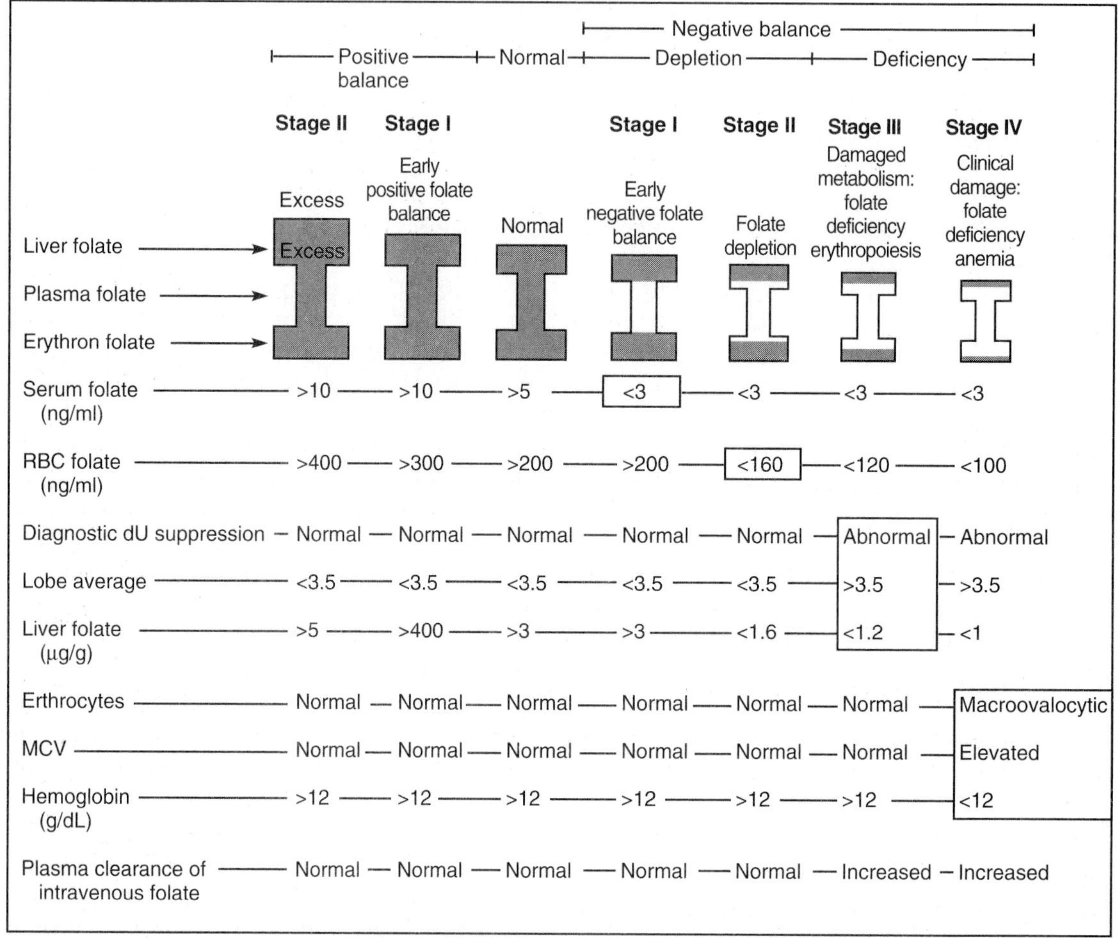

Figure 9-4 Sequential changes in the development of folate deficiency. The shaded areas indicate the relative quantities of folate in each compartment (e.g., in the liver, plasma, and erythrocyte). The sequence of increasingly unshaded areas show its proportional disappearance during successive stages of folate deficiency. The earliest abnormalities in each stage are boxed. RBC = red blood cell; dU = dioxyuridine; MCV = mean corpuscular volume. From Herbert V, Das KC. 1994. Folic acid and vitamin B_{12}. In Shils ME, Olson JA, Shike M, eds. *Modern nutrition in health and disease,* 8th ed. Philadelphia: Lea & Febiger.

tube defects.[85–87] Neural tube defects include spina bifida, encephalocele, and anencephaly.

As shown in Figure 9-4, folate status can be characterized as being in positive balance, normal, or as being in negative balance.[83] Positive folate balance can be divided into two stages: stage I, early positive folate balance and stage II, excess. Figure 9-4 lists several indices of folate status and gives values for these indices during these two stages of positive folate balance, as well as during other times.

Negative folate balance can be divided into four stages, as outlined in Figure 9-4.[83,84,88] Stage I of negative folate balance is called early negative folate balance. The earliest abnormality seen in this stage is a reduction in serum folate to levels

< 3 ng/ml, with all other indices in Figure 9-4 being within normal limits. The earliest abnormalities seen in stage II of negative folate balance, folate depletion, are a less-than-expected red blood cell folate level and abnormally low serum folate levels. As folate status deteriorates, stage III or folate deficiency erythropoiesis follows, as indicated by abnormal values for the deoxyuridine (dU) suppression test, evidence of hypersegmentation of the nuclei of the polymorphonuclear leukocytes (average number of lobes > 3.5), and liver folate < 1.2 μg/g. Stage IV, folate deficiency anemia, is characterized by morphologic changes in erythrocytes (red blood cells become macroovalocytic—MCV increases and the cells become oval in shape) and decreased hemoglobin concentration (anemia).[83,84]

The morphologic changes seen in erythrocytes, leukocytes, and bone marrow cells that accompany folate deficiency are identical to those caused by vitamin B_{12} deficiency. A comparison of values for erythrocyte folate and serum vitamin B_{12} is necessary to differentiate the two deficiencies because folate deficiency can occur as a result of vitamin B_{12} deficiency.[83]

Serum Folate

After about 3 weeks of negative folate balance, serum folate falls below 7 nmol/L (3 ng/ml). This concentration is considered indicative of negative folate balance, but it fails to give useful information on body stores of folate when used alone.[84,89] Serum folate cannot discriminate between a transient fluctuation in serum concentration in response to recent dietary folate intake and chronic deficiency accompanied by depleted body stores and functional changes.[84] Nonnutritional factors that can increase serum folate concentrations include acute renal failure, active liver disease, and hemolysis of red blood cells. Alcohol consumption, cigarette smoking, and possibly oral contraceptive use may lower serum folate levels.[8]

Approaches for measuring serum folate include radioisotope dilution assay and microbiologic assay using *Lactobacillus casei*.[89,90]

Erythrocyte Folate

A reduction in erythrocyte folate stores is considered the best clinical index of depleted tissue stores. Erythrocyte folate levels reflect folate status at the time the erythrocyte was synthesized because only young cells in the bone marrow take up folate.[84,89] Values less than 360 nmol/L (160 ng/ml) are considered indicative of tissue folate depletion.[88] Unlike serum folate, erythrocyte folate is less subject to transient fluctuations in dietary intake. It decreases after tissue stores are depleted because erythrocytes have a 120-day average life span and reflect folate status at the time of their synthesis. It has been shown to correlate with liver folate stores and reflect total body stores.[8]

As with serum folate, erythrocyte folate concentrations can be determined either by the microbiological assay or by radioisotope dilution.[90]

Deoxyuridine Suppression Test

The deoxyuridine (dU) suppression test is a functional indicator of folate status.[84] It is an in vitro biochemical test that not only defines the presence of megaloblastosis but helps identify which nutrient deficiency is responsible (folate or vitamin B_{12}). The dU suppression test is conducted in bone marrow or other DNA-synthesizing cells by measuring the incorporation of radioactive thymidine into DNA in the absence versus the presence of large amounts of deoxyuridine, which should suppress the incorporation of this tracer material to 10% to 20% of the control value.[89] Although the dU suppression test correlates fairly well with plasma and erythrocyte folate concentrations, erythrocyte folate is a superior indicator of folate status.[91]

VITAMIN B_{12}

Vitamin B_{12}, or cobalamin, are terms that include a group of cobalt-containing molecules that can be converted to methylcobalamin or 5′-deoxyadenosylcobalamin, the two coenzyme forms of vitamin B_{12} that are active in human metabolism.[19] Vitamin B_{12} is synthesized by bacteria, fungi, and algae, but not by yeast, plants, or animals. Vitamin B_{12} synthesized by bacteria accumulates in the tissues of animals that are then consumed by humans. Thus animal products serve as the primary dietary source of vitamin B_{12}. Although plants are essentially devoid of vitamin B_{12} (unless they are contaminated by microorganisms or soil containing vitamin B_{12}), foods such as breakfast cereals, soy beverages, and plant-based meat substitutes are sometimes fortified with vitamin B_{12}.[19,83]

The diets of most Americans supply more than adequate amounts of vitamin B_{12}. Data from NHANES III show that mean vitamin B_{12} intake is well above the RDA for all sex-age groups, including pregnant and lactating females.[65] Vegans or strict vegetarians (persons eating no animal products) could become vitamin B_{12} deficient, although this is unlikely because of the above mentioned practice of fortification. Despite these facts, vitamin B_{12} deficiency does occur, although rarely because of a dietary deficiency. More than 95% of the cases of vitamin B_{12} deficiency seen in the United States are due to inadequate absorption of the vitamin, generally because of pernicious anemia caused by inadequate production of intrinsic factor. Because most vitamin B_{12} absorption occurs in the distal ileum, B_{12} malabsorption could also result from surgical resection of the distal ileum or bacterial overgrowth in the small intestine ("blind loop" syndrome) or damage to the ileum from such causes as tropical sprue or regional enteritis.[92]

Intrinsic factor (Castle's intrinsic factor) is a glycoprotein produced by the parietal cells of the gastric glands, located in the body of the stomach. Intrinsic factor (IF) combines with vitamin B_{12} in the upper small intestine. The B_{12}-IF complex is carried to the ileum (the distal part of the small intestine) where it attaches to B_{12}-IF receptors on the brush border of ileal mucosal cells. The B_{12}-IF complex is then taken up by the ileal mucosal cell and makes its way into the blood for distribution to the rest of the body.[83] Under normal circumstances, most vitamin B_{12} is absorbed by this mechanism; however, approximately 1% of ingested vitamin B_{12} can be absorbed through passive diffusion along the entire length of the small intestine.[83] The usual cause of inadequate IF production is atrophy of the gastric mucosa, a condition most often seen in older persons. Thus pernicious anemia is a disease of the elderly, with an average age at diagnosis of 60 years. Other causes of inadequate IF production include total gastrectomy or extensive damage to the gastric mucosa caused by ingestion of corrosive agents.[92]

Clinical features of vitamin B_{12} deficiency involve the blood, the gastrointestinal tract, and the nervous system. An early feature of vitamin B_{12} deficiency is megaloblastic anemia, which is characterized by the presence of abnormally large cells (megaloblasts) in the peripheral blood and a low hemoglobin level. A mean corpuscular volume (MCV) $>$ 100 fL is suggestive of megaloblastic anemia. The tongue may become sore, smooth, and beefy red. Anorexia with moderate weight loss and diarrhea may also be present. The most troublesome consequences of B_{12} deficiency occur in the nervous system. Neurologic manifestations include demyelination and axonal degeneration of the peripheral nerves, spinal cord, and cerebrum. Eventually, irreversible neuronal death can occur in these areas. The earliest symptoms of these changes are numbness and paresthesias (abnormal sensations such as burning, prickling, or the feeling that ants are crawling on the skin) in the extremities. This can progress to weakness, muscular incoordination (ataxia), irritability, forgetfulness, severe dementia, and even psychosis.[92]

As shown in Figure 9-5, vitamin B_{12} status can be characterized as being in positive balance, normal, or as being in negative balance.[83] Positive B_{12} balance can be divided into two stages: stage I, early positive B_{12} balance, and stage II, excess. Figure 9-5 lists several indices of vitamin B_{12} status and gives values for these indices during these two stages of positive B_{12} balance, as well as during other times.

As outlined in Figure 9-5, negative B_{12} balance can be divided into two states of depletion and two stages of deficiency. Stage I of negative B_{12}

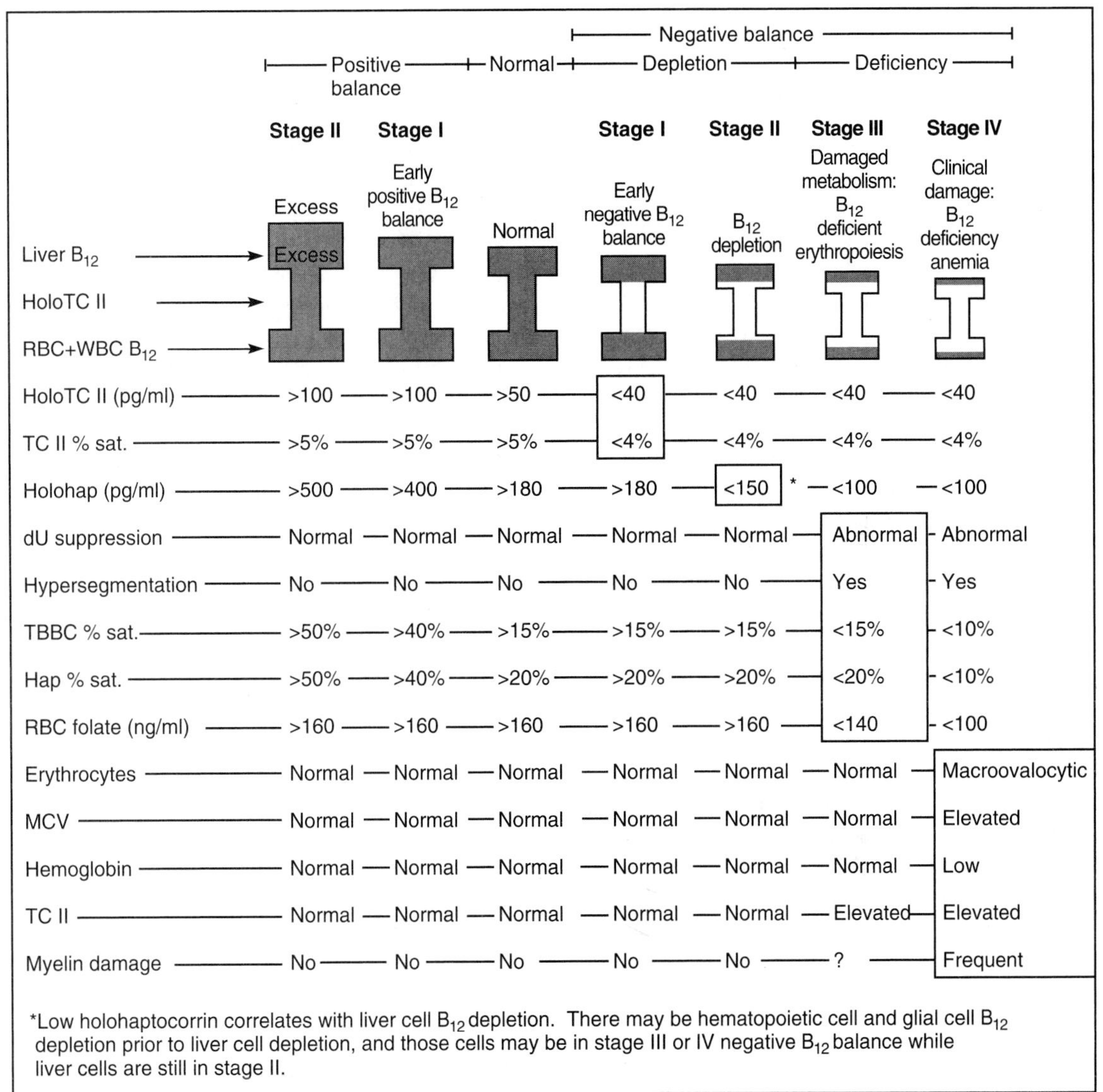

Figure 9-5 Sequential changes in the development of vitamin B_{12} deficiency. The shaded areas indicate the relative quantities of vitamin B_{12} in each compartment (e.g., in the liver, that transported by transcobalamin II, and in the erythrocytes and leukocytes). The sequence of increasingly unshaded areas shows its proportional disappearance during successive stages of vitamin B_{12} deficiency. The earliest abnormalities in each stage are boxed. HoloTC II = the complex of vitamin B_{12} and transcobalamin II; TC II sat. = percent transcobalamin II saturation; holohap = holohaptocorrin; dU = deoxyuridine; TBBC % sat. = total B_{12}-binding capacity percent saturation; hap % sat. = percent saturation of haptocorrin; RBC = red blood cell; MCV = mean corpuscular volume. From Herbert V, Das KC. 1994. Folic acid and vitamin B_{12}. In Shils ME, Olson JA, Shike M, eds. *Modern nutrition in health and disease,* 8th ed. Philadelphia: Lea & Febiger.

balance is called early negative B_{12} balance. The earliest abnormalities in this stage are decreased serum levels of holo-transcobalamin II (vitamin B_{12} complexed with its primary transport protein, transcobalamin II) and decreased saturation of transcobalamin II (a decreased percentage of transcobalamin II that is carrying or is saturated with cobalamin). These occur when decreased vitamin B_{12} absorption depletes the amount of vitamin B_{12} complexed with and carried by its transport protein, transcobalamin II. During this stage, however, total vitamin B_{12} level remains within normal limits. Stage II of negative B_{12} balance is B_{12} depletion. The earliest abnormality seen in this stage is a decreased level of holohaptocorrin (holohap).

Vitamin B_{12} deficiency is represented by stage III and stage IV of negative B_{12} balance. Stage III is known as B_{12} deficient erythropoiesis. This is characterized by abnormal values for the deoxyuridine (dU) suppression test, evidence of hypersegmentation of the nuclei of the polymorphonuclear leukocytes, decreased total B_{12}-binding capacity (TBBC), a lower-than-expected percent saturation of haptocorrin (hap), and decreased levels of folate in erythrocytes or red blood cells (RBC). This is characterized by enlarged erythrocytes (they appear macroovalocytic and have an increased MCV), low hemoglobin, elevated levels of transcobalamin II, and the frequent presence of myelin damage.[83]

Schilling Test

Once vitamin B_{12} deficiency is discovered, the Schilling test can be used to determine its cause.[92,93] In the first stage of the Schilling test, a patient is given an oral dose of vitamin B_{12} labeled with a radioactive isotope of cobalt. A short time later this is followed by an intramuscular or subcutaneous injection of 1 mg of non-labeled vitamin B_{12}. The patient then collects a 24-hour urine specimen. The amount of labeled vitamin B_{12} in the urine specimen is proportional to the amount of vitamin B_{12} absorbed. In pernicious anemia, $<$ 5% of the administered dose of labeled B_{12} should be present in the urine specimen. In the second stage, the patient is given radioactively labeled B_{12} bound to intrinsic factor. Absorption of the vitamin will now approach normal if the patient has pernicious anemia or some other type of intrinsic factor deficiency. Urinary excretion of the labeled vitamin B_{12} should be $>$ 10% of the administered dose. If urinary excretion is still low ($<$ 5% of the administered dose), the patient likely has a defect in vitamin B_{12} absorption due to ileal dysfunction.

In another form of the Schilling test, a fasting patient is given an oral dose of vitamin B_{12} labeled with an isotope of cobalt (^{57}Co), which is bound to intrinsic factor, and, at the same time, a separate oral dose of vitamin B_{12} containing a different isotope of cobalt (^{58}Co), which is not bound to intrinsic factor. In 1 to 2 hours, the patient is given 1 mg of non-labeled vitamin B_{12} by intramuscular or subcutaneous injection. A 24-hour urine specimen is collected. In pernicious anemia, the excretion of ^{58}Co is low (usually $<$ 5% of the administered dose), while excretion of the ^{57}Co that was bound to the intrinsic factor is normal ($>$ 10% of the administered dose). In intestinal malabsorption, excretion of both ^{58}Co and ^{57}Co is low. For the test to be valid, the patient must have a complete 24-hour urine specimen and normal renal function.[93]

BLOOD CHEMISTRY TESTS

Blood chemistry tests include a variety of assays performed on plasma or serum that are useful in the diagnosis and management of disease. They include electrolytes, enzymes, metabolites, and other miscellaneous substances discussed in this section. When run at one time, blood chemistry tests often are known by such names as the *chemistry profile, chemistry panel, chem profile,* or *chem panel.* To perform these tests, clinical laboratories use an automated analyzer capable of performing several thousand blood tests per hour. The patient's plasma or serum sample is placed into the analyzer, which performs the desired tests and provides a printout of the patient's results, including reference ranges and flagged abnormal results. A related series of tests, often known as the *coronary risk profile,* measures levels of triglyceride, total cholesterol, and HDL-C (cholesterol carried by high-density lipoproteins) and calculates LDL-C (cholesterol carried by low-density lipoproteins) and, in some instances, the total cholesterol/HDL-C ratio. These are discussed in Chapter 8.

Following is a brief overview of the major blood chemistry tests. Normal adult serum levels (known as reference ranges) are given. These reference ranges will vary depending on the individual biochemical and analytic method used. It is generally best, however, to use reference ranges suggested by the laboratory performing the analyses.

Alanine Aminotransferase

Alanine aminotransferase (ALT), also known as serum glutamic pyruvic transaminase (SGPT), is an enzyme found in large concentrations in the liver and to a lesser extent in the kidneys, skeletal muscles, and myocardium (heart muscle).[94] Injury to the liver caused by such conditions as hepatitis (viral, alcoholic, and so on), cirrhosis, and bile duct obstruction, or from drugs toxic to the liver is the usual cause of elevated serum ALT levels. Levels may be elevated to a lesser extent in myocardial infarction, musculoskeletal diseases, and acute pancreatitis. Decreased levels may result from chronic renal dialysis.[93] The adult reference range is 0.02 to 0.35 μkat/l (1 to 21 units/l).[94]

Albumin and Total Protein

As discussed earlier in this chapter, albumin is a serum protein produced in the liver. Total protein is the sum of all serum proteins, but the vast majority of total protein is composed of albumin and globulin. Once total protein and albumin are known, an estimate of globulin can be calculated. Levels of albumin and total protein reflect nutritional status, and alterations suggest the need for further diagnostic testing. Factors affecting serum levels of albumin and total protein are discussed earlier in this chapter. The adult reference range for albumin is 35 to 50 g/l (3.5 to 5.0 g/dl), for globulin 23 to 35 g/l (2.3 to 3.5 g/dl), and for total protein 60 to 84 g/l (6.0 to 8.4 g/dl).[94]

Alkaline Phosphatase

Alkaline phosphatase (ALP) is an enzyme found in the liver, bone, placenta, and intestine and is useful in detecting diseases in these organs. Expected values are higher in children, during skeletal growth in adolescents, and during pregnancy.[94] Elevated levels can be seen in conditions involving increased deposition of calcium in bone (hyperparathyroidism, healing fractures, certain bone tumors) and certain liver diseases.[93] Low levels of ALP usually are not clinically significant. The adult reference range is 0.22 to 0.65 μkat/l (13 to 39 units/l).[94]

Aspartate Aminotransferase

Aspartate aminotransferase (AST), also known as serum glutamic oxaloacetic transaminase (SGOT), is an enzyme found in large concentrations in the myocardium, liver, skeletal muscles, kidneys, and pancreas. Within 8 to 12 hours following injury to these organs, AST is released into the blood. Serum levels peak in 24 to 36 hours and then return to normal in about 4 to 6 days following injury.[94] Elevated levels are seen in such conditions as myocardial infarction (blood levels reflect the size of the infarct), liver diseases (for example, acute viral hepatitis), pancreatitis, musculoskeletal injuries, and exposure to drugs toxic to the liver.[93] The adult reference range is 0.12 to 0.45 μkat/l (7 to 27 units/l).[94]

Bilirubin

Bilirubin, the major pigment of bile, is produced by the spleen, liver, and bone marrow from the breakdown of the heme portion of hemoglobin and released into the blood. Most of the bilirubin combines with albumin to form what is called free or unconjugated bilirubin. Free bilirubin then is absorbed by the liver where it is conjugated (joined) to other molecules to form what is called conjugated bilirubin and then excreted into the bile.

Serum bilirubin levels can be reported as direct bilirubin, indirect bilirubin, or total bilirubin. Direct bilirubin is a measure of conjugated bilirubin in serum. Indirect bilirubin is a measure of free or unconjugated bilirubin in serum. Total bilirubin is a measure of both direct and indirect bilirubin.[94]

Serum bilirubin rises when the liver is unable to either conjugate or excrete bilirubin. Elevated conjugated (direct) bilirubin suggests obstruction of bile passages within or near the liver. Elevated free or unconjugated (indirect) bilirubin is indicative of excessive hemolysis (destruction) of red blood cells. Elevated indirect bilirubin also is seen in neonates whose immature livers are unable to adequately conjugate bilirubin. A serum bilirubin concentration greater than about 2 mg/dl results in jaundice. The adult reference ranges for adults are 1.7 to 20.5 μmol/L (0.1 to 1.2 mg/dl) for total, up to 5.1 μmol/L (up to 0.3 mg/dl) for direct (conjugated), and 1.7 to 17.1 μmol/L (0.1 to 1.0 mg/dl) for indirect (unconjugated) bilirubin.[94]

Blood Urea Nitrogen

Urea, the end product of protein metabolism and the primary method of nitrogen excretion, is formed in the liver and excreted by the kidneys in urine. An increased blood urea level usually indicates renal failure, although it may also result from such causes as dehydration, gastrointestinal bleeding, congestive heart failure, high protein intake, insufficient renal blood supply, or blockage of the urinary tract.[94] Blood urea nitrogen (BUN) is more easily measured than urea and is used as an index of blood urea levels. Elevated BUN is referred to as azotemia. Decreased BUN can result from liver disease, overhydration, malnutrition, and anabolic steroid use. Although in the absence of other signs elevated BUN is probably insignificant. The adult reference range is 8 to 25 mg/dl (2.9 to 9.8 mmol/L).[94]

Calcium

Serum levels of calcium, an important cation (positively charged ion), are helpful in detecting disorders of the bones and parathyroid glands, kidney failure, and certain cancers. Calcium is discussed at length earlier in this chapter. The adult reference range for total calcium is 8.5 to 10.5 mg/dl (2.1 to 2.6 mmol/L), and for ionized calcium it is 2.0 to 2.4 mEq/l (1.0 to 1.2 mmol/L).[94]

Carbon Dioxide

Measurement of carbon dioxide (CO_2) in serum helps assess the body's acid-base balance. Elevated CO_2 is seen in metabolic alkalosis, and decreased levels reflect metabolic acidosis. The adult reference range in serum or plasma is 24 to 30 mEq/l (24 to 30 mmol/L).[94]

Chloride

Chloride, an electrolyte, is the primary anion (negatively charged ion) within the extracellular fluid. It works in conjunction with sodium to help regulate acid-base balance, osmotic pressure, and fluid distribution within the body. It often is measured along with sodium, potassium, and carbon dioxide. Low serum chloride levels (hypochloremia) are associated with alkalosis and low serum potassium levels (hypokalemia). Hypokalemia may not accompany hypochloremia if the patient receives a potassium supplement that does not contain chloride or takes a potassium-sparing diuretic. Hyperchloremia (elevated serum chloride) may be seen in kidney disease, overactive thyroid, anemia, and heart disease. The adult reference range is 100 to 106 mEq/l (100 to 106 mmol/L).[94]

Cholesterol

According to the National Cholesterol Education Program, a desirable serum total cholesterol level is < 200 mg/dl (5.17 mmol/L). Chapter 8 discusses recommended levels of serum cholesterol and its relationship to coronary heart disease. Population reference values for serum total cholesterol are shown in Appendix S.

Creatinine

Measurement of serum creatinine, like measurement of blood urea nitrogen, is used for evaluating renal function. Elevated serum levels will be seen when 50% or more of the kidney's nephrons are destroyed. The reference range for adult males is 0.8 to 1.2 mg/dl (70 to 110 µmol/L), and for adult females it is 0.6 to 0.9 mg/dl (50 to 80 µmol/L).[93] Creatinine is discussed in greater detail in Chapter 6.

Glucose

Measurement of serum glucose is of interest in the diagnosis and management of diabetes mellitus. This is discussed in detail in Chapter 8. The adult reference range for fasting serum glucose is 60 to 115 mg/dl (3.3 to 6.4 mmol/L). Use of serum glucose to diagnose diabetes is discussed at length in Chapter 8. Serum glucose can also be used to diagnose hypoglycemia or low blood sugar. Glycosylated hemoglobin (HbA_{1C}), an index of long-term blood sugar control, and the oral glucose tolerance test (OGTT) are also discussed in Chapter 8.

Lactate Dehydrogenase

Lactic dehydrogenase (LDH), an enzyme found in the cells of many organs (skeletal muscles, myocardium, liver, pancreas, spleen, and brain), is released into the blood when cellular damage to these organs occurs. Serum levels of LDH rise 12 to 24 hours following a myocardial infarction and are often measured to determine whether an infarction has occurred. Increased LDH may result from a number of other conditions including hepatitis, cancer, kidney disease, burns, and trauma. Measurement of five different forms of LDH, known as isoenzymes, allows a more definitive diagnosis to be made. Low serum LDH is of no clinical significance. The adult reference range for serum LDH is 45 to 90 units/L (0.75 to 1.50 µkat/L).[93,94]

Phosphorus

The serum level of phosphorus (also known as inorganic phosphorus) is closely correlated with serum calcium level. Elevated serum phosphorus (hyperphosphatemia) is seen in renal failure, hypoparathyroidism, hyperthyroidism, and increased phosphate intake (use of phosphate-containing laxatives and enemas). Low serum phosphorus (hypophosphatemia) can be seen in hyperparathyroidism, rickets, osteomalacia, and chronic use of antacids containing aluminum hydroxide or calcium carbonate, which binds phosphorus in the gastrointestinal tract and prevents its absorption. The adult reference range is 3.0 to 4.5 mg/dl (1.0 to 1.5 mmol/L).[94]

Potassium

Potassium, the major intracellular cation, is involved in maintenance of acid-base balance, the body's fluid balance, and nerve impulse transmission. Elevated serum potassium (hyperkalemia) is most often due to renal failure but also may result from inadequate adrenal gland function (Addison's disease) or severe burns or crushing injuries. Low serum potassium (hypokalemia) can result from a number of causes including use of diuretics or intravenous fluid administration without adequate potassium supplementation, vomiting, diarrhea, and eating disorders.[93,94] The reference range for adults is 3.5 to 5.0 mEq/L (3.5 to 5.0 mmol/L).

Sodium

Sodium, the major extracellular cation, is primarily involved in maintenance of fluid balance and acid-base balance. Elevated serum levels (hypernatremia) are most frequently seen in dehydration resulting from insufficient water intake, excessive water output (for example, severe diarrhea or vomiting, profuse sweating, burns), or loss of antidiuretic hormone control. Hypernatremia suggests the need for water. Hyponatremia may be due to conditions resulting in excessive sodium loss from the body (vomiting, diarrhea, gastric suctioning, diuretic use), conditions resulting in fluid retention (congestive heart failure or renal disease), or water intoxication. The adult reference range is 135 to 145 mEq/L (135 to 145 mmol/L).[94]

Triglyceride

Triglyceride (TG) is a useful indicator of lipid tolerance in patients receiving total parenteral nutrition. Fasting serum TG provides a good estimate of very-low-density lipoprotein levels. Fasting serum levels are increased in liver disease, hypothyroidism, diabetes mellitus, and pancreatitis. Low levels are not clinically significant except in malnutrition. The role of TG in coronary heart disease is controversial. A typical adult reference range for TG is 40 to 150 mg/dl (0.45 to 1.70 mmol/L).[94] A TG level below 250 mg/dl (2.82 mmol/L) in the presence of a desirable serum cholesterol level is generally considered acceptable because there is little evidence that such a level increases the risk of any disease. Chapter 8 contains further details on serum triglyceride. Population reference values for TG are shown in Appendix S.

SUMMARY

1. Biochemical tests to assess nutritional status can be grouped into two general categories: static and functional tests. Static tests are based on measurement of a nutrient or specific metabolite in the blood, urine, or body tissue. Functional tests involve the physiologic processes that rely on the presence of adequate quantities of a nutrient.
2. The value of biochemical tests is limited by nonnutritional factors affecting test results and the occasional inability of tests to identify the nutrient deficiency. Monitoring nutritional status requires the use of several biochemical tests used in conjunction with each other and with data derived from dietary, anthropometric, and clinical methods. Compared with other assessment methods, biochemical tests have the advantage of being somewhat more objective and quantitative.
3. Protein-energy malnutrition can be either primary (insufficient intake of protein and calories) or secondary (resulting from other diseases). When severe, it results in kwashiorkor (principally a protein deficiency), marasmus (predominantly an energy deficiency), or marasmic kwashiorkor (a combination of chronic energy deficit and chronic or acute protein deficiency).
4. Creatinine and 3-methylhistidine are two muscle metabolites excreted in urine used to quantitate muscle mass. Creatinine is excreted in a relatively constant proportion to the body's muscle mass. Muscle mass can be estimated by comparing 24-hour urine creatinine excretion with certain standards. The creatinine-height index is a ratio of a patient's measured 24-hour urinary creatinine excretion and the expected excretion by a reference adult of the same sex and stature expressed as a percent of expected value. The use of creatinine and 3-methylhistidine is limited by problems associated with 24-hour urine collections, the effect of diet on urine concentrations, diurnal variations in excretion of creatinine and 3-methylhistidine, and a variety of other factors affecting their excretion.
5. Included among the serum proteins used to assess protein nutriture are albumin, transferrin, prealbumin, retinol-binding protein, and fibronectin. Considerations in their use include their body pool amount, half-life, and responsiveness to protein and energy depletion and repletion. Other considerations include how serum proteins are affected by nutritional and nonnutritional factors and how they correlate with morbidity and mortality.
6. Because nutrient deficiency often compromises immunity, tests of immunocompetence (e.g., total lymphocyte count and delayed cutaneous hypersensitivity) can be used to assess nutritional status. Although these tests

can detect immune problems associated with general nutritional deficits, they often are unable to identify the specific nutrient that is deficient and are affected by a variety of nonnutritional factors.

7. Iron deficiency is the most common single nutrient deficiency in the United States and the most common cause of anemia. Serum ferritin is the most useful index of the body's iron stores. Hemoglobin is the most widely used screening test for iron-deficiency anemia but is not an early indicator of iron depletion. Hematocrit is defined as the percentage of red blood cells making up the entire volume of whole blood.
8. Models that combine several indicators of iron status are better at predicting the presence of iron deficiency. Among these are the ferritin model, the MCV model, the four-variable model, and the hemoglobin-percentile shift model. These models allow better discrimination between iron-deficiency anemias and those caused by infection, inflammation, and chronic disease than do single measurements. This discrimination is enhanced when nonspecific measures of acute inflammation such as erythrocyte sedimentation rate, zeta-sedimentation rate, or C-reactive protein are included with the models.
9. Biochemical tests for assessing calcium status are hampered by the body's tight control of serum calcium levels. Measurement of urinary calcium, which is more responsive to dietary calcium change than serum calcium, is limited by the need for 24-hour urine samples and several nonnutritional factors that affect results.
10. Despite changes in dietary intake, the body maintains tight metabolic control of zinc status through conservation and redistribution of tissue zinc. Consequently there are no sensitive biochemical or functional indicators of zinc status. Serum zinc level is not reflective of dietary changes and is only a late indicator of the body's exchangeable zinc pool size.
11. Assessing vitamin A status involves static measurements of vitamin levels in serum and liver, and functional tests such as dose-response tests, conjunctival impression cytology, and dark adaptation. Serum measurements are predictive of vitamin A status only when the body's reserves are either critically depleted or overfilled.
12. The relative dose-response test (RDR) is based on the principle that when a person's vitamin A reserves are low, plasma retinol concentration will increase markedly within 5 hours after administration of a dose of vitamin A. The RDR has the ability to identify persons with marginal vitamin A status. It is limited by a 5-hour wait and the need to draw two blood samples.
13. Measurements of vitamin C in serum and leukocytes can be used for assessing vitamin C status. Serum vitamin C is a good indicator of recent vitamin C intake, whereas leukocyte vitamin C better represents cellular stores and the total body pool. There is currently no reliable functional indicator of vitamin C status. Problems with measuring vitamin C in red blood cells, saliva, and urine make these poor indicators.
14. Assays for assessing vitamin B_6 status include measurement of plasma pyridoxal 5′-phosphate (PLP), plasma pyridoxal, plasma total vitamin B_6, erythrocyte PLP, urine 4-pyridoxic acid, and urine total vitamin B_6. Functional measures include determination of erythrocyte transaminase activity, the tryptophan load test, and the methionine load test.
15. Plasma PLP appears to be the single most informative indicator of vitamin B_6 status for healthy persons, but results must sometimes be interpreted with caution because values can be affected by several diseases. Measurement of plasma pyridoxal is recommended in the assessment of B_6 status despite concerns about how well it represents vitamin B_6 status. 4-Pyridoxic acid is the major urinary metabolite of vitamin B_6. It is considered a useful

indicator of immediate dietary intake and of short-term vitamin B_6 status.

16. When vitamin B_6 deficiency exists, unusually high concentrations of xanthurenic acid and cystathionine occur in 24-hour urine collections after administration of tryptophan and methionine, respectively. Direct measures of vitamin B_6 are replacing the tryptophan load test, which historically has been the most widely used indicator of vitamin B_6 status. The methionine load test is used less frequently, and no definitive reference values for urinary cystathionine are available. Both load tests are limited by the need for 24-hour urine collections and by nonnutritional confounders.
17. Erythrocyte alanine transaminase and erythrocyte aspartic acid transaminase are two enzymes whose activity is decreased in vitamin B_6 deficiency. Measurement of their activity before and after in vitro addition of vitamin B_6 can be a useful index of vitamin B_6 status, but the approach has certain limitations.
18. Measures for assessing folate status include measurement of serum folate and erythrocyte folate and the deoxyuridine suppression test. Serum folate is indicative of negative folate balance but cannot discriminate between transient fluctuations in serum folate and chronic deficiency and depleted body stores. Erythrocyte folate is considered to be the best clinical index of depleted tissue stores. The deoxyuridine suppression test is a useful index of plasma and erythrocyte folate concentrations but is not as good an indicator as erythrocyte folate measurement.
19. The primary cause of vitamin B_{12} deficiency is inadequate absorption, usually because of inadequate gastric production of intrinsic factor, although ileal resection or ileal dysfunction can also cause B_{12} malabsorption. Pernicious anemia is characterized by hematologic, gastrointestinal, and nervous system abnormalities. Once vitamin B_{12} deficiency has been diagnosed, the Shilling test is used to determine whether it is due to lack of intrinsic factor production or to some ileal dysfunction.
20. Blood chemistry tests are assays performed on the substances in plasma or serum that are useful in diagnosing and managing disease. They include electrolytes, enzymes, metabolites, and other substances present in serum or plasma. These tests usually are performed using an automated chemistry analyzer capable of performing several thousand blood tests per hour.

REFERENCES

1. Leklem JE. 1990. Vitamin B_6: A status report. *Journal of Nutrition* 120:1503–1507.
2. Benjamin DR. 1989. Laboratory tests and nutritional assessment: Protein-energy status. *Pediatric Clinics of North America* 36:139–161.
3. Underwood BA. 1990. Dose-response tests in field surveys. *Journal of Nutrition* 120:1455–1458.
4. Bingham SA. 1994. The use of 24-h urine samples and energy expenditure to validate dietary assessments. *American Journal of Clinical Nutrition* 59(suppl):227S–231S.
5. Black AE, Prentice SM, Goldberg GR, Jebb SA, Bingham SA, Livingstone MBE, Coward WA. 1993. Measurements of total energy expenditure provide insights into the validity of dietary measurements of energy intake. *Journal of the American Dietetic Association* 93:572–579.
6. Phinney SD. 1981. The assessment of protein nutrition in the hospitalized patient. *Clinics in Laboratory Medicine* 1:767–774.
7. Young VR, Marchini JS, Cortiella J. 1990. Assessment of protein nutritional status. *Journal of Nutrition* 120:1469–1502.
8. Gibson RS. 1990. *Nutritional Assessment.* New York: Oxford University Press.
9. Torun B, Chew F. 1994. Protein-energy malnutrition. In Shils ME, Olson JA, Shike M, eds. *Modern nutrition in health and disease,* 8th ed. Philadelphia: Lea & Febiger.

10. Foster MR, Heppenstall RB, Friedenberg ZB, Hozack WJ. 1990. A prospective assessment of nutritional status and implications in patients with fractures of the hip. *Journal of Orthopedic Trauma* 4:49–57.
11. Bashir Y, Graham TR, Torrence A, Gibson GJ, Corris PA. 1990. Nutritional state of patients with lung cancer undergoing thoracotomy. *Thorax* 45:183–186.
12. Young GA, Kopple JD, Lindholm B, Vonesh EF, et al. 1991. Nutrition assessment of continuous ambulatory peritoneal dialysis patients: An international study. *American Journal of Kidney Diseases* 17:462–471.
13. Henderson CJ, Lovell DJ. 1989. Assessment of protein-energy malnutrition in children and adolescents with juvenile rheumatoid arthritis. *Arthritis Care and Research* 2:108–113.
14. Heymsfield SB, Tighe A, Wang ZM. 1994. Nutritional assessment by anthropometric and biochemical methods. In Shils ME, Olson JA, Shike M, eds. *Modern nutrition in health and disease,* 8th ed. Philadelphia: Lea & Febiger.
15. Rennie MJ, Millward DJ. 1983. 3-Methylhistidine excretion and the urinary 3-methylhistidine/ creatinine ratio are poor indicators of skeletal muscle protein breakdown. *Clinical Science* 65:217–225.
16. Herrmann FR, Safran C, Levkoff SE, Minaker KL. 1992. Serum albumin level on admission as a predictor of death, length of stay, and readmission. *Archives of Internal Medicine* 152:125–130.
17. Tuchschmid Y, Tschantz P. 1992. Complications in gerontologic surgery: Role of nutritional status and serum albumin. *Helvetica Chirurgica Acta* 58:771–774.
18. Kovacevich DS, Braunschweig CL, August DA, eds. 1994. *Parenteral and enteral nutrition manual,* 7th ed. Ann Arbor: University of Michigan Medical Center.
19. Food and Nutrition Board, National Research Council. 1989. *Recommended Dietary Allowances,* 10th ed. Washington, DC: National Academy Press.
20. Unterman TG, Vazquez RM, Slas AJ, Matryn PA, Phillips LS. 1985. Nutrition and somatomedin. XIII. Usefulness of somatomedin-C in nutritional assessment. *American Journal of Medicine* 78:228–234.
21. Sandberg L, VanReken D, Waiwaiku K, Martin-Yeboah P, Weiss C, Updegraff V, Hanson A, Schleman M, Lodhian B. 1985. Plasma fibronectin levels in acute and recovering malnourished children. *Clinical Physiology and Biochemistry* 3:257–264.
22. Yoder MC, Anderson DC, Gopalakrishna GS, Douglas SD, Polin RA. 1987. Comparison of serum fibronectin, prealbumin, and albumin concentrations during nutritional repletion in protein-calorie malnourished infants. *Journal of Pediatric Gastroenterology and Nutrition* 6:84–88.
23. McKone TK, Davis AT, Dean RE. 1985. Fibronectin: A new nutritional parameter. *American Surgeon* 51:336–339.
24. Sandberg LB, Owens AJ, VanReken DE, Horowitz B, Fredell JE, Takyi Y, Troko DM, Horowitz MS, Hanson AP. 1990. Improvement in plasma protein concentrations with fibronectin treatment in severe malnutrition. *American Journal of Clinical Nutrition* 52:651–656.
25. Chandra RK. 1981. Immunodeficiency in undernutrition and overnutrition. *Nutrition Reviews* 39:225–231.
26. Chandra RK. 1991. 1990 McCollum Award Lecture. Nutrition and immunity: Lessons from the past and new insights into the future. *American Journal of Clinical Nutrition* 53:1087–1101.
27. VanDeGraf KM, Fox SI. 1992. *Concepts of human anatomy and physiology.* Dubuque, Iowa: Wm. C. Brown.
28. Chandra RK. 1981. Immunocompetence as a functional index of nutritional status. *British Medical Bulletin* 37:89–94.
29. Myrvik QN. 1994. Immunology and nutrition. In Shils ME, Olson JA, Shike M, eds. *Modern nutrition in health and disease,* 8th ed. Philadelphia: Lea & Febiger.
30. Twomey P, Ziegler D, Rombeau J. 1982. Utility of skin testing in nutritional assessment: A critical review. *Journal of Parenteral and Enteral Nutrition* 6:50–58.
31. Life Sciences Research Office, Federation of American Societies for Experimental Biology. 1989. *Nutrition monitoring in the United States: An update report on nutrition monitoring.* Washington, DC: U.S. Government Printing Office.

32. Johnson MA. 1990. Iron: Nutrition monitoring and nutrition status assessment. *Journal of Nutrition* 120:1486–1491.
33. Expert Scientific Working Group. 1985. Summary of a report on assessment of the iron nutritional status of the United States population. *American Journal of Clinical Nutrition* 42:1318–1330.
34. Fairbanks VF. 1994. Iron in medicine and nutrition. In Shils ME, Olson JA, Shike M, eds. *Modern nutrition in health and disease,* 8th ed. Philadelphia: Lea & Febiger.
35. Ravel R. 1989. *Clinical laboratory medicine: Clinical application of laboratory data,* 5th ed. St Louis: Mosby.
36. Weaver CM. 1990. Assessing calcium status and metabolism. *Journal of Nutrition* 120:1470–1473.
37. Allen LH, Wood RJ. 1994. Calcium and phosphorus. In Shils ME, Olson JA, Shike M, eds. *Modern nutrition in health and disease,* 8th ed. Philadelphia: Lea & Febiger.
38. Nordin BEC, Need AG, Hartley TF, Philcox JC, Wilcox M, Thomas DW. 1989. Improved method for calculating calcium fractions in plasma: Reference values and effects of menopause. *Clinical Chemistry* 35:14–17.
39. McCarron DA. 1982. Low serum concentrations of ionized calcium in patients with hypertension. *New England Journal of Medicine* 307:226–228.
40. Resnick LM, Laragh JH, Sealey LE, Alderman MH. 1983. Divalent cations in essential hypertension: Relations between serum ionized calcium, magnesium, and plasma renin activity. *New England Journal of Medicine* 309:888–891.
41. Kesteloot H, Geboers J. 1982. Calcium and blood pressure. *Lancet* 1:813–815.
42. Robinson D, Bailey AR, Williams PT. 1982. Calcium and blood pressure. *Lancet* 2:1215–1216.
43. Marshall RW, Francis RM, Hodgkinson A. 1982. Plasma total and ionized calcium, albumin, and globulin concentrations in pre- and post-menopausal women and the effects of estrogen administration. *Clinica Chemica Acta* 122:283–287.
44. King JC, Keen CL. 1994. Zinc. In Shils ME, Olson JA, Shike M, eds. *Modern nutrition in health and disease,* 8th ed. Philadelphia: Lea & Febiger.
45. King JC. 1990. Assessment of zinc status. *Journal of Nutrition* 120:1474–1479.
46. Walravens PA, Krebs NF, Hambidge KM. 1983. Linear growth of low income preschool children receiving a zinc supplement. *American Journal of Clinical Nutrition* 38:195–201.
47. Walravens PA, Hambidge KM, Koepfer DM. 1989. Zinc supplementation in infants with a nutritional pattern of failure to thrive: A double-blind, controlled study. *Pediatrics* 83:532–538.
48. Giugliano R, Millward DJ. 1984. Growth and zinc homeostasis in the severely Zn-deficient rat. *British Journal of Nutrition* 52:545–560.
49. Taylor CM, Bacon JR, Aggett PJ, Bremner I. 1991. Homeostatic regulation of zinc absorption and endogenous losses in zinc-deprived men. *American Journal of Clinical Nutrition* 53:755–763.
50. Jackson MJ, Jones DA, Edwards RHT. 1982. Tissue zinc levels as an index of body zinc status. *Clinical Physiology* 2:333–343.
51. Hambidge KM. 1982. Hair analysis: Worthless for vitamins, limited for minerals. *American Journal of Clinical Nutrition* 36:943–949.
52. Taylor A. 1986. Usefulness of measurements of trace elements in hair. *Annals of Clinical Biochemistry* 23:364–378.
53. Jacob RA. 1981. Zinc and copper. *Clinics in Laboratory Medicine* 1:743–766.
54. Davies TS. 1982. Hair analysis and selenium shampoos. *Lancet* 2:935.
55. DeAntonio SM, Katz SA, Scheiner DM, Wood JD. 1982. Anatomically-related variations in trace-metal concentrations in hair. *Clinical Chemistry* 28:2411–2413.
56. Olson JA. 1994. Vitamin A, retinoids, and carotenoids. In Shils ME, Olson JA, Shike M., eds. *Modern nutrition in health and disease,* 8th ed. Philadelphia: Lea & Febiger.
57. Underwood BA. 1990. Methods for assessment of vitamin A status. *Journal of Nutrition* 120:1459–1463.
58. Garry PJ. 1981. Vitamin A. *Clinics in Laboratory Medicine* 1:699–711.
59. Amedee-Manesme O, Mourey MA, Hanck A, Therasse J. 1987. Vitamin A relative dose response test: Validation by intravenous injection in children with liver disease. *American Journal of Clinical Nutrition* 46:286–289.
60. Pilch SM. 1987. Analysis of vitamin A data from the health and nutrition examination surveys. *Journal of Nutrition* 117:636–640.

61. Amedee-Manesme O, Anderson D, Olson JA. 1984. Relation of the relative dose response to liver concentrations of vitamin A in generally well-nourished surgical patients. *American Journal of Clinical Nutrition* 39:898–902.
62. Amedee-Manesme O, Luzeau R, Wittepen JR, Hanck A, Sommer A. 1988. Impression cytology detects subclinical vitamin A deficiency. *American Journal of Clinical Nutrition* 47:875–878.
63. Luzeau R, Carlier C, Ellrodt A, Amedee-Manesme O. 1987. Impression cytology with transfer: An easy method of detection of vitamin A deficiency. *International Journal of Vitamin and Nutrition Research* 58:166–179.
64. Jacob RA. 1990. Assessment of human vitamin C status. *Journal of Nutrition* 120:1480–1485.
65. Alaimo K, McDowell MA, Briefel RR, Bischof AM, Caughman CR, Loria CM, Johnson CL. 1994. Dietary intake of vitamins, minerals, and fiber of persons ages 2 months and over in the United States: Third National Health and Nutrition Examination Survey, Phase 1, 1988–91. *Advance Data from Vital and Health Statistics* No. 258. Hyattsville, Md: U.S. Center for Health Statistics.
66. Sauberlich HW. 1981. Ascorbic acid (vitamin C). *Clinics in Laboratory Medicine* 1:673–684.
67. Solomons NW, Allen LH. 1983. The functional assessment of nutritional status: Principles, practice and potential. *Nutrition Reviews* 41:33–50.
68. Jacob RA. 1994. Vitamin C. In Shils ME, Olson JA, Shike M., eds. *Modern nutrition in health and disease,* 8th ed. Philadelphia: Lea & Febiger.
69. Blanchard J, Conrad KA, Watson RR, Garry PJ, Crawley JD. 1989. Comparison of plasma, mononuclear, and polymorphonuclear leukocyte vitamin C levels in young and elderly women during depletion and supplementation. *European Journal of Clinical Nutrition* 43:97–106.
70. Schaus ES, Kutnink MA, O'Conner DK, Omaye ST. 1986. A comparison of leukocyte ascorbate levels measured by the 2,4-dinitrophenylhydrazine method with high-performance liquid chromatography using electrochemical detection. *Biochemical Medicine and Metabolic Biology* 36:369–376.
71. VanderJagt DJ, Garry PJ, Bhagavan HN. 1989. Ascorbate and dehydroascorbate: Distribution in mononuclear cells of healthy elderly people. *American Journal of Clinical Nutrition* 49:511–516.
72. Omaye ST, Schaus EE, Kutnink MA, Hawkes WC. 1987. Measurement of vitamin C in blood components by high-performance liquid chromatography. Implication in assessing vitamin C status. *Annals of the New York Academy of Science* 498:389–401.
73. Jacob RA, Skala JH, Omaye ST. 1987. Biochemical indices of human vitamin C status. *American Journal of Clinical Nutrition* 46:818–826.
74. Evans RM, Currie L, Campbell A. 1982. The distribution of ascorbic acid between various cellular components of blood in normal individuals, and its relation to the plasma concentration. *British Journal of Nutrition* 47:473–482.
75. Garry PJ, Goodwin JS, Hunt WC, Gilbert BA. 1982. Nutritional status in a healthy elderly population: Vitamin C. *American Journal of Clinical Nutrition* 36:332–339.
76. Schectman G, Byrd JC, Hoffman R. 1991. Ascorbic acid requirements for smokers: Analysis of a population survey. *American Journal of Clinical Nutrition* 53:1466–1470.
77. Sauberlich HE. 1985. Interaction of vitamin B_6 with other nutrients. In Reynolds RD, Leklem JE, eds. *Vitamin B_6: Its role in health and disease.* New York: Alan R. Liss.
78. Leklem JE. 1994. Vitamin B_6. In Shils ME, Olson JA, Shike M, eds. *Modern nutrition in health and disease,* 8th ed. Philadelphia: Lea & Febiger.
79. Leklem JE. 1988. Vitamin B_6 metabolism and function in humans. In Leklem JE, Reynolds RD, eds. *Clinical and physiological applications of vitamin B_6*. New York: Alan R. Liss.
80. Schaumberg H, Kaplan J, Windebank A, Vick N, Rasmus S, Pleasure D, Brown MJ. 1983. Sensory neuropathy from pyridoxine abuse: A new megavitamin syndrome. *New England Journal of Medicine* 309:445–448.
81. Coburn SP, Lewis DLN, Fink WJ, Mahuren JD, Schaltenbrand WD, Costill DL. 1988. Human vitamin B_6 pools estimated through muscle biopsies. *American Journal of Clinical Nutrition* 48:291–294.

82. Leklem JE. 1988. Challenges and directions in the search for clinical applications of vitamin B_6. In Leklem JE, Reynolds RD, eds. *Clinical and physiological applications of vitamin B_6*. New York: Alan R. Liss.
83. Herbert V, Das KC. 1994. Folic acid and vitamin B_{12}. In Shils ME, Olson JA, Shike M., eds. *Modern nutrition in health and disease,* 8th ed. Philadelphia: Lea & Febiger.
84. Bailey LB. 1990. Folate status assessment. *Journal of Nutrition* 120:1508–1511.
85. Reider MJ. 1994. Prevention of neural tube defects with periconceptual folic acid. *Clinical Perinatology* 21:483–503.
86. Rose NC, Mennuti MT. 1994. Periconceptual folate supplementation and neural tube defects. *Clinical Obstetrics and Gynecology* 37:605–620.
87. Rush D. 1994. Periconceptual folate and neural tube defect. *American Journal of Clinical Nutrition* 59(2 suppl):511S–515S.
88. Herbert V. 1987. The 1986 Herman Award Lecture. Nutrition science as a continually unfolding story: The folate and vitamin B_{12} paradigm. *American Journal of Clinical Nutrition* 46:387–402.
89. Colman N. 1981. Laboratory assessment of folate status. *Clinics in Laboratory Medicine* 1:775–796.
90. Wagner C. 1984. Folic acid. In *Present knowledge in nutrition,* 5th ed. Washington, DC: The Nutrition Foundation.
91. Tamura T, Soong SJ, Sauberlich HE, Hatch KD, Cole P, Butterworth CE. 1990. Evaluation of the deoxyuridine suppression test by using whole blood samples from folic acid-supplemented subjects. *American Journal of Clinical Nutrition* 51:80–86.
92. Babior BM, Bunn HF. 1994. Megaloblastic anemias. In Isselbacher KJ, Braunwald E, Wilson JD, Martin JB, Fauci AS, Kasper DL, eds. *Harrison's principles of internal medicine,* 13th ed. New York: McGraw-Hill.
93. Wallach J. 1992. *Interpretation of diagnostic tests,* 5th ed. Boston: Little, Brown.
94. Tilkian SM, Conover MB, Tilkian AG. 1987. *Clinical implications of laboratory tests,* 4th ed. St Louis: Mosby.

Assessment Activity 9-1

VISITING A CLINICAL LABORATORY

Every hospital or clinic has a clinical laboratory where at least some of the facility's biochemical tests are performed. Specimens are sometimes sent to an outside clinical laboratory because it has specialized instruments and expertise or because its automated analyzers allow certain tests to be performed more economically. However, all hospitals have facilities for performing certain basic tests, especially those required in emergency situations. Among these are tests for electrolytes, blood gases, enzymes diagnostic of cardiac or liver disease, and glucose.

We suggest that your class arrange to visit a clinical laboratory to see how some of the tests mentioned in this and other chapters are performed. You may be surprised by the capability of various automated instruments used to perform the chemistry profile and complete blood count on a single specimen of serum or whole blood.

Assessment Activity 9-2

CHEMISTRY PROFILE, COMPLETE BLOOD COUNT, AND CORONARY RISK PROFILE

The chemistry profile, complete blood count (CBC), and coronary risk profile are among the most basic series of tests performed by clinical laboratories. Generally included in the chemistry profile are those tests listed in the section entitled "Blood Chemistry Tests." Included in the CBC are the red blood cell count, white blood cell count, and measurements of hemoglobin, hematocrit, mean corpuscular volume, mean corpuscular hemoglobin, and mean corpuscular hemoglobin concentration. The coronary risk profile measures levels of triglyceride, total cholesterol, and HDL-C (cholesterol carried by high-density lipoproteins) and calculates LDL-C (cholesterol carried by low-density lipoproteins) and the total cholesterol/HDL-C ratio. These tests are discussed in Chapter 8. These measurements are routinely performed using automated instruments capable of performing several thousand tests per hour.

Members of your class may want to have their blood drawn by a qualified venipuncturist and have the sample sent to a clinical laboratory for analysis. Tests that might be performed include the CBC, chemistry profile, and coronary risk profile. One alternative would be to perform some of these tests right in the classroom. A variety of desktop blood analyzers are available, which can perform several different tests. Included among these are the Abbott Vision, the Kodak Ectakem DT 60, and the Boehringer Mannheim Reflotron. You probably have seen one of these used for measuring total cholesterol at a health fair or shopping center. Your school's student health center may have one of these instruments and might be willing to bring it to your classroom for a demonstration.

Another example of a simple test that can be done in the classroom is the hematocrit. The necessary equipment includes a centrifuge, capillary tubes, lancets, alcohol wipes, gloves, and some way of comparing the volume of whole blood in the capillary tube with the volume of packed cells after the tube is spun down. Whatever approach your class takes, compare your test results with the reference values given in this chapter and Chapter 8. Obtain an average value for the class and compare this with the reference values, as well.

Remember, in handling blood specimens or any body fluid, precautions must be taken to protect patients and laboratory staff from infectious agents, especially those causing hepatitis as well as the human immunodeficiency virus (HIV). All body fluids must be regarded as being infectious and handled with the utmost care. All syringes, lancets, needles, tubes, and other materials that have come in contact with blood or other body fluids must be handled safely and disposed of properly. Gloves should be worn whenever drawing blood or handling body fluids.

TEN

Clinical Assessment of Nutritional Status

Outline

INTRODUCTION

Clinical assessment of nutritional status involves a detailed history, a thorough physical examination, and the interpretation of the signs and symptoms associated with malnutrition. Signs are defined as observations made by a qualified examiner of which the patient is usually unaware. Symptoms are clinical manifestations reported by the patient. This chapter discusses clinical assessment of nutritional status and gives some examples of clinical indicators of impaired nutritional status. As a dietitian or nutritionist, you will likely see some of the conditions discussed and illustrated in this chapter. For example, protein-energy malnutrition and severe wasting are common features of certain cancers, acquired immunodeficiency syndrome (AIDS), and advanced disease of the gastrointestinal tract. However, some of the other conditions discussed in this chapter such as clinical signs of advanced nutrient deficiency are rarely seen in developed countries but occur more frequently in less industrialized nations. Despite their rare occurrence, these conditions and their clinical signs are still of interest to students and practitioners of nutrition. Because many of the clinical findings are not specific for a particular nutrient deficiency, they often must be integrated with anthropometric, biochemical, and dietary data before arriving at a definitive diagnosis.

MEDICAL HISTORY

Obtaining a patient's history is the first step in the clinical assessment of nutritional status.[1] A good way to begin is by reviewing the patient's medical record, giving careful attention to the patient's past medical history.[2,3] Components from the medical history to consider in nutritional assessment are shown in Box 10-1.

Essential components of a patient's history include pertinent facts about past and current health and use of medications, and personal and household information.[1,2] A variety of diseases can affect nutritional status. Among these are diabetes, kidney disease, various cancers, coronary heart disease, stroke, liver disease (e.g.,

BOX 10-1

Components of the Medical History to Consider in Nutritional Assessment

- Past and current diagnoses of nutritional consequence
- Diagnostic procedures
- Surgeries
- Chemotherapy and radiation therapy
- History of nutrition-related problems
- Existing nutrient deficiencies
- Medications and their nutrient interactions
- Psychosocial history—alcohol, smoking, finances, social support
- Signs or symptoms suggestive of vitamin deficiency
- Signs or symptoms suggestive of mineral deficiency

Adapted from Phinney SD. 1981. The assessment of protein nutrition in the hospitalized patient. *Clinics in Laboratory Medicine* 1:767–774; McLaren DS. 1992. *A colour atlas and text of diet-related disorders,* 2nd ed. London: Mosby Europe; Jeejeebhoy KN. 1994. Clinical and functional assessments. In Shills ME, Olson, JA, Shike M, eds. *Modern nutrition in health and disease,* 8th ed. Philadelphia: Lea & Febiger.

hepatitis and cirrhosis), gallbladder disease, AIDS, ulcers, and colitis, as well as recent or past surgical procedures. Other conditions affecting nutritional status also should be explored: the ability to chew and swallow; appetite; and the presence of vomiting, diarrhea, constipation, flatulence, belching, and indigestion. An inquiry should be made about the patient's usual weight and any recent changes (gains or losses) in weight. A systematic approach to the detection of deficiency syndromes based on findings from the history is shown in Table 10-1.

Information on the use of medications will provide clues about the patient's actual or perceived medical condition. This will include prescription and over-the-counter medications, vitamin and mineral supplements, and nontraditional medications such as herbal and folk remedies.

Psychosocial factors include the patient's age, occupation, educational level, marital status, income, living arrangements, number of dependents, use of alcohol, tobacco, and illicit drugs, the degree of social and emotional support, and access to and ability to pay for health care. These factors are summarized in Box 10-2.

The necessary detail of the history will vary depending on circumstances and will be influenced by the patient's ability to respond to questioning. In some instances, the necessary information might need to be obtained from a surrogate (a parent, companion, sibling, or other person knowledgeable about the patient's life habits). Much of this information can be obtained from the history and physical examination performed by the admitting physician, from the notes of nurses or social workers, and from previous medical records. Remember that this and all information about the patient should be dealt with in a confidential and strictly professional manner.

DIETARY HISTORY

Included with the history is information about the patient's eating practices. This includes a wide range of information about usual eating pattern (timing and location of meals and snacks), food likes and dislikes, intolerances and allergies, and amount of money available for purchasing food, ability to obtain and prepare food, eligibility for and access to food assistance programs, and use of vitamin, mineral, and other supplements (if not obtained in the history). These and other factors are included in Box 10-2.

TABLE 10-1 Nutritional history screens—a systematic approach to the detection of deficiency syndromes

Mechanism of deficiency	If history of	Suspect deficiency of
Inadequate intake	Alcoholism	Energy, protein, thiamin, niacin, folate, pyridoxine, riboflavin
	Avoidance of fruit, vegetables, grains	Vitamin C, thiamin, niacin, folate
	Avoidance of meat, dairy products, eggs	Protein, vitamin B_{12}
	Constipation, hemorrhoids, diverticulosis	Dietary fiber
	Isolation, poverty, dental disease, food idiosyncrasies	Various nutrients
	Weight loss	Energy, other nutrients
Inadequate absorption	Drugs (especially antacids, anticonvulsants, cholestyramine, laxatives, neomycin, alcohol)	Various nutrients depending on drug/nutrient interaction
	Malabsorption (diarrhea, weight loss, steatorrhea)	Vitamins A, D, K, energy, protein, calcium, magnesium, zinc
	Parasites	Iron, vitamin B_{12} (fish tapeworm)
	Pernicious anemia	Vitamin B_{12}
	Surgery	
	Gastrectomy	Vitamin B_{12}, iron
	Small bowel resection	Vitamin B_{12}, (if distal ileum), others as in malabsorption
Decreased utilization	Drugs (especially anticonvulsants, antimetabolites, oral contraceptives, isoniazid, alcohol)	Various nutrients depending on drug/nutrient interaction
	Inborn errors of metabolism (by family history)	Various nutrients
Increased losses	Alcohol abuse	Magnesium, zinc
	Blood loss	Iron
	Centesis (ascitic, pleural taps)	Protein
	Diabetes, uncontrolled	Energy
	Diarrhea	Protein, zinc, electrolytes
	Draining abscesses, wounds	Protein, zinc
	Nephrotic syndrome	Protein, zinc
	Peritoneal dialysis or hemodialysis	Protein, water-soluble vitamins, zinc
Increased requirements	Fever	Energy
	Hyperthyroidism	Energy
	Physiologic demands (infancy, adolescence, pregnancy, lactation)	Various nutrients
	Surgery, trauma, burns, infection	Energy, protein, vitamin C, zinc
	Tissue hypoxia	Energy (inefficient utilization)
	Cigarette smoking	Vitamin C, folic acid

From Weinsier RL, Morgan SL, Perrin VG. 1993. *Fundamentals of clinical nutrition*. St. Louis: Mosby.

BOX 10-2

Factors to Consider in Taking a Patient's Nutritional History

- Weight changes
- Usual meal pattern
- Appetite
- Satiety
- Discomfort after eating
- Chewing/swallowing ability
- Likes/dislikes
- Taste changes/aversions
- Allergies
- Nausea/vomiting
- Bowel habits—diarrhea, constipation, steatorrhea
- Living conditions
- Snack consumption
- Vitamin/mineral supplement use
- Alcohol/drug use
- Previous diet restrictions
- Surgery/chronic diseases
- Ability to purchase and prepare food
- Access to and ability to pay for health care

Adapted from Phinney SD. 1981. The assessment of protein nutrition in the hospitalized patient. *Clinics in Laboratory Medicine* 1:767–774; McLaren DS. 1992. *A colour atlas and text of diet-related disorders,* 2nd ed. London: Mosby Europe; Jeejeebhoy KN. 1994. Clinical and functional assessments. In Shills ME, Olson, JA, Shike M, eds. *Modern nutrition in health and disease,* 8th ed. Philadelphia: Lea & Febiger.

For example, when inquiring about appetite, satiety, or discomfort, it is important to ask if the patient has experienced any changes in desire for food, if he or she experiences satiety earlier or later than usual, and if there is any pain or discomfort associated with eating. Questions about the ability to chew and swallow food are important. Are there dental or oral problems making it difficult to chew certain foods or to consume adequate energy to support normal body weight? If the patient wears dentures, are they well fitting? If swallowing is painful or difficult, for what foods?

Questioning the patient about bowel habits can often provide information pertinent to the diagnosis of gastrointestinal disease. The patient should be asked about changes in bowel habits such as constipation, diarrhea, or unusual amounts of flatus (gas) and about stool consistency and color. Obviously, the presence of bright red blood in the stool is an important finding. Stools containing digested blood (e.g., from a bleeding peptic ulcer) may appear black or tarry. The finding of frothy, watery, and foul-smelling stools suggests the possibility of fat malabsorption. Table 10-2 gives a listing of clinical findings and links their presence with either an excess or deficiency of various nutrients.

SUBJECTIVE GLOBAL ASSESSMENT

Subjective Global Assessment (SGA) is a clinical technique for assessing the nutritional status of a patient based on features of the patient's history and physical examination.[4] Unlike traditional methods that rely heavily on objective anthropometric and biochemical data, SGA is based on four elements of the patient's history (recent loss of body weight, changes in usual diet, presence of significant gastrointestinal symptoms, and the patient's functional capacity) and three elements of the physical examination (loss of subcutaneous fat, muscle wasting, and presence of edema or ascites).[5] Information obtained from the history and physical examination can be entered into a form such as the one shown in Figure 10-1 to arrive at an SGA rating of nutritional status. Two excellent articles giving detailed descriptions of the approach have been published.[4,5]

Elements of the History

The first of the four elements of the history is the percent and pattern of weight loss within 6 months prior to examination. A weight loss $< 5\%$ is considered small. A 5% to 10% weight loss is

TABLE 10-2 Clinical nutrition examination

Clinical findings	Consider deficiency of	Consider excess of	Frequency
Hair, nails			
Flag sign (traverse depigmentation of hair)	Protein		Rare
Easy pluckable hair	Protein		Common
Sparse hair	Protein, biotin, zinc	Vitamin A	Occasional
Corkscrew hairs and unemerged coiled hairs	Vitamin C		Common
Traverse ridging of nails	Protein		Occasional
Skin			
Scaling	Vitamin A, zinc, essential fatty acids	Vitamin A	Occasional
Cellophane appearance	Protein		Occasional
Cracking (flaky paint or crazy pavement dermatosis)	Protein		Rare
Follicular hyperkeratosis	Vitamins A, C		Occasional
Petechiae (especially perifollicular)	Vitamin C		Occasional
Purpura	Vitamins C, K		Common
Pigmentation, desquamation of sun-exposed areas	Niacin		Rare
Yellow pigmentation-sparing sclerae (benign)		Carotene	Common
Eyes			
Papilledema		Vitamin A	Rare
Night blindness	Vitamin A		Rare
Perioral			
Angular stomatitis	Riboflavin, pyridoxine, niacin		Occasional
Cheilosis (dry, cracking, ulcerated lips)	Riboflavin, pyridoxine, niacin		Rare
Oral			
Atrophic lingual papillae (slick tongue)	Riboflavin, niacin, folate, vitamin B_{12}, protein, iron		Common
Glossitis (scarlet, raw tongue)	Riboflavin, niacin, pyridoxine, folate, vitamin B_{12}		Occasional

Continued

TABLE 10-2 Clinical nutrition examination—cont'd

Clinical findings	Consider deficiency of	Consider excess of	Frequency
Oral—cont'd			
Hypogeusesthesia, hyposmia	Zinc		Occasional
Swollen, retracted, bleeding gums (if teeth are present)	Vitamin C		Occasional
Bones, joints			
Beading of ribs, epiphyseal swelling, bowlegs	Vitamin D		Rare
Tenderness (subperiosteal hemorrhage in child)	Vitamin C		Rare
Neurologic			
Headache		Vitamin A	Rare
Drowsiness, lethargy, vomiting		Vitamins A, D	Rare
Dementia	Niacin, vitamin B_{12}		Rare
Confabulation, disorientation	Thiamin (Korsakoff's psychosis)		Occasional
Ophthalmoplegia	Thiamin, phosphorus		Occasional
Peripheral neuropathy (e.g., weakness, paresthesia, ataxia, and decreased tendon reflexes, fine tactile sense, vibratory sense, and position sense)	Thiamin, pyridoxine, vitamin B_{12}	Pyridoxine	Occasional
Tetany	Calcium, magnesium		Occasional
Other			
Parotid enlargement	Protein (also consider bulimia)		Occasional
Heart failure	Thiamin (wet beriberi), phosphorus		Occasional
Sudden heart failure, death	Vitamin C		Rare
Hepatomegaly	Protein	Vitamin A	Rare
Edema	Protein, thiamin		Common
Poor wound healing, pressure ulcers	Protein, vitamin C, zinc		Common

From Weinsier RL, Morgan SL, Perrin VG. 1993. *Fundamentals of clinical nutrition*. St Louis: Mosby.

HISTORY

1. Weight Change

$$\% \text{ Wt change} = \frac{\text{wt 6 months ago} - \text{current wt}}{\text{wt 6 mos ago}} \times 100$$

Maximum body weight ________

Weight 6 months ago ________

Current weight ________

Overall weight loss in past 6 months ________

Percent weight loss in past 6 months ________

Change in 2 past weeks: ______ increase ______ no change ______ decrease

2. Dietary Intake (relative to normal)

________ No change

________ Change Duration: ________ Weeks

Type: ________ Increased intake

________ Suboptimal solid diet

________ Full liquid diet

________ IV or hypocaloric liquids

________ Starvation

3. Gastrointestinal Symptoms (lasting > 2 weeks)

________ None

________ Nausea ________ Vomiting ________ Diarrhea ________ Anorexia

4. Functional Capacity

________ No dysfunction

________ Dysfunction Duration: ________ weeks

Type: ________ Works suboptimally

________ Ambulatory

________ Bedridden

PHYSICAL EXAMINATION

(For each trait specify: 0 = normal; 1+ = mild; 2+ = moderate; 3+ = severe)

________ Loss of subcutaneous fat (shoulders, triceps, chest, hands)

________ Muscle wasting (quadriceps, deltoids)

________ Ankle edema

________ Ascites

Subjective Global Assessment Rating (select one)

________ A = well nourished

________ B = moderately (or suspected of being) malnourished

________ C = severely malnourished

Figure 10-1 Form for rating nutritional status based on Subjective Global Assessment. From Detsky AS, McLaughlin JR, Baker JP, Johnston N, Whittaker S, Mendelson RA, Jeejeebhoy KN. 1987. What is subjective global assessment of nutritional status? *Journal of Parenteral and Enteral Nutrition*. 11:8–13, Detsky AS, Smalley PS, Change J. 1994. Is this patient malnourished? *Journal of the American Medical Association*. 271:54–58.

considered potentially significant. A weight loss >10% is considered definitely significant. The pattern of weight loss is also important. A patient who has lost 12% of his or her weight in the past 6 months but has recently gained 6% of it back is considered better nourished than a patient who has lost 6% of his or her weight in the past 6 months and continues to lose weight. Information about the patient's maximum weight and what it was 6 months ago can be compared to current weight. Questions about changes in the way clothing fits may confirm reports of weight change. Information about changes in body weight in the past 2 weeks (increase, no change, decrease) should be elicited, as well. These data can be entered or noted in the appropriate places in Figure 10-1.

Dietary intake, the second element of the history, is classified as either normal (i.e., what the patient usually eat) or abnormal (i.e., a change from the patient's usual diet). If abnormal, the duration in weeks is entered, and the appropriate box is checked to indicate the type of dietary intake abnormality (i.e., increased intake, suboptimal solid, full-liquid, IV or hypocaloric liquids, or starvation). The patient can be asked if the amount of food consumed has changed, and if so, by how much and why. If the patient is eating less, it would be valuable to know what happens when he or she tries to eat more. Ask for a description of a typical breakfast, lunch, and dinner and how that compares with what the patient typically ate 6 or 12 months ago.

Information about any gastrointestinal symptoms persisting more than 2 weeks (the third history element) should be elicited and noted on the form. Diarrhea or occasional vomiting lasting only a few days are not considered significant. The presence or absence of any dysfunction in the patient's ability to attend to activities of daily living (the last history element) should also be noted on the form. If a dysfunction is present, its duration and type should be noted.

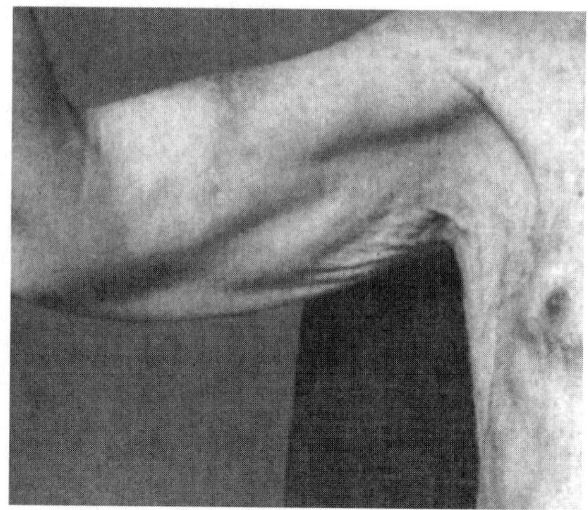

Figure 10-2 An illustration of subcutaneous tissue loss from the arm and chest wall.

Elements of the Physical Examination

The first of the three elements of the physical examination is loss of subcutaneous fat. The four anatomical areas listed in Figure 10-1 (shoulder, triceps, chest, and hands) should be checked for loss of fullness or loose-fitting skin, although the latter may appear in older persons who are not malnourished. Illustrations of subcutaneous fat loss in the arm, chest wall, and hands are shown in Figure 10-2 and Figure 10-3. Loss of subcutaneous fat should be noted as normal (0), mild loss (1+), moderate loss (2+), or severe loss (3+).

According to Detsky, the presence of muscle wasting (the second element of the physical examination) is best assessed by examining the deltoid muscles (located at the sides of the shoulders) and the quadriceps femoris muscles (the muscles of the anterior thigh).[4,5] Loss of subcutaneous fat in the shoulders and deltoid muscle wasting gives the shoulders a squared-off appearance, similar to that shown in Figure 10-4. These areas can be assessed as being normal or mildly, moderately, or severely wasted.

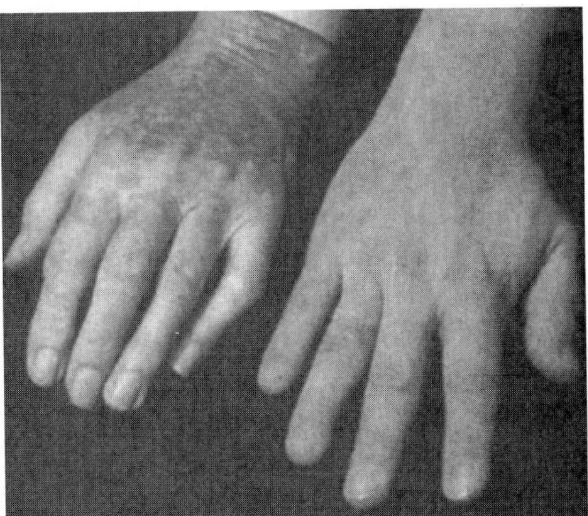

Figure 10-3 Loss of subcutaneous tissue can be clearly seen in the hand on the left compared with the hand of a healthy person on the right.

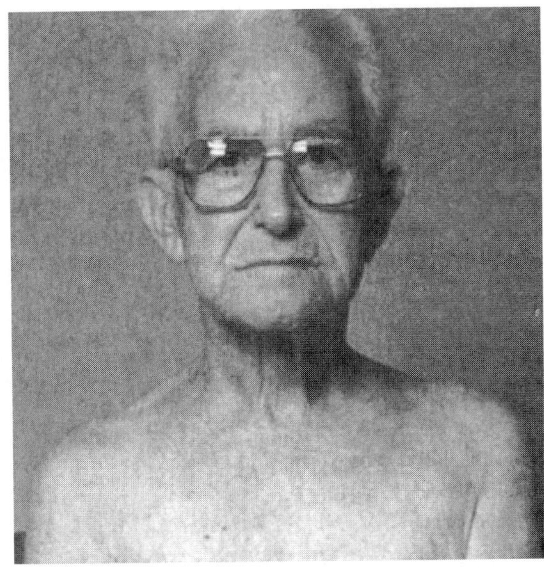

Figure 10-4 The squared-off appearance of the shoulders indicates the loss of subcutaneous tissue and wasting of the deltoid muscle.

The presence of edema at the ankle or sacrum can also be assessed as absent, mild, moderate, or severe. The presence of "pitting" edema can be checked by momentarily pressing the area with a finger and then looking for a persistent depression (more than 5 seconds) where the finger was. Ankle edema and ascites can be assessed as absent, mild, moderate, or severe. When considerable edema or ascites are present, weight loss is a less important variable.

The final step in SGA is arriving at a rating of nutritional assessment. Instead of an explicit numerical weighting scheme (as in the screening form shown in Figure 7-1), SGA depends on the clinician subjectively combining the various elements to arrive at an overall or global assessment. Patients with weight loss >10% that is continuing, poor dietary intake, and severe loss of subcutaneous fat and muscle wasting fall within the severely malnourished category (class C rank). Patients with at least a 5% weight loss, reduced dietary intake, and mild-to-moderate loss of subcutaneous fat and muscle wasting fall within the moderately malnourished category (class B rank). Patients are generally ranked as well nourished when they have had a recent improvement in appetite or the other historical features of SGA. A class A rank would be given to patients having a recent increase in weight (that is not fluid retention) even if their net loss for the past 6 months was between 5% and 10%. Using this approach, very few well-nourished patients are classified as malnourished but some patients with mild-malnutrition may be missed.[4,5]

Despite this subjective nature, clinicians (nurses and residents) trained to use SGA tend to arrive at very similar rankings when comparing their evaluations of a series of 109 patients.[4] The method has also been shown to be a powerful predictor of postoperative complications.[5]

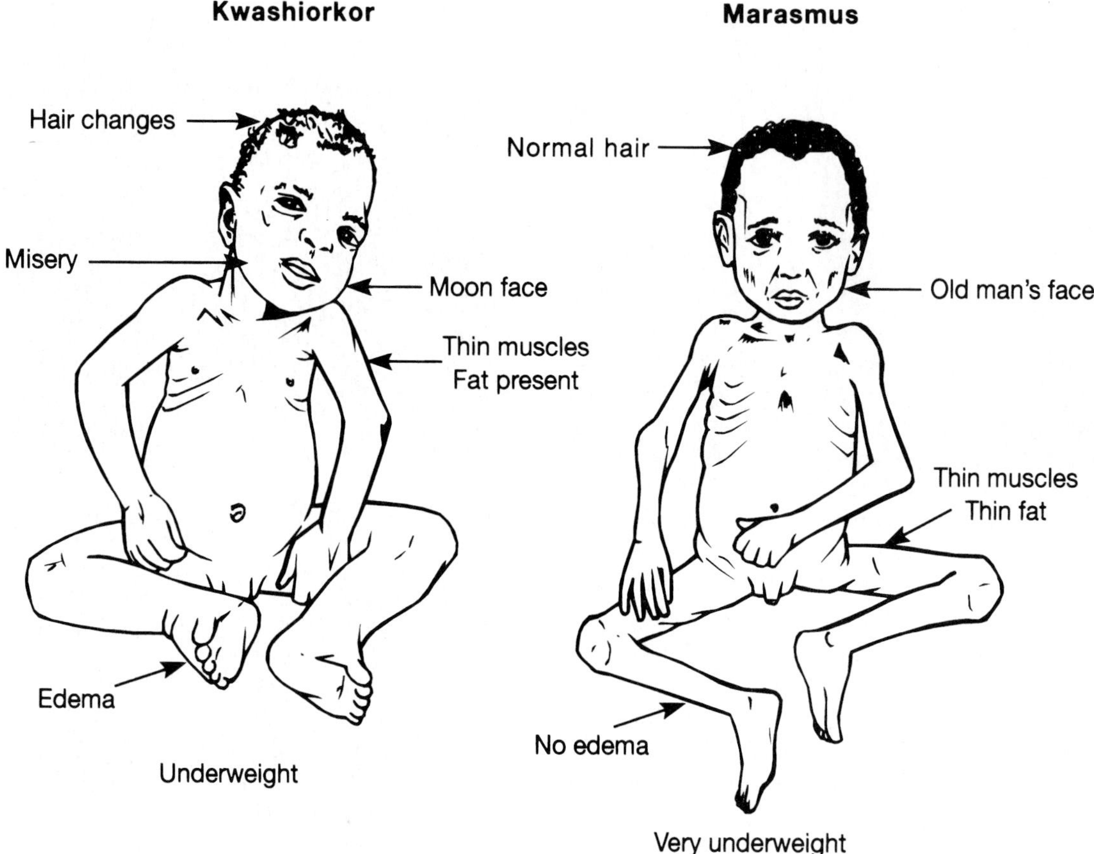

Figure 10-5 Differences in clinical signs between kwashiorkor and marasmus. Adapted from Jellife DB. 1968. *Clinical nutrition in developing countries.* Washington, DC: US Department of Health, Education, and Welfare.

TABLE 10-3 Characteristics of kwashiorkor and marasmus

Variable	Kwashiorkor	Marasmus
Skeletal muscle	No major losses	Significant losses
Serum proteins	Significantly decreased	Relatively normal
Adipose tissue	Preserved	Significant loss
Body weight	Relatively normal	Significant loss
Edema	Pitting edema common	Absent
Predisposing factors	Ample energy with little or no protein	Starvation; lack of both protein and total energy

Data from McLaren DS. 1992. *A colour atlas and text of diet-related disorders,* 2nd ed. London: Mosby Europe; Torún B, Chew F. 1994. Protein-energy malnutrition. In Shils ME, Olson JA, Shike M, eds. *Modern nutrition in health and disease,* 8th ed. Philadelphia: Lea & Febiger; Phinney SD. 1981. The assessment of protein nutrition in the hospitalized patient. *Clinics in Laboratory Medicine* 1:767–774.

CLINICAL SIGNS OF PROTEIN-ENERGY MALNUTRITION

In its most severe states, protein-energy malnutrition (PEM) takes the form of kwashiorkor or marasmus (also discussed in Chapter 9). Kwashiorkor is predominantly a protein deficiency, whereas marasmus is mainly an energy deficiency.[6] Kwashiorkor (Figure 10-5) is characterized by a relatively normal weight, generally intact skeletal musculature, and decreased concentrations of serum proteins.[6–8] A common feature is soft, pitting, painless edema in the feet and legs, extending into the perineum, upper extremities, and face in severe cases. The hair can become dry, brittle, dull, and easily pulled out without pain. The marasmic patient typically presents with significant loss of body weight, skeletal muscle, and adipose tissue mass, but with serum protein concentrations relatively intact. Patients are often seen at 60% or less of their expected weight-for-height, and marasmic children have a marked reduction in their longitudinal growth. Patients are described as having a "skin and bones" appearance. General characteristics of kwashiorkor and marasmus are outlined in Table 10-3.

Although such obvious cases of kwashiorkor and marasmus as illustrated in Figure 10-5 will not often be seen in developed countries, severe cases of protein-energy malnutrition and wasting still occur, especially as a result of AIDS, certain cancers, some gastrointestinal diseases, and alcoholism and other drug abuse. The emaciated condition of the body and general ill health resulting from these and other diseases is also called *cachexia*. Many patients presenting with protein-energy malnutrition and wasting will have diagnostic features in common with either marasmus or kwashiorkor. For example, Figure 10-6 illustrates a case of severe protein-energy malnutrition having several diagnostic features common to marasmus. When this 29-year-old male presented for treatment (A and B), he had lost considerable skeletal muscle, adipose tissue, and body weight.

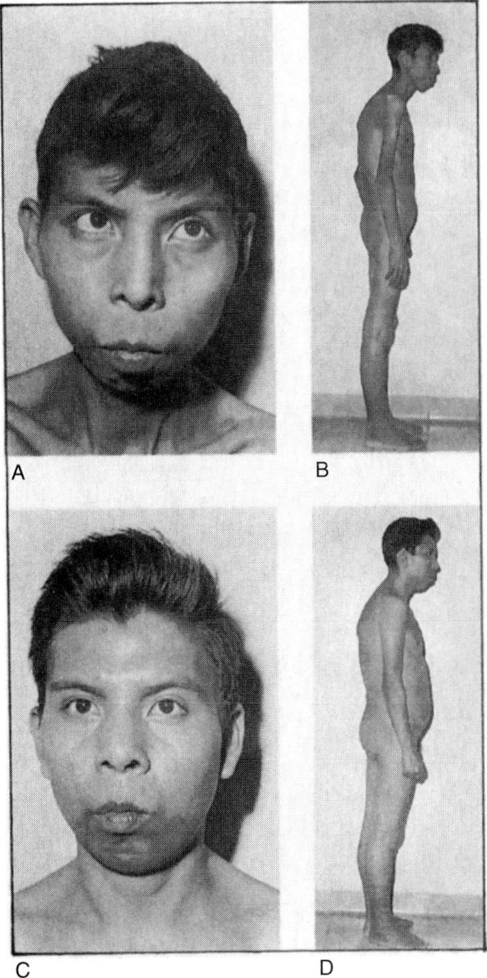

Figure 10-6 Marasmic-like severe protein-energy malnutrition in a 29-year-old male before treatment (**A** and **B**) and after 3 months of nutritional support (**C** and **D**).

There was no edema present. The wasting is particularly apparent in the neck shoulders, and upper arm in A and B. After three months of nutritional support (C and D) there was an obvious increase in skeletal muscle, adipose tissue, and body weight. The face is fuller and there is considerably less wasting apparent in the neck, shoulders, and upper arm.

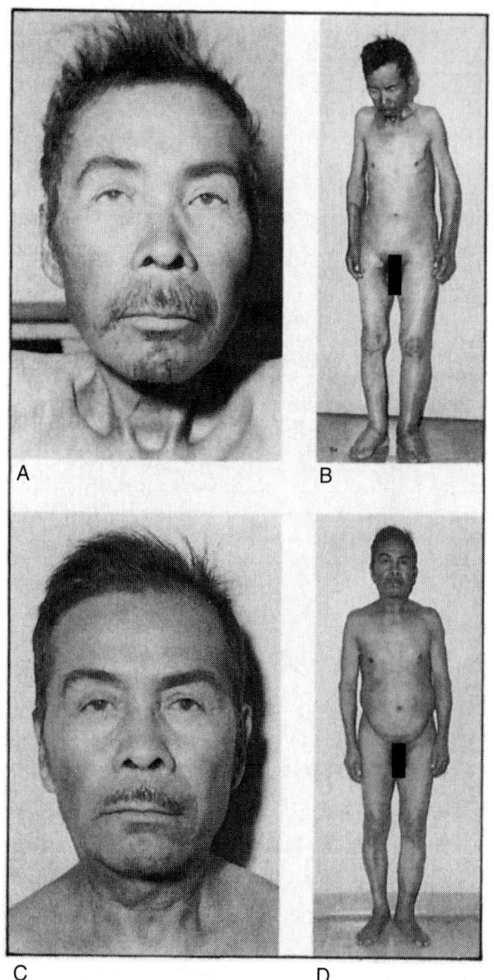

Figure 10-7 Kwashiorkor-like protein-energy malnutrition in a 46-year-old male before treatment (**A** and **B**) and after 3 months of nutritional support (**C** and **D**).

An example of severe protein-energy malnutrition is illustrated in Figure 10-7. As is the case with kwashiorkor, edema can be clearly seen, especially in the legs and feet of this 46-year-old male (A and B). Some wasting can also be seen in the neck, shoulders, and upper arms. After 3 months of treatment (C and D) there is a fuller appearance to the face, neck, shoulders, and upper arms and no apparent edema.

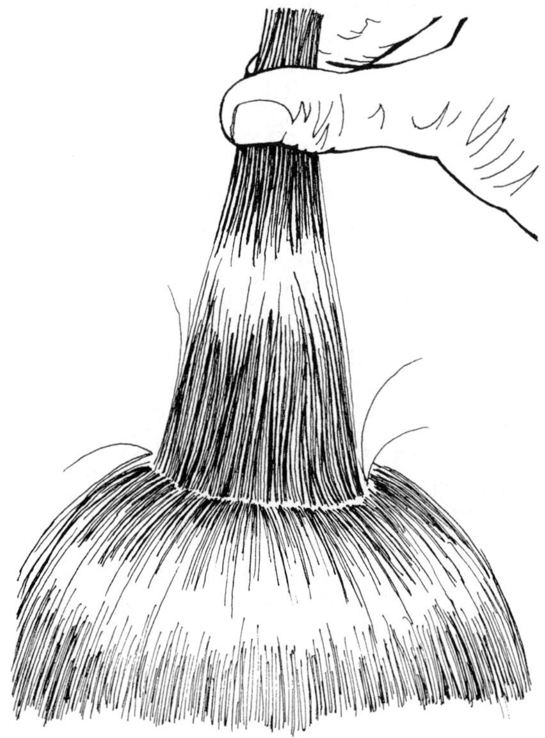

Figure 10-8 The "flag sign" is characterized by bands of depigmented hair that grew during periods of inadequate protein intake. The normally-colored hair grew during periods of relatively adequate protein intake.

Other clinical signs of PEM include the "flag sign" and growth failure. In the flag sign, there are alternating bands of depigmented and normal-colored hair produced by alternating periods of poor and relatively good protein intake. Hair grown during periods of poor protein intake can become depigmented and turn a dull brown, red, or even yellowish white. Hair grown during periods of more adequate protein intake returns to its normal color. The flag sign is especially noticeable in persons with long, dark-colored hair. An example of the flag sign is shown Figure 10-8.

Growth failure (or failure to thrive) is the most common sign of malnutrition in children. It is a failure to gain weight and height at the expected

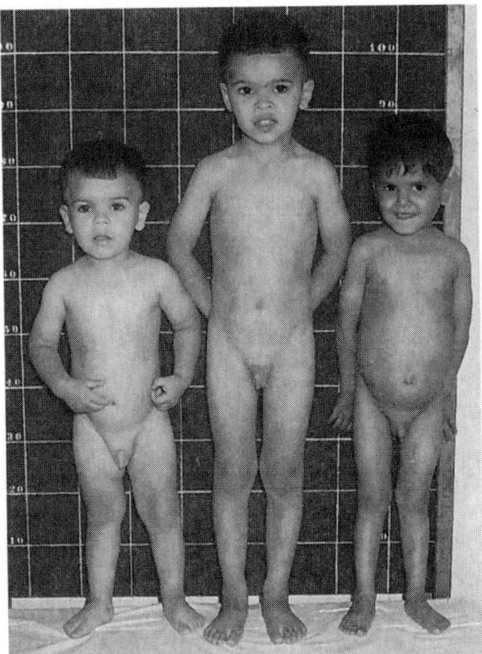

Figure 10-9 An example of growth failure can be seen in the child to the right who is 5.5 years old and yet no more than 5 cm taller than the child on the left who is 2 years old. The child in the middle is 4.5 years old. Less-than-expected height for age (stunting) is the most common evidence of chronic, mild PEM.

rate. Growth failure can result from one or any combination of factors such as inadequate nutrient intake, nutrient malabsorption, failure to utilize nutrients, increased nutrient losses, and increased nutrient requirements. Major contributing factors to growth failure include poverty, inadequate emotional and social nurturing, and infections, especially parasitic gut infestations. Figure 10-9 illustrates growth failure. The ages of the children in this picture are, from left to right, 2, 4.5, and 5.5 years. The children on the left and in the center are of normal size for their age. However, the child on the right has a markedly reduced height-for-age and weight-for-age, although his weight-to-height ratio is normal and there appear to be no other signs of clinical malnutrition. Although he is 3.5 years older than the child on the left, he is less than 5 cm taller.

Classifying Protein-Energy Malnutrition

The severity of PEM in children and adolescents can be classified using records of age and measurements of weight and height or length.[6] From these, weight-for-height (or length) and height-for-age can be calculated. Weight-for-height is a convenient index of current nutritional status, while height-for-age better represents past nutritional status. In this context of classifying the severity of PEM, "wasting" has been suggested as a term for a deficit in weight-for-height and the term "stunting" has been suggested for a deficit in height-for-age. Using these two terms, patients with PEM can be placed in one of four categories: normal; wasted but not stunted (indicating acute PEM); wasted and stunted (indicating acute and chronic PEM); and stunted but not wasted (indicating past PEM with adequate nutrition at present).[6] The severity of wasting can be determined by calculating weight as a percentage of the reference median weight-for-height using the following equation:

$$\%\text{ Weight-for-height} = \frac{\text{actual body weight}}{\text{reference weight for height}} \times 100$$

where reference weight-for-height = the median (or 50th percentile) weight-for-height for the subject's age and sex. To determine the severity of stunting, calculate the height as a percentage of the reference height-for-age using the following equation:

$$\%\text{ Height-for-age} = \frac{\text{actual height or length}}{\text{reference height for age}} \times 100$$

where reference height-for-age = the median (or 50th percentile) height for the subject's age and sex. The values derived from these equations can then be compared with the reference values shown in Table 10-4 to classify the severity of wasting or stunting.

TABLE 10-4 Reference values for classifying deficits in weight-for-height and height-for-age*

Classification	Weight-for-height† (deficit = wasting)	Height-for-age† (deficit = stunting)
Normal	90% to 110%	95% to 105%
Mild deficit	80% to 89%	90% to 94%
Moderate deficit	70% to 79%	85% to 89%
Severe deficit	<70% or with edema	<85%

Adapted from Torún B, Chew F. 1994. Protein-energy malnutrition. In Shills ME, Olson JA, Shike M, eds. *Modern nutrition in health and disease,* 8th ed. Philadelphia: Lea & Febiger.

†Percentage calculated from equations discussed in the text.

*Reference values for classifying the severity of deficits in weight-for-height (wasting) are derived using the percentage of reference median weight-for-height, and deficits in height-for-age (stunting) are derived using the percentage of reference median height-for-age. Median weight-for-height and median height-for-age are derived the NCHS growth charts (see Chapter 6).

TABLE 10-5 Reference values for classifying the severity of protein-energy malnutrition (PEM) in adult males and females and the presence of PEM in adolescent males and females

Subject age	Body Mass Index	PEM
18 yrs and older	<16.0	severe
	16.0–16.9	moderate
	17.0–18.4	mild
	≥18.5	normal
14–17 yrs	<16.5	present
11–13 yrs	<15.0	present

Adapted from Torún B, Chew F. 1994. Protein-energy malnutrition. In Shils ME, Olson JA, Shike M, eds. *Modern nutrition in health and disease,* 8th ed. Philadelphia: Lea & Febiger; Kurtzweil P. 1995. Warding off HIV wasting syndrome. *FDA Consumer.* 29(3):16–20.

A simple approach to assessing the severity of PEM in an adult is to compare his or her body mass index (kg/m^2) (see Chapter 6) with the reference values shown in Table 10-5. The table also gives values for determining the presence of PEM in adolescents but does not allow the severity of PEM in this age group to be assessed.[9] These values can be used for either males or females.

HIV WASTING SYNDROME

Body wasting is a fundamental feature of infection with the human immunodeficiency virus (HIV) and a diagnostic sign that HIV infection has progressed to AIDS. Studies show that 70% to 90% of persons with HIV infection will experience wasting.[10] The U.S. Centers for Disease Control

BOX 10-3

HIV Wasting Syndrome as Defined by the U.S. Centers for Disease Control and Prevention

1. Involuntary weight loss of more than 10% of weight
2. Chronic diarrhea (at least two loose stools a day for 30 days or more) or chronic weakness
3. Constant or intermittent fever for 30 days or more
4. Absence of a condition or illness other than HIV infection that might cause symptoms

From Kurtzweil P. 1995. Warding off HIV wasting syndrome. *FDA Consumer* 29(3):16–20.

and Prevention's definition of HIV wasting syndrome is shown in Box 10-3. Wasting is of considerable concern because of its association with increased morbidity in persons with AIDS.[11,12] It results in physical impairment, psychological stress, decreased tolerance of therapeutic agents, increased susceptibility to infection, and overall diminished quality of life.[11] The known adverse effects of malnutrition on immune function also suggest that wasting may independently affect the progression of AIDS. Prevention of HIV wasting and preservation of body weight (both adipose and lean tissue mass) may enhance survival.[13,14] Although HIV wasting is a multifactorial disease, the causes can be categorized under three general headings: decreased food intake, increased nutrient requirements, and nutrient malabsorption. These major causes and contributing factors of HIV wasting are outlined in Table 10-6. In addition to protein-energy malnutrition, deficiencies of zinc and selenium have been documented in persons with AIDS.[15]

EATING DISORDERS

Anorexia nervosa and bulimia nervosa are conditions in which a disturbance in eating behavior is seen. Both have clinical signs aiding in their diagnosis. Anorexia nervosa is characterized by a refusal to maintain a minimally normal body weight, an intense fear of gaining weight that is not alleviated by losing weight, and a distorted perception of body shape or size in which a person feels overweight (either globally or in certain body areas) despite being markedly underweight.[16] The American Psychiatric Association's diagnostic criteria for anorexia nervosa are shown in Box 10-4. A prominent clinical feature of persons with anorexia nervosa is marked weight loss that in some instances can become extreme and life threatening. Figure 10-10 gives an example of the severe wasting commonly seen in persons with anorexia nervosa.

Bulimia nervosa is characterized by episodes of binging (eating unusually large amounts of food in a discrete period of time) followed by some behavior to prevent weight gain such as purging (usually self-induced vomiting, but also including misuse of laxatives, diuretics, enemas, or other medications), fasting, or excessive exercise.[16] The American Psychiatric Association's diagnostic criteria for bulimia nervosa are shown in Box 10-5. Persons with bulimia nervosa are usually within the normal weight range, although some may be slightly underweight or overweight. Recurrent vomiting may erode the teeth, especially the lingual surfaces of the front teeth, and increase the incidence of dental caries. An example of dental erosion in an 18-year-old female who had, from age 15 years, used vomiting as a purging method is shown in Figure 10-11. There may also be noticeable enlargement of the salivary glands, particularly the parotid glands. An example of asymmetrical hypertrophy of the parotid gland in a 20-year-old female who developed bulimia nervosa at age 17 years is shown in Figure 10-12.

TABLE 10-6 Causes and contributing factors for HIV wasting syndrome

Causes	Contributing factors
Decreased food intake	
Loss of appetite	Nausea, vomiting, medications, altered taste; anorexia caused by the effects of cytokines such as tissue necrosis factor, interleukin-1, and interferon; the presence of undigested micronutrients in ileum and colon may also depress appetite
Difficulty chewing and swallowing	Mouth and throat sores from Kaposi's sarcoma and opportunistic infections such as candidiasis and herpes simplex; esophageal ulcers of viral, mycobacterial, and neoplastic origin; neurologic disease
Decreased interest in eating	Depression, ostracism, isolation, loneliness
Inability to prepare meals	Lack of access to food, poverty, profound weakness, AIDS-induced dementia
Increased nutrient requirements	
Hypermetabolism	Resting metabolic rate is generally increased in persons with AIDS unless severe wasting is present; loss of adipose tissue and negative nitrogen balance are exacerbated by near-normal serum levels of the thyroid hormone triiodothyronine (T_3) that ordinarily fall below normal in the presence of malnutrition and wasting
Fever	Opportunistic infections of viral, mycobacterial, and neoplastic origin
Nutrient malabsorption	
Diarrhea	Occurs in >50% of persons with AIDS; many cases apparently caused by protozoal infections
Inflammation of bowel mucosa	Protozoal infections (cryptosporidiosis and microsporidiosis) appear to result in malabsorption apart from diarrhea; deficiency of lactase and disaccharidase activity seen; HIV alone may affect the structure and function of the small bowel

Data from Oster MH, Enders SR, Samuels SJ, Cone LA, Hooton TM, Browder HP, Flynn NM. 1994. Megestrol acetate in patients with AIDS and cachexia. *Annals of Internal Medicine* 121:400–408; Von Roenn JH, Armstrong D, Kotler DP, Cohn DL, Klimas NG, Tchekmedyian NS, Cone L, Brennan PJ, Weitzman SA. 1994. Megestrol acetate in patients with AIDS-related cachexia. *Annals of Internal Medicine* 121:393–399; Hecker LM, Kotler DP. 1990. Malnutrition in patients with AIDS. *Nutrition Reviews*. 48:393–401; Singer P, Katz DP, Dillon L, Kirvelä O, Lazarus T, Askanazi J. 1992. Nutritional aspects of the acquired immunodeficiency syndrome. *American Journal of Gastroenterology* 87:265–273.

BOX 10-4

The American Psychiatric Association's Diagnostic Criteria for Anorexia Nervosa

A. Refusal to maintain body weight at or above a minimally normal weight for age and height (e.g., weight loss leading to maintenance of body weight less than 85% of that expected or failure to make expected weight gain during period of growth, leading to body weight less than 85% of that expected).

B. Intense fear of gaining weight or becoming fat, even though underweight.

C. Disturbance in the way in which one's body weight or shape is experienced, undue influence of body weight or shape on self-evaluation, or denial of the seriousness of the current low body weight.

D. In postmenarcheal females, amenorrhea, i.e., the absence of at least three consecutive menstrual cycles. (A woman is considered to have amenorrhea if her periods occur only following hormone administration, e.g., estrogen.)

Types of anorexia nervosa:

Restricting type: During the current episode of anorexia nervosa, the person has not regularly engaged in binge-eating or purging behavior (i.e., self-induced vomiting or the misuse of laxatives, diuretics, or enemas).

Binge-eating/purging type: During the current episode of anorexia nervosa, the person has regularly engaged in binge-eating or purging behavior (i.e., self-induced vomiting or the misues of laxatives, diuretics, or enemas).

From American Psychiatric Association. 1994.

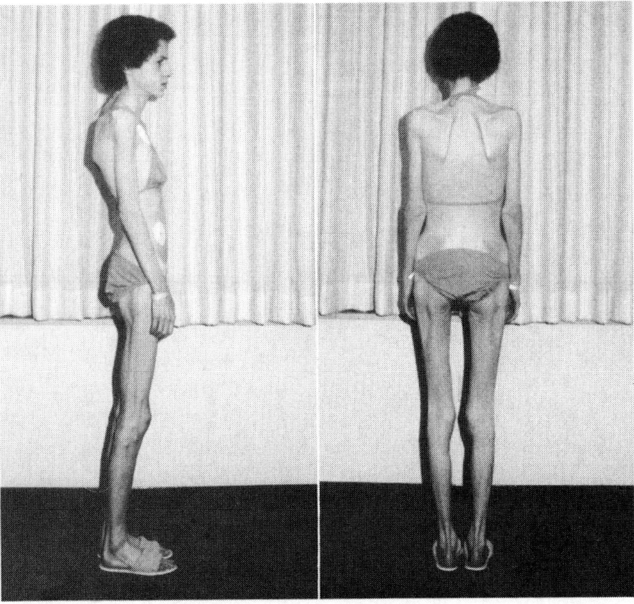

Figure 10-10 An example of severe wasting seen in a person with anorexia nervosa.

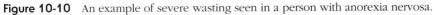

BOX 10-5

The American Psychiatric Association's Diagnostic Criteria for Bulimia Nervosa

A. Recurrent episodes of binge eating. An episode of binge eating is characterized by both of the following:
   (1) Eating, in a discrete period (e.g., within 2-hour period), an amount of food that is definitely larger than most people would eat during a similar period and under similar circumstances.
   (2) A sense of lack of control over eating during the episode (e.g., a feeling that one cannot stop eating or control what or how much one is eating).

B. Recurrent inappropriate compensatory behavior to prevent weight gain, such as self-induced vomiting; misuse of laxatives, diuretics, enemas, or other medications; fasting; or excessive exercise.

C. The binge eating and inappropriate compensatory behaviors both occur, on average, at least twice a week for 3 months.

D. Self-evaluation is unduly influenced by body shape and weight.

E. The disturbance does not occur exclusively during episodes of anorexia nervosa.

Types of anorexia nervosa:

Purging type: During the current episode of bulimia nervosa, the person has regularly engaged in self-induced vomiting or the misuse of laxatives, diuretics, or enemas.

Nonpurging type: During the current episode of bulimia nervosa, the person has used other inappropriate compensatory behaviors, such as fasting or excessive exercise, but has not regularly engaged in self-induced vomiting or the misuse of laxatives, diuretics, or enemas.

From American Psychiatric Association. 1994.

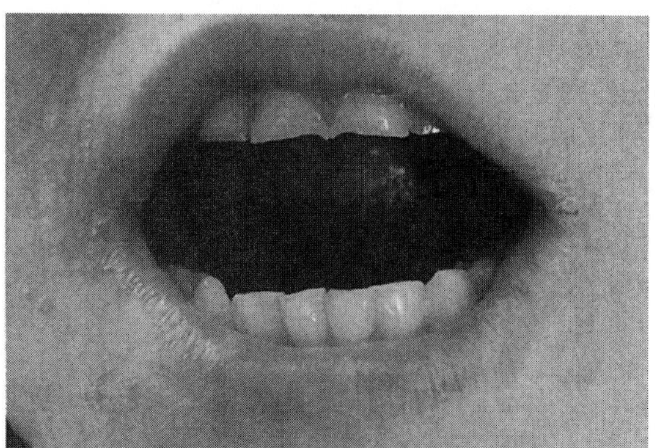

Figure 10-11 An example of dental erosion is an 18-year-old female who had been vomiting to control her weight from the age of 15 years. Note that her top incisors are markedly eroded.

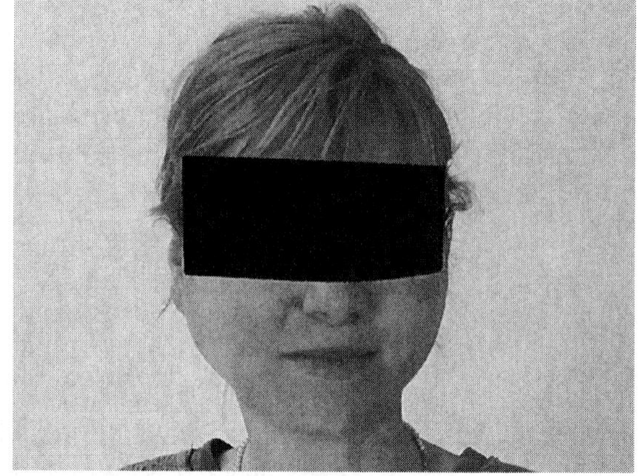

Figure 10-12 An example of asymmetrical parotid gland enlargement in a 20-year-old female who developed bulimia nervosa at the age of 17 years. She was vomiting four times each day.

SUMMARY

1. The first step in the clinical assessment of nutritional status is obtaining a patient's history. This includes pertinent facts about past and current health and use of medications, and personal and household information. Sources include the patient's medical record and data obtained directly from the patient or those familiar with the patient.
2. A diet history is valuable in understanding a patient's nutritional status. This includes information about a patient's usual eating pattern, food likes and dislikes, intolerances and allergies, as well as money available for purchasing food, ability to obtain and prepare food, eligibility for and access to food assistance programs, and use of vitamin, mineral, and other supplements.
3. Subjective global assessment is a clinical technique for assessing the nutritional status of a patient based on features of the patient's history and physical examination rather than relying on more objective measures of nutritional status such as anthropometric and biochemical data.
4. In severe PEM, the conditions known as kwashiorkor and marasmus are seen. Kwashiorkor is predominantly a protein deficiency characterized by a relatively normal weight, generally intact skeletal musculature, decreased concentrations of serum proteins, and edema. Marasmus is mainly an energy deficiency characterized by significant loss of body weight, skeletal muscle, and adipose tissue mass, but with serum protein concentrations relatively intact and no edema.
5. Severe cases of PEM and wasting can result from AIDS, certain cancers, some gastrointestinal diseases, and alcoholism and other drug abuse. The emaciation and general ill health seen in these diseases is sometimes called cachexia.
6. Growth failure and flag sign are two conditions seen in severe PEM. The flag sign is characterized by alternating bands of depigmented and normal-colored hair produced by alternating periods of poor and relatively good protein intake. Growth failure, a failure to gain weight and height at the expected rate, is the most common sign of malnutrition in children.
7. The severity of PEM in children and adolescents can be assessed by calculating weight as a percentage of reference median weight-for-height and by calculating height as a percentage of reference height-for-age. These two values can then be compared with published guidelines. The severity of PEM in an adult can be assessed by comparing body mass index (kg/m^2) with the reference values.
8. Body wasting is a fundamental feature of HIV infection and a diagnostic sign that HIV infection has progressed to AIDS. Wasting is of considerable concern because of its association with increased morbidity in persons with AIDS.[10] The primary causes of this wasting can be categorized under three general headings: decreased food intake, increased nutrient requirements, and nutrient malabsorption.
9. Anorexia nervosa is characterized by a refusal to maintain a minimally normal body weight, an intense fear of gaining weight, and a distorted perception of body shape or size. Bulimia nervosa is characterized by episodes of binging followed by some behavior to prevent weight gain such as purging, fasting, or excessive exercise.

REFERENCES

1. Ireton-Jones CS, Hasse JM. 1992. Comprehensive nutritional assessment: The dietitian's contribution to the team effort. *Nutrition* 8:75–81.
2. Hopkins B. 1993. Assessment of nutritional status. In Gottschlich MM, Matarese LE, Shronts EP, eds. *Nutrition support dietetics core curriculum,* 2nd ed. Silver Spring, Md: American Society for Parenteral and Enteral Nutrition.

3. Jeejeebhoy KN. 1994. Clinical and functional assessments. In Shils ME, Olson JA, Shike M, eds. *Modern nutrition in health and disease,* 8th ed. Philadelphia: Lea & Febiger.
4. Detsky AS, McLaughlin JR, Baker JP, Johnston N, Whittaker S, Mendelson RA, Jeejeebhoy KN. 1987. What is subjective global assessment of nutritional status? *Journal of Parenteral and Enteral Nutrition* 11:8–13.
5. Detsky AS, Smalley PS, Change J. 1994. Is this patient malnourished? *Journal of the American Medical Association* 271:54–58.
6. Torún B, Chew F. 1994. Protein-energy malnutrition. In Shils ME, Olson JA, Shike M, eds. *Modern nutrition in health and disease,* 8th ed. Philadelphia: Lea & Febiger.
7. Phinney SD. 1981. The assessment of protein nutrition in the hospitalized patient. *Clinics in Laboratory Medicine* 1:767–774.
8. McLaren DS. 1992. *A colour atlas and text of diet-related disorders,* 2nd ed. London: Mosby Europe.
9. James WPT, Ferro-Luzzi A, Waterlow JC. 1988. Definition of chronic energy deficiency in adults. Report of a working party of the International Dietary Energy Consultative Group. *European Journal of Clinical Nutrition* 42:969–981.
10. Kurtzweil P. 1995. Warding off HIV wasting syndrome. *FDA Consumer* 29(3):16–20.
11. Oster MH, Enders SR, Samuels SJ, Cone LA, Hooton TM, Browder HP, Flynn NM. 1994. Megestrol acetate in patients with AIDS and cachexia. *Annals of Internal Medicine* 121: 400–408.
12. Von Roenn JH, Armstrong D, Kotler DP, Cohn DL, Klimas NG, Tchekmedyian NS, Cone L, Brennan PJ, Weitzman SA. 1994. Megestrol Acetate in patients with AIDS-related cachexia. *Annals of Internal Medicine* 121:393–399.
13. Kotler DP, Tierney AR, Wang J, Pierson RN. 1989. Magnitude of body-cell-mass depletion and the timing of death from wasting in AIDS. *American Journal of Clinical Nutrition* 50:444–447.
14. Hecker LM, Kotler DP. 1990. Malnutrition in patients with AIDS. *Nutrition Reviews* 48:393–401.
15. Singer P, Katz DP, Dillon L, Kirvelä O, Lazarus T, Askanazi J. 1992. Nutritional aspects of the acquired immunodeficiency syndrome. *American Journal of Gastroenterology* 87:265–273.
16. American Psychiatric Association. 1994. *Diagnostic and statistical manual of mental disorders,* 4th ed. Washington, DC: American Psychiatric Association.

Assessment Activity 10-1

USING SUBJECTIVE GLOBAL ASSESSMENT

This Assessment Activity gives you an opportunity to practice using Subjective Global Assessment (SGA), a clinical technique for assessing nutritional status using data from a patient's history and physical examination, both of which can be found in a patient's medical record. Begin by making two photocopies of the SGA rating form found in Figure 10-1. Then, using the information from each of the two cases below, complete the chart and arrive at an SGA rating of each patient's nutritional status. You may find it helpful to review the section in this chapter which explains SGA.

The cases below are straightforward; and you and your classmates should arrive at the same rating for each case. However, because of the subjective nature of this approach, there may be an occasional instance when two or more health professionals do not arrive at the same rating of one patient's nutritional status. This should not necessarily detract from the usefulness of SGA because clinicians generally arrive at decisions by carefully evaluating the available evidence in light of professional knowledge and past experiences. Thus health care is not only a science but also an art.

Case 1

A 73-year-old female is admitted to the hospital complaining of loss of appetite and rapid onset of satiety for 6 weeks. For the past 3 days she has vomited practically all food and beverages consumed. She is ambulatory but has felt weak and has been unable to carry out her activities of daily living for the past 2 weeks. On physical examination the woman looks somewhat wasted with moderate loss of subcutaneous tissue in the upper arms, shoulders, and thoracic regions. There is moderate edema in the ankles but no ascites present. For the past 10 years or so her body weight has been stable at approximately 147 lb (66.8 kg). However, in the past 4 months or so she has steadily lost weight. Her current weight is 123 lb (55.9 kg). Using SGA, how would you rate her nutritional status?

Case 2

A 61-year-old male is admitted to the hospital for resection of his sigmoid colon and rectum, following discovery of a mass in the sigmoid colon by his physician during a flexible sigmoidoscopy. The patient originally complained of bright red blood in his bowel movements. He reported no significant gastrointestinal symptoms other than the bleeding. He denies any change in his functional capacity. His maximum weight was 167 lb (75.9 kg) at age 46 years. In his late 40s he lost about 15 lb (6.8 kg) and for the past 12 years he has maintained his weight at about 152 lb (69.1 kg). Between 2 and 6 months before admission his appetite had been less than normal and he gradually lost 13 lb (5.9 kg). In the past 2 months before admission his appetite improved and he gained 5 lb (2.3 kg). On physical examination there is no evidence of subcutaneous tissue loss, muscle wasting, edema, or ascites.

ELEVEN

COUNSELING THEORY AND TECHNIQUE

OUTLINE

INTRODUCTION

Awareness of nutritional status and dietary practices obtained through nutritional assessment often is followed by attempts to change dietary practices. This chapter provides a brief introduction to several counseling theories that provide a variety of useful techniques for initiating and maintaining dietary change.

The purpose of this chapter is *not* to teach you how to be a therapist. It is intended to briefly introduce you to those theories that we believe are most pertinent to nutritional counseling and to acquaint you with some fundamental approaches to counseling your clients. The most effective counselors are those who adapt techniques from several counseling theories to suit their needs and those of their individual clients. As you study this chapter, note the different counseling theories and techniques. Then, based on your professional judgment, use those techniques you feel are best suited to you and the needs of your clients.

Because communication lies at the foundation of interviewing and counseling, the first part of this chapter deals with fundamentals of communication theory and basic skills necessary for effective listening and interviewing. The chapter ends with a practical plan for initiating and maintaining dietary change.

Finally, as important as good nutrition is to health, do not lose sight of the fact that other practices such as smoking and alcohol and drug use have a profound impact on health. Cigarette smoking, for example, has been called "the chief, single, avoidable cause of death in our society and the most important health issue of our time."[1] We encourage you to be a model of good health habits, not only those relating to diet, but in all areas. By so doing, you will be most effective in helping your clients to achieve better health.

COMMUNICATION

Communication is the process of sending and receiving messages. It lies at the foundation of all efforts to interview, counsel, educate, and change behavior. Although we all communicate (or at least attempt to) and have a basic idea of what it involves, communication is a complex process and is not easily defined. The simplified communication model in Figure 11-1 shows the major components of human communication: sender, receiver, message, feedback, and interference.

The *sender* is the one initiating the communication, the first person to speak. The *message* is the communication. It contains components that are both verbal (what is spoken) and nonverbal (what is implied by the emotional tone of the sender's voice, facial expression, posture, diction, pronunciation, choice of words, dress, and the environment in which the communication occurs).[2] Verbal and nonverbal communication occur simultaneously. The *receiver* is the listener, the one to whom the message is sent. *Feedback* is the response the receiver gives to messages after interpreting them. Feedback distinguishes one-way communication from two-way communication.[2] The absence of feedback or making no provision for it will likely result in distorted communication because the sender is unable to determine how the message was received. As with the message, feedback is both verbal and nonverbal.

Interference is anything adversely affecting transmission or interpretation of the message. It can arise from the environment or the emotional or physiologic state of either the sender or receiver. Noise, lack of privacy, interruptions, an office that is too hot or too cold, and uncomfortable seating are examples of environmental factors that may cause interference. Emotional factors leading to interference include fear of disease or death, loneliness, grief, prejudice, and bias. Physiologic factors such as pain, deficits of hearing or vision, or difficulty in speaking can often be sources of interference.

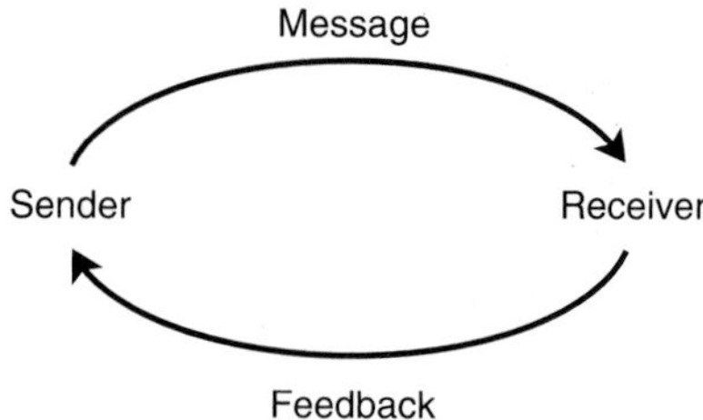

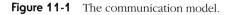

Figure 11-1 The communication model.

BOX 11-1

Guidelines to More Supportive Communication

Description rather than evaluation
Problem orientation rather than manipulation
Equality rather than superiority
Empathy rather than neutrality
Provisionalism rather than certainty

From Gibb JR. 1961. Defensive communication. *Journal of Communication* 11:141–148.

Verbal Communication

Dietary counseling generally involves some type of behavioral change on the receiver's part. The receiver may perceive attempts to change lifelong habits or practices he or she enjoys as a potential threat. Thus the receiver may become defensive, which interferes with good communication. The receiver's defensive reactions can be prevented or minimized through the use of the guidelines to supportive communication outlined in Box 11-1 and the following paragraphs. The more supportive communication is, the less the receiver perceives it as a threat and the more he or she is able to concentrate on the structure, content, and meaning of the message.[2,3]

Describe behavior rather than evaluate it. Discussing a client's behavior in a judgmental or evaluative way will likely cause the client to become defensive. The client will then be thinking of ways to defend himself or herself rather than concentrating on the counselor's message. Evaluating or judging behavior can lead to an argument. Instead, the counselor can present the facts or seek information in objective, nonjudgmental ways that do not imply guilt or ask the client to change his or her behavior.

For example, in an attempt to raise awareness of the seriousness of the problem at hand, a counselor may accuse a client with poorly controlled diabetes of being "irresponsible" or "committing suicide." A better approach would be to objectively discuss the client's blood sugar levels and nonjudgmentally discuss factors that may be affecting them.

Use problem orientation rather than manipulation. Much of our speech is an attempt to persuade others to alter their behavior, attitudes, or activities. Often when we want people to see things our way, we lead them through a series of questions until they arrive at the "correct conclusion." This is a form of manipulation and implies that the person being directed is inadequate or inferior. This is likely to result in a defensive response that interferes with communication. Problem orientation, on the other hand, is the antithesis of persuasion. The sender communicates a desire to work with the receiver in defining a mutual problem and seeking a workable solution. The sender implies that he or she has no prearranged answer or viewpoint and no hidden agenda to exert control over the receiver. Thus the receiver arrives at his or her own conclusions and establishes goals and objectives to which there will be greater adherence.

Communicate equality rather than superiority. A sender can promote supportive communication by considering himself or herself a collaborator with or an equal to the receiver. When treated with respect and trust and involved in participative problem solving, the receiver will feel more obligated to the success of any agreed-on solution. If the sender communicates superiority, the receiver will likely become defensive. Although clients often need and appreciate the reassurance of a dietitian's nutritional expertise, dietitians should avoid urging a particular plan of action based primarily on their superior knowledge or ability.

Empathize rather than remain neutral. Communication conveying compassion and respect for others is supportive and defense reducing. Particularly reassuring is a sender who identifies with the problems and shares in the feelings of the receiver. Communication conveying neutrality may indicate a lack of concern for the receiver's welfare. Attempts to reassure the receiver that he or she is overly anxious or need not feel rejected or bad deny the legitimacy of the receiver's emotions and suggest a lack of acceptance.

Be receptive rather than dogmatic. A willingness to hold one's own attitudes as provisional, to examine other ideas rather than take sides, and to solve problems rather than debate issues gives listeners a sense of participation in and control over the problem-solving process. On the other hand, persons who seem to know all the answers or who regard themselves as teachers rather than team players tend to put others on guard and stifle supportive communication.

Nonverbal Communication

As shown in Figure 11-1, communication occurs simultaneously on two levels—verbal and nonverbal. Sometimes referred to as *body language,* nonverbal communication in the form of gestures, posture, facial expressions, and tone of voice is sometimes a more reliable indicator of the client's feelings and attitudes than are his or her words.[4] Verbal communication is generally under conscious control and is subject to censorship. It can be used to persuade, mislead, or cover facts a client wishes to hide. Nonverbal communication, on the other hand, is not as easily controlled by conscious thought and often can be a more reliable indicator of a person's dominant emotions than his or her words.[2,4] Lack of congruence or agreement between verbal and nonverbal communication can be an important indicator that a client is consciously or unconsciously omitting something.

Facial expressions are an important source of nonverbal communication. Sadness often can be seen in the face of a distressed client through a downturned mouth or quivering lip. Unusually prolonged and intense eye contact may indicate anger. Guilt, insecurity, or fear may be indicated by failure to maintain eye contact, especially when this occurs during discussion of a particularly sensitive topic.[4]

Posture may indicate a person's feelings. A client seated with arms relaxed at the sides and slightly slouched in the chair can communicate openness, whereas a client may communicate a distrustful, defensive attitude by sitting up very straight with arms tightly crossed over the chest. A client who leans away from the counselor or moves his chair to distance himself may indicate defensiveness or distrust. One leaning closer to the counselor may express a desire for greater intimacy.[4] Cultural differences exist in what is considered to be a comfortable distance between two communicating persons. In general, people from Latin cultures prefer being closer, whereas those from North America and parts of Europe favor a somewhat greater distance.

The tone of voice is an important indicator, as well. A client asked about her diet may warmly and pleasantly respond "It's going well," and mean just that. The same words uttered in a mechanistic and toneless way may indicate a problem with the diet.

Nonverbal communication also facilitates the dietitian's communication to clients. Appropriate eye contact, gestures, facial expressions, and posture assure the client of the dietitian's attention, interest, acceptance, and support. The astute dietitian should carefully note the client's nonverbal cues and their possible significance and use nonverbal communication to respond to the client in a supportive way.[2]

Promoting Effective Communication

Effective communication requires consideration of several factors. It is important that messages and feedback be transmitted in ways that are understandable to both sender and receiver. When talking with clients or providing instruction, health professionals should use understandable language and minimize use of medical terminology. Feedback should be encouraged, and the receiver should be given ample opportunity to ask questions and clarify any potential misunderstandings. Both sender and receiver should be aware of their nonverbal communication so that it supports, rather than interferes with, effective communication.

The environment in which communication takes place should be comfortable, conducive to good communication, and as free as possible of interferences that can adversely affect communication. Adequate time for counseling and client instruction is necessary before clients can even begin to change lifelong habits and adopt new ones. Awareness of the client's abilities, concerns, and fears is also important to effective communication. The dietitian also should be aware of his or her own concerns and limitations and avoid allowing these to interfere with the communication process.

Consider a dietitian seated at the bedside of a patient in whom diabetes has been recently diagnosed. The dietitian is giving the patient some last-minute instructions on the diabetic exchange system before the patient is discharged. Environmental interference can come from the roommate's television, interruptions from a nurse or physician, a phone call, or the arrival of a visitor. The patient's fear about having diabetes, concerns about being able to manage a new diet, worries about hospitalization costs, and thoughts about what the future holds may preoccupy his mind and interfere with the instruction. The dietitian

TABLE 11-1 The six steps of listening

Hearing	The reception of sound waves by the ear
Attending	Mentally focusing on a specific sound
Understanding	Interpretation of the message and assignment of meaning by the brain
Remembering	Storage of message for later use
Evaluating	Making an evaluative judgment about the message
Responding	A verbal and/or nonverbal response to the message

From Samovar LA, Mills J. 1992. *Oral communication: Message and response,* 8th ed. Dubuque, Iowa: Wm. C. Brown.

also may be preoccupied with concerns of her own, such as other patients needing assessment and instruction, and these can interfere with the communication process. This is obviously not an ideal situation for communication or instruction, but unfortunately it is one commonly encountered in real life. Awareness of these and other impediments to good communication, however, is necessary before they can be addressed and effectively dealt with.

LISTENING

Communication is a two-way process. It not only involves *sending* messages but *receiving* them as well. Listening, therefore, is essential to the interviewing and counseling process. In some instances, the best help a counselor can give a client is to simply listen attentively and nonjudgmentally. It is also an excellent way to establish good rapport with a client.[5] As important as listening is, most of us are not very good at it.[6] Listening is a highly active process demanding concentration and attention. It involves several steps (Table 11-1).[6]

A number of misconceptions exist about listening.[6] For example, some people believe that *hearing* and *listening* are the same activity. Listening is a process involving much more than simply hearing sounds such as music or voices. It is mistakenly assumed that when several people hear the same sound (for example, a person talking), they all receive the same message. Quite the opposite is true. Listening is a highly subjective experience, and the interpretations placed on what is heard can vary widely from person to person.

Listening Skills

Some people believe that listening is a passive activity, when in reality it is an active process requiring concentration and specific skills that can be learned if one wants to be a better listener.[6–8] Listening skills can be grouped under four categories: openness, concentration, attention, and comprehension.[7]

Openness or objectivity involves a willingness to investigate new ideas and interact with others with minimal internal distortion from personal prejudices. Openness does not necessarily mean acceptance or approval of another's ideas but simply a willingness to "hear a person out." It requires the listener to set aside his or her personal biases, which may interfere with effective listening.[5–7]

Concentration entails focusing the mind on what the speaker is saying. It is made easier when environmental distractions and interferences are minimized. Counseling should take place in a room that is quiet, comfortable, and private.

It is estimated that people with normal intelligence think about five times faster than they talk.[2] Thus while listening to another person talk, our mind can simultaneously be thinking other things. Unfortunately, many people have allowed this to become a major barrier to effective listening. Rather than focusing the mind on critical and careful listening, we often take mental excursions ranging from thinking about the speaker's hair style to daydreaming.[6] A good listener will use this extra mental capacity to analyze and understand the speaker's verbal and nonverbal messages.

The counselor should indicate that the client has his or her full attention and acceptance by maintaining good eye contact with the client and having an empathic facial expression and relaxed posture. The counselor should give the client ample opportunity for expression without interruption while at the same time providing occasional, brief verbal and nonverbal responses indicating reception of the message. Appropriately timed nods or verbal responses such as "I understand" or "I see" will help assure the client of the counselor's attentive listening.

Comprehension not only involves attaching meaning to information but correctly interpreting the meaning of the client's communication. The counselor's comprehension of the client's message can be enhanced through use of such techniques as reflection, paraphrasing, clarification, and probing.[7] Reflection is restating the affective or emotional part of the client's words. This gives the client opportunity to hear what she just said and to elaborate on her emotions. A client may say, "I feel depressed about my lack of progress." The affective part of this message is the statement "I feel depressed." In reflection, the counselor simply restates the client's words: "You say you feel depressed." This gives the client opportunity to elaborate on her feelings.[7,9] In paraphrasing, the client's message is restated or rephrased in the counselor's own words. This helps ensure that the counselor has correctly interpreted the client's message. Clarification is simply asking the client to repeat or restate what was just said. Probing is asking the client to provide greater detail on some specific point. It is often used when collecting a 24-hour dietary recall.

INTERVIEWING

Interviewing can be defined as a guided communication process between two persons or parties with the predetermined purpose of obtaining or exchanging specific information through the asking and answering of questions.[2,8] The goal of the interview is obtaining specific information from the client while maintaining an interpersonal environment conducive to disclosure by the client.[2] Of the several types of interviews that exist, the nutrition counselor is primarily concerned with interviews to gather information from clients, give information to clients, and deal with client problems.[8]

Interviewing Skills

As in communication and listening, there are several basic conditions or skills that increase a person's effectiveness as an interviewer. Among these are physical surroundings, freedom from interruption and interference, privacy, establishing good rapport, attentiveness, openness, and the client's context.[2] Factors to consider in the physical surroundings are the comfort of both the client and the interviewer, the seating arrangement, distance between the interviewer and client, and the presence of physical barriers separating them.

It is best to conduct an interview in a location free of interruptions and interferences. In an office setting, the counselor should arrange to have phone calls held. In a hospital, interviews should not be scheduled during the time of physicians' rounds, nursing or other care, or visiting hours. A convenient time should be arranged with nursing and other staff. When held in the patient's room, arrangements can be made with nursing staff to avoid unnecessary interruptions, the patient's door can be closed, televisions and radios can be turned down or off, and visitors can be kindly asked to step outside.[2,4,8] Parents, spouses, partners, and siblings can be important sources of information about the patient. The counselor may want to have them present during the interview or available for questions later.

Early establishment of good rapport is essential to an effective interview. Establishing good client rapport will place the client at ease and make him or her more willing to share important information.[2] A counselor should begin the interview with a pleasant greeting. She should introduce herself and briefly give the reason for the interview. If the counselor is late, she should apologize for any inconvenience and explain why.[8]

Attentiveness, already mentioned in the context of listening, is also an important interviewing skill. Nonverbal and verbal expressions of attention, such as appropriate eye contact, posture, facial expressions, well-timed nods, or relevant verbal responses will help assure the client of the counselor's interest and attention. Openness or interviewer objectivity, previously discussed in relation to listening, is an important interviewing skill.

The client's emotional context—his or her beliefs, attitudes, feelings, and values—is also an important consideration when interviewing. Fears about health, concerns about death, feelings of loneliness or grief may preoccupy a client's thoughts and interfere with his or her ability to participate in the interview. Putting apprehensive clients at ease and allowing them to express their feelings can help alleviate their fears and facilitate the interviewing process.

BOX 11-2

Examples of Different Types of Questions

Open questions
"Tell me about yourself."
"Tell me about your eating habits."
"What have you been doing to lower your blood cholesterol level?"

Closed questions
"Do you smoke?"
"Do you salt your food at the table?"
"Do you eat chicken with or without the skin?"

Neutral questions
"What is the first thing you have to eat or drink after waking up in the morning?"
"What kind of milk do you drink?"
"How many times a week do you eat ice cream?"

Leading questions
"What do you eat for breakfast?"
"You don't use whole milk, do you?"
"Do you eat ice cream *every* evening?"

Obtaining Information

Before the interview, the counselor should review the client's medical record for pertinent information. This provides the counselor with considerable background information on the client and allows the interview to be more directed and concise. Using the "funnel sequence" is suggested. This begins with more general, open questions and gradually narrows to more specific inquiries using closed questions.[8]

Open questions invite rather than demand answers and provide clients substantial freedom in determining the amount and type of information to give.[2,8] Open questions let the client talk and offer information that he or she feels is important. They are generally easy to answer and pose little threat to the client. They give the counselor the opportunity to listen and observe. They have the disadvantage of consuming large amounts of time if clients dwell on irrelevant information.[8] Examples of open questions are given in Box 11-2.

Closed questions, on the other hand, are restrictive in nature and allow the counselor to control answers and ask for specific information. They often provide too little information and fail to reveal why a client has a particular attitude.[8] Examples of closed questions are given in Box 11-2.

Questions also can be classified as neutral or leading (Box 11-2).[8] *Neutral questions* allow the client to answer without pressure or direction from the counselor. In *leading questions,* the counselor makes implicit or explicit suggestions about the expected or desired answer. In answering leading questions, the client merely agrees with what the counselor is apparently suggesting. Counselors should avoid leading clients either by verbal or nonverbal means. When clients respond to their questions, counselors must avoid such expressions as surprise, agreement, disagreement, or disgust, which can suggest expected or desired answers.[2]

When information is sought from or provided to clients, counselors should use understandable language. Health care professionals often make the mistake of assuming that clients understand the technical language used daily in hospitals and other health care organizations. Or they assume that if a client does not understand something, he or she will simply ask what a word means. Many clients are so overwhelmed by the unfamiliar or intimidated by the authority of health care professionals that they fail to seek answers to their questions. Thus a counselor should avoid using technical language with clients and not assume that clients will understand medical terminology even if it is explained to them.

COUNSELING THEORIES

Several counseling theories and techniques have been developed and are currently in use today. Our purpose in writing this section is not to teach you how to be a therapist; that takes considerable professional training and practice. Rather, our purpose is to briefly introduce you to those theories we believe are most pertinent to nutritional counseling and to acquaint you with some fundamental approaches to counseling your clients.

Each counseling theory discussed in the following pages has something of value to offer the dietetic practitioner. Each also has certain limitations or drawbacks. We believe that an awareness of these theories and an ability to adapt their more fundamental and benign counseling techniques to suit each unique counseling situation will greatly enhance your ability as a helping professional.

Person-Centered Approach

The person-centered approach to counseling is based primarily on the work of psychologist Carl Rogers.[10–12] Rogers taught that if people could experience human relationships characterized by respect and trust they would develop in a positive and constructive manner. He objected to the idea that people need to be instructed, punished, rewarded, and managed by others who are in a superior and "expert" position. He believed that people possess an innate ability to move away from maladjustment to psychological health. The primary responsibility for this rests with the client rather than with an authority who directs a passive client.[13]

Rogers advocated three qualities of counselors that create a growth-promoting climate in which persons advance to become what they are capable of becoming. These counselor qualities are genuineness or realness, unconditional positive regard and acceptance of the client, and deep understanding of the client's feelings. According to Rogers, if a counselor communicates these attitudes, clients will become less defensive, more open to experiences within themselves and the world, and able to relate to others in social and constructive ways.[13] Rogers wrote, "If I can provide a certain type of relationship, the other person will discover within himself the capacity to use that relationship for growth and change, and personal development will occur."[10]

The client's personality change is brought about by the counselor's attitudes instead of by certain techniques, theories, or knowledge. The counselor's primary role is providing a therapeutic climate in which the client feels free to explore areas of his or her life that are currently distorted or denied to awareness. Within this climate, the client is then able to lose his or her "defenses and rigid perceptions and move to a higher level of personal functioning."[13]

The counselor's "genuineness or realness" is the congruence between what is expressed to the client and what is experienced within the counselor's mind. Through genuineness, the counselor serves as a model of a human struggling toward greater awareness and personal functioning.[13]

Unconditional positive regard and acceptance allows the client to be accepted as he or she is and to express feelings and attitudes without risk of losing the counselor's acceptance. While the client's *feelings* are accepted, not all *overt behavior* is approved or accepted. According to Rogers, the greater the counselor's degree of positive regard and acceptance of the client, the greater will be the success of therapy.[13]

As the counselor develops a deep understanding of the client's feelings and experiences, he or she is able to sense the client's feelings as if they were his or her own. This permits the counselor to expand the client's awareness and understanding of these feelings and help the client to resolve internal conflicts and to become more the person the client wishes to become.[13]

The person-centered approach has the advantage of being a safer approach to counseling than other models that place the counselor in a directive position of making interpretations, forming diagnoses, and attempting more drastic personality changes. Its core skills of listening, understanding, caring, and acceptance are needed by all counselors. No matter what counseling approach they use, counselors lacking in these core skills will not be effective in carrying out their treatment. These skills are also valuable for others in the helping professions. Although people in crisis do not necessarily need answers, they do need someone willing to really listen, care, and understand, and on whom they can "unload" their feelings and experiences without fear of rejection. The presence of a caring, listening, understanding person can do much to promote healing.[13]

Counselors using the person-centered approach have been criticized for merely giving support to clients without challenging them. Rogers has suggested, therefore, that counselors include more "caring confrontations." Counselors using "caring confrontation" are more active in suggesting topics for exploration, interpreting behavior, helping clients set goals, and giving advice.[13]

Behavior Modification

Behavior modification (also known as behavior therapy) attempts to alter previously learned human behavior or to encourage the development of new behavior through a variety of action-oriented methods as opposed to changing feelings or thoughts.[13–15] A major premise of behavior modification is that "all behavior, normal or abnormal, is acquired and maintained according to certain definable principles."[16] Behaviors resulting in positive consequences tend to be repeated, and those behaviors not followed by favorable consequences tend not to be repeated.[15]

Early or "radical" behaviorists viewed human behavior as almost totally the result of positive reinforcements (the addition of something such as praise or money as a consequence of behavior) or negative reinforcements (the removal of unpleasant stimuli once a certain behavior is performed). Currently, behaviorists view humans as both the *product* of environmental influences as well as the *producer* of their environment. Early behaviorists viewed humans as lacking freedom and self-determination. Modern behaviorists, on the other hand, acknowledge the presence of freedom and self-determination. They attempt to increase clients' freedom and control by assisting them in overcoming crippling behaviors and becoming freer to choose from options that were previously not available to them.[13]

Antecedents and Consequences

Behaviorists view actions as being preceded by antecedents and followed by consequences.[14,17] For example, eating is generally preceded by some antecedent or stimulus such as smelling or seeing food, coming home from work or school, sitting down to study or watch television, seeing an advertisement for food on television or in a magazine, or experiencing anxiety, boredom, or loneliness. Behavior modification holds that when antecedents to behaviors are recognized, they can be modified or controlled to decrease the occurrence of negative behaviors and increase the occurrence of positive behaviors. This is referred to as stimulus control. Examples of stimulus control include eating before grocery shopping, preparing a shopping list and only purchasing items on the list, storing food out of sight, and avoiding the purchase of ready-to-eat foods.

Consequences reinforce the behavior they follow. They may be positive, negative, or neutral. When consequences are positive, behavior is more likely to be repeated. Behavior followed by negative consequences is less likely to be repeated. The delicious tastes and feelings of satiety accompanying a meal are examples of positive consequences that reinforce or reward the practice of eating. Behaviorists also believe that positive consequences are more effective in promoting behavioral change than are negative consequences.[14]

Self-Monitoring

A valuable behavior modification technique is self-monitoring or record keeping—the careful observation and accurate recording of the behavior to be controlled.[13,16,18] If the behavior is eating, for example, clients carefully observe their eating and record its occurrence along with comments about relevant antecedents and consequences related to their eating. Self-monitoring has several functions:[18]

- It provides information about eating habits and the factors influencing them.
- It involves clients in observing and analyzing their dietary habits.
- It increases clients' awareness of their diets and behavior as it happens.
- It gives the counselor and client something to review objectively and impartially. For example, they focus on specific problem behaviors in the record, not in the client.
- It increases the clients' skills in manipulating their diets to achieve desired results (for example, finding suitable low-fat entrees to replace others that are high in total fat and saturated fat or finding acceptable low-calorie snack foods to replace high-calorie snacks).
- It increases counselor-client interaction.
- It allows client and counselor to monitor behavior over time and track client progress.

Various forms have been developed for self-monitoring.[18] One example is shown in Appendix T. In general, forms for self-monitoring eating behavior should allow the recording of such information as the food eaten, how food was prepared, the amount eaten, where and when the food was eaten, what happened or how the client felt before eating, what happened or how the client felt after eating, and whether the food was eaten alone or with someone else and with whom.

For monitoring behaviors related to a specific goal (for example, substitution of high-calorie snacks with low-calorie snacks), the client can record the day, time, type of snack eaten, and amount eaten on a pocket-sized card that he or she can carry.

To be successful, the self-monitoring method ought to be easy to use, convenient, and readily available when the behavior occurs; be clearly understood by the client; be relevant to the dietary problem; and be used for observational purposes rather than to judge the problem.

Goals and Self-Contracts

Behaviorists believe that feelings result from behavior.[13,15] Consequently, the focus of attention in counseling is changing behavior and not altering feelings or delving into past experiences. Goals are of central importance in behavior modification and are expressed in terms of altering overt behavior in ways that are both specific and measurable. Therefore, the goals of therapy must be clear, specific, measurable, attainable, and agreed on by both the client and the counselor. The client selects counseling goals at the beginning of the counseling process.

For example, a client may want to decrease his elevated total cholesterol level to less than 200 mg/dl. Having been taught by the counselor that total cholesterol levels are related to saturated fat intake, the client, with the counselor's assistance, may decide to use soft tub margarine instead of butter at home and remove the skin from chicken before eating it. The client's progress then can be evaluated objectively in terms of goal attainment and other measurable ways. For example, the client's self-monitoring records can demonstrate adherence to the goals, and measurements of total serum cholesterol may indicate overall progress in lowering serum cholesterol.

Once goals are identified, the counselor can help the client write a self-contract. This is an agreement the client enters into with himself or herself to help build commitment to the goal for change.[15,17,18] The contract should clearly state the goal in terms of a specific time frame and detail the reward for successfully achieving the goal. As an option, it may state the punishment, if any, for not reaching the goal. An example of a self-contract is shown in Figure 11-2.

Self-contract

____
Name

____
Period of time

____
Specific behavior goal

____
Reward when successful

________________ ________
Signature Date

________________ ________
Signature Date

Figure 11-2 An example of a self-contract.

Modeling

In addition to learning through positive or negative reinforcements, behaviorists hold that people learn through the process of modeling.[13,14,17,18] Also known as observational learning or imitation, modeling is "the process by which the behavior of an individual or a group (the model) acts as a stimulus for similar thoughts, attitudes, and behaviors on the part of observers."[13] Through modeling, clients develop new behaviors without trial-and-error learning. Clients, for example, can learn new behaviors by observing the success of other group members or through others' success stories shared by the counselor.[14]

Modeling can take place by observing a live model (for example, counselors demonstrate the behavior they hope clients will acquire), symbolic models (the client observes the desired behavior performed on videotape or film), or multiple models (new skills are learned as successful peers within the group demonstrate the desired behavior).[13] Modeling is more likely to be successful when the model is similar to the client in age, sex, race, and attitudes than when the model is unlike the client. The likelihood that behaviors will be imitated by clients is increased when models are competent in performing the behavior, exhibit warmth, and possess a realistic degree of prestige and status.

Reinforcers

According to behavior modification, behavior is maintained and strengthened when followed by positive reinforcers.[13,16,17] Thus a positive reinforcer is any consequence that maintains and strengthens behavior by its presence; in other words the positive reinforcer makes the behavior more likely to recur.[17] A negative reinforcer is an unpleasant consequence that maintains and strengthens behavior by its being removed from the situation.[17] Reinforcers are often referred to as rewards. Rewards that are effective in reinforcing behavior can take many forms and vary from client to client.

If rewards are used, the counselor must identify rewards likely to effectively reinforce desired behaviors and set up a reinforcement system. As an

BOX 11-3

Examples of Rewards Used in Behavior Modification

Spending money on appropriate things
Reading a book
Watching television
Making a long-distance call
Taking an afternoon or day off
Visiting a friend
Spending time at a favorite hobby
Relaxing or taking a nap

example, consider a client on a weight-control program. The counselor and client can set up a system that allows the client to receive a reward for having lost a certain amount of weight. The weight-loss goal may be set rather low to make it easily attainable at the beginning of counseling. As counseling progresses and the client develops skill in managing his behavior, successive goals can be somewhat more difficult to attain. Rewards can include money or material items (an amount of money or a certain purchase for each goal reached), activities (doing something the client especially enjoys each time a goal is reached), or social interaction (visiting someone special or making a phone call when a goal is attained).[14,17] Examples of rewards are shown in Box 11-3.

Behavior Modification Techniques Summarized

Behavior modification uses a number of techniques. The major ones employed in weight management are outlined in Table 11-2.[16] Some of these techniques were not originally developed by behaviorists but were adapted from other approaches or disciplines and incorporated into behavior modification programs to increase the success of behavioral change. Among these are nutrition education, physical activity, and cognitive restructuring. Cognitive restructuring will be discussed in the section on rational-emotive therapy.

Behavior modification has contributed a variety of specific behavioral techniques to nutritional counseling and treatment of diet-related problems. Its emphasis on changing problem behaviors rather than merely talking about problems and gathering insights allows counselors to focus on assisting clients in formulating a specific plan of action. However, in its attempt to deal with problem solving and changing certain behaviors, it has been criticized for deemphasizing the role of feelings and emotions in counseling.[13]

Rational-Emotive Therapy

Unlike behavior modification, which primarily focuses on the relationship between our environment and behavior, rational-emotive therapy (RET) deals with the effects that our thoughts have on our behavior.[2] The major premise of RET is that emotional disturbances are largely the product of irrational thinking.[13] RET holds that our emotions are mainly the product of our beliefs, evaluations, interpretations, and reactions to life situations.[13]

RET views humans as having the potential for both rational thinking and irrational thinking. It views humans as engaging in considerable self-talk and self-evaluation, much of which is irrational and self-denigrating and can result in emotional disturbances. Rather than factors outside of ourselves being the main determinants of behavior, RET holds that our irrational beliefs about ourselves primarily determine our behavior, emotions, and the resulting consequences. In other words, "men are disturbed not by things, but by the view which they take of them."[13] Thus RET focuses on disputing irrational beliefs and helping people change the irrational beliefs that directly result in disturbed emotions and dysfunctional behavior.[13]

Cognitive Restructuring

A client's self-talk can be viewed as positive, neutral, or negative. Positive self-talk supports

TABLE 11-2 Examples of behavior modification techniques used in weight-control programs

Stimulus control	Reward
Shopping	Solicit help from family and friends
Shop for food after eating	Have family and friends provide help in the form of praise and material reward
Shop from a list	Use self-monitoring records as basis for rewards
Avoid ready-to-eat foods	Plan specific rewards for specific behaviors (behavioral contracts)
Do not carry more cash than needed for shopping	**Self-monitoring**
Plans	Keep diet diary that includes:
Plan to limit food intake	Time and place of eating
Substitute exercise for snacking	Type and amount of food
Eat meals and snacks at scheduled times	Who is present
Do not accept food offered by others	How you feel
Activities	**Nutrition education**
Store food out of sight	Use diet diary to identify problem areas
Eat all food in the same place	Make small changes that you can continue
Remove food from inappropriate storage areas in the house	Learn nutritional values of foods
Keep serving dishes off the table	Decrease fat intake; increase intake of complex carbohydrates
Use smaller dishes and utensils	**Physical activity**
Avoid being the food server	Routine activity
Leave table immediately after eating	Increase routine activity
Do not save leftovers	Increase use of stairs
Holidays and parties	Keep record of distance walked daily
Drink fewer alcoholic beverages	Exercise
Plan eating habits before parties	Begin a very mild exercise program
Eat a low-calorie snack before parties	Keep a record of daily exercise
Practice polite ways to decline food	Increase the exercise very gradually
Do not get discouraged by occasional setback	**Cognitive restructuring**
Eating behavior	Avoid setting unreasonable goals
Put fork down between mouthfuls	Think about progress, not shortcomings
Chew thoroughly before swallowing	Avoid imperatives like "always" and "never"
Prepare foods one portion at a time	Counter negative thoughts with rational statements
Leave some food on the plate	Set weight goals
Pause in the middle of the meal	
Do nothing else while eating (read, watch television)	

From Stunkard AJ, Berthold HC. 1985. What is behavior therapy? A very short description of behavioral weight control. *American Journal of Clinical Nutrition* 41:821–823.

TABLE 11-3 Identifying and disputing irrational and destructive thoughts

Irrational thought	Rational, self-defensive statement
"I can't believe I ate six of those cookies! I've blown it. Oh well, I may as well go ahead and finish the rest of the bag."	"I *did* slip by eating those six cookies, but I *did not* blow my program. The best thing for me to do now is to stop eating them. I *can* do better."
"I ate half a bag of potato chips! I'm an absolute failure."	"My success or failure at anything is not based on one incident. I'm human. It's okay to make mistakes once in awhile. I don't have to be perfect."
"The way she's looking at me, she must think my idea is stupid."	"I can't read other people's minds. The way to find out what she thinks is to just ask. Besides, not everyone has to like my idea."

behavior change whereas negative self-talk opposes change. Consider a client beginning a weight-management program. An example of positive self-talk would be the client silently observing, "I'm going to like this program." Negative self-talk would be the thoughts, "I don't think I can handle this" or "I'm no good at dieting; I'll never succeed at this program." According to RET, the likelihood of successful behavioral change is considerably less when people view themselves as failing as compared to when they see themselves succeeding. In addition, persons viewing themselves as failing at weight management are less likely to begin addressing their behavioral problems and, when faced with difficult challenges (for example, the urging of friends to eat fattening food at a party), they are more likely to slip from their program and potentially give it up altogether.[13,14]

Although our irrational beliefs may have begun through early indoctrination by our parents or significant others ("You're never going to amount to anything!"), it is primarily our own repetition of these irrational thoughts that keeps these dysfunctional attitudes alive and operative within us. Thus RET teaches that we are largely responsible for creating our own problems, that we have the ability to change, that we must identify our irrational beliefs, and that we must dispute these irrational beliefs using the process of cognitive restructuring.[13]

A first step in cognitive restructuring is becoming aware of negative self-talk.[2,13,19,20] One approach is asking the client to record his or her irrational and destructive internal messages on a form similar to the one shown in Table 11-3.[20] Once an irrational internal message is identified, it can be disputed by substituting it with a rational, self-defensive statement. This can also be recorded on the form shown in Table 10-6.

Clients can be led to dispute their irrational self-talk and beliefs by encouraging them to ask such questions as: "What is the factual evidence in support of my thoughts?" "Why do I assume I am a rotten person because of the way I behave?" "Would it really be catastrophic if my worst fears were to come true?" "What can I say in defense of myself?"[13,19] As clients learn to recognize and dispute their irrational self-criticisms, they then can be encouraged to substitute negative self-talk with positive, self-affirming statements.

Other RET techniques include changing one's language, cognitive rehearsal, and thought stopping.[2,13,17,19,20] An example of changing one's language is avoiding negative self-fulfilling statements ("I will fail, look like a pig, and no one will like me"). People telling themselves that they will fail may actually increase the probability of failure. Cognitive rehearsal (also known as rational-emotive imagery) involves clients thinking, feeling, and behaving the way they would like to in real life. As clients see themselves overcoming in their thoughts, the likelihood of them overcoming in real life is increased. Thought stopping is a two-step process. First, whenever a negative thought enters the client's mind, he or she says "Stop!" either out loud or very clearly within the mind. This is followed by substituting a positive, rational thought for the negative, irrational thought. Again, the basis of these exercises is that our language (either audible or silent) influences our thoughts, which in turn influence our emotions and behavior.

Reality Therapy

The central premises of reality therapy are that individuals are responsible for their behavior and that if a person's current behavior is not meeting his or her needs, steps can be taken to change behavior so that personal needs are met.[13,21] Reality therapy is based primarily on the work of psychiatrist William Glasser, who abandoned traditional psychoanalysis early in his career and went on to develop his own counseling approach. According to Glasser, every person's behavior is an attempt to fulfill his or her basic human needs. "It is always what we want at the time that causes our behavior."[22] Rather than being determined by outside forces (as is taught by behaviorists), he views behavior as completely driven from within the person by the necessity to fulfill five innate needs: survival, love, power, fun, and freedom.[22] "All of our lives we must attempt to live in a way that will best satisfy one or more of these needs."[22]

Glasser teaches that each of us creates our own inner world from which we view the world outside of ourselves. Each person is responsible for the kind of inner world he or she creates. Instead of external factors depressing or angering us, we anger or depress ourselves. "Neurotic" and "psychotic" behavior does not just happen to us, it is something we choose in an attempt to control our world. If a client complains of anxiety, the counselor may ask what behavior is causing the anxiety. The focus is not on the anxiety but on whatever behavior is causing the anxiety. According to Glasser, once people acknowledge and act on the reality that their behavior is the result of their choices, change occurs.[13]

Reality therapy begins by the counselor's establishing an accepting and supportive relationship with the client. The client is then led to examine and evaluate his own behavior to determine if it is contributing to his problems. Once the client acknowledges he is not getting what he wants from his behavior, the counselor helps the client develop an action plan for changing his behavior so that it contributes to his success. The plan should have goals that are simple, specific, clear, attainable, and involve something the client will do soon and on a daily basis. The counselor then helps the client make a commitment to follow through with the plan and refuse to give up. The counselor makes it clear to the client that she will neither accept excuses nor use punishment to coerce the client.

Many people tend to blame other individuals or circumstances for their problems. Reality therapy asserts that people are responsible for their own behavior and attacks the excuses many people make for their actions in an attempt to evade responsibility.[23] A client who runs to the refrigerator every time she feels anxious, for example, may benefit from acknowledging that her behavior does not depend on some outside stimulus (in this case the "anxiety") but on her own conscious choice. The client should be helped to recognize that she has a variety of options for dealing with her anxiety. Then, under the guidance of a counselor, the client can select from her options and develop a plan to deal with her problematic behavior in positive ways.[23]

INITIATING AND MAINTAINING DIETARY CHANGE: A PRACTICAL PLAN

From the previous discussion of counseling theories, a number of counselor characteristics and behavioral change techniques can be identified. These characteristics and techniques are effective in initiating and maintaining nutrition behavior, but their use does not guarantee success. Each nutrition counselor will want to integrate them into a total program with which he or she feels comfortable. The counselor will also want to consider clients' needs, resources, and social support, as well as the skill level of support staff.

No single counseling approach can be recommended for all clients. Rather, counselors are encouraged to use an eclectic approach—that is, one composed of elements drawn from a variety of approaches. An effective behavioral change program would selectively incorporate several techniques into a multicomponent program that is suitable to both the counselor and the client. However, it is neither necessary nor wise to use all the counseling techniques at one's disposal.

Motivation

No counselor can motivate a client. Motivation only comes from within the client. A counselor can only create a climate that will help clients to motivate themselves. People tend to be motivated by challenge, growth, achievement, promotion, and recognition. Emphasis should be placed on providing a proper environment for self-growth by challenging clients, giving them responsibility and encouragement, and giving full range to individual strength.

Characteristics of Effective Counselors

From this discussion of counseling theories, it is possible to identify several characteristics of effective counselors. By practicing good communication, listening, and counseling skills, one of the first steps in initiating behavioral change can take place—establishing good rapport with the client. The following are characteristics of effective counselors:[24]

- Empathy—the ability to climb into the world of the client and communicate back feelings of understanding.
- Respect—a deep and genuine appreciation for the worth of a client, separate and apart from his or her behavior. The strength and ability of the client to overcome and adjust is appreciated.
- Warmth—communication of concern and appropriate affection.
- Genuineness—being freely and deeply one's self. One is congruent and not just playing a role.
- Concreteness—essential ideas and elements are ferreted out.
- Self-disclosure—information about self is revealed for the benefit of the client at the appropriate time.
- Potency and self-actualization—one is dynamic, in command, conveys feelings of trust and warmth, is competent, inner directed, creative, sensitive, nonjudgmental, productive, serene, satisfied. This comes across to the client in a helpful way.

Initial Assessment

The initial assessment of the client serves several important functions.[18]

- It makes the counselor and client aware of the client's dietary habits, health history, and related factors.
- It provides baseline information from which to gauge progress.
- It alerts the counselor and client to the various demands being placed on the client so that realistic priorities can be set.
- It gives the counselor and client ideas for making dietary changes.
- It gives the counselor an opportunity to develop rapport and a sense of partnership with the client.
- It enables the counselor to develop a plan of gradual change suitable to the client's way of living.

As discussed in Chapters 3 and 8, a variety of techniques can be used for obtaining dietary information. In addition to this data, however, information should be collected on the client's current health status, health history, and past and present health habits.

Initiating Dietary Change

Counselors and clients should have reasonable expectations about what changes should be undertaken, the extent of change, and the rate at which change is made. Clients should be carefully guided in what benefits they can reasonably expect from dietary change and the amount of change necessary to realize those benefits.[18,25]

Goals can be set by the client under the guidance of the counselor. Goals should be specific, measurable, reasonable, and attainable. Whatever the final behavioral goal is, most people will not be able to master it at the first effort or in one step. Behavioral change should be approached gradually with a number of small, easily attained goals that collectively lead to the final goal. A client can never begin too low and the steps upward can never be too small.[17] Short-term goals spanning 1 to 2 weeks are more effective than long-term goals covering months.[25] Because obstacles and setbacks will be encountered, goals should have some flexibility. One approach to building a client's commitment to attaining goals can be through a written self-contract.

Reinforcers or rewards can help promote maintenance of behavioral change, especially at the beginning of a program. If they are used, counselors will need to work with each individual client (and possibly with a key individual providing social support for the client) to identify reinforcers providing ample incentive to goal attainment. At this time the use of other behavior modification strategies (see Table 10-5) can be discussed with the client. Serious consideration should be given to using stimulus control, self-monitoring, and cognitive restructuring in ways suitable to both counselor and client.

Maintaining Dietary Change

Although counselors can assist clients in making dietary changes (for example, in learning about nutrition, setting realistic goals, and managing the antecedents to behaviors), it is ultimately the client's responsibility to change dietary habits. To be permanently successful, clients will need to be guided toward self-sufficiency.[18]

A key element in self-sufficiency is the client's involvement in the change process.[18] The client should be asked, "What changes can *you* make?" "What can *you* say when someone offers you another serving of dessert?" "What steps can *you* take to avoid overeating at a party?" The more the client "owns" the program, the more successful he or she will be at maintaining dietary change.

Four areas where counselors can help clients increase self-control over eating habits are maintaining commitment, record keeping, environmental restructuring, and use of reinforcers or rewards.[18] At first, most clients are enthusiastic about behavioral change. After several days or weeks, however, this enthusiasm begins to wane. Some suggestions for strengthening commitment to dietary change include the following:[18]

- Praise the client for his or her successful experiences and attribute success to the client's abilities.
- Encourage the client to tell family members and friends about his or her dietary goals. After making a public commitment to dietary change, adherence to the program is more likely.
- Ask the client to state the kinds of problems he or she will likely encounter. Problems will occur, but they will be less likely to derail the client's progress when they are anticipated and planned for.
- Concentrate on foods the client can eat, rather than those to be avoided. Help clients realize that healthy eating is not synonymous with deprivation.

Record keeping provides information on the client's performance, aids the client in observing and analyzing his or her environment, and helps in recognizing the antecedents or cues to eating behavior. Record keeping can range from marking a 3×5-inch card every time a between-meal snack is declined to keeping elaborate food records.[18]

Some researchers think that restructuring the environment is the most important technique in maintaining change. Counselors can ask clients to identify specific changes that can be made in their physical, social, and cognitive (mental) environments to promote long-term dietary change.

A client may associate some event such as sitting in a favorite chair reading the newspaper or watching television with eating high-calorie foods. The presence of inappropriate foods at home also can be a deterrent to successful change. Altering the arrangement of furniture in the room where television is watched or the newspaper is read can help promote and maintain change. Purchasing healthful foods to substitute for inappropriate items can be helpful as well.

The counselor should ask the client to identify social situations that promote poor eating habits. How is the client's eating behavior affected by various social functions or what family and friends say to the client? The counselor should explore with the client ways that social interactions can be supportive of dietary change. What could family and friends say to promote the client's success? Through role playing, the client can develop skill in asking for support from others.[18] In dealing with the mental environment, the client should be encouraged to use some of the cognitive restructuring techniques discussed earlier in this chapter. Use of reinforcers or rewards and self-contracts also is discussed earlier in this chapter.

Relapse Prevention

For the purposes of behavioral change, a relapse can be defined as the resumption of an unwanted habit or behavior that one has, for a period of time, overcome or turned from.[17,26] Consider a man with the habit of eating a half-pint of premium butter-pecan ice cream every evening. For several weeks he has limited himself to only 1 cup of nonfat frozen dessert 4 evenings a week. When he returns to 2 cups of butter-pecan ice cream every evening for several weeks, he has relapsed. However, if he merely indulges once or twice in butter-pecan ice cream while spending a weekend with relatives and then returns to 1 cup of the nonfat variety 4 evenings a week, he has only experienced a lapse. A lapse can be defined as "a single event, a reemergence of a previous habit, which may or may not lead to a state of relapse."[26] Thus a lapse is a temporary fall, a slip, or a mistake. When a lapse occurs, corrective action can be taken to prevent a relapse—a total loss of control—from occurring.[26]

A key to relapse prevention is to prepare clients for the occurrence of lapses and to help them cope in ways that prevent a relapse.[25] If counselors and clients have previously discussed the likelihood of lapses occurring, clients will be better prepared when they do occur, and the risk of lapses leading to full-blown relapses will be minimized. Clients should be taught to anticipate situations likely to produce lapses, such as illness, travel, live-in visitors, overwork, emotional distress, and schedule changes.[25]

Counselors should help clients to view lapses for what they really are—merely a temporary fall, a slip, a mistake. A counselor and client can discuss what corrective actions the client can take to recover from the lapse and to prevent a relapse from occurring. Techniques such as modeling, role playing, cognitive rehearsal, and direct instruction can help in this.[2] A client needs to be assured that if a relapse does occur, it is not "the end of the world." The client has suffered a setback, but prompt action can limit the relapse to a temporary setback.

KNOWING ONE'S LIMITS

When working with clients, it is important that counselors know the limits of their abilities to help people and when they need to refer a client to more experienced help. Emotional problems are common, and from time to time nutrition counselors encounter individuals needing psychological counseling. If a client indicates that she is having emotional problems, a nutrition counselor may very gently and tactfully ask if she would like assistance in getting psychological counseling from a local mental health clinic or professional. The counselor may help her in calling and making an appointment with an appropriate agency or person.[13,25]

Some individuals may not be ready or willing to change certain habits. Circumstances in a person's life may not be conducive to change at the particular time he is seeing a counselor. It may be necessary to suggest that a client postpone weight loss or control of mildly elevated serum cholesterol until *after* he deals with a more pressing problem like separation, divorce, bankruptcy, or substance abuse.

This chapter has offered a very brief overview of dietary counseling. It is meant to be only an introduction to the topic. Readers interested in developing the skill of nutritional counseling are encouraged to take course work and study other sources for further information. Other excellent resources include the following:

Raab C, Tillotson JL. 1985. *Heart to heart: A manual on nutrition counseling for the reduction of cardiovascular disease risk factors.* Bethesda, Md: U.S. Department of Health and Human Services, Public Health Service; National Institutes of Health.

Holli BB, Calabrese RJ. 1991. *Communication and education skills: The dietitian's guide,* 2nd ed. Philadelphia: Lea & Febiger.

Watson DL, Tharp RG. 1989. *Self-directed behavior: Self-modification for personal adjustment,* 5th ed. Pacific Grove, Calif: Brooks/Cole.

SUMMARY

1. Communication, the process of sending and receiving messages, lies at the foundation of all efforts to interview, counsel, educate, and change diet. The basic components of human communication are the sender, receiver, message, feedback, and interference.
2. A counselor's attempts to help bring about dietary change may elicit a defensive reaction from the receiver or client. When this occurs, the receiver fails to concentrate on the structure, content, and meaning of the message. This is one source of interference to communication. When communication is supportive of the receiver, this defensive reaction can be prevented, and the interference to communication can be minimized.
3. Communication occurs simultaneously at both the verbal and nonverbal level. Nonverbal communication involves gestures, posture, facial expressions, and tone of voice. It is sometimes a more reliable indicator of a person's true feelings than are words. Unlike verbal communication, which is generally under conscious control and subject to censorship, nonverbal communication is not as easily controlled by conscious thought. It is also an effective way for the counselor to communicate to the client.
4. Effective communication is promoted by proper use of feedback, language that is understandable to both counselor and client, an environment that is conducive to good communication, and awareness of the physical and psychological barriers to communication.
5. Listening is an important part of interviewing and counseling and an excellent way to establish rapport. Despite its importance, most people are not good listeners. Listening involves six steps: hearing, attending, understanding, remembering, evaluating, and responding.
6. Rather than being a passive activity, listening is a highly active process demanding concentration and attention. It is also a skill that can be learned. Listening skills can be grouped under four categories: openness, concentration, attention, and comprehension.
7. Interviewing is a guided communication process between two persons for the purpose of obtaining or exchanging specific information through the asking and answering of questions. The goal of the interview is obtaining specific information from the client while maintaining an interpersonal environment conducive to disclosure by the client. Conditions that increase interviewing effectiveness

include comfortable physical surroundings, freedom from interruption and interference, and privacy. Counselor qualities that contribute to a successful interview include the ability to establish good rapport, attentiveness, openness, and an understanding of the client's situation.

8. Several types of questions can be used in the interview. Open questions invite rather than demand answers and give the client substantial freedom in determining the amount and type of information to give. Closed questions are restrictive and allow the counselor to control answers and ask for specific information. Neutral questions allow the client to answer without pressure or direction from the counselor. Leading questions contain implicit or explicit suggestions about the expected or desired answer.
9. The person-centered approach to counseling is largely based on the idea that if people experience human relationships characterized by respect and trust they will develop in a positive and constructive manner. Three counselor qualities that create a growth-promoting climate for the client are genuineness or realness, unconditional positive regard and acceptance of the client, and deep understanding of the client's feelings. Within this climate, the client is then able to lose his or her "defenses and rigid perceptions and move to a higher level of personal functioning."[10]
10. The main contribution of person-centered therapy is its core skills: listening, understanding, caring, and acceptance. Regardless of the approach used, counselors deficient in these skills will lack efficiency in carrying out their treatment. The presence of a caring, listening, understanding person can do much to promote healing in a person experiencing a crisis.
11. Behavior modification attempts to alter previously learned human behavior or encourage the learning of new behavior through a variety of action-oriented methods, as opposed to changing feelings or thoughts. Although early behaviorists viewed human behavior as almost totally the result of reinforcements, modern behaviorists view humans as both the product of environmental influences and the producer of their environment.
12. Behaviorists view actions as being preceded by antecedents and followed by consequences. The modification or control of antecedents to decrease the occurrence of negative behaviors and increase the occurrence of positive behaviors is referred to as stimulus control. Other techniques of behavior modification include self-monitoring or record keeping, modeling, cognitive restructuring, education, physical activity, and the use of goals, self-contracts, and reinforcers.
13. The major premise of rational-emotive therapy (RET) is that emotional disturbances are largely the product of irrational thinking. RET holds that our emotions are mainly the product of our beliefs, evaluations, interpretations, and reactions to life situations. Rather than factors outside of ourselves being the main determinants of behavior, RET holds that our irrational beliefs about ourselves primarily determine our behavior, emotions, and the resulting consequences.
14. A major technique of RET is cognitive restructuring, which focuses on helping people dispute their irrational beliefs and change the thoughts that directly result in disturbed emotions and dysfunctional behavior. RET also uses such techniques as cognitive rehearsal and thought stopping.
15. Reality therapy views every person's behavior as an attempt to fulfill his or her basic human needs. Reality therapy views behavior as being driven, not by outside forces but from within the person by the necessity to fulfill the need for survival, love, power, fun, and freedom. Each individual is responsible for his or her behavior, and if current behavior is not meeting a person's needs, he or she can

take steps to change behavior so that personal needs are met.

16. In reality therapy, the counselor begins by establishing an accepting and supportive relationship with a client. The client is then led to examine and evaluate his behavior to determine if it is contributing to his problems. Once the client acknowledges he is not getting what he wants from his behavior, the counselor helps the client develop an action plan for changing his behavior so that it contributes to his success.
17. No single counseling approach can be recommended for all clients. Counselors are encouraged to use an eclectic approach—one composed of elements drawn from a variety of methods. An effective behavioral change program would selectively incorporate several techniques into a multicomponent program that is suitable to both the counselor and the client.
18. In addition to having good communication and listening skills, effective counselors convey empathy, respect, warmth, genuineness, concreteness, openness, potency, and self-actualization.
19. It is important for counselors and clients to have reasonable expectations about what changes should be undertaken, the extent of change, and the rate at which change is made. Goals set by the client under the guidance of the counselor should be specific, measurable, reasonable, and attainable. Behavioral change will be more successful when achieved through a number of small steps. Short-term goals spanning 1 to 2 weeks are more effective than long-term goals covering months.
20. If rewards or reinforcers are used, counselors will need to work with each individual client to identify those providing ample incentive to goal attainment. Serious consideration also should be given to using stimulus control, self-monitoring, and cognitive restructuring in ways suitable to both counselor and client.
21. It is ultimately the client's responsibility to change dietary habits. To be permanently successful, clients need to be guided toward self-sufficiency. Four areas where counselors can help clients develop self-sufficiency in dietary change are maintaining commitment, record keeping, environmental restructuring, and use of reinforcers or rewards.
22. A relapse can be defined as the resumption of an unwanted habit or behavior that one has, for a period of time, overcome or turned from. A lapse can be defined as a temporary fall, a slip, a mistake, or a reemergence of a previous habit, which may or may not lead to a state of relapse. Counselors should prepare clients for the occurrence of lapses and help them cope in ways that will prevent a relapse. Clients should be taught to anticipate situations likely to produce lapses, such as illness, travel, live-in visitors, overwork, emotional distress, and schedule changes.
23. Counselors should know the limits of their abilities and when they need to refer clients needing psychological counseling to more experienced help. Some individuals may not be ready or willing to change certain habits. It may be necessary to suggest that a client postpone dietary change until after his or her more pressing problems have been resolved.

REFERENCES

1. U.S. Department of Health and Human Services. 1984. *The health consequences of smoking: Chronic obstructive lung disease, a report of the Surgeon General.* Rockville, Md: Office on Smoking and Health.
2. Holli BB, Calabrese RJ. 1991. *Communication and education skills: The dietitian's guide,* 2nd ed. Philadelphia: Lea & Febiger.
3. Gibb JR. 1961. Defensive communication. *Journal of Communication* 11:141–148.
4. Enelow AJ, Swisher SN. 1979. *Interviewing and patient care,* 2nd ed. New York: Oxford University Press.

5. Bartley KC. 1987. *Dietetic practitioner skills: Nutrition education, counseling, and business management.* New York: Macmillan.
6. Samovar LA, Mills J. 1992. *Oral communication: Message and response,* 8th ed. Dubuque, Iowa: Wm. C. Brown.
7. Curry-Bartley KR. 1986. The art and science of listening. *Topics in Clinical Nutrition* 1:14–24.
8. Stewart CJ, Cash WB. 1991. *Interviewing: Principles and practices,* 6th ed. Dubuque, Iowa: Wm. C. Brown.
9. Snetselaar LG. 1983. *Nutrition counseling skills: Assessment, treatment, and evaluation.* Rockville, Md: Aspen.
10. Rogers C. 1961. *On becoming a person.* Boston: Houghton Mifflin.
11. Rogers C. 1970. *Carl Rogers on encounter groups.* New York: Harper & Row.
12. Rogers C. 1977. *Carl Rogers on personal power: Inner strength and its revolutionary impact.* New York: Delacorte.
13. Corey G. 1991. *Theory and practice of counseling and psychotherapy,* 4th ed. Pacific Grove, Calif: Brooks/Cole.
14. Williams AB. 1991. Behavior modification. In Holli BB, Calabrese RJ. *Communication and education skills: The dietitian's guide,* 2nd ed. Philadelphia: Lea & Febiger.
15. Hodges PAM, Vickery CE. 1989. *Effective counseling: Strategies for dietary management.* Rockville, Md: Aspen.
16. Stunkard AJ, Berthold HC. 1985. What is behavior therapy? A very short description of behavioral weight control. *American Journal of Clinical Nutrition* 41:821–823.
17. Watson DL, Tharp RG. 1989. *Self-directed behavior: Self-modification for personal adjustment,* 5th ed. Pacific Grove, Calif: Brooks/Cole Publishing.
18. Raab C, Tillotson JL. 1985. *Heart to heart: A manual on nutrition counseling for the reduction of cardiovascular disease risk factors.* Bethesda, Md: U.S. Department of Health and Human Services, Public Health Service; National Institutes of Health.
19. Burns DD. 1981. *Feeling good: The new mood therapy.* New York: Signet.
20. Burns DD. 1990. *The feeling good handbook: Using the new mood therapy in everyday life.* New York: New American Library/Dutton.
21. Glasser W. 1984. *Take effective control of your life.* New York: Harper & Row.
22. Glasser W. 1990. *The quality school: Managing students without coercion.* New York: Harper & Row.
23. Hoeltzel KE. 1986. Counseling methods for dietitians. *Topics in clinical nutrition* 1:33–42.
24. Nieman DC. 1990. *Fitness and sports medicine: An introduction.* Palo Alto, Calif: Bull.
25. American College of Sports Medicine. 1991. *Guidelines for exercise testing and prescription,* 4th ed. Philadelphia: Lea & Febiger.
26. Brownell KD, Marlatt GA, Lichtenstein E, Wilson GT. 1986. Understanding and preventing relapse. *American Psychologist* 41:765–782.

Assessment Activity 11-1

COUNSELING PRACTICE

Becoming an effective counselor requires considerable skill and practice. This activity is designed to help you "get your feet wet."

Members of your class should divide into groups of two students each. You should take the 3-day food record that you completed in Assessment Activity 3-2 and the result of the computerized analysis of that food record obtained in Assessment Activity 5-1 and give these to your partner.

Review your partner's food record and computerized analysis. Study the Competency Checklist for Nutrition Counselors shown in Appendix U. Use this as a guide for your counseling session and to evaluate yourself after you have counseled your partner.

Using techniques discussed in this chapter, assist your partner in identifying one specific, measurable, and attainable goal that will improve his or her diet. Guide your partner in developing a simple action plan for attaining the goal he or she has decided on.

Videotape (or audiotape) the counseling session and view (or listen to) it alone later to see how you did. Look for what you did right and note improvements you can make next time. Use the Competency Checklist for Nutrition Counselors in Appendix U to evaluate your counseling skills.

If time allows, repeat this exercise.

APPENDIX A

DIETARY REFERENCE VALUES FOR FOOD ENERGY AND NUTRIENTS FOR THE UNITED KINGDOM

From Department of Health. 1991. Report on Health and Social Subjects No. 41: *Dietary reference values for food energy and nutrients for the United Kingdom*. London: Her Majesty's Stationery Office.

Dietary reference values for fat and carbohydrate for adults as a percentage of daily total energy intake (percentage of food energy)

	Individual minimum	Population average	Individual maximum
Saturated fatty acids		10 (11)	
Cis-polyunsaturated fatty acids		6 (6.5)	10
	n−3 0.2		
	n−6 1.0		
Cis-monounsaturated fatty acids		12 (13)	
Trans fatty acids		2 (2)	
Total fatty acids		30 (32.5)	
Total fat		33 (35)	
Non-milk extrinsic sugars	0	10 (11)	
Intrinsic and milk sugars and starch		37 (39)	
Total carbohydrate		47 (50)	
Non-starch polysaccharide (g/d)	12	18	24

The average percentage contribution to total energy does not total 100% because figures for protein and alcohol are excluded. Protein intakes average 15% of total energy which is above the RNI. It is recognized that many individuals will derive some energy from alcohol, and this has been assumed to average 5% approximating to current intakes. However the Panel allowed that some groups might not drink alcohol and that for some purposes nutrient intakes as a proportion of food energy (without alcohol) might be useful. Therefore, average figures are given as percentages both of total energy and, in parenthesis, of food energy.

Reference nutrient intakes for protein

Age	Reference nutrient intake* (g/day)	
0–3 months	12.5†	
4–6 months	12.7	
7–9 months	13.7	
10–12 months	14.9	
1–3 years	14.5	
4–6 years	19.7	
7–10 years	28.3	
Males		
11–14 years	42.1	
15–18 years	55.2	
19–50 years	55.5	
50+ years	53.3	
Females		
11–14 years	41.2	
15–18 years	45.0	
19–50 years	45.0	
50+ years	46.5	
Pregnancy‡		+ 6
Lactation‡		
0–4 months		+11
4+ months		+ 8

*These figures, based on egg and milk protein, assume complete digestibility.
†No values for infants 0–3 months are given by WHO. The RNI is calculated from the recommendations of COMA.
‡To be added to adult requirement through all stages of pregnancy and lactation.

Reference nutrient intakes for minerals (SI units)

Age	Calcium mmol/day	Phosphorus[1] mmol/day	Magnesium mmol/day	Sodium mmol/day	Potassium mmol/day	Chloride[4] mmol/day	Iron µmol/day	Zinc µmol/day	Copper µmol/day	Selenium µmol/day	Iodine µmol/d
0–3 months	13.1	13.1	2.2	9	20	9	30	60	5	0.1	0.4
4–6 months	13.1	13.1	2.5	12	22	12	80	60	5	0.2	0.5
7–9 months	13.1	13.1	3.2	14	18	14	140	75	5	0.1	0.5
10–12 months	13.1	13.1	3.3	15	18	15	140	75	5	0.1	0.5
1–3 years	8.8	8.8	3.5	22	20	22	120	75	6	0.2	0.6
4–6 years	11.3	11.3	4.8	30	28	30	110	100	9	0.3	0.8
7–10 years	13.8	13.8	8.0	50	50	50	160	110	11	0.4	0.9
Males											
11–14 years	25.0	25.0	11.5	70	80	70	200	140	13	0.6	1.0
15–18 years	25.0	25.0	12.3	70	90	70	200	145	16	0.9	1.0
19–50 years	17.5	17.5	12.3	70	90	70	160	145	19	0.9	1.0
50+ years	17.5	17.5	12.3	70	90	70	160	145	19	0.9	1.0
Females											
11–14 years	20.0	10.0	11.5	70	80	70	260[5]	140	13	0.6	1.0
15–18 years	20.0	20.0	12.3	70	90	70	260[5]	110	16	0.8	1.1
19–50 years	17.5	17.5	10.9	70	90	70	260[5]	110	19	0.8	1.1
50+ years	17.5	17.5	10.9	70	90	70	160	110	19	0.8	1.1
Pregnancy	*	*	*	*	*	*	*	*	*	*	*
Lactation:											
0–4 months	+14.3	+14.3	+2.1	*	*	*	*	+90	+5	+0.2	*
4+ months	+14.3	+14.3	+2.1	*	*	*	*	+40	+5	+0.2	*

Age	Calcium mg/day	Phosphorus[1] mg/day	Magnesium mg/day	Sodium mg/day[2]	Potassium mg/day[3]	Chloride[4] mg/day	Iron mg/day	Zinc mg/day	Copper mg/day	Selenium µg/day	Iodine µg/day
0–3 months	525	400	55	210	800	320	1.7	4.0	0.2	10	50
4–6 months	525	400	60	280	850	400	4.3	4.0	0.3	13	60
7–9 months	525	400	75	320	700	500	7.8	5.0	0.3	10	60
10–12 months	525	400	80	350	700	500	7.8	5.0	0.3	10	60
1–3 years	350	270	85	500	800	800	6.9	5.0	0.4	15	70
4–6 years	450	350	120	700	1,100	1,100	6.1	6.5	0.6	20	100
7–10 years	550	450	200	1,200	2,000	1,800	8.7	7.0	0.7	30	110
Males											
11–14 years	1,000	775	280	1,600	3,100	2,500	11.3	9.0	0.8	45	130
15–18 years	1,000	775	300	1,600	3,500	2,500	11.3	9.5	1.0	70	140
19–50 years	700	550	300	1,600	3,500	2,500	8.7	9.5	1.2	75	140
50+ years	700	550	300	1,600	3,500	2,500	8.7	9.5	1.2	75	140
Females											
11–14 years	800	625	280	1,600	3,100	2,500	14.8[5]	9.0	0.8	45	130
15–18 years	800	625	300	1,600	3,500	2,500	14.8[5]	7.0	1.0	60	140
19–50 years	700	550	270	1,600	3,500	2,500	14.8[5]	7.0	1.2	60	140
50+ years	700	550	270	1,600	3,500	2,500	8.7	7.0	1.2	60	140
Pregnancy	*	*	*	*	*	*	*	*	*	*	*
Lactation:											
0–4 months	+550	+440	+50	*	*	*	*	+6.0	+0.3	+15	*
4+ months	+550	+440	+50	*	*	*	*	+2.5	+0.3	+15	*

*No increment

[1]Phosphorus RNI is set equal to calcium in molar terms

[2]1 mmol sodium = 23 mg

[3]1 mmol potassium = 39 mg

[4]Corresponds to sodium 1 mmol = 35.5 mg

[5]Insufficient for women with high menstrual losses where the most practical way of meeting iron requirements is to take iron supplements.

Reference nutrient intakes for vitamins

Age	Thiamin mg/day	Riboflavin mg/day	Niacin (nicotinic acid equivalent) mg/day	Vitamin B_6 mg/day§	Vitamin B_{12} µg/day	Folate µg/day	Vitamin C mg/day	Vitamin A µg/day	Vitamin D µg/day
0–3 months	0.2	0.4	3	0.2	0.3	50	25	350	8.5
4–6 months	0.2	0.4	3	0.2	0.3	50	25	350	8.5
7–9 months	0.2	0.4	4	0.3	0.4	50	25	350	7
10–12 months	0.3	0.4	5	0.4	0.4	50	25	350	7
1–3 years	0.5	0.6	8	0.7	0.5	70	30	400	7
4–6 years	0.7	0.8	11	0.9	0.8	100	30	500	—
7–10 years	0.7	1.0	12	1.0	1.0	150	30	500	—
Males									
11–14 years	0.9	1.2	15	1.2	1.2	200	35	600	—
15–18 years	1.1	1.3	18	1.5	1.5	200	40	700	—
19–50 years	1.0	1.3	17	1.4	1.5	200	40	700	—
50+ years	0.9	1.3	16	1.4	1.5	200	40	700	†
Females									
11–14 years	0.7	1.1	12	1.0	1.2	200	35	600	—
15–18 years	0.8	1.1	14	1.2	1.5	200	40	600	—
19–50 years	0.8	1.1	13	1.2	1.5	200	40	600	—
50+ years	0.8	1.1	12	1.2	1.5	200	40	600	†
Pregnancy	+0.1‡	+0.3	*	*	*	+100	+10	+100	10
Lactation:									
0–4 months	+0.2	+0.5	+2	*	+0.5	+60	+30	+350	10
4+ months	+0.2	+0.5	+2	*	+0.5	+60	+30	+350	10

*No increment †After age 65 the RNI is 10 µg/d for men and women ‡For last trimester only §Based on protein providing 14.7% of EAR for energy

Safe intakes

Nutrient	Safe intake
Vitamins:	
Pantothenic acid	
Adults	3–7 mg/day
Infants	1.7 mg/day
Biotin	10–200 μg/day
Vitamin E	
Men	above 4 mg/day
Women	above 3 mg/day
Infants	0.4 mg/g polyunsaturated fatty acids
Vitamin K	
Adults	1 μg/kg/day
Infants	10 μg/day
Minerals:	
Manganese	
Adults	1.4 mg (26 μmol)/day
Infants and children	16 μg (0.3 μmol)/day
Molybdenum	
Adults	50–400 μg/day
Infants, children and adolescents	0.5–1.5 μg/kg/day
Chromium	
Adults	25 μg (0.5 μmol)/day
Children and adolescents	0.1–1.0 μg (2–20 μmol)/kg/day
Fluoride (for infants only)	0.05 mg (3 μmol)/kg/day

APPENDIX B

RECOMMENDED NUTRIENT INTAKES FOR CANADIANS

From Health and Welfare Canada. 1990. *Nutrition Recommendations.* Ottawa: Canadian Government Publishing Centre. Health and Welfare Canada, reproduced with permission of the Minister of Supply and Services Canada, 1991.

Summary of examples of recommended nutrients based on energy expressed as daily rates

Age	Sex	Energy kcal	Thiamin mg	Riboflavin mg	Niacin NE*	n-3 PUFA† g	n-6 PUFA g
Months							
0–4	Both	600	0.3	0.3	4	0.5	3
5–12	Both	900	0.4	0.5	7	0.5	3
Years							
1	Both	1100	0.5	0.6	8	0.6	4
2–3	Both	1300	0.6	0.7	9	0.7	4
4–6	Both	1800	0.7	0.9	13	1.0	6
7–9	M	2200	0.9	1.1	16	1.2	7
	F	1900	0.8	1.0	14	1.0	6
10–12	M	2500	1.0	1.3	18	1.4	8
	F	2200	0.9	1.1	16	1.1	7
13–15	M	2800	1.1	1.4	20	1.4	9
	F	2200	0.9	1.1	16	1.2	7
16–18	M	3200	1.3	1.6	23	1.8	11
	F	2100	0.8	1.1	15	1.2	7
19–24	M	3000	1.2	1.5	22	1.6	10
	F	2100	0.8	1.1	15	1.2	7
25–49	M	2700	1.1	1.4	19	1.5	9
	F	2000	0.8	1.0	14	1.1	7
50–74	M	2300	0.9	1.3	16	1.3	8
	F	1800	0.8‡	1.0‡	14‡	1.1‡	7‡
75+	M	2000	0.8	1.0	14	1.0	7
	F§	1700	0.8‡	1.0‡	14‡	1.1‡	7‡
Pregnancy (additional)							
1st Trimester		100	0.1	0.1	0.1	0.05	0.3
2nd Trimester		300	0.1	0.3	0.2	0.16	0.9
3rd Trimester		300	0.1	0.3	0.2	0.16	0.9
Lactation (additional)		450	0.2	0.4	0.3	0.25	1.5

*Niacin Equivalents
†PUFA, polyunsaturated fatty acids
‡Level below which intake should not fall
§Assumes moderate physical activity

Summary examples of recommended nutrient intake based on age and body weight expressed as daily rates

Age	Sex	Weight kg	Protein g	Vit. A RE*	Vit. D µg	Vit. E mg	Vit. C mg	Folate µg	Vit. B_{12} µg	Calcium mg	Phosphorus mg	Magnesium mg	Iron mg	Iodine µg	Zinc mg
Months															
0–4	Both	6.0	12†	400	10	3	20	50	0.3	250‡	150	20	0.3§	30	2§
5–12	Both	9.0	12	400	10	3	20	50	0.3	400	200	32	7	40	3
Years															
1	Both	11	19	400	10	3	20	65	0.3	500	300	40	6	55	4
2–3	Both	14	22	400	5	4	20	80	0.4	550	350	50	6	65	4
4–6	Both	18	26	500	5	5	25	90	0.5	600	400	65	8	85	5
7–9	M	25	30	700	2.5	7	25	125	0.8	700	500	100	8	110	7
	F	25	30	700	2.5	6	25	125	0.8	700	500	100	8	95	7
10–12	M	34	38	800	2.5	8	25	170	1.0	900	700	130	8	125	9
	F	36	40	800	5	7	25	180	1.0	1100	800	135	8	110	9
13–15	M	50	50	900	5	9	30	150	1.5	1100	900	185	10	160	12
	F	48	42	800	5	7	30	145	1.5	1000	850	180	13	160	9
16–18	M	62	55	1000	5	10	40‖	185	1.9	900	1000	230	10	160	12
	F	53	43	800	2.5	7	30‖	160	1.9	700	850	200	12	160	9
19–24	M	71	58	1000	2.5	10	40‖	210	2.0	800	1000	240	9	160	12
	F	58	43	800	2.5	7	30‖	175	2.0	700	850	200	13	160	9
25–49	M	74	61	1000	2.5	9	40‖	220	2.0	800	1000	250	9	160	12
	F	59	44	800	2.5	6	30‖	175	2.0	700	850	200	13	160	9
50–74	M	73	60	1000	5	7	40‖	220	2.0	800	1000	250	9	160	12
	F	63	47	800	5	6	30‖	190	2.0	800	850	210	8	160	9
75+	M	69	57	1000	5	6	40‖	205	2.0	800	1000	230	9	160	12
	F	64	47	800	5	5	30‖	190	2.0	800	850	210	8	160	9
Pregnancy (additional)															
1st Trimester			5	100	2.5	2	0	300	1.0	500	200	15	0	25	6
2nd Trimester			20	100	2.5	2	10	300	1.0	500	200	45	5	25	6
3rd Trimester			24	100	2.5	2	10	300	1.0	500	200	45	10	25	6
Lactation (additional)			20	400	2.5	3	25	100	0.5	500	200	65	0	50	6

*Retinol Equivalents

†Protein is assumed to be from breast milk and must be adjusted for infant formula.

‡Infant formula with high phosphorus should contain 375 mg calcium.

§Breast milk is assumed to be the source of the mineral.

APPENDIX C

THE U.S. RECOMMENDED DAILY ALLOWANCES (U.S. RDAs)

From Federal Register, July 19, 1990, page 29477.

Vitamins and minerals	Unit of measurement	Infants	Children under 4 years of age	Adults and children 4 or more years of age	Pregnant or lactating women
Vitamin A	International units	1500	2500	5000	8000
Vitamin D	International units	400	400	400	400
Vitamin E	International units	5	10	30	30
Vitamin C	Milligrams	35	40	60	60
Folic acid	Milligrams	.1	.2	.4	.8
Thiamine	Milligrams	.5	.7	1.5	1.7
Riboflavin	Milligrams	.6	.8	1.7	2
Niacin	Milligrams	8	9	20	20
Vitamin B_6	Milligrams	.4	.7	2	2.5
Vitamin B_{12}	Micrograms	2	3	6	8
Biotin	Milligrams	.05	.15	.30	.30
Pantothenic acid	Milligrams	3	5	10	10
Calcium	Grams	.6	.8	1	1
Phosphorus	Grams	.6	.8	1	1
Iodine	Micrograms	45	70	150	150
Iron	Milligrams	15	10	18	18
Magnesium	Milligrams	70	200	400	450
Copper	Milligrams	.6	1	2	2
Zinc	Milligrams	5	8	15	15

APPENDIX D

1987–88 Nationwide Food Consumption Survey 24-Hour Recall Form

From the Human Nutrition Information Serivce, USDA.

NATIONAL ANALYSTS
A Division of Booz·Allen
& Hamilton Inc.

Study #: 09010-067-001
OMB #: 0586-0020
Expires: 12/31/1988

Interviewing Period

Spring	1
Summer	2
Fall	3
Winter	4

Segment #: [ ][ ][ ][ ][ ][ ][ ]

Housing Unit #: [ ][ ][ ]

Person (line) #: [ ][ ]

Interviewer #: [ ][ ][ ]

FOR INTERVIEWER'S USE ONLY

Time began:________ AM 1 / PM 2

Time ended:________ AM 1 / PM 2

NATIONWIDE FOOD CONSUMPTION SURVEY
(NFCS 1987)
UNITED STATES DEPARTMENT OF AGRICULTURE
Individual Intake Record

DAY ONE

This record is for: ________________________________
PERSON'S FIRST NAME

This person's date of birth is: [ ][ ] MONTH [ ][ ] DAY [ ][ ][ ][ ] YEAR

DAY ONE is from 12:00 AM to 11:59 PM yesterday. That date was:

(CIRCLE NUMBER FOR DAY OF WEEK)

Sunday	1
Monday	2
Tuesday	3
Wednesday	4
Thursday	5
Friday	6
Saturday	7

[ ][ ] MONTH [ ][ ] DAY [1][9][8][ ] YEAR

Your cooperation is entirely voluntary. This information will be used to estimate the types and amounts of foods and beverages consumed by people like you. Results will be used to help ensure an adequate and safe food supply for all. This survey is authorized by law. **(IF ASKED, SAY: National Agricultural Research, Extension and Teaching Policy Act of 1977, Section 1428, 7 U.S.C. 3178.)**

All information will be kept confidential and will be reported as statistics only.

DAY 1 ANSWER SHEET

ANSWER ONCE FOR EACH OCCASION					USE A NEW LINE FOR EACH ITEM. USE FIB AND MEASURING UTENSILS				
Q.1			Q.2	Q.3		Q.4	Q.5	Q.6a	Q.6b
When									
Time	A M	P M	What Called	With Whom	Line #	Name of Food/Drink	Complete Description	Quantity Consumed	How Esti-mated
	1	2			101				
	1	2			102				
	1	2			103				
	1	2			104				
	1	2			105				
	1	2			106				
	1	2			107				
	1	2			108				
	1	2			109				
	1	2			110				
	1	2			111				
	1	2			112				
	1	2			113				
	1	2			114				
	1	2			115				
	1	2			116				
	1	2			117				
	1	2			118				
	1	2			119				
	1	2			120				

DAY 1 ANSWER SHEET											
ANSWER FOR EACH ITEM				ANSWER IF MAIN MEAL PLANNER/ PREPARER **AND** "1" OR "2" IN Q.7						ANSWER ONLY IF "3" IN Q.7	ANSWER ONLY IF "1" IN Q.12
Q.7			Q.8	Q.9				Q.10		Q.11	Q.12
FOOD SOURCE				(a)	(b)		(c)				
From Home		Not From Home	SOURCE OF HOME ITEMS	Fat in Preparation	Fat Used	No Fat Used	Fat Type	Salt Used in Preparation	No Salt Used in Preparation	Where Obtained	Added/ Changed Item
1	2	3			1	2		1	2		1
1	2	3			1	2		1	2		1
1	2	3			1	2		1	2		1
1	2	3			1	2		1	2		1
1	2	3			1	2		1	2		1
1	2	3			1	2		1	2		1
1	2	3			1	2		1	2		1
1	2	3			1	2		1	2		1
1	2	3			1	2		1	2		1
1	2	3			1	2		1	2		1
1	2	3			1	2		1	2		1
1	2	3			1	2		1	2		1
1	2	3			1	2		1	2		1
1	2	3			1	2		1	2		1
1	2	3			1	2		1	2		1
1	2	3			1	2		1	2		1
1	2	3			1	2		1	2		1
1	2	3			1	2		1	2		1
1	2	3			1	2		1	2		1
1	2	3			1	2		1	2		1

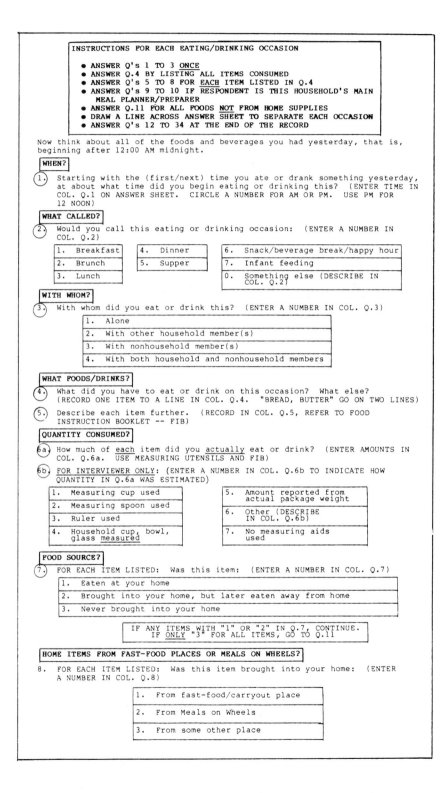

INSTRUCTIONS FOR EACH EATING/DRINKING OCCASION

- **ANSWER Q's 1 TO 3 ONCE**
- **ANSWER Q.4 BY LISTING ALL ITEMS CONSUMED**
- **ANSWER Q's 5 TO 8 FOR EACH ITEM LISTED IN Q.4**
- **ANSWER Q's 9 TO 10 IF RESPONDENT IS THIS HOUSEHOLD'S MAIN MEAL PLANNER/PREPARER**
- **ANSWER Q.11 FOR ALL FOODS NOT FROM HOME SUPPLIES**
- **DRAW A LINE ACROSS ANSWER SHEET TO SEPARATE EACH OCCASION**
- **ANSWER Q's 12 TO 34 AT THE END OF THE RECORD**

Now think about all of the foods and beverages you had yesterday, that is, beginning after 12:00 AM midnight.

WHEN?

1. Starting with the (first/next) time you ate or drank something yesterday, at about what time did you begin eating or drinking this? (ENTER TIME IN COL. Q.1 ON ANSWER SHEET. CIRCLE A NUMBER FOR AM OR PM. USE PM FOR 12 NOON)

WHAT CALLED?

2. Would you call this eating or drinking occasion: (ENTER A NUMBER IN COL. Q.2)

1. Breakfast	4. Dinner	6. Snack/beverage break/happy hour
2. Brunch	5. Supper	7. Infant feeding
3. Lunch		0. Something else (DESCRIBE IN COL. Q.2)

WITH WHOM?

3. With whom did you eat or drink this? (ENTER A NUMBER IN COL. Q.3)

1. Alone
2. With other household member(s)
3. With nonhousehold member(s)
4. With both household and nonhousehold members

WHAT FOODS/DRINKS?

4. What did you have to eat or drink on this occasion? What else? (RECORD ONE ITEM TO A LINE IN COL. Q.4. "BREAD, BUTTER" GO ON TWO LINES)

5. Describe each item further. (RECORD IN COL. Q.5, REFER TO FOOD INSTRUCTION BOOKLET -- FIB)

QUANTITY CONSUMED?

6a. How much of each item did you actually eat or drink? (ENTER AMOUNTS IN COL. Q.6a. USE MEASURING UTENSILS AND FIB)

6b. FOR INTERVIEWER ONLY: (ENTER A NUMBER IN COL. Q.6b TO INDICATE HOW QUANTITY IN Q.6a WAS ESTIMATED)

1. Measuring cup used	5. Amount reported from actual package weight
2. Measuring spoon used	6. Other (DESCRIBE IN COL. Q.6b)
3. Ruler used	
4. Household cup, bowl, glass measured	7. No measuring aids used

FOOD SOURCE?

7. FOR EACH ITEM LISTED: Was this item: (ENTER A NUMBER IN COL. Q.7)

1. Eaten at your home
2. Brought into your home, but later eaten away from home
3. Never brought into your home

IF ANY ITEMS WITH "1" OR "2" IN Q.7, CONTINUE. IF ONLY "3" FOR ALL ITEMS, GO TO Q.11

HOME ITEMS FROM FAST-FOOD PLACES OR MEALS ON WHEELS?

8. FOR EACH ITEM LISTED: Was this item brought into your home: (ENTER A NUMBER IN COL. Q.8)

1. From fast-food/carryout place
2. From Meals on Wheels
3. From some other place

- **IF RESPONDENT IS THIS HOUSEHOLD'S MAIN MEAL PLANNER/PREPARER AND ANY ITEMS FOR THIS OCCASION ARE "1" OR "2" IN Q.7, CONTINUE**
- **IF RESPONDENT IS NOT THE MAIN MEAL PLANNER/PREPARER OR ALL ITEMS FOR THIS OCCASION ARE "3" IN Q.7, GO TO INSTRUCTIONS BEFORE Q.11**

FAT USED IN PREPARATION?

9a. Think about the preparation of the foods/drinks you consumed on this occasion. By preparation, I mean the seasoning or cooking of the foods/drinks before they were brought to the table. Were any fats or oils used in preparing any of these items? (ENTER A NUMBER IN COL. Q.9a ONCE FOR THIS OCCASION)

1. Yes	2. No (GO TO Q.10)

9b. For which items from your home food supplies did you use fats or oils in the preparation? (IN COL. Q.9b CIRCLE THE APPROPRIATE NUMBER)

9c. FOR EACH ITEM WHERE FAT/OIL WAS USED: What type of fat or oil was used for this item? (ENTER A NUMBER IN COL. Q.9c)

1. Olive oil	6. Any diet margarine
2. Corn, cottonseed, safflower or sunflower oil	7. Margarine blend
3. Soybean oil or other vegetable oil (include nut oils)	8. Butter
4. Regular tub or liquid margarine	9. Animal shortening (meat/bacon drippings)
5. Regular stick margarine	10. Vegetable shortening
	11. Don't know/remember

SALT USED IN PREPARATION?

10. For which items from your home food supplies did you use salt in the preparation? (IN COL. Q.10 CIRCLE THE APPROPRIATE NUMBER)

- **REFER TO Q.7. IF ANY ITEM FOR THIS OCCASION IS "3," CONTINUE**
- **IF NO ITEM IS "3," DRAW LINE ACROSS ANSWER PAGES AND ANSWER Q's 1 TO 11 FOR NEXT OCCASION. WHEN ALL OCCASIONS HAVE BEEN RECORDED, GO TO Q.12 ON NEXT PAGE**

WHERE OBTAINED/SERVICE?

11. Where did you get this food/beverage which was not from your home food supplies?

1.	Restaurant with waiter/waitress service at a table or counter
2.	Cafeteria or self-serve buffet restaurant
3.	Restaurant where food was ordered and picked up at a counter or drive-up window (include fast-food places)
4.	School
5.	Day-care center or summer day camp
6.	Community feeding program (include those for senior citizens, disabled, or needy persons)
7.	Vending machine (MUST RECORD ADDITIONAL NUMBER FOR LOCATION)
8.	Store
9.	At someone else's home
10.	Some other place? (DESCRIBE IN COL. Q.11)

DRAW LINE ACROSS ANSWER PAGES AND ANSWER Q's 1 TO 11 UNTIL ALL EATING/DRINKING OCCASIONS HAVE BEEN RECORDED. IF ALL FOOD/DRINKS RECORDED, GO TO Q.12 ON NEXT PAGE

(12.) (SHOW CARD I) Some food and drink items consumed at home or away from home are often forgotten in surveys like this. Have you forgotten any: (CIRCLE NUMBER FOR EACH)

(IF ANY ITEM HAS BEEN FORGOTTEN ("1" CIRCLED), COMPLETE Q's 1 TO 11 AND CIRCLE "1" IN COL. Q.12 FOR EACH SUCH ITEM)

(READ)	Yes	No
Snacks/desserts Chips, fruits, candy, nuts, cheese, cookies	1	2
Nonalcoholic drinks at meals or as snacks Coffee, tea, soft drinks, juice, other drinks	1	2
Alcoholic beverages Beer, wine, cocktails, other drinks	1	2
Accessory foods added to other foods at meals or snacks Butter/margarine, sugar/sweetener, salad dressing, sauce/gravy, mustard/ketchup, relish, cream/milk, jam/jelly/syrup	1	2
Side dishes Crackers, bread/rolls	1	2
Foods eaten or tasted while preparing meals or cleaning up	1	2
Other items	1	2
FOR OFFICE USE ONLY		

TIME Q.12 ENDED:___________

AM	1
PM	2

(13a.) About how many fluid ounces of water did you drink yesterday other than in coffee, tea, fruitade, and the like? (IF NONE, ENTER "0" AND GO TO Q.13c)

_______________FLUID OUNCES

13b. How much of the water you drank yesterday was from your home supplies? Would you say:

None,	1
Some,	2
Most, or	3
All?	4

(13c.) About how many fluid ounces of water do you usually drink in a 24-hour period?

__________FLUID OUNCES

(14a.) Would you say the amount of food and drink you had yesterday was:

	Less than usual,	1
(GO TO Q.15)	Usual, or	2
	More than usual for this day of the week?	3

14b. IF LESS OR MORE: Which one of the following reasons best describes why it was different?

Sick or ill	1
Short of money	2
Traveling	3
At a social occasion or on a special day	4
On holiday or vacation	5
Too little time or too busy	6
Not hungry or very hungry	7
Dieting	8
Some other reason? (DESCRIBE) ____________________________	0

15. In general, would you say the healthfulness of your diet is:

Excellent,	1
Very good,	2
Good,	3
Fair, or	4
Poor?	5

16a. How often do you add salt to your food at the table? Would you say:

(GO TO Q.17a)	Never,	1
	Sometimes,	2
	Often, or	3
	Always (almost always)?	4

16b. Would you say that the amount of salt you usually add to foods at the table is:

Light,	1
Moderate, or	2
Heavy?	3

16c. When you use salt at the table, is it:

Regular salt,	1
Lite salt,	2
Salt substitute, or	3
Some other kind (DESCRIBE)? ______	4

16d. Do you usually use iodized salt?

Yes	1
No	2
Don't know	3

17a. Are you on a special diet?

	Yes	1
(GO TO Q.18)	No	2

17b. (SHOW CARD J) What type of special diet are you on?

(CIRCLE AS MANY AS APPLY)

Low calorie/weight loss diet	1
Low fat/cholesterol diet	2
Low salt diet	3
Low sugar/sugar free diet	4
Diabetic diet	5
Other diet (DESCRIBE) ______	0

18. Do you consider yourself to be a vegetarian?

Yes	1
No	2

19. How often, if at all, do you take any vitamin or mineral supplements by mouth, such as a pill or liquid? Would you say:

	Every day,	1
(CONTINUE)	Almost every day,	2
	Every so often, or	3
(GO TO Q.21)	Not at all?	4

20. Do you usually take a:

(CIRCLE AS MANY AS APPLY)

Multivitamin,	1
Multivitamin with iron or other minerals,	2
Combination of Vitamin C and iron,	3
Other combination of vitamins and minerals,	4
Vitamin C,	5
Iron,	6
Calcium, or	7
Other single vitamins/minerals?	8

21. About how much do you weigh without shoes?

______ POUNDS

22. How tall are you without shoes?

______ FEET ______ INCHES

23. In general, would you say your health is:

Excellent,	1
Very good,	2
Good,	3
Fair, or	4
Poor?	5

24. Do you have any disability or handicap that limits your activities?

Yes	1
No	2

25. Has a doctor ever told you that you have: (CIRCLE A NUMBER FOR EACH)

	Yes	No
Diabetes?	1	2
High blood pressure (hypertension)?	1	2
Heart disease?	1	2
Cancer?	1	2
Osteoporosis?	1	2

26. Do you have trouble biting or chewing food?

	Yes	1
(GO TO INSTRUCTIONS AT BOTTOM OF THIS COLUMN)	No	2

27. Do you have this trouble because of: (CIRCLE A NUMBER FOR EACH)

	Yes	No
Poor fitting dentures?	1	2
Loss of teeth, dentures or replacement?	1	2
Other reasons?	1	2

- **IF RESPONDENT IS 18 YEARS OF AGE OR OLDER, CONTINUE**
- **IF RESPONDENT IS UNDER 18 YEARS OF AGE, THIS RECORD IS COMPLETED; GO TO Q.35**

28. Think now about how you usually spend your leisure time, that is, other than at your job or doing housework. Would you say your usual level of physical activity is:

(READ UNDERLINED WORDS)

	Heavy/Rigorous (running, playing tennis, swimming, doing heavy gardening, etc., three or more times per week),	1
	Moderate (doing rigorous activities one or two times per week or doing steady walking, or other moderate activities three or more times per week), or	2
	Light (playing golf, taking a stroll, or doing nonrigorous activities occasionally)?	3
(GO TO Q.31)	Bedridden	4

29. Do you exercise or play sports regularly?

	Yes	1
(GO TO Q.31)	No	2

30. For how long have you exercised or played sports regularly?

#______ WEEKS OR #______ MONTHS OR #______ YEARS

31. Have you smoked 100 or more cigarettes during your entire life?

	Yes	1
(GO TO Q.36)	No	2

32. Do you smoke cigarettes now?

	Yes	1
(GO TO Q.34)	No	2

33. On the average, how many cigarettes per day do you smoke?

#______ PER DAY

GO TO Q.36

34. How long has it been since you smoked cigarettes regularly?

#______ YEARS

Less than one year	00
Never smoked regularly	98

GO TO Q.36

INTERVIEWER COMMENTS

35. IF INTAKE IS FOR CHILD UNDER 12 YEARS OF AGE:

Circle a code for the main respondent in Col. a and for all persons who assisted in responding in Col. b.

	Main Resp.	Others
	Col. a	Col. b
Child's mother	1	1
Child's father	2	2
Child's sister	3	3
Child's brother	4	4
Child's grandparent	5	5
Child	6	6
Other person (DESCRIBE) ______	0	0

36. IF INTAKE IS FOR PERSON 12 YEARS OF AGE OR OLDER

Circle a code for the main respondent in Col. a and for all persons who assisted in responding in Col. b.

	Main Resp.	Others
	Col. a	Col. b
Sample person	1	1
Mother	2	2
Father	3	3
Sister	4	4
Brother	5	5
Grandparent	6	6
Other person (DESCRIBE) ______	0	0

(37.) Were the descriptions of foods/beverages consumed yesterday difficult for the respondent to answer?

	Yes	1
(GO TO Q.39)	No	2

38. What were the reasons for this difficulty?

______

______

______

______

(39.) Were the amounts of foods/beverages consumed yesterday difficult for the respondent to answer?

	Yes	1
(TERMINATE)	No	2

40. What were the reasons for this difficulty?

______

______

______

______

APPENDIX E

Food Record Recording Form

7 - Day Food Diary

Name ______________________________ Age __________

Address ______________________________ City __________

State ______________ Zip __________ Phone __________

Height __________ Weight __________ Sex __________

Physician/Dietitian ______________________________ Phone __________

For Females Only: Are you pregnant? __________

Are you breast-feeding? __________

Directions for Using the Food Diary

1. Keep your food diary current. List foods immediately after they are eaten. **Please Print all entries**.
2. Record only one food item per line in this record booklet.
3. Be as specific as possible when describing the food item eaten: the way it was cooked (if it was cooked) and the amount that was eaten.
4. Include brand names whenever possible.
5. Report only the food portion that was actually eaten — for example: **T-bone steak, 4 oz. broiled.** (do not include the bones.)
6. Record amounts in household measures — for example: **ounces, tablespoons, cups, slices** or **units**, as in one cup nonfat milk, two slices of wheat toast, or one raw apple.
7. Include method that was used to prepare food item — for example: **fresh, frozen, stewed, fried, baked, canned, broiled, raw**, or **braised**.
8. For canned foods, include the liquid in which it was canned — for example: **sliced peaches in heavy syrup, fruit cocktail in light syrup,** or tuna in water.
9. Foods items listed without specific amounts eaten will be analyzed using portion sizes.
10. Do not alter your normal diet during the period you keep this diary.
11. Remember to record the amounts of visible fats (oils, butter, salad dressings, margarine, and so on) you eat or use in cooking.

* The following are examples of the way to list food items and amounts.

Time	Food Item and Method of Preparation	Amount Eaten
7 am	Apple, raw, fresh	1 medium
12 pm	Beef Stew	10 oz portion
12 pm	Bread, whole wheat, fresh	2 Slices
3 pm	Cereal, Corn Flakes	2 Cups
	with sugar	2 Tbs.
	with milk, non fat	½ cup
7 pm	Chicken, fried	2 legs
7 pm	Coleslaw, with mayo	1 cup
7 pm	Eggs, Chicken (fried in butter)	2 large
7 pm	Fish, salmon, baked	10 oz

Name ______________________________ Date ______________

Time	Food Item and Method of Preparation	Amount Eaten

APPENDIX F

THIRD NATIONAL HEALTH AND NUTRITION EXAMINATION SURVEY DIET QUESTIONNAIRE FOR AGES 17+ YEARS

From National Center for Health Statistics. 1990. National Health and Nutrition Examination Survey III Data Collection Forms. National Center for Health Statistics, Centers for Disease Control and Prevention, Public Health Service; U.S. Department of Health and Human Services.

Courtesy of the National Center for Health Statistics; Centers for Disease Control and Prevention.

DIET (AGES 17+ YEARS)	
M1. CHECK ITEM. REFER TO AGE OF SP.	1 ☐ UNDER 60 YEARS (M4) 2 ☐ 60+ YEARS (M2)
Now I'm going to ask you some general questions about your eating habits. M2. Some cities, churches, and other organizations provide meals for senior citizens. Do you receive meals from any such programs?	1 ☐ Y 2 ☐ N (M4)
M3. Are these meals ever delivered to your home, such as Meals on Wheels?	1 ☐ Y 2 ☐ N
M4. How often do you eat <u>breakfast</u> - every day, on some days, rarely, never, on weekends only?	1 ☐ every day 2 ☐ some days 3 ☐ rarely 4 ☐ never 5 ☐ weekends only
M5. How tall are you without shoes?	______ feet/ ______ inches or ______ centimeters 999 ☐ DK
M6. How much do you weigh without clothes or shoes? FEMALES: IF CURRENTLY PREGNANT, ASK: About how much did you weigh <u>before</u> your pregnancy?	______ pounds or ______ kilograms 999 ☐ DK
M7. CHECK ITEM. REFER TO AGE OF SP.	1 ☐ 25 YEARS OR LESS (M10) 2 ☐ 26 YEARS THROUGH 35 YEARS (M9) 3 ☐ 36 YEARS AND OLDER
M8. How much did you weigh <u>10 years ago</u>?	______ pounds or ______ kilograms 999 ☐ DK
M9. How much did you weigh when you were <u>25 years old</u>?	______ pounds or ______ kilograms 999 ☐ DK
M10. Up to the present time, what is the most you have ever weighed? (FEMALES): Do not include any times when you were pregnant.	______ pounds or ______ kilograms 999 ☐ DK

M11. Do you consider yourself now to be overweight, underweight, or about the right weight?	1 ☐ overweight 2 ☐ underweight 3 ☐ about the right weight
M12. Would you like to weigh more, less, or stay about the same?	1 ☐ more 2 ☐ less 3 ☐ stay about the same
M13. During the past 12 months, have you tried to lose weight?	1 ☐ Y 2 ☐ N
M14. During the past 12 months, have you changed what you eat because of any medical reason or health condition?	1 ☐ Y 2 ☐ N (N1)
M15. What was the medical reason or health condition that caused you to change what you eat? MARK ALL THAT APPLY.	01 ☐ OVERWEIGHT/OBESITY 02 ☐ HIGH BLOOD PRESSURE/HYPERTENSION 03 ☐ HIGH BLOOD CHOLESTEROL 04 ☐ DIABETES 05 ☐ HEART DISEASE 06 ☐ ALLERGY 07 ☐ ULCER 08 ☐ OTHER 10 ________ SPECIFY 99 ☐ DK

FOOD FREQUENCY (AGES 17+ YEARS)

HAND CARD HAQ-5. Now I'm going to ask you how often you usually eat certain foods. When answering think about your usual diet over the past month. Tell me how often you usually ate or drank these foods per day, per week, per month, or not at all.	Times / Day / Week / Month / Never / DK _ _ per 1 ☐ D 2 ☐ W 3 ☐ M or 4 ☐ N 9 ☐ DK
N1. MILK AND MILK PRODUCTS First are milk and milk products. Do not include their use in cooking. a. How often did you have chocolate milk and hot cocoa?	_ _ per 1 ☐ D 2 ☐ W 3 ☐ M or 4 ☐ N 9 ☐ DK
b. How often did you have milk to drink or on cereal? Do not count small amounts of milk added to coffee or tea.	_ _ per 1 ☐ D 2 ☐ W 3 ☐ M or 4 ☐ N 9 ☐ DK
c. CHECK ITEM. REFER TO RESPONSES IN N1a AND N1b.	1 ☐ "NEVER" IN BOTH N1a AND N1b (N1e) 2 ☐ OTHER
d. What type of milk was it? Was it usually whole, 2%, 1%, skim, nonfat, or some other type? IF SP CANNOT PROVIDE USUAL TYPE, MARK ALL THAT APPLY.	01 ☐ whole/regular 02 ☐ 2%/low fat 03 ☐ 1% 04 ☐ skim/nonfat 05 ☐ buttermilk 06 ☐ evaporated 07 ☐ other 08 ________ specify 99 ☐ DK
e. Yogurt and frozen yogurt	_ _ per 1 ☐ D 2 ☐ W 3 ☐ M or 4 ☐ N 9 ☐ DK
f. Ice cream, ice milk , and milkshakes	_ _ per 1 ☐ D 2 ☐ W 3 ☐ M or 4 ☐ N 9 ☐ DK
g. Cheese, all types including American, Swiss, cheddar, and cottage cheese	_ _ per 1 ☐ D 2 ☐ W 3 ☐ M or 4 ☐ N 9 ☐ DK
h. Pizza, calzone, and lasagna	_ _ per 1 ☐ D 2 ☐ W 3 ☐ M or 4 ☐ N 9 ☐ DK
i. Cheese dishes such as macaroni and cheese, cheese nachos, cheese enchiladas, and quesadillas	_ _ per 1 ☐ D 2 ☐ W 3 ☐ M or 4 ☐ N 9 ☐ DK

	Times	Day	Week	Month		Never	DK
N2. <u>MAIN DISHES, MEAT, FISH, CHICKEN, AND EGGS</u> Next are main dishes, meat, fish, chicken, and eggs.	_ _ per	1☐ D	2☐ W	3☐ M	or	4☐ N	9☐ DK
a. How often did you eat any type of stew, or soup containing <u>vegetables</u>, including minestrone, tomato, and split pea?	_ _ per	1☐ D	2☐ W	3☐ M	or	4☐ N	9☐ DK
b. Spaghetti and pasta with tomato sauce	_ _ per	1☐ D	2☐ W	3☐ M	or	4☐ N	9☐ DK
c. Bacon, sausage (chorizo) and luncheon meats such as hot dogs, salami, and bologna	_ _ per	1☐ D	2☐ W	3☐ M	or	4☐ N	9☐ DK
d. Liver and other organ meats such as heart, kidney, tongue, and tripe (menudo)	_ _ per	1☐ D	2☐ W	3☐ M	or	4☐ N	9☐ DK
e. Beef, including hamburger, steaks, roast beef, and meatloaf	_ _ per	1☐ D	2☐ W	3☐ M	or	4☐ N	9☐ DK
f. Pork and ham, including roast pork, pork chops, and spare ribs	_ _ per	1☐ D	2☐ W	3☐ M	or	4☐ N	9☐ DK
g. Shrimp, clams, oysters, crab, and lobster	_ _ per	1☐ D	2☐ W	3☐ M	or	4☐ N	9☐ DK
h. Fish including fillets, fish sticks, fish sandwiches, and tuna fish	_ _ per	1☐ D	2☐ W	3☐ M	or	4☐ N	9☐ DK
i. Chicken, all types, including baked, fried, chicken nuggets, and chicken salad. Include turkey.	_ _ per	1☐ D	2☐ W	3☐ M	or	4☐ N	9☐ DK
j. How often did you have eggs including scrambled, fried, omelettes, hard-boiled eggs, and egg salad?	_ _ per	1☐ D	2☐ W	3☐ M	or	4☐ N	9☐ DK
N3. <u>FRUIT AND FRUIT JUICES</u> Next are fruit juices and fruit. Include all forms - fresh, frozen, canned, and dried.							
a. How often did you have orange juice, grapefruit juice, and tangerine juice?	_ _ per	1☐ D	2☐ W	3☐ M	or	4☐ N	9☐ DK
b. Other fruit juices such as grape juice, apple juice, cranberry juice, and fruit nectars	_ _ per	1☐ D	2☐ W	3☐ M	or	4☐ N	9☐ DK
c. Citrus fruits including oranges, grapefruits, and tangerines	_ _ per	1☐ D	2☐ W	3☐ M	or	4☐ N	9☐ DK
d. Melons including cantaloupe, honeydew, and watermelon	_ _ per	1☐ D	2☐ W	3☐ M	or	4☐ N	9☐ DK
e. Peaches, nectarines, apricots, guava, mango, and papaya	_ _ per	1☐ D	2☐ W	3☐ M	or	4☐ N	9☐ DK
f. How often did you have any other fruits such as apples, bananas, pears, berries, cherries, grapes, plums, and strawberries? (Include plantains.)	_ _ per	1☐ D	2☐ W	3☐ M	or	4☐ N	9☐ DK

N4. VEGETABLES These next questions are about vegetables. Please remember to include fresh, raw, frozen, canned, and cooked vegetables.	Times: __ per · Day: 1 ☐ D · Week: 2 ☐ W · Month: 3 ☐ M · or · Never: 4 ☐ N · DK: 9 ☐ DK
a. How often did you have carrots and vegetable mixtures containing carrots?	__ per 1 ☐ D 2 ☐ W 3 ☐ M or 4 ☐ N 9 ☐ DK
b. Broccoli	__ per 1 ☐ D 2 ☐ W 3 ☐ M or 4 ☐ N 9 ☐ DK
c. Brussels sprouts and cauliflower	__ per 1 ☐ D 2 ☐ W 3 ☐ M or 4 ☐ N 9 ☐ DK
d. White potatoes, including baked, mashed, boiled, french-fries, and potato salad	__ per 1 ☐ D 2 ☐ W 3 ☐ M or 4 ☐ N 9 ☐ DK
e. Sweet potatoes, yams, and orange squash including acorn, butternut, hubbard, and pumpkin	__ per 1 ☐ D 2 ☐ W 3 ☐ M or 4 ☐ N 9 ☐ DK
f. Tomatoes including fresh and stewed tomatoes, tomato juice, and salsa	__ per 1 ☐ D 2 ☐ W 3 ☐ M or 4 ☐ N 9 ☐ DK
g. Spinach, greens, collards, and kale	__ per 1 ☐ D 2 ☐ W 3 ☐ M or 4 ☐ N 9 ☐ DK
h. Tossed salad	__ per 1 ☐ D 2 ☐ W 3 ☐ M or 4 ☐ N 9 ☐ DK
i. Cabbage, cole slaw, and sauerkraut	__ per 1 ☐ D 2 ☐ W 3 ☐ M or 4 ☐ N 9 ☐ DK
j. Hot red chili peppers. Do not count ground red chili peppers.	__ per 1 ☐ D 2 ☐ W 3 ☐ M or 4 ☐ N 9 ☐ DK
k. Peppers including green, red, and yellow peppers	__ per 1 ☐ D 2 ☐ W 3 ☐ M or 4 ☐ N 9 ☐ DK
l. Any other vegetables such as green beans, corn, peas, mushrooms, and zucchini	__ per 1 ☐ D 2 ☐ W 3 ☐ M or 4 ☐ N 9 ☐ DK
N5. BEANS, NUTS, CEREALS, AND GRAIN PRODUCTS	
a. How often did you have beans, lentils, and (chickpeas/garbanzos)? Include kidney, pinto, refried, black, and baked beans.	__ per 1 ☐ D 2 ☐ W 3 ☐ M or 4 ☐ N 9 ☐ DK
b. Peanuts, peanut butter, other types of nuts, and seeds	__ per 1 ☐ D 2 ☐ W 3 ☐ M or 4 ☐ N 9 ☐ DK
Now I'm going to ask how often you ate certain cereals. c. How about All-Bran, All-Bran Extra Fiber, 100% Bran, and Fiber One?	__ per 1 ☐ D 2 ☐ W 3 ☐ M or 4 ☐ N 9 ☐ DK
d. Total, Product 19, Most, and Just Right	__ per 1 ☐ D 2 ☐ W 3 ☐ M or 4 ☐ N 9 ☐ DK

	Times / Day / Week / Month / Never / DK
N5. BEANS, NUTS, CEREALS, AND GRAIN PRODUCTS (cont.)	__ per 1☐D 2☐W 3☐M or 4☐N 9☐DK
e. All other cold-cereals like corn flakes, Cheerios, Rice Krispies, and presweetened cereals	__ per 1☐D 2☐W 3☐M or 4☐N 9☐DK
f. Cooked, hot cereals like oatmeal, cream of wheat, cream of rice, and grits	__ per 1☐D 2☐W 3☐M or 4☐N 9☐DK
Now let's talk about white bread products only. I'll ask about dark breads next.	
g. How often did you have white bread, rolls, bagels, biscuits, English muffins, and crackers? Include those used for sandwiches.	__ per 1☐D 2☐W 3☐M or 4☐N 9☐DK
h. Dark breads and rolls, including whole wheat, rye, and pumpernickel	__ per 1☐D 2☐W 3☐M or 4☐N 9☐DK
i. Corn bread, corn muffins, and corn tortillas	__ per 1☐D 2☐W 3☐M or 4☐N 9☐DK
j. Flour tortillas	__ per 1☐D 2☐W 3☐M or 4☐N 9☐DK
k. Rice	__ per 1☐D 2☐W 3☐M or 4☐N 9☐DK
l. Salted snacks such as potato chips, taco chips, corn chips, and salted pretzels and popcorn	__ per 1☐D 2☐W 3☐M or 4☐N 9☐DK
N6. DESSERTS, SWEETS, AND BEVERAGES	
a. How often did you have cakes, cookies, brownies, pies, doughnuts, and pastries?	__ per 1☐D 2☐W 3☐M or 4☐N 9☐DK
b. Chocolate candy and fudge	__ per 1☐D 2☐W 3☐M or 4☐N 9☐DK
Next are hot and iced beverages.	
c. How often did you have Hi-C, Tang, Hawaiian Punch, Koolaid, and other drinks with added vitamin C?	__ per 1☐D 2☐W 3☐M or 4☐N 9☐DK
d. Diet colas, diet sodas, and diet drinks such as Crystal Light	__ per 1☐D 2☐W 3☐M or 4☐N 9☐DK
e. Regular colas and sodas, not diet	__ per 1☐D 2☐W 3☐M or 4☐N 9☐DK
f. Regular coffee with caffeine	__ per 1☐D 2☐W 3☐M or 4☐N 9☐DK
g. Regular tea with caffeine	__ per 1☐D 2☐W 3☐M or 4☐N 9☐DK
h. Beer and lite beer	__ per 1☐D 2☐W 3☐M or 4☐N 9☐DK
i. Wine, wine coolers, sangria, and champagne	__ per 1☐D 2☐W 3☐M or 4☐N 9☐DK
j. Hard liquor such as tequila, gin, vodka, scotch, rum, whiskey and liqueurs, either alone or mixed	__ per 1☐D 2☐W 3☐M or 4☐N 9☐DK

	Times	Day	Week	Month		Never	DK
N7. FATS How often were these items added to your foods after preparation? For example, this would include on top of vegetables or baked potatoes, or as a spread on bread.	__ per	1 ☐ D	2 ☐ W	3 ☐ M	or	4 ☐ N	9 ☐ DK
a. Margarine	__ per	1 ☐ D	2 ☐ W	3 ☐ M	or	4 ☐ N	9 ☐ DK
b. Butter	__ per	1 ☐ D	2 ☐ W	3 ☐ M	or	4 ☐ N	9 ☐ DK
c. Oil and vinegar, mayonnaise and salad dressings such as Italian and Thousand Island, including those added to salads and sandwiches	__ per	1 ☐ D	2 ☐ W	3 ☐ M	or	4 ☐ N	9 ☐ DK

N8. Have I missed any other foods or beverages that you had at least once per week in the past month?

1. ☐ Y (specify) → 2. ☐ N (N9)

PROBE: How often did you eat . . . in the past month?

a. 1 ______	__ per	1 ☐ D	2 ☐ W	3 ☐ M	or	4 ☐ N	9 ☐ DK
b. 1 ______	__ per	1 ☐ D	2 ☐ W	3 ☐ M	or	4 ☐ N	9 ☐ DK
c. 1 ______	__ per	1 ☐ D	2 ☐ W	3 ☐ M	or	4 ☐ N	9 ☐ DK
d. 1 ______	__ per	1 ☐ D	2 ☐ W	3 ☐ M	or	4 ☐ N	9 ☐ DK
e. 1 ______	__ per	1 ☐ D	2 ☐ W	3 ☐ M	or	4 ☐ N	9 ☐ DK
f. 1 ______	__ per	1 ☐ D	2 ☐ W	3 ☐ M	or	4 ☐ N	9 ☐ DK

N9. CHECK ITEM. REFER TO AGE OF SP.

1 ☐ UNDER 20 YEARS (P1)

2 ☐ 20 + YEARS

N10. REFER TO AGE OF SP. HAND CARD HAQ-6.
READ RESPONSE CATEGORIES TO SP IF NECESSARY.

Now I am going to ask how often you drank milk over your lifetime. Try to remember whether you were a milk drinker or a non-milk drinker during different times in your life. Then think of certain events that might have occurred during each time period, for example, were you in school, at home with children, on a farm, or in the service.

How often did you drink any type of milk, including milk added to cereal, when you were a ________? Do not count small amounts of milk added to coffee or tea.

Time period (age)	more than once per day	once per day	less than once per day but more than once per week	once per week	less than once per week	never	don't know
a. Child (5–12)	1 ☐	2 ☐	3 ☐	4 ☐	5 ☐	0 ☐	9 ☐
b. Teenager (13–17)	1 ☐	2 ☐	3 ☐	4 ☐	5 ☐	0 ☐	9 ☐
c. Young adults (18–35)	1 ☐	2 ☐	3 ☐	4 ☐	5 ☐	0 ☐	9 ☐
d. Middle-aged adult (36–65)	1 ☐	2 ☐	3 ☐	4 ☐	5 ☐	0 ☐	9 ☐
e. Older adult (over 65)	1 ☐	2 ☐	3 ☐	4 ☐	5 ☐	0 ☐	9 ☐

APPENDIX G

Database and Age- and Sex-Specific Portion Sizes for Food Items on Screening Questionnaire for Fat Intake Shown in Chapter 3

From National Cancer Institute, Division of Cancer Prevention and Control, National Institutes of Health.

Age- and sex-specific portion sizes* for food items on screening questionnaire

		Age- and Sex-Specific portion sizes (g)					
		Females			Males		
		Small	Medium	Large	Small	Medium	Large
Hamburgers, cheeseburgers							
Age	19–29	56.0	84.0	134.0	70.0	100.0	168.0
	30–60	56.0	84.0	111.0	67.0	100.0	168.0
	61+	50.0	70.0	84.0	53.0	84.0	126.0
Beef steaks, roasts							
Age	19–29	63.0	108.0	168.0	84.0	126.0	210.0
	30–60	60.0	85.0	157.0	84.0	126.0	168.0
	61+	50.0	84.0	126.0	70.0	112.0	168.0
Pork, incl. chops, roasts							
Age	19–29	53.0	84.0	126.0	70.0	112.0	168.0
	30–60	54.0	84.0	126.0	67.0	100.0	168.0
	61+	42.0	84.0	105.0	56.0	84.0	126.0
Hot dogs							
Age	19–29	44.0	88.0	132.0	45.0	90.0	135.0
	30–60	44.0	88.0	132.0	44.0	88.0	132.0
	61+	44.0	88.0	132.0	45.0	90.0	135.0

Continued

Age- and sex-specific portion sizes* for food items on screening questionnaire—*cont'd*

		Age- and Sex-Specific portion sizes (g)					
		Females			Males		
		Small	Medium	Large	Small	Medium	Large
Ham, lunch meats							
Age	19–29	28.0	56.0	84.0	28.0	56.0	112.0
	30–60	28.0	56.0	84.0	28.0	56.0	84.0
	61+	28.0	56.0	84.0	28.0	56.0	84.0
Whole milk							
Age	19–29	150.0	270.0	330.0	226.0	270.0	330.0
	30–60	150.0	270.0	330.0	150.0	270.0	330.0
	61+	150.0	270.0	330.0	150.0	270.0	330.0
Doughnuts, cookies, cake							
Age	19–29	21.0	42.0	64.0	36.0	49.0	84.0
	30–60	28.0	42.0	63.0	31.0	48.0	84.0
	61+	24.0	42.0	53.0	23.0	42.0	64.0
White bread, rolls, etc.							
Age	19–29	28.0	46.0	56.0	40.0	56.0	92.0
	30–60	28.0	46.0	56.0	40.0	56.0	92.0
	61+	23.0	46.0	69.0	28.0	46.0	69.0
Eggs							
Age	19–29	50.0	100.0	150.0	50.0	100.0	128.0
	30–60	50.0	100.0	150.0	50.0	100.0	150.0
	61+	50.0	100.0	150.0	50.0	100.0	150.0
Cheese, excluding cottage							
Age	19–29	28.0	56.0	84.0	28.0	56.0	84.0
	30–60	28.0	56.0	84.0	28.0	56.0	84.0
	61+	28.0	56.0	69.0	28.0	56.0	84.0
Margarine, butter							
Age	19–29	5.5	11.0	16.0	5.5	11.0	16.0
	30–60	5.5	11.0	16.0	5.5	11.0	16.0
	61+	5.5	11.0	16.0	5.5	11.0	16.0
Mayonnaise, salad dressing							
Age	19–29	9.0	15.0	24.0	9.0	15.0	28.0
	30–60	9.0	18.0	28.0	9.0	15.0	28.0
	61+	9.0	18.0	28.0	9.0	18.0	28.0
French fries							
Age	19–29	52.0	115.0	126.0	52.0	126.0	252.0
	30–60	52.0	126.0	144.0	52.0	126.0	178.0
	61+	52.0	60.0	126.0	52.0	126.0	157.0

*Portion sizes are those used in the database developed by Gladys Block of the National Cancer Institute. They derive ultimately from portion sizes actually reported by respondents, using three-dimensional abstract models, in the NHANES II data. However, many of the items on this screener are unitary (e.g., one or two eggs, one or two pats of butter), and the portion sizes for unitary items were modified in some instances to correspond to those units.

Food list and database for screening questionnaire for fat intake*†

	Portion sizes (g)			Nutrient content			
	Small	Medium	Large	Total fat (g) per 100 g	Saturated Fat (g) per 100 g‡	Oleic acid (g) per 100 g‡	Linoleic acid (g) per 100 g‡
Hamburgers, cheeseburgers	43	85	128	20.3	9.7	8.9	0.4
Beef steaks, roasts	56	112	168	10.2	4.9	4.5	0.2
Pork, incl. chops, roast	44	88	132	15.4	5.5	6.5	1.4
Hot dogs	44	88	132	29.0	12.9	13.0	0.9
Ham, lunch meats	28	56	84	25.0	9.0	10.0	1.5
Whole milk (as a beverage)	122	244	366	3.5	1.9	1.2	0.1
Doughnuts, cookies, cake, pastry	24	42	63	16.8	4.5	8.0	2.2
White bread, rolls, bagels, etc., including sandwiches	25	50	75	4.0	0.7	1.5	0.8
Eggs	50	100	150	12.9	4.4	5.1	0.8
Cheese, excluding cottage	28	56	84	25.0	15.4	7.8	0.6
Margarine or butter	5	10	15	80.7	17.2§	35.0§	26.0§
Salad dressing, mayonnaise	8	16	24	60.0	10.7	13.6	31.2
French fries	51	102	153	8.4	2.1	1.8	4.2

Do you eat these every day?‖

Dark bread, such as whole wheat, rye, pumpernickel? Yes/No

Breakfast cereal? Yes/No

*Foods are listed in the order in which they might be used in an actual questionnaire with a respondent, *not* in order of their importance as nutrient sources. The two categorical variables are not important sources of fat at all, but are to be used only as behavioral markers.

†Fat scores would be calculated as follows:

Algorithm for 13-item list: Use foods 1–13. "Times" = No. of times, in the "How often" column; "Factor" indicates the time unit: Day = 7; Week = 1; Month = 0.2333; Year = 0.01923. Calculate sum of (Times × Factor × Reported portion size/100 × fat per 100 g). After adding all the foods, divide by 7 for daily estimate. Divide resulting distribution at midpoint, for above and below median. (Midpoint of the screener distribution among this population of mostly white, health-conscious women aged 45–69 years was 21.3 g.) Quintile cut-points were 1–11.9, 12–19.5, 19.6–23.9, 24–36.9, 37 or higher.

Algorithm for 13-item augmented list: for the sum, use foods 1–13; calculate as in Algorithm 1. Include in the questionnaire, but not in the sum, food 14 ("Dark bread such as whole wheat, rye, pumpernickel") and food 15 ("Breakfast cereal"). Then the algorithm for categorizing as "high" or "low" on percent of calories from fat is as follows: If below screener median (calculated from foods 1–13), then categorize as "low"; if above screener median, categorize as "high"; if above screener median *and* eats dark bread every day *and* eats breakfast cereal every day, then move from "high" to "low."

‡Saturated fat and oleic acid (monounsaturated fat) are not used in calculating the screener estimate used to identify respondents with a high (or low) mean percent of calories from fat. They are provided here for investigators who may wish to use the instrument to rank respondents on gram intake of these nutrients. Linoleic acid is provided for the same reason, but it should be noted that the questionnaire was not designed to assess this nutrient, and a better screening instrument could probably be developed using the linoleic acid table from reference 3. Since its correlation with reference data was tolerable, some investigators may wish to calculate linoleic in studies in which the main purpose is to assess one of the other fats.

§Values are for margarine. Butter has 44.6 g saturated fat, 26.7 g oleic acid, 2.4 g linoleic acid. If linoleic and oleic acids are of central importance to a proposed study, rather than total fat, consider asking butter and margarine separately.

‖Included as a categorical variable, but not included in the grams-of-fat calculation.

APPENDIX H

MEDFICTS Dietary Assessment Questionnaire

From National Cholesterol Education Program. 1993. *Second Report of the Expert Panel on Detection, Evaluation, and Treatment of High Blood Cholesterol in Adults.* Bethesda, MD: U.S. Department of Health and Human Services: Public Health Service; National Institutes of Health; National Heart, Lung, and Blood Institute.

Name ____________
Date ____________

MEDFICTS: Dietary Assessment Questionnaire

(**M**eats, **E**ggs, **D**airy, **F**ried foods, **I**n baked goods, **C**onvenience foods, **T**able fats, **S**nacks)

Directions: For each food category for both Group 1 and Group 2 listings: Please check a box in the "Weekly Consumption" column and in the "Serving Size" column. If patient rarely or never eats the food listed, please check only the "Weekly Consumption" box.

FOOD CATEGORY	WEEKLY CONSUMPTION				SERVING SIZE			SCORE
	Rarely/ Never	3 or less serv/wk	4 or more serv/wk		Small	Average	Large	For office use
M Meats • Average amount per day: 6 oz (equal in size to 2 decks of playing cards) • Base your estimate on the food you consume the most of								
Group 1 **Beef**: Ribs, Steak, Chuck blade, Brisket, Ground Beef, Meatloaf, Corned Beef. **Processed meats**: Regular hamburger, Fast food hamburger, Bacon, Lunchmeat, Sausage, Hot dogs, Knockworst. **Pork & Others**: Pork shoulder, Pork chops, roast, Pork ribs, Ground pork, Regular ham, Lamb steaks, ribs, chops, Organ meats, Poultry with skin	☐	3 pts	7 pts	x	1 pts	2 pts	3 pts	= ____
Group 2 **Lean Cuts of Beef**: Sirloin tip, Flank steak, Round steak, Rump roast, Chuck arm roast. **Low-fat Processed Meats**: Low-fat lunchmeat, Low-fat hot dogs, Canadian bacon. **Poultry, Fish, Meat**: Poultry without skin, Fish, seafood, Lamb flank, leg-shank, sirloin, roast, Lean ham cured and fresh, Pork loin chops, tenderloin, Veal chops, cutlets, roast, Venison	☐	☐	☐		☐	☐	6 pts +	= ____
E Eggs • Weekly consumption is expressed as <u>times</u>/week					How many eggs do you eat each time?			
Group 1 Whole eggs, Yolks	☐	3 pts	7 pts	x	≤1 1 pts	2 2 pts	≥3 3 pts	= ____
Group 2 Egg whites, Egg substitutes (1/2 cup = 2 eggs)	☐	☐	☐		≤1	2	≥3	
D Dairy								
Milk • Average serving: 1 cup								
Group 1 Whole milk, 2% milk, 2% buttermilk, Yogurt (whole milk)	☐	3 pts	7 pts	x	1 pts	2 pts	3 pts	= ____
Group 2 Skim milk, 1% milk, Skim milk-buttermilk, Yogurt (nonfat & low-fat)	☐	☐	☐		☐	☐	☐	
Cheese • Average serving: 1 oz.								
Group 1 Cream cheese, Cheddar, Monterey Jack, Colby, Swiss, American processed, Blue cheese, Regular cottage cheese and Ricotta (1/2 cup)	☐	3 pts	7 pts	x	1 pts	2 pts	3 pts	= ____
Group 2 Low-fat & fat-free cheeses, Skim milk mozzarella, String cheese, Low-fat & fat-free cottage cheese, and Skim milk ricotta (1/2 C)	☐	☐	☐		☐	☐	☐	
Frozen Desserts • Average serving: 1/2 cup								
Group 1 Ice cream, Milk shakes	☐	3 pts	7 pts	x	1 pts	2 pts	3 pts	= ____
Group 2 Ice milk, Frozen yogurt	☐	☐	☐		☐	☐	☐	

+ Score 6 points if this box is checked.

Comments: ________________________

Total ______

(OVER)

MEDFICTS

FOOD CATEGORY	WEEKLY CONSUMPTION			SERVING SIZE			SCORE
	Rarely/ Never	3 or less serv/wk	4 or more serv/wk	Small	Average	Large	For office use
F Fried Foods • Average serving: see below							
Group 1 French fries, Fried vegetables: (1/2 cup) *Fried chicken, fish, and meat: (3 oz.) *Check meat category also		3 pts	7 pts	x 1 pts	2 pts	3 pts	=
Group 2 Vegetables, - not deep fried Meat, Poultry, or fish - prepared by baking, broiling, grilling, poaching, roasting, stewing							
I In Baked Goods Average serving: 1 serving							
Group 1 Doughnuts, Biscuits, Butter rolls, Muffins, Croissants, Sweet rolls, Danish, Cakes, Pies, Coffee cakes, Cookies		3 pts	7 pts	x 1 pts	2 pts	3 pts	=
Group 2 Fruit bars, Low-fat cookies/cakes/pastries, Angel food cake, Homemade baked goods with vegetable oils							
C Convenience Foods • Average Serving: see below							
Group 1 Canned, Packaged, or Frozen dinners; e.g., Pizza (1 slice), Macaroni & cheese (about 1 cup), Pot pie (1), Cream soups (1 cup)		3 pts	7 pts	x 1 pts	2 pts	3 pts	=
Group 2 Diet/Reduced calorie or reduced fat dinners (1 dinner)							
T Table Fats • Average serving: see below							
Group 1 Butter, Stick magarine: 1 pat Regular salad dressing or mayonnaise, Sour cream: 1 - 2 Tbsp		3 pts	7 pts	x 1 pts	2 pts	3 pts	=
Group 2 Diet and tub magarine, Low-fat & fat-free salad dressings Low-fat & fat-free mayonnaise							
S Snacks • Average serving: see below							
Group 1 Chips (poptato, corn, taco), Cheese puffs, Snack mix, Nuts, Regular crackers, Regular popcorn, Candy (milk chocolate, caramel, coconut)		3 pts	7 pts	x 1 pts	2 pts	3 pts	=
Group 2 Air-popped or low-fat popcorn, Low-fat crackers, Hard candy, Licorice, Fruit rolls, Bread sticks, Pretzels, Fat-free chips Fruit							

Directions for scoring:
Multiply Weekly Consumption points (3 or 7) by Serving Size points (1, 2, 3) for Group 1 foods only except for a large serving of Group 2 meats

Example: 3 pts, 7 pts ✔, 1 pts, 2 pts, 3 pts ✔

3 x 7 = 21 points

Add score on page 1 and page 2 to get Final Score

Key
40 - 70 - Step I Diet
less than 40 - Step II Diet

(shaded box) = Foods high in fat, saturated fat, and/or cholesterol

Total ________

Score from page 1 + ________

Final Score ________

Comments: ____________________
(Note frequent use of foods high in fat or saturated fat, e.g. coffeee creamer, whipped topping)

APPENDIX I

THE 131-ITEM WILLETT FOOD FREQUENCY QUESTIONNAIRE

From Dr. Walter Willett, Department of Nutrition, School of Public Health, Harvard University.

DIET ASSESSMENT

ID:

1. Do you currently take multiple vitamins? (Please report individual vitamins under question 2.)

○ No ○ Yes → If yes, a) How many do you take per week? → ○ 2 or less ○ 3-5 ○ 6-9 ○ 10 or more

b) What specific brand do you usually use? → Specify exact brand and type

2. Not counting multiple vitamins, do you take any of the following preparations:

a) Vitamin A? ○ No ○ Yes, seasonal only ○ Yes, most months — If Yes,

How many years? →	○ 0-1 yr.	○ 2-4 yrs.	○ 5-9 yrs.	○ 10+ yrs.	○ Don't know
What dose per day? →	○ Less than 8,000 IU	○ 8,000 to 12,000 IU	○ 13,000 to 22,000 IU	○ 23,000 IU or more	○ Don't know

b) Vitamin C? ○ No ○ Yes, seasonal only ○ Yes, most months — If Yes,

How many years? →	○ 0-1 yr.	○ 2-4 yrs.	○ 5-9 yrs.	○ 10+ yrs.	○ Don't know
What dose per day? →	○ Less than 400 mg.	○ 400 to 700 mg.	○ 750 to 1250 mg.	○ 1300 mg. or more	○ Don't know

c) Vitamin B_6? ○ No ○ Yes → If yes,

How many years? →	○ 0-1 yr.	○ 2-4 yrs.	○ 5-9 yrs.	○ 10+ yrs.	○ Don't know
What dose per day? →	○ Less than 10 mg.	○ 10 to 39 mg.	○ 40 to 79 mg.	○ 80 mg. or more	○ Don't know

d) Vitamin E? ○ No ○ Yes → If yes,

How many years? →	○ 0-1 yr.	○ 2-4 yrs.	○ 5-9 yrs.	○ 10+ yrs.	○ Don't know
What dose per day? →	○ Less than 100 IU	○ 100 to 250 IU	○ 300 to 500 IU	○ 600 IU or more	○ Don't know

e) Selenium? ○ No ○ Yes → If yes,

How many years? →	○ 0-1 yr.	○ 2-4 yrs.	○ 5-9 yrs.	○ 10+ yrs.	○ Don't know
What dose per day? →	○ Less than 80 mcg.	○ 80 to 130 mcg.	○ 140 to 250 mcg.	○ 260 mcg. or more	○ Don't know

f) Iron? ○ No ○ Yes → If yes,

How many years? →	○ 0-1 yr.	○ 2-4 yrs.	○ 5-9 yrs.	○ 10+ yrs.	○ Don't know
What dose per day? →	○ Less than 51 mg.	○ 51 to 200 mg.	○ 201 to 400 mg.	○ 401 mg. or more	○ Don't know

g) Zinc? ○ No ○ Yes → If yes,

How many years? →	○ 0-1 yr.	○ 2-4 yrs.	○ 5-9 yrs.	○ 10+ yrs.	○ Don't know
What dose per day? →	○ Less than 25 mg.	○ 25 to 74 mg.	○ 75 to 100 mg.	○ 101 mg. or more	○ Don't know

h) Calcium? (Include Calcium in Dolomite.) ○ No ○ Yes → If yes,

How many years? →	○ 0-1 yr.	○ 2-4 yrs.	○ 5-9 yrs.	○ 10+ yrs.	○ Don't know
What dose per day? →	○ Less than 400 mg.	○ 400 to 900 mg.	○ 901 to 1300 mg.	○ 1301 mg. or more	○ Don't know

i) Are there other supplements that you take on a regular basis? Please mark if yes:

○ Folic acid ○ Vitamin D ○ B-Complex Vitamins ○ Cod liver Oil ○ Omega-3 Fatty-acids ○ Iodine ○ Copper ○ Brewer's Yeast ○ Beta-Carotene ○ Magnesium ○ Other (please specify):

3. For each food listed, fill in the circle indicating how often on average you have used the amount specified during the past year.

DAIRY FOODS	Never, or less than once per month	1-3 per mo.	1 per week	2-4 per week	5-6 per week	1 per day	2-3 per day	4-5 per day	6+ per day
	AVERAGE USE LAST YEAR								
Skim or low fat milk (8 oz. glass)	○	○	Ⓦ	○	○	Ⓓ	○	○	○
Whole milk (8 oz. glass)	○	○	Ⓦ	○	○	Ⓓ	○	○	○
Cream, e.g. coffee, whipped (Tbs)	○	○	Ⓦ	○	○	Ⓓ	○	○	○
Sour cream (Tbs)	○	○	Ⓦ	○	○	Ⓓ	○	○	○
Non-dairy coffee whitener (tsp.)	○	○	Ⓦ	○	○	Ⓓ	○	○	○
Sherbet or ice milk (½ cup)	○	○	Ⓦ	○	○	Ⓓ	○	○	○
Ice cream (½ cup)	○	○	Ⓦ	○	○	Ⓓ	○	○	○
Yogurt (1 cup)	○	○	Ⓦ	○	○	Ⓓ	○	○	○
Cottage or ricotta cheese (½ cup)	○	○	Ⓦ	○	○	Ⓓ	○	○	○
Cream cheese (1 oz.)	○	○	Ⓦ	○	○	Ⓓ	○	○	○
Other cheese, e.g. American, cheddar, etc., plain or as part of a dish (1 slice or 1 oz. serving)	○	○	Ⓦ	○	○	Ⓓ	○	○	○
Margarine (pat), added to food or bread; exclude use in cooking	○	○	Ⓦ	○	○	Ⓓ	○	○	○
Butter (pat), added to food or bread; exclude use in cooking	○	○	Ⓦ	○	○	Ⓓ	○	○	○

Please turn to page 2

Page 2

3. (Continued) Please fill in your average use, during the past year, of each specified food.

Please try to average your seasonal use of foods over the entire year. For example, if a food such as cantaloupe is eaten 4 times a week during the approximate 3 months that it is in season, then the average use would be once per week.

FRUITS	Never, or less than once per month	1-3 per mo.	1 per week	2-4 per week	5-6 per week	1 per day	2-3 per day	4-5 per day	6+ per day
Raisins (1 oz. or small pack) or grapes	○	○	Ⓦ	○	○	Ⓓ	○	○	○
Prunes (½ cup)	○	○	Ⓦ	○	○	Ⓓ	○	○	○
Bananas (1)	○	○	Ⓦ	○	○	Ⓓ	○	○	○
Cantaloupe (¼ melon)	○	○	Ⓦ	○	○	Ⓓ	○	○	○
Watermelon (1 slice)	○	○	Ⓦ	○	○	Ⓓ	○	○	○
Fresh apples or pears (1)	○	○	Ⓦ	○	○	Ⓓ	○	○	○
Apple juice or cider (small glass)	○	○	Ⓦ	○	○	Ⓓ	○	○	○
Oranges (1)	○	○	Ⓦ	○	○	Ⓓ	○	○	○
Orange juice (small glass)	○	○	Ⓦ	○	○	Ⓓ	○	○	○
Grapefruit (½)	○	○	Ⓦ	○	○	Ⓓ	○	○	○
Grapefruit juice (small glass)	○	○	Ⓦ	○	○	Ⓓ	○	○	○
Other fruit juices (small glass)	○	○	Ⓦ	○	○	Ⓓ	○	○	○
Strawberries, fresh, frozen or canned (½ cup)	○	○	Ⓦ	○	○	Ⓓ	○	○	○
Blueberries, fresh, frozen or canned (½ cup)	○	○	Ⓦ	○	○	Ⓓ	○	○	○
Peaches, apricots or plums (1 fresh, or ½ cup canned)	○	○	Ⓦ	○	○	Ⓓ	○	○	○

VEGETABLES	Never, or less than once per month	1-3 per mo.	1 per week	2-4 per week	5-6 per week	1 per day	2-3 per day	4-5 per day	6+ per day
Tomatoes (1)	○	○	Ⓦ	○	○	Ⓓ	○	○	○
Tomato juice (small glass)	○	○	Ⓦ	○	○	Ⓓ	○	○	○
Tomato sauce (½ cup) e.g. spaghetti sauce	○	○	Ⓦ	○	○	Ⓓ	○	○	○
Red chili sauce (1 Tbs)	○	○	Ⓦ	○	○	Ⓓ	○	○	○
Tofu or soybeans (3-4 oz.)	○	○	Ⓦ	○	○	Ⓓ	○	○	○
String beans (½ cup)	○	○	Ⓦ	○	○	Ⓓ	○	○	○
Broccoli (½ cup)	○	○	Ⓦ	○	○	Ⓓ	○	○	○
Cabbage or cole slaw (½ cup)	○	○	Ⓦ	○	○	Ⓓ	○	○	○
Cauliflower (½ cup)	○	○	Ⓦ	○	○	Ⓓ	○	○	○
Brussels sprouts (½ cup)	○	○	Ⓦ	○	○	Ⓓ	○	○	○
Carrots, raw (½ carrot or 2-4 sticks)	○	○	Ⓦ	○	○	Ⓓ	○	○	○
Carrots, cooked (½ cup)	○	○	Ⓦ	○	○	Ⓓ	○	○	○
Corn (1 ear or ½ cup frozen or canned)	○	○	Ⓦ	○	○	Ⓓ	○	○	○
Peas, or lima beans (½ cup fresh, frozen, canned)	○	○	Ⓦ	○	○	Ⓓ	○	○	○
Mixed vegetables (½ cup)	○	○	Ⓦ	○	○	Ⓓ	○	○	○
Beans or lentils, baked or dried (½ cup)	○	○	Ⓦ	○	○	Ⓓ	○	○	○
Yellow (winter) squash (½ cup)	○	○	Ⓦ	○	○	Ⓓ	○	○	○
Eggplant, zucchini, or other summer squash (½ cup)	○	○	Ⓦ	○	○	Ⓓ	○	○	○
Yams or sweet potatoes (½ cup)	○	○	Ⓦ	○	○	Ⓓ	○	○	○
Spinach, cooked (½ cup)	○	○	Ⓦ	○	○	Ⓓ	○	○	○
Spinach, raw as in salad	○	○	Ⓦ	○	○	Ⓓ	○	○	○
Kale, mustard or chard greens (½ cup)	○	○	Ⓦ	○	○	Ⓓ	○	○	○
Iceberg or head lettuce (serving)	○	○	Ⓦ	○	○	Ⓓ	○	○	○
Romaine or leaf lettuce (serving)	○	○	Ⓦ	○	○	Ⓓ	○	○	○
Celery (4" stick)	○	○	Ⓦ	○	○	Ⓓ	○	○	○
Beets (½ cup)	○	○	Ⓦ	○	○	Ⓓ	○	○	○
Alfalfa sprouts (½ cup)	○	○	Ⓦ	○	○	Ⓓ	○	○	○
Garlic, fresh or powdered (1 clove or shake)	○	○	Ⓦ	○	○	Ⓓ	○	○	○

EGGS, MEAT, ETC.	Never, or less than once per month	1-3 per mo.	1 per week	2-4 per week	5-6 per week	1 per day	2-3 per day	4-5 per day	6+ per day
Eggs (1)	○	○	Ⓦ	○	○	Ⓓ	○	○	○
Chicken or turkey, with skin (4-6 oz.)	○	○	Ⓦ	○	○	Ⓓ	○	○	○
Chicken or turkey, without skin (4-6 oz.)	○	○	Ⓦ	○	○	Ⓓ	○	○	○
Bacon (2 slices)	○	○	Ⓦ	○	○	Ⓓ	○	○	○
Hot dogs (1)	○	○	Ⓦ	○	○	Ⓓ	○	○	○

Please go to page 3

Mark Reflex by NCS EP-45448:654 A9101 Printed in U.S.A. Page 3

3. (Continued) Please fill in your <u>average</u> use, <u>during the past year</u>, of each specified food.

MEATS (CONTINUED)	Never, or less than once per month	1-3 per mo.	1 per week	2-4 per week	5-6 per week	1 per day	2-3 per day	4-5 per day	6+ per day
Processed meats, e.g. sausage, salami, bologna, etc. (piece or slice)	○	○	Ⓦ	○	○	Ⓓ	○	○	○
Liver (3-4 oz.)	○	○	Ⓦ	○	○	Ⓓ	○	○	○
Hamburger (1 patty)	○	○	Ⓦ	○	○	Ⓓ	○	○	○
Beef, pork, or lamb as a sandwich or mixed dish, e.g. stew, casserole, lasagne, etc.	○	○	Ⓦ	○	○	Ⓓ	○	○	○
Beef, pork, or lamb as a main dish, e.g. steak, roast, ham, etc. (4-6 oz.)	○	○	Ⓦ	○	○	Ⓓ	○	○	○
Canned tuna fish (3-4 oz.)	○	○	Ⓦ	○	○	Ⓓ	○	○	○
Dark meat fish, e.g. mackerel, salmon, sardines, bluefish, swordfish (3-5 oz.)	○	○	Ⓦ	○	○	Ⓓ	○	○	○
Other fish (3-5 oz.)	○	○	Ⓦ	○	○	Ⓓ	○	○	○
Shrimp, lobster, scallops as a main dish	○	○	Ⓦ	○	○	Ⓓ	○	○	○

BREADS, CEREALS, STARCHES	Never, or less than once per month	1-3 per mo.	1 per week	2-4 per week	5-6 per week	1 per day	2-3 per day	4-5 per day	6+ per day
Cold breakfast cereal (1 cup)	○	○	Ⓦ	○	○	Ⓓ	○	○	○
Cooked oatmeal (1 cup)	○	○	Ⓦ	○	○	Ⓓ	○	○	○
Other cooked breakfast cereal (1 cup)	○	○	Ⓦ	○	○	Ⓓ	○	○	○
White bread (slice), including pita bread	○	○	Ⓦ	○	○	Ⓓ	○	○	○
Dark bread (slice)	○	○	Ⓦ	○	○	Ⓓ	○	○	○
English muffins, bagels, or rolls (1)	○	○	Ⓦ	○	○	Ⓓ	○	○	○
Muffins or biscuits (1)	○	○	Ⓦ	○	○	Ⓓ	○	○	○
Brown rice (1 cup)	○	○	Ⓦ	○	○	Ⓓ	○	○	○
White rice (1 cup)	○	○	Ⓦ	○	○	Ⓓ	○	○	○
Pasta, e.g. spaghetti, noodles, etc. (1 cup)	○	○	Ⓦ	○	○	Ⓓ	○	○	○
Other grains, e.g. bulgar, kasha, couscous, etc. (1 cup)	○	○	Ⓦ	○	○	Ⓓ	○	○	○
Pancakes or waffles (serving)	○	○	Ⓦ	○	○	Ⓓ	○	○	○
French fried potatoes (4 oz.)	○	○	Ⓦ	○	○	Ⓓ	○	○	○
Potatoes, baked, boiled (1) or mashed (1 cup)	○	○	Ⓦ	○	○	Ⓓ	○	○	○
Potato chips or corn chips (small bag or 1 oz.)	○	○	Ⓦ	○	○	Ⓓ	○	○	○
Crackers, Triskets, Wheat Thins (1)	○	○	Ⓦ	○	○	Ⓓ	○	○	○
Pizza (2 slices)	○	○	Ⓦ	○	○	Ⓓ	○	○	○

		BEVERAGES	Never, or less than once per month	1-3 per mo.	1 per week	2-4 per week	5-6 per week	1 per day	2-3 per day	4-5 per day	6+ per day
CARBONATED BEVERAGES Consider the serving size as 1 glass, bottle or can for these carbonated beverages.	Low Calorie (sugar-free) types	Low calorie cola, e.g. Tab with caffeine	○	○	Ⓦ	○	○	Ⓓ	○	○	○
		Low calorie caffeine-free cola, e.g. Pepsi Free	○	○	Ⓦ	○	○	Ⓓ	○	○	○
		Other low calorie carbonated beverage, e.g. Fresca, Diet 7-Up, diet ginger ale	○	○	Ⓦ	○	○	Ⓓ	○	○	○
	Regular types (not sugar-free)	Coke, Pepsi, or other cola with sugar	○	○	Ⓦ	○	○	Ⓓ	○	○	○
		Caffeine Free Coke, Pepsi, or other cola with sugar	○	○	Ⓦ	○	○	Ⓓ	○	○	○
		Other carbonated beverage with sugar, e.g. 7-Up, ginger ale	○	○	Ⓦ	○	○	Ⓓ	○	○	○
OTHER BEVERAGES		Hawaiian Punch, lemonade, or other non-carbonated fruit drinks (1 glass, bottle, can)	○	○	Ⓦ	○	○	Ⓓ	○	○	○
		Decaffeinated coffee (1 cup)	○	○	Ⓦ	○	○	Ⓓ	○	○	○
		Coffee (1 cup)	○	○	Ⓦ	○	○	Ⓓ	○	○	○
		Tea (1 cup), not herbal teas	○	○	Ⓦ	○	○	Ⓓ	○	○	○
		Beer (1 glass, bottle, can)	○	○	Ⓦ	○	○	Ⓓ	○	○	○
		Red wine (4 oz. glass)	○	○	Ⓦ	○	○	Ⓓ	○	○	○
		White wine (4 oz. glass)	○	○	Ⓦ	○	○	Ⓓ	○	○	○
		Liquor, e.g. whiskey, gin, etc. (1 drink or shot)	○	○	Ⓦ	○	○	Ⓓ	○	○	○

Please turn to page 4

Page 4

ID:

3. (Continued) Please fill in your average use during the past year, of each specified food.

SWEETS, BAKED GOODS, MISCELLANEOUS	Never, or less than once per month	1-3 per mo.	1 per week	2-4 per week	5-6 per week	1 per day	2-3 per day	4-5 per day	6+ per day
Chocolate (bars or pieces) e.g. Hershey's, M&M's	○	○	Ⓦ	○	○	Ⓓ	○	○	○
Candy bars, e.g. Snickers, Milky Way, Reeses	○	○	Ⓦ	○	○	Ⓓ	○	○	○
Candy without chocolate (1 oz.)	○	○	Ⓦ	○	○	Ⓓ	○	○	○
Cookies, home baked (1)	○	○	Ⓦ	○	○	Ⓓ	○	○	○
Cookies, ready made (1)	○	○	Ⓦ	○	○	Ⓓ	○	○	○
Brownies (1)	○	○	Ⓦ	○	○	Ⓓ	○	○	○
Doughnuts (1)	○	○	Ⓦ	○	○	Ⓓ	○	○	○
Cake, home baked (slice)	○	○	Ⓦ	○	○	Ⓓ	○	○	○
Cake, ready made (slice)	○	○	Ⓦ	○	○	Ⓓ	○	○	○
Sweet roll, coffee cake or other pastry, home baked (serving)	○	○	Ⓦ	○	○	Ⓓ	○	○	○
Sweet roll, coffee cake or other pastry, ready made (serving)	○	○	Ⓦ	○	○	Ⓓ	○	○	○
Pie, homemade (slice)	○	○	Ⓦ	○	○	Ⓓ	○	○	○
Pie, ready made (slice)	○	○	Ⓦ	○	○	Ⓓ	○	○	○
Jams, jellies, preserves, syrup, or honey (1 Tbs)	○	○	Ⓦ	○	○	Ⓓ	○	○	○
Peanut butter (Tbs)	○	○	Ⓦ	○	○	Ⓓ	○	○	○
Popcorn (1 cup)	○	○	Ⓦ	○	○	Ⓓ	○	○	○
Nuts (small packet or 1 oz.)	○	○	Ⓦ	○	○	Ⓓ	○	○	○
Bran, added to food (1 Tbs)	○	○	Ⓦ	○	○	Ⓓ	○	○	○
Wheat germ (1 Tbs)	○	○	Ⓦ	○	○	Ⓓ	○	○	○
Chowder or cream soup (1 cup)	○	○	Ⓦ	○	○	Ⓓ	○	○	○
Oil and vinegar dressing, e.g. Italian (1 Tbs)	○	○	Ⓦ	○	○	Ⓓ	○	○	○
Mayonnaise or other creamy salad dressing (1 Tbs)	○	○	Ⓦ	○	○	Ⓓ	○	○	○
Mustard, dry or prepared (1 tsp)	○	○	Ⓦ	○	○	Ⓓ	○	○	○
Pepper (1 shake)	○	○	Ⓦ	○	○	Ⓓ	○	○	○
Salt (1 shake)	○	○	Ⓦ	○	○	Ⓓ	○	○	○

4. How much of the visible fat on your meats do you remove before eating?
○ Remove all visible fat ○ Remove small part of fat
○ Remove majority ○ Remove none
○ (Don't eat meat)

5. What kind of fat do you usually use for frying and sautéing? (Exclude "Pam"-type spray)
○ Real butter ○ Vegetable oil ○ Lard
○ Margarine ○ Vegetable shortening

6. What kind of fat do you usually use for baking?
○ Real butter ○ Vegetable oil ○ Lard
○ Margarine ○ Vegetable shortening

7. What form of margarine do you usually use?
○ None ○ Stick ○ Tub ○ Spread
○ Low-calorie stick ○ Low-calorie tub

8. How often do you eat food that is fried at home? (Exclude the use of "Pam"-type spray)
○ Daily ○ 4-6 times per week
○ 1-3 times per week ○ Less than once a week

9. How often do you eat fried food away from home? (e.g. french fries, fried chicken, fried fish)
○ Daily ○ 4-6 times per week
○ 1-3 times per week ○ Less than once a week

10. How many teaspoons of sugar do you add to your beverages or food each day? → ______ tsp.

11. What type of cooking oil do you usually use? → ______ Specify type and brand

12. What kind of cold breakfast cereal do you usually use? → ______ Specify type and brand

13. Are there any other important foods that you usually eat at least once per week?

Include for example: paté, tortillas, yeast, cream sauce, custard, horseradish, parsnips, rhubarb, radishes, fava beans, carrot juice, coconut, avocado, mango, papaya, dried apricots, dates, figs.

(Do not include dry spices and do not list something that has been listed in the previous sections.)

	Other foods that you usually use at least once per week	Usual serving size	Servings per week
(a)			
(b)			
(c)			
(d)			

APPENDIX J

The Youth/Adolescent Questionnaire, a Food Frequency Questionnaire Designed by Researchers at Brigham and Women's Hospital and Harvard University for Assessing the Dietary Intake of Older Children and Adolescents

From Helaine R. H. Rockett, MS, RD, FADA, Department of Medicine, Channing Laboratory, 180 Longwood Avenue, Boston, MA 02115.

PAGE ONE EATING SURVEY K-93-1 HARVARD MEDICAL SCHOOL

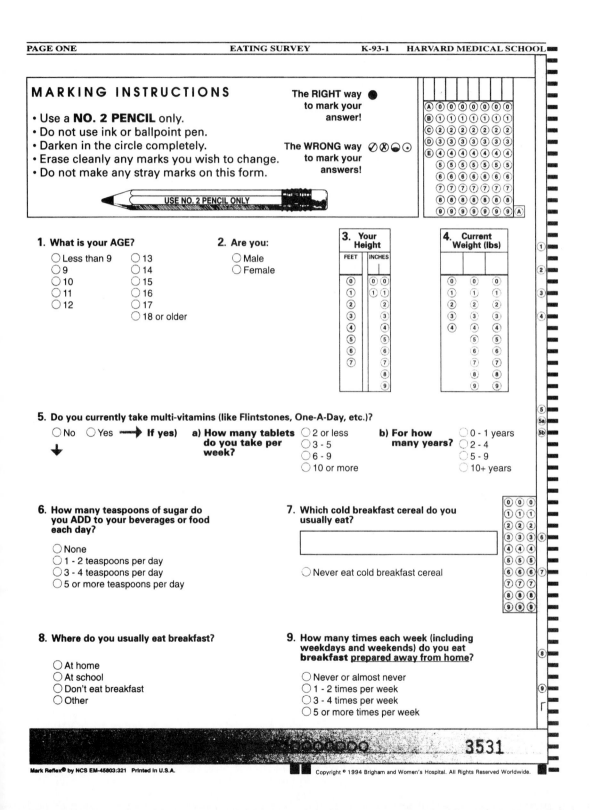

MARKING INSTRUCTIONS

- Use a **NO. 2 PENCIL** only.
- Do not use ink or ballpoint pen.
- Darken in the circle completely.
- Erase cleanly any marks you wish to change.
- Do not make any stray marks on this form.

The RIGHT way to mark your answer! ●

The WRONG way to mark your answers! ⊘ ⊗ ◒ ⊙

USE NO. 2 PENCIL ONLY

1. What is your AGE?

○ Less than 9 ○ 9 ○ 10 ○ 11 ○ 12 ○ 13 ○ 14 ○ 15 ○ 16 ○ 17 ○ 18 or older

2. Are you:

○ Male ○ Female

3. Your Height

FEET: 0 1 2 3 4 5 6 7

INCHES: 0 1 / 0 1 2 3 4 5 6 7 8 9

4. Current Weight (lbs)

0 1 2 3 4 / 0–9 / 0–9

5. Do you currently take multi-vitamins (like Flintstones, One-A-Day, etc.)?

○ No ○ Yes → **If yes)**

a) How many tablets do you take per week? ○ 2 or less ○ 3 - 5 ○ 6 - 9 ○ 10 or more

b) For how many years? ○ 0 - 1 years ○ 2 - 4 ○ 5 - 9 ○ 10+ years

6. How many teaspoons of sugar do you ADD to your beverages or food each day?

○ None
○ 1 - 2 teaspoons per day
○ 3 - 4 teaspoons per day
○ 5 or more teaspoons per day

7. Which cold breakfast cereal do you usually eat?

○ Never eat cold breakfast cereal

8. Where do you usually eat breakfast?

○ At home
○ At school
○ Don't eat breakfast
○ Other

9. How many times each week (including weekdays and weekends) do you eat breakfast prepared away from home?

○ Never or almost never
○ 1 - 2 times per week
○ 3 - 4 times per week
○ 5 or more times per week

3531

Mark Reflex® by NCS EM-45803:321 Printed in U.S.A.

10. How many times each week (including weekdays and weekends) do you eat lunch prepared away from home?

- ○ Never or almost never
- ○ 1 - 2 times per week
- ○ 3 - 4 times per week
- ○ 5 or more times per week

11. How many times each week do you eat after-school snacks or foods prepared away from home?

- ○ Never or almost never
- ○ 1 - 2 times per week
- ○ 3 - 4 times per week
- ○ 5 or more times per week

12. How many times each week (weekdays and weekends) do you eat dinner prepared away from home?

- ○ Never or almost never
- ○ 1 - 2 times per week
- ○ 3 - 4 times per week
- ○ 5 or more times per week

13. How many times per week do you prepare dinner for yourself (and/or others in your house)?

- ○ Never or almost never
- ○ Less than once per week
- ○ 1 - 2 times per week
- ○ 3 - 4 times per week
- ○ 5 or more times per week

14. How often do you have dinner that is ready made, like frozen dinners, Spaghetti-O's, etc.

- ○ Never
- ○ 1 - 2 times per week
- ○ 3 - 4 times per week
- ○ 5'or more times per week

15. How many times each week (including weekdays and weekends) do you eat late night snacks prepared away from home?

- ○ Never
- ○ 1 - 2 times per week
- ○ 3 - 4 times per week
- ○ 5 or more times per week

16. How often do you eat food that is fried at home, like fried chicken?

- ○ Less than once per week
- ○ 1 - 3 times per week
- ○ 4 - 6 times per week
- ○ Daily

17. How often do you eat fried food away from home (like french fries, fried chicken)?

- ○ Less than once per week
- ○ 1 - 3 times per week
- ○ 4 - 6 times per week
- ○ Daily

DIETARY INTAKE

Estimate how often you eat the following foods:

Example 1 **If you drink one can of diet soda 2 - 3 times per week, then your answer should look like this:**

E1. Diet soda (1 can or glass)

- ○ Never
- ○ 1 - 3 cans per month
- ○ 1 can per week
- ● 2 - 6 cans per week
- ○ 1 can per day
- ○ 2 or more cans per day

PAGE THREE HARVARD MEDICAL SCHOOL

BEVERAGES

FILL OUT ONE BUBBLE FOR EACH FOOD ITEM

18. Diet soda (1 can or glass)
- ○ Never
- ○ 1 - 3 cans per month
- ○ 1 can per week
- ○ 2 - 6 cans per week
- ○ 1 can per day
- ○ 2 or more cans per day

19. Soda - not diet (1 can or glass)
- ○ Never
- ○ 1 - 3 cans per month
- ○ 1 can per week
- ○ 2 - 6 cans per week
- ○ 1 can per day
- ○ 2 or more cans per day

20. Hawaiian Punch, lemonade, Koolaid or other non-carbonated fruit drink (1 glass)
- ○ Never
- ○ 1 - 3 glasses per month
- ○ 1 glass per week
- ○ 2 - 4 glasses per week
- ○ 5 - 6 glasses per week
- ○ 1 glass per day
- ○ 2 or more glasses per day

21. Iced Tea - sweetened (1 glass)
- ○ Never
- ○ 1 - 3 glasses per month
- ○ 1 - 4 glasses per week
- ○ 5 or more glasses per week

22. Tea (1 cup)
- ○ Never
- ○ 1 - 3 cups per month
- ○ 1 - 2 cups per week
- ○ 3 - 6 cups per week
- ○ 1 or more cups per day

23. Coffee - not decaf. (1 cup)
- ○ Never
- ○ 1 - 3 cups per month
- ○ 1 - 2 cups per week
- ○ 3 - 6 cups per week
- ○ 1 or more cups per day

24. Beer (1 glass, bottle or can)
- ○ Never
- ○ 1 - 3 cans per month
- ○ 1 can per week
- ○ 2 or more cans per week

25. Wine or wine coolers (1 glass)
- ○ Never
- ○ 1 - 3 glasses per month
- ○ 1 glass per week
- ○ 2 or more glasses per week

26. Liquor, like vodka or rum (1 drink or shot)
- ○ Never
- ○ 1 - 3 drinks per month
- ○ 1 drink per week
- ○ 2 or more drinks per week

Example 2 If you eat:

2 pats of margarine on toast
1 - 2 pats of margarine on sandwich
1 pat of margarine on vegetables

5 - 6 pats total all day

then answer this way →

E2. Margarine (1 pat) - not butter
- ○ Never
- ○ 1 - 3 pats per month
- ○ 1 pat per week
- ○ 2 - 6 pats per week
- ○ 1 pat per day
- ○ 2 - 4 pats per day
- ● 5 or more pats per day

DAIRY PRODUCTS

27. What TYPE of milk do you usually drink?
- ○ Whole milk
- ○ 2% milk
- ○ 1% milk
- ○ Skim/nonfat milk
- ○ Don't know
- ○ Don't drink milk

28. Milk (glass or with cereal)
- ○ Never
- ○ 1 glass per week or less
- ○ 2 - 6 glasses per week
- ○ 1 glass per day
- ○ 2 - 3 glasses per day
- ○ 4+ glasses per day

29. Chocolate milk (glass)
- ○ Never
- ○ 1 - 3 glasses per month
- ○ 1 glass per week
- ○ 2 - 6 glasses per week
- ○ 1 - 2 glasses per day
- ○ 3 or more glasses per day

3531

30. Instant Breakfast Drink (1 packet)
- ◯ Never
- ◯ 1 - 3 times per month
- ◯ Once per week
- ◯ 2 - 4 times per week
- ◯ 5 or more times per week

31. Whipped cream
- ◯ Never
- ◯ 1 - 3 times per month
- ◯ Once per week
- ◯ 2 - 4 times per week
- ◯ 5 or more times per week

32. Yogurt (1 cup) - Not frozen
- ◯ Never
- ◯ 1 - 3 cups per month
- ◯ 1 cup per week
- ◯ 2 - 6 cups per week
- ◯ 1 cup per day
- ◯ 2 or more cups per day

33. Cottage or ricotta cheese
- ◯ Never
- ◯ 1 - 3 times per month
- ◯ Once per week
- ◯ 2 or more times per week

34. Cheese (1 slice)
- ◯ Never
- ◯ 1 - 3 slices per month
- ◯ 1 slice per week
- ◯ 2 - 6 slices per week
- ◯ 1 slice per day
- ◯ 2 or more slices per day

35. Cream cheese
- ◯ Never
- ◯ 1 - 3 times per month
- ◯ Once per week
- ◯ 2 or more times per week

36. What TYPE of yogurt, cottage cheese & dairy products (besides milk) do you use mostly?
- ◯ Nonfat/Skim
- ◯ Lowfat
- ◯ Regular
- ◯ Don't know

37. Butter (1 pat) - NOT margarine
- ◯ Never
- ◯ 1 - 3 pats per month
- ◯ 1 pat per week
- ◯ 2 - 6 pats per week
- ◯ 1 pat per day
- ◯ 2 - 4 pats per day
- ◯ 5 or more pats per day

38. Margarine (1 pat) - NOT butter
- ◯ Never
- ◯ 1 - 3 pats per month
- ◯ 1 pat per week
- ◯ 2 - 6 pats per week
- ◯ 1 pat per day
- ◯ 2 - 4 pats per day
- ◯ 5 or more pats per day

39. What FORM and BRAND of margarine does your family usually use?
- ◯ None
- ◯ Stick
- ◯ Tub
- ◯ Squeeze (liquid)

⓪ ① ② ③ ④ ⑤ ⑥ ⑦ ⑧ ⑨
⓪ ① ② ③ ④ ⑤ ⑥ ⑦ ⑧ ⑨
⓪ ① ② ③ ④ ⑤ ⑥ ⑦ ⑧ ⑨

WHAT SPECIFIC BRAND AND TYPE (LIKE "PARKAY CORN OIL SPREAD")?

Leave blank if you don't know.

40. What TYPE of oil does your family use at home?
- ◯ Canola oil
- ◯ Corn oil
- ◯ Safflower oil
- ◯ Olive oil
- ◯ Vegetable oil
- ◯ Don't know

MAIN DISHES

41. Cheeseburger (1)
- ◯ Never
- ◯ 1 - 3 per month
- ◯ One per week
- ◯ 2 - 4 per week
- ◯ 5 or more per week

42. Hamburger (1)
- ◯ Never
- ◯ 1 - 3 per month
- ◯ One per week
- ◯ 2 - 4 per week
- ◯ 5 or more per week

43. Pizza (2 slices)
- ◯ Never
- ◯ 1 - 3 times per month
- ◯ Once per week
- ◯ 2 - 4 times per week
- ◯ 5 or more times per week

44. Tacos/burritos (1)
- ◯ Never
- ◯ 1 - 3 per month
- ◯ One per week
- ◯ 2 - 4 per week
- ◯ 5 or more per week

45. Which taco filling do you usually have:
- ◯ Beef & beans
- ◯ Beef
- ◯ Chicken
- ◯ Beans

46. Chicken nuggets (6)
- ◯ Never
- ◯ 1 - 3 times per month
- ◯ Once per week
- ◯ 2 - 4 times per week
- ◯ 5 or more times per week

PAGE FIVE HARVARD MEDICAL SCHOOL

47. Hot dogs (1)
- ○ Never
- ○ 1 - 3 per month
- ○ One per week
- ○ 2 - 4 per week
- ○ 5 or more per week

48. Peanut butter sandwich (1) (plain or with jelly, fluff, etc.)
- ○ Never
- ○ 1 - 3 per month
- ○ One per week
- ○ 2 - 4 per week
- ○ 5 or more per week

49. Chicken or turkey sandwich (1)
- ○ Never
- ○ 1 - 3 per month
- ○ One per week
- ○ 2 or more per week

50. Roast beef or ham sandwich (1)
- ○ Never
- ○ 1 - 3 per month
- ○ One per week
- ○ 2 or more per week

51. Salami, bologna, or other deli meat sandwich (1)
- ○ Never
- ○ 1 - 3 per month
- ○ One per week
- ○ 2 or more per week

52. Tuna sandwich (1)
- ○ Never
- ○ 1 - 3 per month
- ○ One per week
- ○ 2 or more per week

53. Chicken or turkey as main dish (1 serving)
- ○ Never
- ○ 1 - 3 times per month
- ○ Once per week
- ○ 2 - 4 times per week
- ○ 5 or more times per week

54. Fish sticks, fish cakes or fish sandwich (1 serving)
- ○ Never
- ○ 1 - 3 times per month
- ○ Once per week
- ○ 2 or more times per week

55. Fresh fish as main dish (1 serving)
- ○ Never
- ○ 1 - 3 times per month
- ○ Once per week
- ○ 2 - 4 times per week
- ○ 5 or more times per week

56. Beef (steak, roast) or lamb as main dish (1 serving)
- ○ Never
- ○ 1 - 3 times per month
- ○ Once per week
- ○ 2 - 4 times per week
- ○ 5 or more times per week

57. Pork or ham as main dish (1 serving)
- ○ Never
- ○ 1 - 3 times per month
- ○ Once per week
- ○ 2 - 4 times per week
- ○ 5 or more times per week

58. Meatballs or meatloaf (1 serving)
- ○ Never
- ○ 1 - 3 times per month
- ○ Once per week
- ○ 2 - 4 times per week
- ○ 5 or more times per week

59. Lasagna/baked ziti (1 serving)
- ○ Never
- ○ 1 - 3 times per month
- ○ Once per week
- ○ 2 or more times per week

60. Macaroni and cheese (1 serving)
- ○ Never
- ○ 1 - 3 times per month
- ○ Once per week
- ○ 2 or more times per week

61. Spaghetti with tomato sauce (1 serving)
- ○ Never
- ○ 1 - 3 times per month
- ○ Once per week
- ○ 2 - 4 times per week
- ○ 5 or more times per week

62. Eggs (1)
- ○ Never
- ○ 1 - 3 eggs per month
- ○ One egg per week
- ○ 2 - 4 eggs per week
- ○ 5 or more eggs per week

63. Liver: beef, calf, or pork (1 serving)
- ○ Never
- ○ Less than once per month
- ○ Once per month
- ○ 2 - 3 times per month
- ○ Once per week or more

64. Shrimp, lobster, scallops (1 serving)
- ○ Never
- ○ 1 - 3 times per month
- ○ Once per week
- ○ 2 or more times per week

3531

MISCELLANEOUS FOODS

65. Brown gravy
- ○ Never
- ○ Once per week or less
- ○ 2 - 6 times per week
- ○ Once per day
- ○ 2 or more times per day

66. Ketchup
- ○ Never
- ○ 1 - 3 times per month
- ○ Once per week
- ○ 2 - 4 times per week
- ○ 5 or more times per week

67. Clear soup (with rice, noodles, vegetables) 1 bowl
- ○ Never
- ○ 1 - 3 bowls per month
- ○ 1 bowl per week
- ○ 2 or more bowls per week

68. Cream (milk) soups or chowder (1 bowl)
- ○ Never
- ○ 1 - 3 bowls per month
- ○ 1 bowl per week
- ○ 2 - 6 bowls per week
- ○ 1 or more bowls per day

69. Mayonnaise
- ○ Never
- ○ 1 - 3 times per month
- ○ Once per week
- ○ 2 - 6 times per week
- ○ Once per day

70. Low calorie salad dressing
- ○ Never
- ○ 1 - 3 times per month
- ○ Once per week
- ○ 2 - 6 times per week
- ○ Once or more per day

71. Salad dressing (not low calorie)
- ○ Never
- ○ 1 - 3 times per month
- ○ Once per week
- ○ 2 - 6 times per week
- ○ Once or more per day

72. Salsa
- ○ Never
- ○ 1 - 3 times per month
- ○ Once per week
- ○ 2 - 6 times per week
- ○ Once or more per day

73. How much fat on your beef, pork, or lamb do you eat?
- ○ Eat all
- ○ Eat some
- ○ Eat none
- ○ Don't eat meat

74. Do you eat the skin of the chicken or turkey?
- ○ Yes
- ○ No
- ○ Sometimes

BREADS & CEREALS

75. Cold breakfast cereal (1 bowl)

- ○ Never
- ○ 1 - 3 bowls per month
- ○ 1 bowl per week
- ○ 2 - 4 bowls per week
- ○ 5 - 7 bowls per week
- ○ 2 or more bowls per day

76. Hot breakfast cereal, like oatmeal, grits (1 bowl)

- ○ Never
- ○ 1 - 3 bowls per month
- ○ 1 bowl per week
- ○ 2 - 4 bowls per week
- ○ 5 - 7 bowls per week
- ○ 2 or more bowls per day

77. White bread, pita bread, or toast (1 slice)

- ○ Never
- ○ 1 slice per week or less
- ○ 2 - 4 slices per week
- ○ 5 - 7 slices per week
- ○ 2 - 3 slices per day
- ○ 4+ slices per day

78. Dark bread (1 slice)

- ○ Never
- ○ 1 slice per week or less
- ○ 2 - 4 slices per week
- ○ 5 - 7 slices per week
- ○ 2 - 3 slices per day
- ○ 4+ slices per day

79. English muffins or bagels (1)

- ○ Never
- ○ 1 - 3 per month
- ○ 1 per week
- ○ 2 - 4 per week
- ○ 5 or more per week

80. Muffin (1)

- ○ Never
- ○ 1 - 3 muffins per month
- ○ 1 muffin per week
- ○ 2 - 4 muffins per week
- ○ 5 or more muffins per week

81. Cornbread (1 square)

- ○ Never
- ○ 1 - 3 times per month
- ○ Once per week
- ○ 2 - 4 times per week
- ○ 5 or more per week

82. Biscuit/roll (1)

- ○ Never
- ○ 1 - 3 per month
- ○ 1 per week
- ○ 2 - 4 per week
- ○ 5 or more per week

83. Rice

- ○ Never
- ○ 1 - 3 times per month
- ○ Once per week
- ○ 2 - 4 times per week
- ○ 5 or more times per week

84. Noodles, pasta

- ○ Never
- ○ 1 - 3 times per month
- ○ Once per week
- ○ 2 - 4 times per week
- ○ 5 or more times per week

85. Tortilla - no filling (1)

- ○ Never
- ○ 1 - 3 per month
- ○ 1 per week
- ○ 2 - 4 per week
- ○ 5 or more per week

86. Other grains, like kasha, couscous, bulgar

- ○ Never
- ○ 1 - 3 times per month
- ○ Once per week
- ○ 2 or more times per week

87. Pancakes (2) or waffles (1)

- ○ Never
- ○ 1 - 3 times per month
- ○ Once per week
- ○ 2 or more times per week

88. French fries (large order)

- ○ Never
- ○ 1 - 3 orders per month
- ○ 1 order per week
- ○ 2 - 4 orders per week
- ○ 5 or more orders per week

89. Potatoes - baked, boiled, mashed

- ○ Never
- ○ 1 - 3 times per month
- ○ Once per week
- ○ 2 - 4 times per week
- ○ 5 or more times per week

FRUITS & VEGETABLES

90. Raisins (small pack)
- ○ Never
- ○ 1 - 3 times per month
- ○ 1 per week
- ○ 2 - 4 times per week
- ○ 5 or more times per week

91. Grapes (bunch)
- ○ Never
- ○ 1 - 3 times per month
- ○ Once per week
- ○ 2 - 4 times per week
- ○ 5 or more times per week

92. Bananas (1)
- ○ Never
- ○ 1 - 3 per month
- ○ 1 per week
- ○ 2 - 4 per week
- ○ 5 or more per week

93. Cantaloupe, melons (1/4 melon)
- ○ Never
- ○ 1 - 3 times per month
- ○ 1 per week
- ○ 2 or more times per week

94. Apples (1) or applesauce
- ○ Never
- ○ 1 - 3 per month
- ○ 1 per week
- ○ 2 - 6 per week
- ○ 1 or more per day

95. Pears (1)
- ○ Never
- ○ 1 - 3 per month
- ○ 1 per week
- ○ 2 - 6 per week
- ○ 1 or more per day

96. Oranges (1), grapefruit (1/2)
- ○ Never
- ○ 1 - 3 per month
- ○ 1 per week
- ○ 2 - 6 per week
- ○ 1 or more per day

97. Strawberries
- ○ Never
- ○ 1 - 3 times per month
- ○ Once per week
- ○ 2 or more times per week

98. Peaches, plums, apricots (1)
- ○ Never
- ○ 1 - 3 per month
- ○ 1 per week
- ○ 2 or more per week

99. Orange juice (1 glass)
- ○ Never
- ○ 1 - 3 glasses per month
- ○ 1 glass per week
- ○ 2 - 6 glasses per week
- ○ 1 glass per day
- ○ 2 or more glasses per day

100. Apple juice and other fruit juices (1 glass)
- ○ Never
- ○ 1 - 3 glasses per month
- ○ 1 glass per week
- ○ 2 - 6 glasses per week
- ○ 1 glass per day
- ○ 2 or more glasses per day

101. Tomatoes (1)
- ○ Never
- ○ 1 - 3 per month
- ○ 1 per week
- ○ 2 - 6 per week
- ○ 1 or more per day

102. Tomato/spaghetti sauce
- ○ Never
- ○ 1 - 3 times per month
- ○ Once per week
- ○ 2 - 4 times per week
- ○ 5 or more times per week

103. Tofu
- ○ Never
- ○ 1 - 3 times per month
- ○ Once per week
- ○ 2 - 4 times per week
- ○ 5 or more times per week

104. String beans
- ○ Never
- ○ 1 - 3 times per month
- ○ Once per week
- ○ 2 - 4 times per week
- ○ 5 or more times per week

PAGE NINE **HARVARD MEDICAL SCHOOL**

105. Broccoli
- ○ Never
- ○ 1 - 3 times per month
- ○ Once per week
- ○ 2 - 4 times per week
- ○ 5 or more times per week

106. Beets (not greens)
- ○ Never
- ○ Once per week or less
- ○ 2 or more times per week

107. Corn
- ○ Never
- ○ 1 - 3 times per month
- ○ Once per week
- ○ 2 - 4 times per week
- ○ 5 or more times per week

108. Peas or lima beans
- ○ Never
- ○ 1 - 3 times per month
- ○ Once per week
- ○ 2 - 4 times per week
- ○ 5 or more times per week

109. Mixed vegetables
- ○ Never
- ○ 1 - 3 times per month
- ○ Once per week
- ○ 2 - 4 times per week
- ○ 5 or more times per week

110. Spinach
- ○ Never
- ○ 1 - 3 times per month
- ○ Once a week
- ○ 2 - 4 times per week
- ○ 5 or more times per week

111. Greens/kale
- ○ Never
- ○ 1 - 3 times per month
- ○ Once per week
- ○ 2 - 4 times per week
- ○ 5 or more times per week

112. Green/red peppers
- ○ Never
- ○ 1 - 3 times per month
- ○ Once a week
- ○ 2 - 4 times per week
- ○ 5 or more times per week

113. Yams/sweet potatoes (1)
- ○ Never
- ○ 1 - 3 times per month
- ○ Once a week
- ○ 2 - 4 times per week
- ○ 5 or more times per week

114. Zucchini, summer squash, eggplant
- ○ Never
- ○ 1 - 3 times per month
- ○ Once per week
- ○ 2 - 4 times per week
- ○ 5 or more times per week

115. Carrots, cooked
- ○ Never
- ○ 1 - 3 times per month
- ○ Once per week
- ○ 2 - 4 times per week
- ○ 5 or more times per week

116. Carrots, raw
- ○ Never
- ○ 1 - 3 times per month
- ○ Once per week
- ○ 2 - 4 times per week
- ○ 5 or more times per week

117. Celery
- ○ Never
- ○ 1 - 3 times per month
- ○ Once per week
- ○ 2 - 4 times per week
- ○ 5 or more times per week

118. Lettuce/tossed salad
- ○ Never
- ○ 1 - 3 times per month
- ○ Once per week
- ○ 2 - 6 times per week
- ○ One or more per day

119. Coleslaw
- ○ Never
- ○ 1 - 3 times per month
- ○ Once per week
- ○ 2 or more times per week

120. Potato salad
- ○ Never
- ○ 1 - 3 times per month
- ○ Once per week
- ○ 2 or more times per week

121. Beans/lentils/soybeans
- ○ Never
- ○ Once per week or less
- ○ 2 - 6 times per week
- ○ Once per day

SNACK FOODS/DESSERTS

122. Fill in the number of snacks (food or drinks) eaten on school days and weekends/vacation days.

Snacks	School Days					Vacation/Weekend Days				
	NONE	1	2	3	4 OR MORE	NONE	1	2	3	4 OR MORE
Between breakfast and lunch	○	○	○	○	○	○	○	○	○	○
After lunch, before dinner	○	○	○	○	○	○	○	○	○	○
After dinner	○	○	○	○	○	○	○	○	○	○

Think about your usual snacks. Estimate how often you eat each type of snack food.

Example 3 If you eat poptarts rarely (about 6 per year) then your answer should look like this:

E3. Poptarts (1)
- ● Never/less than 1 per month
- ○ 1 - 3 per month
- ○ 1 - 6 per week
- ○ 1 or more per day

123. Potato chips (1 small bag)
- ○ Never/less than 1 per month
- ○ 1 - 3 small bags per month
- ○ One small bag per week
- ○ 2 - 6 small bags per week
- ○ 1 or more small bags per day

124. Corn chips/Doritos (small bag)
- ○ Never/less than 1 per month
- ○ 1 - 3 small bags per month
- ○ One small bag per week
- ○ 2 - 6 small bags per week
- ○ 1 or more small bags per day

125. Nachos with cheese (1 serving)
- ○ Never/less than 1 per month
- ○ 1 - 3 times per month
- ○ Once per week
- ○ 2 or more times per week

126. Popcorn (1 small bag)
- ○ Never/less than 1 per month
- ○ 1 - 3 small bags per month
- ○ 1 - 4 small bags per week
- ○ 5 or more small bags per week

127. Pretzels (1 small bag)
- ○ Never/less than 1 per month
- ○ 1 - 3 small bags per month
- ○ 1 small bags per week
- ○ 2 or more small bags per week

128. Peanuts, nuts (1 small bag)
- ○ Never/less than 1 per month
- ○ 1 - 3 small bags per month
- ○ 1 - 4 small bags per week
- ○ 5 or more small bags per week

129. Fun fruit (1 pack)
- ○ Never/less than 1 per month
- ○ 1 - 3 packs per month
- ○ 1 - 4 packs per week
- ○ 5 or more packs per week

130. Graham crackers
- ○ Never/less than 1 per month
- ○ 1 - 3 times per month
- ○ 1 - 4 times per week
- ○ 5 or more times per week

131. Crackers, like saltines or wheat thins
- ○ Never/less than 1 per month
- ○ 1 - 3 times per month
- ○ 1 - 4 times per week
- ○ 5 or more times per week

45803-2/3

132. Poptarts (1)
- ○ Never/less than 1 per month
- ○ 1 - 3 poptarts per month
- ○ 1 - 6 poptarts per week
- ○ 1 or more poptarts per day

133. Cake (1 slice)
- ○ Never/less than 1 per month
- ○ 1 - 3 slices per month
- ○ 1 slice per week
- ○ 2 or more slices per week

134. Snack cakes, Twinkies (1 package)
- ○ Never/less than 1 per month
- ○ 1 - 3 per month
- ○ Once per week
- ○ 2 - 6 per week
- ○ 1 or more per day

135. Danish, sweetrolls, pastry (1)
- ○ Never/less than 1 per month
- ○ 1 - 3 per month
- ○ 1 per week
- ○ 2 - 4 per week
- ○ 5 or more per week

136. Donuts (1)
- ○ Never/less than 1 per month
- ○ 1 - 3 donuts per month
- ○ 1 donut per week
- ○ 2 - 6 donuts per week
- ○ 1 or more donuts per day

137. Cookies (1)
- ○ Never/less than 1 per month
- ○ 1 - 3 cookies per month
- ○ 1 cookie per week
- ○ 2 - 6 cookies per week
- ○ 1 - 3 cookies per day
- ○ 4 or more cookies per day

138. Brownies (1)
- ○ Never/less than 1 per month
- ○ 1 - 3 per month
- ○ 1 per week
- ○ 2 - 4 per week
- ○ 5 or more per week

139. Pie (1 slice)
- ○ Never/less than 1 per month
- ○ 1 - 3 slices per month
- ○ 1 slice per week
- ○ 2 or more slices per week

140. Chocolate (1 bar or packet) like Hershey's or M & M's
- ○ Never/less than 1 per month
- ○ 1 - 3 per month
- ○ 1 per week
- ○ 2 - 6 per week
- ○ 1 or more per day

141. Other candy bars (Milky Way, Snickers)
- ○ Never/less than 1 per month
- ○ 1 - 3 candy bars per month
- ○ 1 candy bar per week
- ○ 2 - 4 candy bars per week
- ○ 5 or more candy bars per week

142. Other candy without chocolate (mints, Lifesavers) (1 pack)
- ○ Never/less than 1 per month
- ○ 1 - 3 times per month
- ○ Once per week
- ○ 2 - 4 times per week
- ○ 5 or more times per week

143. Jello
- ○ Never/less than 1 per month
- ○ 1 - 3 times per month
- ○ Once per week
- ○ 2 - 4 times per week
- ○ 5 or more times per week

144. Pudding
- ○ Never/less than 1 per month
- ○ 1 - 3 times per month
- ○ Once per week
- ○ 2 - 4 times per week
- ○ 5 or more times per week

145. Frozen yogurt
- ○ Never/less than 1 per month
- ○ 1 - 3 times per month
- ○ Once per week
- ○ 2 - 4 times per week
- ○ 5 or more times per week

146. Ice cream
- ○ Never/less than 1 per month
- ○ 1 - 3 times per month
- ○ Once per week
- ○ 2 - 4 times per week
- ○ 5 or more times per week

147. Milkshake or frappe (1)
- ○ Never/less than 1 per month
- ○ 1 - 3 per month
- ○ 1 per week
- ○ 2 or more per week

148. Popsicles
- ○ Never/less than 1 per month
- ○ 1 - 3 popsicles per month
- ○ 1 popsicle per week
- ○ 2 - 4 popsicles per week
- ○ 5 or more popsicles per week

149. Please list any other important foods that you usually eat at least once per week that are not listed (for example, coconut, hummus, falafel, eggrolls, chili, plantains, mangoes, etc. . .)

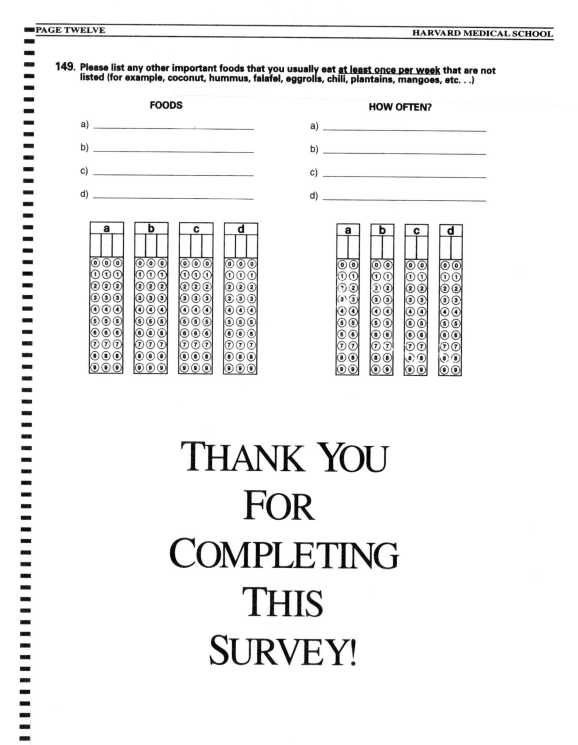

FOODS	HOW OFTEN?
a) ______________	a) ______________
b) ______________	b) ______________
c) ______________	c) ______________
d) ______________	d) ______________

a	b	c	d
0 0 0	0 0 0	0 0 0	0 0 0
1 1 1	1 1 1	1 1 1	1 1 1
2 2 2	2 2 2	2 2 2	2 2 2
3 3 3	3 3 3	3 3 3	3 3 3
4 4 4	4 4 4	4 4 4	4 4 4
5 5 5	5 5 5	5 5 5	5 5 5
6 6 6	6 6 6	6 6 6	6 6 6
7 7 7	7 7 7	7 7 7	7 7 7
8 8 8	8 8 8	8 8 8	8 8 8
9 9 9	9 9 9	9 9 9	9 9 9

a	b	c	d
0 0	0 0	0 0	0 0
1 1	1 1	1 1	1 1
2 2	2 2	2 2	2 2
3 3	3 3	3 3	3 3
4 4	4 4	4 4	4 4
5 5	5 5	5 5	5 5
6 6	6 6	6 6	6 6
7 7	7 7	7 7	7 7
8 8	8 8	8 8	8 8
9 9	9 9	9 9	9 9

THANK YOU FOR COMPLETING THIS SURVEY!

APPENDIX K

HEALTH HABITS AND HISTORY QUESTIONNAIRE

From Health Habits and History Questionnaire: Diet History and Other Risk Factors. National Cancer Institute, Division of Cancer Prevention and Control, National Institutes of Health.
Courtesy of the National Cancer Institute, Division of Cancer Prevention and Control, National Institutes of Health.

FOOD QUESTIONNAIRE

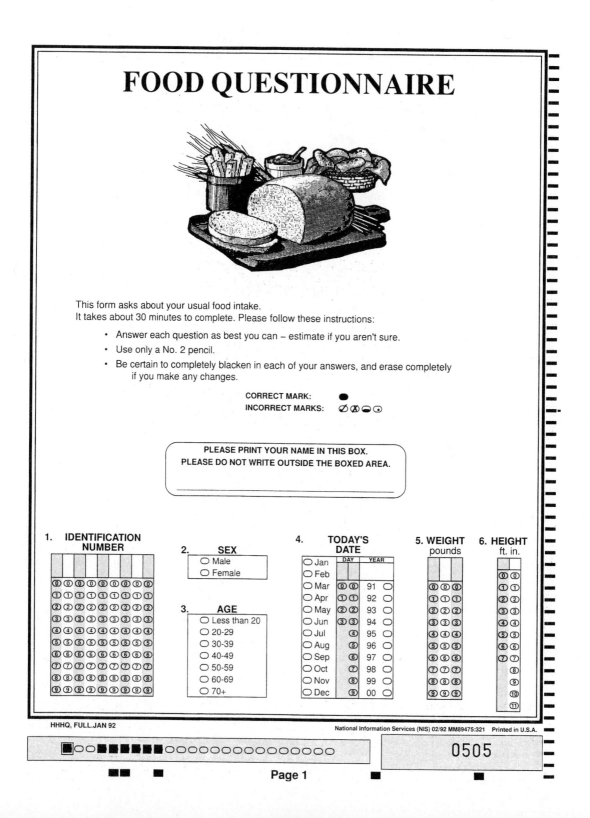

This form asks about your usual food intake.
It takes about 30 minutes to complete. Please follow these instructions:

- Answer each question as best you can – estimate if you aren't sure.
- Use only a No. 2 pencil.
- Be certain to completely blacken in each of your answers, and erase completely if you make any changes.

CORRECT MARK: ●
INCORRECT MARKS: ⊘ ⊗ ⊖ ⊙

PLEASE PRINT YOUR NAME IN THIS BOX.
PLEASE DO NOT WRITE OUTSIDE THE BOXED AREA.

1. IDENTIFICATION NUMBER

0	0	0	0	0	0	0	0	0
1	1	1	1	1	1	1	1	1
2	2	2	2	2	2	2	2	2
3	3	3	3	3	3	3	3	3
4	4	4	4	4	4	4	4	4
5	5	5	5	5	5	5	5	5
6	6	6	6	6	6	6	6	6
7	7	7	7	7	7	7	7	7
8	8	8	8	8	8	8	8	8
9	9	9	9	9	9	9	9	9

2. SEX

- ○ Male
- ○ Female

3. AGE

- ○ Less than 20
- ○ 20-29
- ○ 30-39
- ○ 40-49
- ○ 50-59
- ○ 60-69
- ○ 70+

4. TODAY'S DATE

Month	DAY		YEAR
○ Jan			
○ Feb			
○ Mar	0	0	91 ○
○ Apr	1	1	92 ○
○ May	2	2	93 ○
○ Jun	3	3	94 ○
○ Jul		4	95 ○
○ Aug		5	96 ○
○ Sep		6	97 ○
○ Oct		7	98 ○
○ Nov		8	99 ○
○ Dec		9	00 ○

5. WEIGHT pounds

0	0	0
1	1	1
2	2	2
3	3	3
4	4	4
5	5	5
6	6	6
7	7	7
8	8	8
9	9	9

6. HEIGHT ft. in.

ft.	in.
0	0
1	1
2	2
3	3
4	4
5	5
6	6
7	7
	8
	9
	10
	11

HHHQ, FULL.JAN 92

National Information Services (NIS) 02/92 MM89475:321 Printed in U.S.A.

0505

7. Do you smoke cigarettes now?

○ No
○ Yes **IF YES, on the average, about how many cigarettes a day do you smoke now?**
○ 1 - 5 ○ 6 - 14 ○ 15 - 24 ○ 25 - 34 ○ 35 or more

8. About how many times have you gone on a diet to lose weight?

○ Never ○ 1 - 2 ○ 3 - 5 ○ 6 - 8 ○ 9 - 11 ○ 12 or more

9. During the past year have you taken any vitamins or minerals?

○ No ○ Yes, fairly regularly ○ Yes, but not regularly

IF YES, what do you take fairly regularly?

VITAMIN TYPE	NUMBER OF TABLETS								FOR HOW MANY YEARS?				
	NONE	1-3 PER WEEK	4-6 PER WEEK	1 PER DAY	2 PER DAY	3 PER DAY	4 PER DAY	5+ PER DAY	LESS THAN 1 YR	1-2 YEARS	3-5 YEARS	6-9 YEARS	10+ YEARS
Multiple Vitamins													
Stress-tabs type	○	○	○	○	○	○	○	○	○	○	○	○	○
Therapeutic, Theragran type	○	○	○	○	○	○	○	○	○	○	○	○	○
One-a-day type	○	○	○	○	○	○	○	○	○	○	○	○	○
Other Vitamins													
Vitamin A	○	○	○	○	○	○	○	○	○	○	○	○	○
Vitamin E	○	○	○	○	○	○	○	○	○	○	○	○	○
Calcium or Tums	○	○	○	○	○	○	○	○	○	○	○	○	○
Vitamin C	○	○	○	○	○	○	○	○	○	○	○	○	○

10. If you take Vitamin E or Vitamin C:

How many units per Vitamin E tablet? ○ 100 ○ 200 ○ 400 ○ 1000 ○ Don't know
How many milligrams per Vitamin C tablet? ○ 100 ○ 250 ○ 500 ○ 1000 ○ Don't know

11. Do you regularly take pills containing any of these nutrients?

○ No or don't know ○ Iron ○ Beta-carotene
○ Zinc ○ Selenium ○ ________________

12. What kinds of fat do you *usually* use in cooking (to fry, stir-fry, or saute)? Mark only one or two.

○ Don't know or don't cook ○ Lard, fatback, baconfat ○ Pam or no oil ○ Crisco
○ Stick margarine ○ Butter ○ Soft tub margarine ○ Oil
○ 1/2 butter, 1/2 margarine ○ Low calorie margarine

13. What kinds of fat do you *usually* add to vegetables, potatoes, etc.? Mark only one or two.

○ Don't add fat ○ Lard, fatback, baconfat ○ Low calorie margarine
○ Stick margarine ○ Soft tub margarine ○ 1/2 butter, 1/2 margarine
○ Butter ○ Whipped butter ○ Crisco

14. When you eat the following foods, how often do you eat a low-fat or non-fat version of that food?

CHEESE ○ Always low-fat ○ Sometimes ○ Rarely low-fat
ICE CREAM/YOGURT ○ Always low-fat ○ Sometimes ○ Rarely low-fat
SALAD DRESSING ○ Always low-fat ○ Sometimes ○ Rarely low-fat

Page 2

15.	SELDOM/NEVER	SOMETIMES	OFTEN/ALWAYS
a. How often do you add salt to your food?	○	○	○
b. How often do you add pepper to your food?	○	○	○
c. How often do you eat the skin on chicken?	○	○	○
d. How often do you eat the fat on meat?	○	○	○

16. About how often do you eat the following foods from restaurants or carry-outs? Remember to think about all meals (breakfast, lunch, dinner or snacks).

RESTAURANT FOOD	NUMBER OF VISITS LAST YEAR						
	NEVER IN PAST YEAR	1-4 TIMES PAST YEAR	5-11 TIMES PAST YEAR	1-3 TIMES A MONTH	ONCE A WEEK	2-4 TIMES A WEEK	ALMOST EVERY DAY
Fried chicken	○	○	○	○	○	○	○
Burgers	○	○	○	○	○	○	○
Pizza	○	○	○	○	○	○	○
Chinese food	○	○	○	○	○	○	○
Mexican food	○	○	○	○	○	○	○
Fried fish	○	○	○	○	○	○	○

17. This section is about your *usual* eating habits over the past year.

FIRST: Mark the column to show how often, on the average, you ate the food during the past year. Please BE CAREFUL which column you put your answer in.

SECOND: Mark whether your usual serving size is small, medium or large. Please DO NOT OMIT serving size.

ADDITIONAL COMMENTS:

- Please DO NOT SKIP any foods. If you never eat a food, mark "Never or less than once a month."

- A small serving is about one-half the medium serving size shown, or less.
- A large serving is about one-and-a-half times the medium serving size shown, or more.

SAMPLE: This person ate a medium serving of rice about twice per month and never ate squash.

TYPE OF FOOD	HOW OFTEN									HOW MUCH			
	NEVER OR LESS THAN ONCE PER MONTH	1 PER MON	2-3 PER MON	1 PER WEEK	2 PER WEEK	3-4 PER WEEK	5-6 PER WEEK	1 PER DAY	2+ PER DAY	MEDIUM SERVING	YOUR SERVING SIZE		
											S	M	L
Rice	○	○	●	○	○	○	○	○	○	3/4 cup	○	●	○
Winter squash, baked squash	●	○	○	○	○	○	○	○	○	1/2 cup	○	○	○

0505

TYPE OF FOOD	HOW OFTEN									HOW MUCH			
	NEVER OR LESS THAN ONCE PER MONTH	1 PER MON	2-3 PER MON	1 PER WEEK	2 PER WEEK	3-4 PER WEEK	5-6 PER WEEK	1 PER DAY	2+ PER DAY	MEDIUM SERVING	YOUR SERVING SIZE S	M	L
FRUITS AND JUICES													
EXAMPLE: Apples, etc.	○	○	○	●	○	○	○	○	○	1 medium or 1/2 cup	○	●	○
Apples, applesauce, pears	○	○	○	○	○	○	○	○	○	1 medium or 1/2 cup	○	○	○
Bananas	○	○	○	○	○	○	○	○	○	1 medium	○	○	○
Peaches, apricots (fresh or canned	○	○	○	○	○	○	○	○	○	1 medium or 1/2 cup	○	○	○
Cantaloupe (in season)	○	○	○	○	○	○	○	○	○	1/4 medium	○	○	○
Cantaloupe (rest of year)	○	○	○	○	○	○	○	○	○	1/4 medium	○	○	○
Watermelon (in season)	○	○	○	○	○	○	○	○	○	1 slice	○	○	○
Strawberries (in season)	○	○	○	○	○	○	○	○	○	1/2 cup	○	○	○
Oranges	○	○	○	○	○	○	○	○	○	1 medium	○	○	○
Grapefruit	○	○	○	○	○	○	○	○	○	1/2 medium	○	○	○
Orange juice or grapefruit juice	○	○	○	○	○	○	○	○	○	6 ounce glass	○	○	○
Fruit drinks with added vitamin C, such as Hi-C	○	○	○	○	○	○	○	○	○	6 ounce glass	○	○	○
Any other fruit, including berries, fruit cocktail, grapes	○	○	○	○	○	○	○	○	○	1/2 cup	○	○	○
BREAKFAST FOODS													
High fiber, bran or granola cereals, shredded wheat	○	○	○	○	○	○	○	○	○	1 medium bowl	○	○	○
Highly fortified cereals, such as Total, Just Right or Product 19	○	○	○	○	○	○	○	○	○	1 medium bowl	○	○	○
Other cold cereals, such as corn flakes, Rice Krispies	○	○	○	○	○	○	○	○	○	1 medium bowl	○	○	○
Cooked cereal, or grits	○	○	○	○	○	○	○	○	○	1 medium bowl	○	○	○
Milk on cereal	○	○	○	○	○	○	○	○	○	1/2 cup	○	○	○
Sugar added to cereal	○	○	○	○	○	○	○	○	○	2 teasp	○	○	○
Eggs	○	○	○	○	○	○	○	○	○	1 egg=sml 2 eggs=med	○	○	○
Bacon	○	○	○	○	○	○	○	○	○	2 slices	○	○	○
Sausage	○	○	○	○	○	○	○	○	○	2 patties or links	○	○	○

0505

TYPE OF FOOD	HOW OFTEN									HOW MUCH			
	NEVER OR LESS THAN ONCE PER MONTH	1 PER MON	2-3 PER MON	1 PER WEEK	2 PER WEEK	3-4 PER WEEK	5-6 PER WEEK	1 PER DAY	2+ PER DAY	MEDIUM SERVING	YOUR SERVING SIZE		
											S	M	L
VEGETABLES													
String beans, green beans	○	○	○	○	○	○	○	○	○	1/2 cup	○	○	○
Peas	○	○	○	○	○	○	○	○	○	1/2 cup	○	○	○
Chili with beans	○	○	○	○	○	○	○	○	○	3/4 cup	○	○	○
Other beans such as baked beans, pintos, kidney, limas, and lentils	○	○	○	○	○	○	○	○	○	3/4 cup	○	○	○
Corn	○	○	○	○	○	○	○	○	○	1/2 cup	○	○	○
Winter squash/baked squash	○	○	○	○	○	○	○	○	○	1/2 cup	○	○	○
Tomatoes, tomato juice	○	○	○	○	○	○	○	○	○	1 medium or 6 oz. glass	○	○	○
Red chili sauce, taco sauce, salsa picante	○	○	○	○	○	○	○	○	○	2 tablesp	○	○	○
Broccoli	○	○	○	○	○	○	○	○	○	1/2 cup	○	○	○
Cauliflower or brussels sprouts	○	○	○	○	○	○	○	○	○	1/2 cup	○	○	○
Spinach (raw)	○	○	○	○	○	○	○	○	○	3/4 cup	○	○	○
Spinach (cooked)	○	○	○	○	○	○	○	○	○	1/2 cup	○	○	○
Mustard greens, turnip greens, collards	○	○	○	○	○	○	○	○	○	1/2 cup	○	○	○
Cole slaw, cabbage, sauerkraut	○	○	○	○	○	○	○	○	○	1/2 cup	○	○	○
Carrots, or mixed vegetables containing carrots	○	○	○	○	○	○	○	○	○	1/2 cup	○	○	○
Green salad	○	○	○	○	○	○	○	○	○	1 medium bowl	○	○	○
Regular salad dressing & mayonnaise, including on sandwiches or on potato salad, etc.	○	○	○	○	○	○	○	○	○	2 tablesp	○	○	○
French fries and fried potatoes	○	○	○	○	○	○	○	○	○	3/4 cup	○	○	○
Sweet potatoes, yams	○	○	○	○	○	○	○	○	○	1/2 cup	○	○	○
Other potatoes, including boiled, baked, mashed & potato salad	○	○	○	○	○	○	○	○	○	1 medium or 1/2 cup	○	○	○
Rice	○	○	○	○	○	○	○	○	○	3/4 cup	○	○	○
Any other vegetable, including cooked onions, summer squash	○	○	○	○	○	○	○	○	○	1/2 cup	○	○	○
Butter, margarine or other fat added to veg., potatoes, etc.	○	○	○	○	○	○	○	○	○	2 pats	○	○	○

TYPE OF FOOD	HOW OFTEN									HOW MUCH			
											YOUR SERVING SIZE		
	NEVER OR LESS THAN ONCE PER MONTH	1 PER MON	2-3 PER MON	1 PER WEEK	2 PER WEEK	3-4 PER WEEK	5-6 PER WEEK	1 PER DAY	2+ PER DAY	MEDIUM SERVING	S	M	L
MEAT, FISH, POULTRY, LUNCH ITEMS													
Hamburgers, cheeseburgers, meatloaf, beef burritos, tacos	○	○	○	○	○	○	○	○	○	1 medium or 4 oz.	○	○	○
Beef, (steaks, roasts, etc., including sandwiches)	○	○	○	○	○	○	○	○	○	4 ounces	○	○	○
Beef stew or pot pie with carrots or other vegetables	○	○	○	○	○	○	○	○	○	1 cup	○	○	○
Liver, including chicken livers	○	○	○	○	○	○	○	○	○	4 ounces	○	○	○
Pork, including chops, roasts	○	○	○	○	○	○	○	○	○	2 chops or 4 ounces	○	○	○
Fried chicken	○	○	○	○	○	○	○	○	○	2 small or 1 large pce	○	○	○
Chicken or turkey (roasted, stewed or broiled, including on sandwiches)	○	○	○	○	○	○	○	○	○	2 small or 1 large pce	○	○	○
Fried fish or fish sandwich	○	○	○	○	○	○	○	○	○	4 ounces or 1 sandwich	○	○	○
Tuna, tuna salad, tuna casserole	○	○	○	○	○	○	○	○	○	1/2 cup	○	○	○
Oysters	○	○	○	○	○	○	○	○	○	5 pieces, 1/4 cup or 3 oz.	○	○	○
Shell fish, (shrimp, crab, lobster, etc.)	○	○	○	○	○	○	○	○	○	5 pieces, 1/4 cup or 3 oz.	○	○	○
Other fish (broiled or baked)	○	○	○	○	○	○	○	○	○	2 pieces or 4 ounces	○	○	○
Spaghetti, lasagna, other pasta with tomato sauce	○	○	○	○	○	○	○	○	○	1 cup	○	○	○
Pizza	○	○	○	○	○	○	○	○	○	2 slices	○	○	○
Mixed dishes with cheese (such as macaroni and cheese)	○	○	○	○	○	○	○	○	○	1 cup	○	○	○
Liverwurst	○	○	○	○	○	○	○	○	○	2 slices	○	○	○
Hot dogs	○	○	○	○	○	○	○	○	○	2 hot dogs	○	○	○
Ham, bologna, salami and other lunch meats	○	○	○	○	○	○	○	○	○	2 slices or 2 ounces	○	○	○
Vegetable and tomato soups, including vegetable beef, minestrone	○	○	○	○	○	○	○	○	○	1 medium bowl	○	○	○
Other soups	○	○	○	○	○	○	○	○	○	1 medium bowl	○	○	○

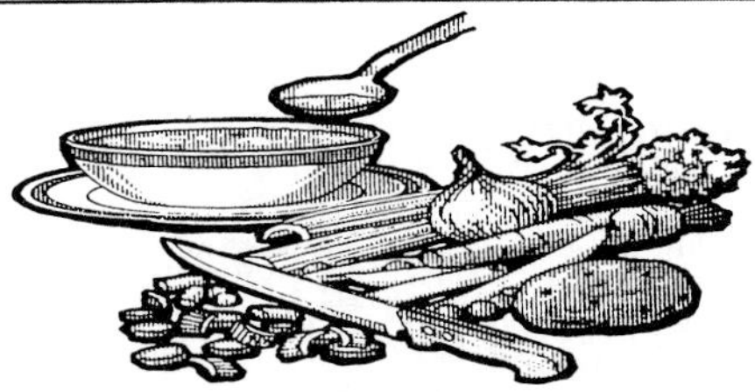

TYPE OF FOOD	HOW OFTEN									HOW MUCH			
	NEVER OR LESS THAN ONCE PER MONTH	1 PER MON	2-3 PER MON	1 PER WEEK	2 PER WEEK	3-4 PER WEEK	5-6 PER WEEK	1 PER DAY	2+ PER DAY	MEDIUM SERVING	YOUR SERVING SIZE S	M	L
BREADS, SNACKS, SPREADS													
Biscuits, muffins, (including fast foods)	○	○	○	○	○	○	○	○	○	1 medium piece	○	○	○
White bread (including sandwiches, bagels, burger rolls, French or Italian bread	○	○	○	○	○	○	○	○	○	2 slices	○	○	○
Dark bread, such as wheat, rye, pumpernickel, (including sandwiches)	○	○	○	○	○	○	○	○	○	2 slices	○	○	○
Corn bread, corn muffins, corn tortillas	○	○	○	○	○	○	○	○	○	1 medium piece	○	○	○
Salty snacks, such as potato chips, corn chips, popcorn	○	○	○	○	○	○	○	○	○	2 handfuls or 1 cup	○	○	○
Peanuts, peanut butter	○	○	○	○	○	○	○	○	○	2 tablesp	○	○	○
Margarine on bread or rolls	○	○	○	○	○	○	○	○	○	2 pats	○	○	○
Butter on bread or rolls	○	○	○	○	○	○	○	○	○	2 pats	○	○	○
Gravies made with meat drippings, or white sauce	○	○	○	○	○	○	○	○	○	2 tablesp	○	○	○
DAIRY PRODUCTS													
Cottage cheese	○	○	○	○	○	○	○	○	○	1/2 cup	○	○	○
Other cheeses and cheese spreads	○	○	○	○	○	○	○	○	○	2 slices or 2 ounces	○	○	○
Flavored yogurt, frozen yogurt	○	○	○	○	○	○	○	○	○	1 cup	○	○	○
SWEETS													
Ice cream	○	○	○	○	○	○	○	○	○	1 scoop or 1/2 cup	○	○	○
Doughnuts, cookies, cake, pastry	○	○	○	○	○	○	○	○	○	1 piece or 3 cookies	○	○	○
Pumpkin pie, sweet potato pie	○	○	○	○	○	○	○	○	○	1 medium slice	○	○	○
Other pies	○	○	○	○	○	○	○	○	○	1 medium slice	○	○	○
Chocolate candy	○	○	○	○	○	○	○	○	○	1 small bar or 1 oz	○	○	○
Other candy, jelly, honey, brown sugar	○	○	○	○	○	○	○	○	○	3 pieces or 1 tblsp.	○	○	○

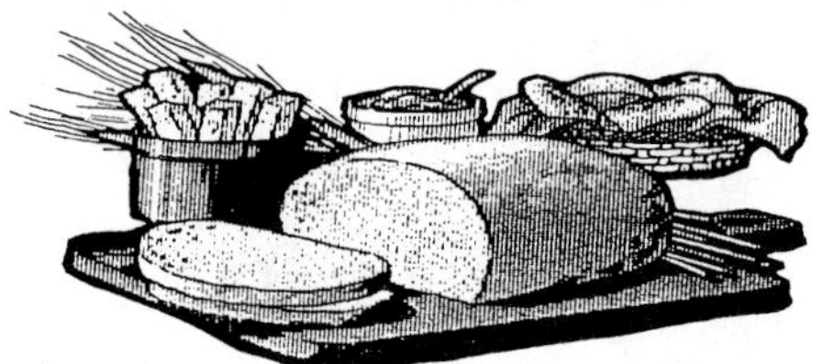

TYPE OF FOOD	HOW OFTEN: NEVER OR LESS THAN ONCE PER MONTH	1-3 PER MON	1 PER WEEK	2-4 PER WEEK	5-6 PER WEEK	1 PER DAY	2-3 PER DAY	4-5 PER DAY	6+ PER DAY	HOW MUCH: MEDIUM SERVING	YOUR SERVING SIZE: S	M	L
BEVERAGES (Please note that the categories for these columns are different.)													
Whole milk and beverages with whole milk (not incl. on cereal)										8 oz. glass			
2% milk and beverages with 2% milk (not including on cereal)										8 oz. glass			
Skim milk, 1% milk or buttermilk (not including on cereal)										8 oz. glass			
Regular soft drinks (not diet soda)										12 oz can or bottle			
Beer										12 oz can or bottle			
Wine or wine coolers										1 medium glass			
Liquor										1 shot			
Coffee, regular or decaf										1 medium cup			
Tea (hot or iced)										1 medium cup			
Lemon in tea										1 teasp			
Non-dairy creamer in coffee or tea										1 tablesp			
Cream (real) or Half-and-Half in coffee or tea										1 tablesp			
Milk in coffee or tea										1 tablesp			
Sugar in coffee or tea										2 teaspoons			
Glasses of water										8 oz. glass			

18.

SUMMARY QUESTIONS	AVERAGE USE LAST YEAR: LESS THAN ONCE PER WEEK	1-2 PER WEEK	3-4 PER WEEK	5-6 PER WEEK	1 PER DAY	1 1/2 PER DAY	2 PER DAY	3 PER DAY	4+ PER DAY
a. How often do you use fat or oil in cooking?									
b. About how many servings of vegetables do you eat, not counting salad or potatoes?									
c. About how many servings of fruit do you eat, not counting juices?									
d. About how many servings of cold cereal do you eat?									

THANK YOU VERY MUCH FOR TAKING THE TIME TO FILL OUT THIS QUESTIONNAIRE.

Please take a moment to fill in any questions you may have skipped.

0505

APPENDIX L

FOOD COMPOSITION TABLES

From Adams CF, and Richardson M. 1981. Nutritive value of foods, *Home and Garden Bulletin No. 72,* U.S. Department of Agriculture, Washington, D.C.: U.S. Government Printing Office.

Foods, Approximate Measures, Units, and Weight	(g)	Water (%)	Food Energy (cal)	Protein (g)	Fat (g)	Fatty Acids: Saturated (total) (g)	Fatty Acids: Unsaturated: Oleic (g)	Fatty Acids: Unsaturated: Linoleic (g)
Dairy products (cheese, cream, imitation cream, milk; related products)								
Cheese:								
Natural:								
Blue, 1 oz	28	42	100	6	8	5.3	1.9	.2
Camembert (3 wedges per 4 oz container), 1 wedge	38	52	115	8	9	5.8	2.2	.2
Cheddar:								
Cut pieces, 1 oz	28	37	115	7	9	6.1	2.1	.2
1 cu in	17.2	37	70	4	6	3.7	1.3	.1
Shredded, 1 cup	113	37	455	28	37	24.2	8.5	.7
Cottage (curd not pressed down):								
Creamed (cottage cheese, 4% fat):								
Large curd, 1 cup	225	79	235	28	10	6.4	2.4	.2
Small curd, 1 cup	210	79	220	26	9	6.0	2.2	.2
Low fat (2%), 1 cup	226	79	205	31	4	2.8	1.0	.1
Low fat (1%), 1 cup	226	82	165	28	2	1.5	.5	.1
Uncreamed (cottage cheese dry curd, less than ½% fat, 1 cup)	145	80	125	25	1	.4	.1	Tr
Cream, 1 oz	28	54	100	2	10	6.2	2.4	.2
Mozzarella, made with—								
Whole milk, 1 oz	28	48	90	6	7	4.4	1.7	.2
Part skim milk, 1 oz	28	49	80	8	5	3.1	1.2	.1
Parmesan, grated:								
Cup, not pressed down, 1 cup	100	18	455	42	30	19.1	7.7	.3
Tablespoon, 1 tbsp	5	18	25	2	2	1.0	.4	Tr
Ounce, 1 oz	28	18	130	12	9	5.4	2.2	.1
Provolone, 1 oz	28	41	100	7	8	4.8	1.7	.1
Ricotta, made with—								
Whole milk, 1 cup	246	72	430	28	32	20.4	7.1	.7
Part skim milk, 1 cup	246	74	340	28	19	12.1	4.7	.5
Romano, 1 oz	28	31	110	9	8	—	—	—
Swiss, 1 oz	28	37	105	8	8	5.0	1.7	.2
Pasteurized process cheese:								
American, 1 oz	28	39	105	6	9	5.6	2.1	.2
Swiss, 1 oz	28	42	95	7	7	4.5	1.7	.1

Blanks indicate no data available.
Tr. Trace.
For notes, see end of table.

Nutrients in Indicated Quantity

Carbohydrate (g)	Calcium (mg)	Phosophorus (mg)	Iron (mg)	Potassium (mg)	Vitamin A Value (IU)	Thiamin (mg)	Riboflavin (mg)	Niacin (mg)	Ascorbic Acid (mg)
1	150	110	.1	73	200	.01	.11	.3	0
Tr	147	132	.1	71	350	.01	.19	.2	0
Tr	204	145	.2	28	300	.01	.11	Tr	0
Tr	124	88	.1	17	180	Tr	.06	Tr	0
1	815	579	.8	111	1200	.03	.42	.1	0
6	135	297	.3	190	370	.05	.37	.3	Tr
6	126	277	.3	177	340	.04	.34	.3	Tr
8	155	340	.4	217	160	.05	.42	.3	Tr
6	138	302	.3	193	80	.05	.37	.3	Tr
3	46	151	.3	47	40	.04	.21	.2	0
1	23	30	.3	34	400	Tr	.06	Tr	0
1	163	117	.1	21	260	Tr	.08	Tr	0
1	207	149	.1	27	180	.01	.10	Tr	0
4	1376	807	1.0	107	700	.05	.39	.3	0
Tr	69	40	Tr	5	40	Tr	.02	Tr	0
1	390	229	.3	30	200	.01	.11	.1	0
1	214	141	.1	39	230	.01	.09	Tr	0
7	509	389	.9	257	1210	.03	.48	.3	0
13	669	449	1.1	308	1060	.05	.46	.2	0
1	302	215	—	—	160	—	.11	Tr	0
1	272	171	Tr	31	240	.01	.10	Tr	0
Tr	174	211	.1	46	340	.01	.10	Tr	0
1	219	216	.2	61	230	Tr	.08	Tr	0

Foods, Approximate Measures, Units, and Weight	(g)	Water (%)	Food Energy (cal)	Protein (g)	Fat (g)	Fatty Acids: Saturated (total) (g)	Fatty Acids: Unsaturated: Oleic (g)	Fatty Acids: Unsaturated: Linoleic (g)
Pasteurized process cheese food, American, 1 oz	28	43	95	6	7	4.4	1.7	.1
Pasteurized process cheese spread, American, 1 oz	28	48	80	5	6	3.8	1.5	.1
Cream, sweet:								
Half-and-half								
(cream and milk), 1 cup	242	81	315	7	28	17.3	7.0	.6
1 tbsp	15	81	20	Tr	2	1.1	.4	Tr
Light, coffee, or table, 1 cup	240	74	470	6	46	28.8	11.7	1.0
1 tbsp	15	74	30	Tr	3	1.8	.7	.1
Whipping, unwhipped (volume about double when whipped):								
Light, 1 cup	239	64	700	5	74	46.2	18.3	1.5
1 tbsp	15	64	45	Tr	5	2.9	1.1	.1
Heavy, 1 cup	238	58	820	5	88	54.8	22.2	2.0
1 tbsp	15	58	80	Tr	6	3.5	1.4	.1
Whipped topping								
(pressurized), 1 cup	60	61	155	2	13	8.3	3.4	.3
1 tbsp	3	61	10	Tr	1	.4	.2	Tr
Cream, sour, 1 cup	230	71	495	7	48	30.0	12.1	1.1
1 tbsp	12	71	25	Tr	3	1.6	.6	.1
Cream products, imitation (made with vegetable fat):								
Sweet:								
Creamers:								
Liquid (frozen), 1 cup	245	77	335	2	24	22.8	.3	Tr
1 tbsp	15	77	20	Tr	1	1.4	Tr	0
Powdered, 1 cup	94	2	515	5	33	30.6	.9	Tr
1 tsp	2	2	10	Tr	1	.7	Tr	0
Whipped topping:								
Frozen, 1 cup	75	50	240	1	19	16.3	1.0	.2
1 tbsp	4	50	15	Tr	1	.9	.1	Tr
Powdered, made with whole milk, 1 cup	80	67	150	3	10	8.5	.6	.1
1 tbsp	4	67	10	Tr	Tr	.4	Tr	Tr
Pressurized, 1 tbsp	4	60	10	Tr	1	.8	.1	Tr
Sour dressing (imitation sour cream) made with nonfat dry milk								
1 cup	235	75	415	8	39	31.2	4.4	1.1
1 tbsp	12	75	20	Tr	2	1.6	.2	.1
Milk:								
Fluid:								
Whole (3.3% fat), 1 cup	244	88	150	8	8	5.1	2.1	.2
Lowfat (2%):								
No milk solids added, 1 cup	244	89	120	8	5	2.9	1.2	.1

For notes, see end of table.

Nutrients in Indicated Quantity

Carbohydrate (g)	Calcium (mg)	Phosophorus (mg)	Iron (mg)	Potassium (mg)	Vitamin A Value (IU)	Thiamin (mg)	Riboflavin (mg)	Niacin (mg)	Ascorbic Acid (mg)
2	163	130	.2	79	260	.01	.13	Tr	0
2	159	202	.1	69	220	.01	.12	Tr	0
10	254	230	.2	314	260	.08	.36	.2	2
1	16	14	Tr	19	20	.01	.02	Tr	Tr
9	231	192	.1	292	1730	.08	.36	.1	2
1	14	12	Tr	18	110	Tr	.02	Tr	Tr
7	166	146	.1	231	2690	.06	.30	.1	1
Tr	10	9	Tr	15	170	Tr	.02	Tr	Tr
7	154	149	.1	179	3500	.05	.26	.1	1
Tr	10	9	Tr	11	220	Tr	.02	Tr	Tr
7	61	54	Tr	88	550	.02	.04	Tr	0
Tr	3	3	Tr	4	30	Tr	Tr	Tr	0
10	268	195	.1	331	1820	.08	.34	.2	2
1	14	10	Tr	17	90	Tr	.02	Tr	Tr
28	23	157	.1	467	220[1]	0	0	0	0
2	1	10	Tr	29	10[1]	0	0	0	0
52	21	397	.1	763	190[1]	0	.16[1]	0	0
1	Tr	8	Tr	16	Tr[1]	0	Tr[1]	0	0
17	5	6	.1	14	650[1]	0	0	0	0
1	Tr	Tr	Tr	1	30[1]	0	0	0	0
13	72	69	Tr	121	290[1]	.02	.09	Tr	1
1	4	3	Tr	6	10[1]	Tr	Tr	Tr	Tr
1	Tr	1	Tr	1	20[1]	0	0	0	0
11	266	205	.1	380	20[1]	.09	.38	.2	2
1	14	10	Tr	19	Tr	.01	.02	Tr	Tr
11	291	228	.1	370	310[2]	.09	.40	.2	2
12	297	232	.1	377	500	.10	.40	.2	2

Foods, Approximate Measures, Units, and Weight	(g)	Water (%)	Food Energy (cal)	Protein (g)	Fat (g)	Fatty Acids: Saturated (total) (g)	Unsaturated: Oleic (g)	Unsaturated: Linoleic (g)
Lowfat (1%)								
No milk solids added, 1 cup	244	90	100	8	3	1.6	.7	.1
Nonfat (skim):								
No milk solids added, 1 cup	245	91	85	8	Tr	.3	.1	Tr
Buttermilk, 1 cup	245	90	100	8	2	1.3	.5	Tr
Canned:								
Evaporated, unsweetened:								
Whole milk, 1 cup	252	74	340	17	19	11.6	5.3	0.4
Skim milk, 1 cup	255	79	200	19	1	.3	.1	Tr
Sweetened, condensed, 1 cup	306	27	980	24	27	16.8	6.7	.7
Dried:								
Buttermilk, 1 cup	120	3	465	41	7	4.3	1.7	.2
Nonfat instant:								
Envelope, net wt, 3.2 oz[5], 1 envelope	91	4	325	32	1	.4	.1	Tr
Cup[7], 1 cup	68	4	245	24	Tr	.3	.1	Tr
Milk beverages:								
Chocolate milk (commercial):								
Regular, 1 cup	250	82	210	8	8	5.3	2.2	.2
Lowfat (2%), 1 cup	250	84	180	8	5	3.1	1.3	.1
Lowfat (1%), 1 cup	250	85	160	8	3	1.5	.7	.1
Eggnog (commercial), 1 cup	254	74	340	10	19	11.3	5.0	.6
Malted milk, home-prepared with 1 cup of whole milk and 2 to 3 heaping tsp of malted milk powder (about ¾ oz):								
Chocolate, 1 cup of milk plus ¾ oz of powder	265	81	235	9	9	5.5	—	—
Natural, 1 cup of milk plus ¾ oz of powder	265	81	235	11	10	6.0	—	—
Shakes, thick:[8]								
Chocolate, container, net wt, 10.6 oz, 1 container	300	72	355	9	8	5.0	2.0	.2
Vanilla, container, net wt, 11 oz, 1 container	313	74	350	12	9	5.9	2.4	.2
Milk desserts, frozen:								
Ice cream:								
Regular (about 11% fat):								
Hardened, ½ gal	1064	61	2155	38	115	71.3	28.8	2.6
1 cup	133	61	270	5	14	8.9	3.6	.3
3 fl oz container	50	61	100	2	5	3.4	1.4	.1
Soft serve (frozen custard), 1 cup	173	60	375	7	23	13.5	5.9	.6

Nutrients in Indicated Quantity

For notes, see end of table.

Nutrients in Indicated Quantity

Carbohydrate (g)	Calcium (mg)	Phosophorus (mg)	Iron (mg)	Potassium (mg)	Vitamin A Value (IU)	Thiamin (mg)	Riboflavin (mg)	Niacin (mg)	Ascorbic Acid (mg)
12	300	235	.1	381	500	.10	.41	.2	2
12	302	247	.1	406	500	.09	.34	.2	2
12	285	219	.1	371	80[3]	.08	.38	.1	2
25	657	510	.5	764	610[3]	.12	.80	.5	5
29	738	497	.7	845	1000[4]	.11	.79	.4	3
166	868	775	.6	1136	1000[3]	.28	1.27	.6	8
59	1421	1119	.4	1910	260[3]	.47	1.90	1.1	7
47	1120	896	.3	1552	2160[6]	.38	1.59	.8	5
35	837	670	.2	1160	1610[6]	.28	1.19	.6	4
26	280	251	.6	417	3003	.09	.41	.3	2
26	284	254	.6	422	500	.10	.42	.3	2
26	287	257	.6	426	500	.10	.40	.2	2
34	330	278	.5	420	890	.09	.48	.3	4
29	304	265	.5	500	330	.14	.43	.7	2
27	347	307	.3	529	380	.20	.54	1.3	2
63	396	378	.9	672	260	.14	.67	.4	0
56	457	361	.3	572	360	.09	.61	.5	0
254	1406	1075	1.0	2052	4340	.42	2.63	1.1	6
32	176	134	.1	257	540	.05	.33	.1	1
12	66	51	Tr	96	200	.02	.12	.1	Tr
38	236	199	.4	338	790	.08	.45	.2	1

Foods, Approximate Measures, Units, and Weight	(g)	Water (%)	Food Energy (cal)	Protein (g)	Fat (g)	Fatty Acids: Saturated (total) (g)	Fatty Acids: Unsaturated: Oleic (g)	Fatty Acids: Unsaturated: Linoleic (g)
Rich (about 16% fat),								
hardened, ½ gal	1188	59	2805	33	190	118.3	47.8	4.3
1 cup	148	59	350	4	24	14.7	6.0	.5
Ice milk:								
Hardened								
(about 4.3% fat), ½ gal	1048	69	1470	41	45	28.1	11.3	1.0
1 cup	131	69	185	5	6	3.5	1.4	.1
Soft serve								
(about 2.6% fat), 1 cup	175	70	225	8	5	2.9	1.2	0.1
Sherbet								
(about 2% fat), ½ gal	1542	66	2160	17	31	19.0	7.7	.7
1 cup	193	66	270	2	4	2.4	1.0	.1
Milk desserts, other:								
Custard, baked, 1 cup	265	77	305	14	15	6.8	5.4	.7
Puddings:								
From home recipe:								
Starch base:								
Chocolate, 1 cup	260	66	385	8	12	7.6	3.3	.3
Vanilla (blancmange), 1 cup	255	76	285	9	10	6.2	2.5	.2
Tapioca cream, 1 cup	165	72	220	8	8	4.1	2.5	.5
From mix (chocolate) and milk:								
Regular (cooked), 1 cup	260	70	320	9	8	4.3	2.6	.2
Instant, 1 cup	260	69	325	8	7	3.6	2.2	.3
Yogurt:								
With added milk solids:								
Made with lowfat milk:								
Fruit-flavored[9], 1 container,								
net wt 8 oz	227	75	230	10	3	1.8	.6	.1
Plain, 1 container, net wt 8 oz	227	85	145	12	4	2.3	.8	.1
Made with nonfat milk,								
1 container, net wt 8 oz	227	85	125	13	Tr	.3	.1	Tr
Without added milk solids:								
Made with whole milk,								
1 container, net wt 8 oz	227	88	140	8	7	4.8	1.7	.1
Eggs								
Eggs, large (24 oz per dozen):								
Raw:								
Whole, without shell, 1 egg	50	75	80	6	6	1.7	2.0	.6
White, 1 white	33	88	15	3	Tr	0	0	0
Yolk, 1 yolk	17	49	65	3	6	1.7	2.1	.6
Cooked:								
Fried in butter, 1 egg	46	72	85	5	6	2.4	2.2	.6

For notes, see end of table.

Nutrients in Indicated Quantity

Carbohydrate (g)	Calcium (mg)	Phosophorus (mg)	Iron (mg)	Potassium (mg)	Vitamin A Value (IU)	Thiamin (mg)	Riboflavin (mg)	Niacin (mg)	Ascorbic Acid (mg)
256	1213	927	.8	1771	7200	.36	2.27	.9	5
32	151	115	.1	221	900	.04	.28	.1	1
232	1409	1035	1.5	2117	1710	.61	2.78	.9	6
29	176	129	.1	265	210	.08	.35	.1	1
38	274	202	.3	412	180	.12	.54	.2	1
469	827	594	2.5	1585	1480	.26	.71	1.0	31
59	103	74	.3	198	190	.03	.09	.1	4
29	297	310	1.1	387	930	.11	.50	.3	1
67	250	255	1.3	445	390	.05	.36	.3	1
41	298	232	Tr	352	410	.08	.41	.3	2
28	173	180	.7	223	480	.07	.30	.2	2
59	265	247	.8	354	340	.05	.39	.3	2
63	374	237	1.3	335	340	.08	.39	.3	2
42	343	269	.2	439	120[10]	.08	.40	.2	1
16	415	326	.2	531	150[10]	.10	.49	.3	2
17	452	355	.2	579	20[10]	.11	.53	.3	2
11	274	215	.1	351	280	.07	.32	.2	1
1	28	90	1.0	65	260	.04	.15	Tr	0
Tr	4	4	Tr	45	0	Tr	.09	Tr	0
Tr	26	86	.9	15	310	.04	.07	Tr	0
1	26	80	.9	58	290	.03	.13	Tr	0

Foods, Approximate Measures, Units, and Weight	(g)	Water (%)	Food Energy (cal)	Protein (g)	Fat (g)	Fatty Acids: Saturated (total) (g)	Unsaturated: Oleic (g)	Unsaturated: Linoleic (g)
Hard-cooked, shell removed, 1 egg	50	75	80	6	6	1.7	2.0	.6
Poached, 1 egg	50	74	80	6	6	1.7	2.0	.6
Scrambled (milk added) in butter; also omelet, 1 egg	64	76	95	6	7	2.8	2.3	.6
Fats, Oils; Related Products								
Butter:								
Regular (1 brick or 4 sticks per lb):								
Stick (½ cup), 1 stick	113	16	815	1	92	57.3	23.1	2.1
Tablespoon (about ⅛ stick), 1 tbsp	14	16	100	Tr	12	7.2	2.9	.3
Pat (1-in square, ⅓ in high; 90 per lb), 1 pat	5	16	35	Tr	4	2.5	1.0	.1
Whipped (6 sticks or two 8 oz containers per lb)								
Stick (½ cup), 1 stick	76	16	540	1	61	38.2	15.4	1.4
Tablespoon (about ⅛ stick), 1 tbsp	9	16	65	Tr	8	4.7	1.9	.2
Pat (1¼ in square, ⅓ in high; 120 per lb), 1 pat	4	16	25	Tr	3	1.9	.8	.1
Fats, cooking (vegetable shortenings), 1 cup	200	0	1770	0	200	48.8	88.2	48.4
1 tbsp	13	0	110	0	13	3.2	5.7	3.1
Lard 1 tbsp	13	0	115	0	13	5.1	5.3	1.3
Margarine:								
Regular (1 brick or 4 sticks per lb):								
Stick (½ cup), 1 stick	113	16	815	1	92	16.7	42.9	24.9
Tablespoon (about ⅛ stick), 1 tbsp	14	16	100	Tr	12	2.1	5.3	3.1
Pat (1-in square, ⅓ in high; 90 per lb), 1 pat	5	16	35	Tr	4	.7	1.9	1.1
Soft, two 8 oz containers per lb, 1 container	227	16	1635	1	184	32.5	71.5	65.4
1 tbsp	14	16	100	Tr	12	2.0	4.5	4.1
Whipped (6 sticks per lb):								
Stick (½ cup), 1 stick	76	16	545	Tr	61	11.2	28.7	16.7
Tablespoon (about ⅛ stick), 1 tbsp	9	16	70	Tr	8	1.4	3.6	2.1
Oils, salad or cooking:								
Corn, 1 cup	218	0	1925	0	218	27.7	53.6	125.1
1 tbsp	14	0	120	0	14	1.7	3.3	7.8

For notes, see end of table.

Nutrients in Indicated Quantity

Carbohydrate (g)	Calcium (mg)	Phosophorus (mg)	Iron (mg)	Potassium (mg)	Vitamin A Value (IU)	Thiamin (mg)	Riboflavin (mg)	Niacin (mg)	Ascorbic Acid (mg)
1	28	90	1.0	65	260	.04	.14	Tr	0
1	28	90	1.0	65	260	.04	.13	Tr	0
1	47	97	.9	85	310	.04	.16	Tr	0
Tr	27	26	.2	29	3470[11]	.01	.04	Tr	0
Tr	3	3	Tr	4	430[11]	Tr	Tr	Tr	0
Tr	1	1	Tr	1	150[11]	Tr	Tr	Tr	0
Tr	18	17	.1	20	2310[11]	Tr	.03	Tr	0
Tr	2	2	Tr	2	290[11]	Tr	Tr	Tr	0
Tr	1	1	Tr	1	120[11]	0	Tr	Tr	0
0	0	0	0	0	—	0	0	0	0
0	0	0	0	0	—	0	0	0	0
0	0	0	0	0	0	0	0	0	0
Tr	27	26	.2	29	3750[12]	.01	.04	Tr	0
Tr	3	3	Tr	4	470[12]	Tr	Tr	Tr	0
Tr	1	1	Tr	1	170[12]	Tr	Tr	Tr	0
Tr	53	53	.4	59	7500[12]	.01	.08	.1	0
Tr	3	3	Tr	4	470[12]	Tr	Tr	Tr	0
Tr	18	17	.1	20	2500[12]	Tr	.03	Tr	0
Tr	2	2	Tr	2	310[12]	Tr	Tr	Tr	0
0	0	0	0	0	—	0	0	0	0
0	0	0	0	0	—	0	0	0	0

Foods, Approximate Measures, Units, and Weight	(g)	Nutrients in Indicated Quantity							
						Fatty Acids			
						Saturated	Unsaturated		
		Water (%)	Food Energy (cal)	Protein (g)	Fat (g)	(total) (g)	Oleic (g)	Linoleic (g)	
Olive, 1 cup	216	0	1910	0	216	30.7	154.4	17.7	
1 tbsp	14	0	120	0	14	1.9	9.7	1.1	
Peanut, 1 cup	216	0	1910	0	216	37.4	98.5	67.0	
1 tbsp	14	0	120	0	14	2.3	6.2	4.2	
Safflower, 1 cup	218	0	1925	0	218	20.5	25.9	159.8	
1 tbsp	14	0	120	0	14	1.3	1.6	10.0	
Soybean oil, hydrogenated (partially hardened), 1 cup	218	0	1925	0	218	31.8	93.1	75.6	
1 tbsp	14	0	120	0	14	2.0	5.8	4.7	
Soybean-cottonseed oil blend hydrogenated, 1 cup	218	0	1925	0	218	38.2	63.0	99.6	
1 tbsp	14	0	120	0	14	2.4	3.9	6.2	
Salad dressings:									
Commercial:									
Blue cheese:									
Regular, 1 tbsp	15	32	75	1	8	1.6	1.7	3.8	
Low calorie (5 cal per tsp), 1 tbsp	16	84	10	Tr	1	.5	.3	Tr	
French:									
Regular, 1 tbsp	16	39	65	Tr	6	1.1	1.3	3.2	
Low calorie (5 cal per tsp), 1 tbsp	16	77	15	Tr	1	.1	.1	.4	
Italian:									
Regular, 1 tbsp	15	28	85	Tr	9	1.6	1.9	4.7	
Low calorie (5 cal per tsp), 1 tbsp	15	90	10	Tr	1	.1	.1	.4	
Mayonnaise, 1 tbsp	14	15	100	Tr	11	2.0	2.4	5.6	
Mayonnaise type:									
Regular, 1 tbsp	15	41	65	Tr	6	1.1	1.4	3.2	
Low calorie (8 cal per tsp), 1 tbsp	16	81	20	Tr	2	.4	.4	1.0	
Tartar sauce, regular, 1 tbsp	14	34	75	Tr	8	1.5	1.8	4.1	
Thousand Island:									
Regular, 1 tbsp	16	32	80	Tr	8	1.4	1.7	4.0	
Low calorie (10 cal per tsp), 1 tbsp	15	68	25	Tr	2	.4	.4	1.0	
From home recipe:									
Cooked type[13], 1 tbsp	16	68	25	1	2	.5	.6	.3	

Fish, Shellfish, Meat, Poultry, Related Products

Foods, Approximate Measures, Units, and Weight	(g)	Water (%)	Food Energy (cal)	Protein (g)	Fat (g)	Saturated (total) (g)	Oleic (g)	Linoleic (g)
Fish and shellfish:								
Bluefish, baked with butter or margarine, 3 oz	85	68	135	22	4	—	—	—

For notes, see end of table.

Nutrients in Indicated Quantity

Carbohydrate (g)	Calcium (mg)	Phosophorus (mg)	Iron (mg)	Potassium (mg)	Vitamin A Value (IU)	Thiamin (mg)	Riboflavin (mg)	Niacin (mg)	Ascorbic Acid (mg)
0	0	0	0	0	—	0	0	0	0
0	0	0	0	0	—	0	0	0	0
0	0	0	0	0	—	0	0	0	0
0	0	0	0	0	—	0	0	0	0
0	0	0	0	0	—	0	0	0	0
0	0	0	0	0	—	0	0	0	0
0	0	0	0	0	—	0	0	0	0
0	0	0	0	0	—	0	0	0	0
0	0	0	0	0	—	0	0	0	0
0	0	0	0	0	—	0	0	0	0
1	12	11	Tr	6	30	Tr	.02	Tr	Tr
1	10	8	Tr	5	30	Tr	.01	Tr	Tr
3	2	2	.1	13	—	—	—	—	—
2	2	2	.1	13	—	—	—	—	—
1	2	1	Tr	2	Tr	Tr	Tr	Tr	—
Tr	Tr	1	Tr	2	Tr	Tr	Tr	Tr	—
Tr	3	4	.1	5	40	Tr	.01	Tr	—
2	2	4	Tr	1	30	Tr	Tr	Tr	—
2	3	4	Tr	1	40	Tr	Tr	Tr	—
1	3	4	.1	11	30	Tr	Tr	Tr	Tr
2	2	3	.1	18	50	Tr	Tr	Tr	Tr
2	2	3	.1	17	50	Tr	Tr	Tr	Tr
2	14	15	.1	19	80	.01	.03	Tr	Tr
0	25	244	.6	—	40	.09	.08	1.6	—

Foods, Approximate Measures, Units, and Weight	(g)	Water (%)	Food Energy (cal)	Protein (g)	Fat (g)	Fatty Acids: Saturated (total) (g)	Unsaturated: Oleic (g)	Unsaturated: Linoleic (g)
Clams:								
Raw, meat only, 3 oz	85	82	65	11	1	—	—	—
Canned, solids and liquid, 3 oz	85	86	45	7	1	.2	Tr	Tr
Crabmeat (white or king), canned, not pressed, 1 cup down	135	77	135	24	3	.6	0.4	0.1
Fish sticks, breaded, cooked, frozen (stick, 4 × 1 fish stick or 1 × ½ in), 1 oz	28	66	50	5	3	—	—	—
Haddock, breaded, fried[14], 3 oz	85	66	140	17	5	1.4	2.2	1.2
Ocean perch, breaded, fried[14], 1 fillet	85	59	195	16	11	2.7	4.4	2.3
Oysters, raw, meat only (13-19 medium Selects) 1 cup	240	85	160	20	4	1.3	.2	.1
Salmon, pink, canned, solids and liquid, 3 oz	85	71	120	17	5	.9	.8	.1
Sardines, Atlantic, canned in oil, drained solids, 3 oz	85	62	175	20	9	3.0	2.5	.5
Scallops, frozen, breaded, fried, reheated, 6 scallops	90	60	175	16	8	—	—	—
Shad, baked with butter or margarine, bacon, 3 oz	85	64	170	20	10	—	—	—
Shrimp:								
Canned meat, 3 oz	85	70	100	21	1	.1	.1	Tr
French fried[16], 3 oz	85	57	190	17	9	2.3	3.7	2.0
Tuna, canned in oil, drained solids, 3 oz	85	61	170	24	7	1.7	1.7	.7
Tuna salad[17], 1 cup	205	70	350	30	22	4.3	6.3	6.7
Meat and meat products:								
Bacon (20 slices per lb, raw), broiled or fried, 2 slices crisp	15	8	85	4	8	2.5	3.7	.7
Beef, cooked:[18]								
Cuts braised, simmered, or pot roasted:								
Lean and fat (piece, 2½ × 2½ × ¾ in), 3 oz	85	53	245	23	16	6.8	6.5	.4
Lean only from item directly above, 2.5 oz	72	62	140	22	5	2.1	1.8	.2
Ground beef, broiled:								
Lean with 10% fat, 3 oz or patty 3 × ⅝ in	85	60	185	23	10	4.0	3.9	.3
Lean with 21% fat, 2.9 oz or patty 3 × ⅝ in	82	54	235	20	17	7.0	6.7	.4

For notes, see end of table.

Nutrients in Indicated Quantity

Carbohydrate (g)	Calcium (mg)	Phosophorus (mg)	Iron (mg)	Potassium (mg)	Vitamin A Value (IU)	Thiamin (mg)	Riboflavin (mg)	Niacin (mg)	Ascorbic Acid (mg)
2	59	138	5.2	154	90	.08	.15	1.1	8
2	47	116	3.5	119	—	.01	.09	.9	—
1	61	246	1.1	149	—	.11	.11	2.6	—
2	3	47	.1	—	0	.01	.02	.5	—
5	34	210	1.0	296	—	.03	.06	2.7	2
6	28	192	1.1	242	—	.10	.10	1.6	—
8	226	343	13.2	290	740	.34	.43	6.0	—
0	167[15]	243	.7	307	60	.03	.16	6.8	—
0	372	424	2.5	502	190	.02	.17	4.6	—
9	—	—	—	—	—	—	—	—	—
0	20	266	.5	320	30	.11	.22	7.3	—
1	96	224	2.6	104	50	.01	.03	1.5	—
9	61	162	1.7	195	—	.03	.07	2.3	—
0	7	199	1.6	—	70	.04	.10	10.1	—
7	41	291	2.7	—	590	.08	.23	10.3	2
Tr	2	34	.5	35	0	.08	.05	.8	—
0	10	114	2.9	184	30	.04	.18	3.6	—
0	10	108	2.7	176	10	.04	.17	3.3	—
0	10	196	3.0	261	20	.08	.20	5.1	—
0	9	159	2.6	221	30	.07	.17	4.4	—

		Nutrients in Indicated Quantity						
						Fatty Acids		
						Saturated	Unsaturated	
Foods, Approximate Measures, Units, and Weight	**(g)**	**Water (%)**	**Food Energy (cal)**	**Protein (g)**	**Fat (g)**	**(total) (g)**	**Oleic (g)**	**Linoleic (g)**
Roast, oven cooked, no liquid added:								
Relatively fat, such as rib:								
Lean and fat (2 pieces 4⅛ × 2¼ × ¼ in), 3 oz	85	40	375	17	33	14.0	13.6	.8
Lean only, 1.8 oz	51	57	125	14	7	3.0	2.5	.3
Relatively lean, such as heel of round:								
Lean and fat (2 pieces, 4⅛ × 2¼ × ¼ in), 3 oz	85	62	165	25	7	2.8	2.7	.2
Lean only, 2.8 oz	78	65	125	24	3	1.2	1.0	0.1
Steak:								
Relatively lean sirloin, broiled:								
Lean and fat (piece, 2½ × 2½ × ¾ in), 3 oz	85	44	330	20	27	11.3	11.1	6
Lean only, 2.0 oz	56	59	115	18	4	1.8	1.6	2
Relatively lean-round, braised:								
Lean and fat (piece, 4⅛ × 2¼ × ½ in) 3 oz	85	55	220	24	13	5.5	5.2	4
Lean only, 2.4 oz	68	61	130	21	4	1.7	1.5	2
Beef, canned:								
Corned beef, 3 oz	85	59	185	22	10	4.9	4.5	2
Corned beef hash, 1 cup	220	67	400	19	25	11.9	10.9	5
Beef, dried, chipped, 2½ oz jar	71	48	145	24	4	2.1	2.0	.1
Beef and vegetable stew, 1 cup	245	82	220	16	11	4.9	4.5	.2
Beef potpie (home recipe), baked (piece, ⅓ of 9-in diameter pie)[19], 1 piece	210	55	515	21	30	7.9	12.8	6.7
Chili con carne with beans, canned, 1 cup	255	72	340	19	16	7.5	6.8	.3
Chop suey with beef and pork (home recipe), 1 cup	250	75	300	26	17	8.5	6.2	.7
Heart, beef, lean, braised, 3 oz	85	61	160	27	5	1.5	1.1	.6
Lamb, cooked:								
Chop, rib (cut 3 per lb with bone), broiled:								
Lean and fat, 3.1 oz 89	43	360	18	32	14.8	12.1	1.2	
Lean only, 2 oz	57	60	120	16	6	2.5	2.1	.2
Leg, roasted:								
Lean and fat (2 pieces, 4⅛ × 2¼ × ¼ in), 3 oz	85	54	235	22	16	7.3	6.0	.6
Lean only, 2.5 oz	71	62	130	20	5	2.1	1.8	.2

For notes, see end of table.

Nutrients in Indicated Quantity									
Carbohydrate (g)	Calcium (mg)	Phosophorus (mg)	Iron (mg)	Potassium (mg)	Vitamin A Value (IU)	Thiamin (mg)	Riboflavin (mg)	Niacin (mg)	Ascorbic Acid (mg)
0	8	158	2.2	189	70	.05	.13	3.1	—
0	6	131	1.8	161	10	.04	.11	2.6	—
0	11	208	3.2	279	10	.06	.19	4.5	—
0	10	199	3.0	268	Tr	.06	.18	4.3	—
0	9	162	2.5	220	50	.05	.15	4.0	—
0	7	146	2.2	202	10	.05	.14	3.6	—
0	10	213	3.0	272	20	.07	.19	4.8	—
0	9	182	2.5	238	10	.05	.16	4.1	—
0	17	90	3.7	—	—	.01	.20	2.9	—
24	29	147	4.4	440	—	.02	.20	4.6	—
0	14	287	3.6	142	—	.05	.23	2.7	0
15	29	184	2.9	613	2400	.15	.17	4.7	17
39	29	149	3.8	334	1720	.30	.30	5.5	6
31	82	321	4.3	594	150	.08	.18	3.3	—
13	60	248	4.8	425	600	.28	.38	5.0	33
1	5	154	5.0	197	20	.21	1.04	6.5	1
0	8	139	1.0	200	—	.11	.19	4.1	—
0	6	121	1.1	174	—	.09	.15	3.4	—
0	9	177	1.4	241	—	.13	.23	4.7	—
0	9	169	1.4	227	—	.12	.21	4.4	—

Foods, Approximate Measures, Units, and Weight	(g)	Water (%)	Food Energy (cal)	Protein (g)	Fat (g)	Fatty Acids: Saturated (total) (g)	Fatty Acids: Unsaturated: Oleic (g)	Fatty Acids: Unsaturated: Linoleic (g)
Shoulder, roasted:								
Lean and fat (3 pieces, 2½ × 2½ × ¼ in), 3 oz	85	50	285	18	23	10.8	8.8	.9
Lean only, 2.3 oz	64	61	130	17	6	3.6	2.3	.2
Liver, beef, fried (slice, 6½ × 2⅜ × ⅜ in)[20], 3 oz	85	56	195	22	9	2.5	3.5	.9
Pork, cured, cooked:								
Ham, light cure, lean and fat, roasted (2 pieces, 4⅛ × 2¼ × ¼ in)[22], 3 oz	85	54	245	18	19	6.8	7.9	1.7
Luncheon meat:								
Boiled ham, slice (8 per 8 oz pkg), 1 oz	28	59	65	5	5	1.7	2.0	.4
Canned, spiced or unspiced:								
Slice, approx. 3 × 2 × ½ in, 1 slice	60	55	175	9	15	5.4	6.7	1.0
Pork, fresh, cooked:[18]								
Chop, loin (cut 3 per lb with bone), broiled:								
Lean and fat, 2.7 oz	78	42	305	19	25	8.9	10.4	2.2
Lean only, 2 oz	56	53	150	17	9	3.1	3.6	.8
Roast, oven cooked, no liquid added:								
Lean and fat (piece, 2½ × 2½ × ¾ in), 3 oz	85	46	310	21	24	8.7	10.2	2.2
Lean only, 2.4 oz	68	55	175	20	10	3.5	4.1	.8
Shoulder cut, simmered:								
Lean and fat (3 pieces, 2½ × 2½ × ¼ in), 3 oz	85	46	320	20	26	9.3	10.9	2.3
Lean only, 2.2 oz	63	60	135	18	6	2.2	2.6	.6
Sausages (see also Luncheon meat):								
Bologna, slice (8 per 8 oz pkg), 1 slice	28	56	85	3	8	3.0	3.4	.5
Braunschweiger, slice (6 per 6 oz pkg), 1 slice	28	53	90	4	8	2.6	3.4	.8
Brown and serve (10–11 per 8 oz pkg), browned, 1 link	17	40	70	3	6	2.3	2.8	.7
Deviled ham, canned, 1 tbsp	13	51	45	2	4	1.5	1.8	.4
Frankfurter (8 per 1 lb pkg), cooked (reheated), 1 frankfurter	56	57	170	7	15	5.6	6.5	1.2
Meat, potted (beef, chicken, turkey), canned, 1 tbsp	13	61	30	2	2	—	—	—
Pork link (16 per 1 lb pkg), cooked, 1 link	13	35	60	2	6	2.1	2.4	.5

For notes, see end of table.

Nutrients in Indicated Quantity

Carbohydrate (g)	Calcium (mg)	Phosphorus (mg)	Iron (mg)	Potassium (mg)	Vitamin A Value (IU)	Thiamin (mg)	Riboflavin (mg)	Niacin (mg)	Ascorbic Acid (mg)
0	9	146	1.0	206	—	.11	.20	4.0	—
0	8	140	1.0	193	—	.10	.18	3.7	—
5	9	405	7.5	323	45,390[21]	.22	3.56	14.0	23
0	8	146	2.2	199	0	.40	.15	3.1	—
0	3	47	.8	—	0	.12	.04	.7	—
1	5	65	1.3	133	0	.19	.13	1.8	—
0	9	209	2.7	216	0	.75	.22	4.5	—
0	7	181	2.2	192	0	.63	.18	3.8	—
0	9	218	2.7	233	0	.78	.22	4.8	—
0	9	211	2.6	224	0	.73	.21	4.4	—
0	9	118	2.6	158	0	.46	.21	4.1	—
0	8	111	2.3	146	0	.42	.19	3.7	—
Tr	2	36	.5	65	—	.05	.06	.7	—
1	3	69	1.7	—	1850	.05	.41	2.3	—
Tr	—	—	—	—	—	—	—	—	—
0	1	12	.3	—	0	.02	.01	.2	—
1	3	57	.8	—	—	.08	.11	1.4	—
0	—	—	—	—	—	Tr	.03	.2	—
Tr	1	21	.3	35	0	.10	.04	.5	—

Foods, Approximate Measures, Units, and Weight	(g)	Water (%)	Food Energy (cal)	Protein (g)	Fat (g)	Fatty Acids: Saturated (total) (g)	Unsaturated: Oleic (g)	Unsaturated: Linoleic (g)
Salami:								
Dry type, slice (12 per 4 oz pkg) 1 slice	10	30	45	2	4	1.6	1.6	.1
Cooked type, slice (8 per 8 oz pkg) 1 slice	28	51	90	5	7	3.1	3.0	.2
Vienna sausage (7 per 4 oz can) 1 sausage	16	63	40	2	3	1.2	1.4	.2
Veal, medium fat, cooked, bone removed:								
Cutlet (4⅛ × 2¼ × ½ in), braised or broiled, 3 oz	85	60	185	23	9	4.0	3.4	.4
Rib (2 pieces, 4⅛ × 2¼ × ¼ in), roasted, 3 oz	85	55	230	23	14	6.1	5.1	.6
Poultry and poultry products:								
Chicken, cooked:								
Breast, fried, bones removed, ½ breast (3.3 oz with bones)[23], 2.8 oz	79	58	160	26	5	1.4	1.8	1.1
Drumstick, fried, bones removed (2 oz with bones)[23], 1.3 oz	38	55	90	12	4	1.1	1.3	.9
Half broiler, broiled, bones removed (10.4 oz, 6.2 oz with bones)	176	71	240	42	7	2.2	2.5	1.3
Chicken, canned, boneless, 3 oz	85	65	170	18	10	3.2	3.8	2.0
Chicken a la king, cooked (home recipe), 1 cup	245	68	470	27	34	12.7	14.3	3.3
Chicken and noodles, cooked (home recipe), 1 cup	240	71	365	22	18	5.9	7.1	3.5
Chicken chow mein:								
Canned, 1 cup	250	89	95	7	Tr	—	—	—
From home recipe, 1 cup	250	78	255	31	10	2.4	3.4	3.1
Chicken potpie (home recipe), baked, piece (⅓ of 9-in diameter pie)[19] 1 piece	232	57	545	23	31	11.3	10.9	5.6
Turkey, roasted, flesh without skin:								
Dark meat, piece, 2½ × 1⅝ × ¼ in 4 pieces	85	61	175	26	7	2.1	1.5	1.5
Light meat, piece, 4 × 2 × ¼ in 2 pieces	85	62	150	28	3	.9	.6	.7
Light and dark meat:								
Chopped or diced, 1 cup	140	61	265	44	9	2.5	1.7	1.8
Pieces (1 slice white meat, 4 × 2 × ¼ in 3 pieces with 2 slices dark meat, 2½ × 1⅝ × ¼ in)	85	61	160	27	5	1.5	1.0	1.1

For notes, see end of table.

Nutrients in Indicated Quantity									
Carbohydrate (g)	Calcium (mg)	Phosophorus (mg)	Iron (mg)	Potassium (mg)	Vitamin A Value (IU)	Thiamin (mg)	Riboflavin (mg)	Niacin (mg)	Ascorbic Acid (mg)
Tr	1	28	.4	—	—	.04	.03	.5	—
Tr	3	57	.7	—	—	.07	.07	1.2	—
Tr	1	24	.3	—	—	.01	.02	.4	—
0	9	196	2.7	258	—	.06	.21	4.6	—
0	10	211	2.9	259	—	.11	.26	6.6	—
1	9	218	1.3	—	70	.04	.17	11.6	—
Tr	6	89	.9	—	50	.03	.15	2.7	—
0	16	355	3.0	483	160	.09	.34	15.5	—
0	18	210	1.3	117	200	.03	.11	3.7	3
12	127	358	2.5	404	1130	.10	.42	5.4	12
26	26	247	2.2	149	430	.05	.17	4.3	Tr
18	45	85	1.3	418	150	.05	.10	1.0	13
10	58	293	2.5	473	280	.08	.23	4.3	10
42	70	232	3.0	343	3090	.34	.31	5.5	5
0	—	—	2.0	338	—	.03	.20	3.6	—
0	—	—	1.0	349	—	.04	.12	9.4	—
0	11	351	2.5	514	—	.07	.25	10.8	—
0	7	213	1.5	312	—	.04	.15	6.5	—

Foods, Approximate Measures, Units, and Weight	(g)	Nutrients in Indicated Quantity: Water (%)	Food Energy (cal)	Protein (g)	Fat (g)	Fatty Acids: Saturated (total) (g)	Unsaturated: Oleic (g)	Linoleic (g)
Fruits and Fruit Products								
Apples, raw, unpeeled, without cores:								
2¾-in diameter (about 3 per lb with cores), 1 apple	138	84	80	Tr	1	—	—	—
3¼-in diameter (about 2 per lb with cores), 1 apple	212	84	125	Tr	1	—	—	—
Applejuice, bottled or canned[24], 1 cup	248	88	120	Tr	Tr	—	—	—
Applesauce, canned:								
Sweetened, 1 cup	255	76	230	1	Tr	—	—	—
Unsweetened, 1 cup	244	89	100	Tr	Tr	—	—	—
Apricots:								
Raw, without pits (about 12 per lb with pits), 3 apricots	107	85	55	1	Tr	—	—	—
Canned in heavy syrup (halves and syrup), 1 cup	258	77	220	2	Tr	—	—	—
Dried:								
Uncooked (28 large or 37 medium halves per cup, 1 cup)	130	25	340	7	1	—	—	—
Cooked, unsweetened, fruit and liquid, 1 cup	250	76	215	4	1	—	—	—
Apricot nectar, canned, 1 cup	251	85	145	1	Tr	—	—	—
Avocados, raw, whole, without skins and seeds:								
California, mid- and late-winter (with skin and seed, 3⅛-in diameter; wt 10 oz) 1 avocado	216	74	370	5	37	5.5	22.0	3.7
Florida, late summer and fall (with skin and seed, 3⅝-in diameter; wt 1 lb) 1 avocado	304	78	390	4	33	6.7	15.7	5.3
Banana without peel (about 2.6 per lb with peel) 1 banana	119	76	100	1	Tr	—	—	—
Banana flakes 1 tbsp	6	3	20	Tr	Tr	—	—	—
Blackberries, raw 1 cup	144	85	85	2	1	—	—	—
Blueberries, raw 1 cup	145	83	90	1	1	—	—	—
Cantaloupe; see muskmelons								
Cherries:								
Sour (tart), red, pitted, canned, water pack 1 cup	244	88	105	2	Tr	—	—	—
Sweet, raw, without pits and stems 10 cherries	68	80	45	1	Tr	—	—	—
Cranberry juice cocktail, bottled, sweetened 1 cup	253	83	165	Tr	Tr	—	—	—

For notes, see end of table.

Nutrients in Indicated Quantity									
Carbohydrate (g)	Calcium (mg)	Phosophorus (mg)	Iron (mg)	Potassium (mg)	Vitamin A Value (IU)	Thiamin (mg)	Riboflavin (mg)	Niacin (mg)	Ascorbic Acid (mg)
20	10	14	.4	152	120	.04	.03	.1	6
31	15	21	.6	233	190	.06	.04	.2	8
30	15	22	1.5	250	—	.02	.05	.2	2[25]
61	10	13	1.3	166	100	.05	.03	.1	3[26]
26	10	12	1.2	190	100	.05	.02	.1	2[26]
14	18	25	.5	301	2890	.03	.04	.6	11
57	28	39	.8	604	4490	.05	.05	1.0	10
86	87	140	7.2	1273	14,170	.01	.21	4.3	16
54	55	88	4.5	795	7500	.01	.13	2.5	8
37	23	30	.5	379	2380	.03	.03	.5	36[26]
13	22	91	1.3	1303	630	.24	.43	3.5	30
27	30	128	1.8	1836	880	.33	.61	4.9	43
26	10	31	.8	440	230	.06	.07	.8	12
5	2	6	.2	92	50	.01	.01	.2	Tr
19	46	27	1.3	245	290	.04	.06	.6	30
22	22	19	1.5	117	150	.04	.09	.7	20
26	37	32	.7	317	1660	.07	.05	.5	12
12	15	13	.3	129	70	.03	.04	.3	7
42	13	8	.8	25	Tr	.03	.03	.1	81

Foods, Approximate Measures, Units, and Weight	(g)	Water (%)	Food Energy (cal)	Protein (g)	Fat (g)	Fatty Acids: Saturated (total) (g)	Fatty Acids: Unsaturated: Oleic (g)	Fatty Acids: Unsaturated: Linoleic (g)
Cranberry sauce, sweetened, canned, strained 1 cup	277	62	405	Tr	1	—	—	—
Dates:								
Whole, without pits, 10 dates	80	23	220	2	Tr	—	—	—
Chopped, 1 cup	178	23	490	4	1	—	—	—
Fruit cocktail, canned, in heavy syrup 1 cup	255	80	195	1	Tr	—	—	—
Grapefruit:								
Raw, medium, 3¾-in diameter (about 1 lb 1 oz):								
Pink or red, ½ grapefruit with peel[28]	241	89	50	1	Tr	—	—	—
White, ½ grapefruit with peel[28]	241	89	45	1	Tr	—	—	—
Canned, sections with syrup, 1 cup	254	81	180	2	Tr	—	—	—
Grapefruit juice:								
Raw, pink, red, or white 1 cup	246	90	95	1	Tr	—	—	—
Canned, white:								
Unsweetened, 1 cup	247	89	100	1	Tr	—	—	—
Sweetened, 1 cup	250	86	135	1	Tr	—	—	—
Frozen, concentrate, unsweetened:								
Undiluted, 6 fl oz can, 1 can	207	62	300	4	1	—	—	—
Diluted with 3 parts water by volume, 1 cup	247	89	100	1	Tr	—	—	—
Dehydrated crystals, prepared with water (1 lb yields about 1 gal), 1 cup	247	90	100	1	Tr	—	—	—
Grapes, European type (adherent skin), raw:								
Thompson seedless, 10 grapes	50	81	35	Tr	Tr	—	—	—
Tokay and Emperor, seeded types, 10 grapes[30]	60	81	40	Tr	Tr	—	—	—
Grapejuice:								
Canned or bottled, 1 cup	253	83	165	1	Tr	—	—	—
Frozen concentrate, sweetened:								
Undiluted, 6 fl oz can, 1 can	216	53	395	1	Tr	—	—	—
Diluted with 3 parts water by volume, 1 cup	250	86	135	1	Tr	—	—	—
Grape drink, canned, 1 cup	250	86	135	Tr	Tr	—	—	—
Lemon, raw, size 165, without peel and seeds (about 4 per lb with peels and seeds), 1 lemon	74	90	20	1	Tr	—	—	—

For notes, see end of table.

Nutrients in Indicated Quantity

Carbohydrate (g)	Calcium (mg)	Phosophorus (mg)	Iron (mg)	Potassium (mg)	Vitamin A Value (IU)	Thiamin (mg)	Riboflavin (mg)	Niacin (mg)	Ascorbic Acid (mg)
104	17	11	.6	83	60	.03	.03	.1	6
58	47	50	2.4	518	40	.07	.08	1.8	0
130	105	112	5.3	1153	90	.16	.18	3.9	0
50	23	31	1.0	411	360	.05	.03	1.0	5
13	20	20	.5	166	540	.05	.02	.2	44
12	19	19	.5	159	10	.05	.02	.2	44
45	33	36	.8	343	30	.08	.05	.5	76
23	22	37	.5	399	([29])	.10	.05	.5	93
24	20	35	1.0	400	20	.07	.05	.5	84
32	20	35	1.0	405	30	.08	.05	.5	78
72	70	124	.8	1250	60	.29	.12	1.4	286
24	25	42	.2	420	20	.10	.04	.5	96
24	22	40	.2	412	20	.10	.05	.5	91
9	6	10	.2	87	50	.03	.02	.2	2
10	7	11	.2	99	60	.03	.02	.2	2
42	28	30	.8	293	—	.10	.05	.5	Tr[25]
100	22	32	.9	255	40	.13	.22	1.5	32[31]
33	8	10	.3	85	10	.05	.08	.5	10[31]
35	8	10	.3	88	—	.03[32]	03[32]	.3	([32])
6	19	12	.4	102	10	03	01	.1	39

Foods, Approximate Measures, Units, and Weight	(g)	Water (%)	Food Energy (cal)	Protein (g)	Fat (g)	Fatty Acids: Saturated (total) (g)	Fatty Acids: Unsaturated: Oleic (g)	Fatty Acids: Unsaturated: Linoleic (g)
Lemon juice:								
Raw, 1 cup	244	91	60	1	Tr	—	—	—
Canned or bottled, unsweetened, 1 cup	244	92	55	1	Tr	—	—	—
Frozen, single strength, unsweetened, 1 can 6 fl oz can	183	92	40	1	Tr	—	—	—
Lemonade concentrate, frozen:								
Undiluted, 6 fl oz can, 1 can	219	49	425	Tr	Tr	—	—	—
Diluted with 4⅓ parts water by volume, 1 cup	248	89	105	Tr	Tr	—	—	—
Limeade concentrate, frozen:								
Undiluted, 6 fl oz can, 1 can	218	50	410	Tr	Tr	—	—	—
Diluted with 4⅓ parts water by volume, 1 cup	247	89	100	Tr	Tr	—	—	—
Limejuice:								
Raw, 1 cup	246	90	65	1	Tr	—	—	—
Canned, unsweetened, 1 cup	246	90	65	1	Tr	—	—	—
Muskmelons, raw, with rind, without seed cavity:								
Cantaloupe, orange-fleshed (with rind and seed cavity, 5-in diameter, 2⅓ lb), ½ melon with rind[33]	477	91	80	2	Tr	—	—	—
Honeydew (with rind and seed cavity, 6½-in diameter, 5¼ lb) ⅒ melon with rind[33]	226	91	50	1	Tr	—	—	—
Oranges, all commercial varieties, raw:								
Whole, 2⅝-in diameter, without peel and seeds (about 2½ per lb with peel and seeds), 1 orange	131	86	65	1	Tr	—	—	—
Sections without membranes, 1 cup	180	86	90	2	Tr	—	—	—
Orange juice:								
Raw, all varieties, 1 cup	248	88	110	2	Tr	—	—	—
Canned, unsweetened, 1 cup	249	87	120	2	Tr	—	—	—
Frozen concentrate:								
Undiluted, 6 fl oz can, 1 can	213	55	360	5	Tr	—	—	—
Diluted with 3 parts water by volume, 1 cup	249	87	120	2	Tr	—	—	—
Dehydrated crystals, prepared with water (1 lb yields about 1 gal), 1 cup	248	88	115	1	Tr	—	—	—

For notes, see end of table.

Nutrients in Indicated Quantity									
Carbohydrate (g)	Calcium (mg)	Phosophorus (mg)	Iron (mg)	Potassium (mg)	Vitamin A Value (IU)	Thiamin (mg)	Riboflavin (mg)	Niacin (mg)	Ascorbic Acid (mg)
20	17	24	.5	344	50	07	02	.2	112
19	17	24	.5	344	50	07	02	.2	102
13	13	16	.5	258	40	05	02	.2	81
112	9	13	.4	153	40	.05	06	7	66
28	2	3	.1	40	10	.01	02	.2	17
108	11	13	.2	129	Tr	.02	.02	.2	26
27	3	3	Tr	32	Tr	Tr	Tr	Tr	6
22	22	27	.5	256	20	.05	.02	.2	79
22	22	27	.5	256	20	.05	.02	.2	52
20	38	44	1.1	682	9240	.11	.08	1.6	90
11	21	24	.6	374	60	.06	.04	.9	34
16	54	26	.5	263	260	.13	.05	.5	66
22	74	36	.7	360	360	.18	.07	.7	90
26	27	42	.5	496	500	.22	.07	1.0	124
28	25	45	1.0	496	500	.17	.05	.7	100
87	75	126	.9	1500	1620	.68	.11	2.8	360
29	25	42	.2	503	540	.23	.03	.9	120
27	25	40	.5	518	500	.20	.07	1.0	109

Foods, Approximate Measures, Units, and Weight	(g)	Water (%)	Food Energy (cal)	Protein (g)	Fat (g)	Fatty Acids: Saturated (total) (g)	Unsaturated: Oleic (g)	Unsaturated: Linoleic (g)
Orange and grapefruit juice:								
Frozen concentrate:								
Undiluted, 6 fl oz can, 1 can	210	59	330	4	1	—	—	—
Diluted with 3 parts water by volume, 1 cup	248	88	110	1	Tr	—	—	—
Papayas, raw, ½-in cubes, 1 cup	140	89	55	1	Tr	—	—	—
Peaches:								
Raw:								
Whole, 2½-in diameter, peeled, pitted (about 4 per lb with peels and pits), 1 peach	100	89	40	1	Tr	—	—	—
Sliced, 1 cup	170	89	65	1	Tr	—	—	—
Canned, yellow-fleshed, solids and liquid (halves or slices):								
Syrup pack, 1 cup	256	79	200	1	Tr	—	—	—
Water pack, 1 cup	244	91	75	1	Tr	—	—	—
Dried:								
Uncooked, 1 cup	160	25	420	5	1	—	—	—
Cooked, unsweetened, halves and juice, 1 cup	250	77	205	3	1	—	—	—
Frozen, sliced, sweetened:								
10-oz container, 1 container	284	77	250	1	Tr	—	—	—
Cup, 1 cup	250	77	220	1	Tr	—	—	—
Pears:								
Raw, with skin, cored:								
Bartlett, 2½-in diameter (about 2½ per lb with cores and stems), 1 pear	164	83	100	1	1	—	—	—
Bosc, 2½-in diameter (about 3 per lb with cores and stems), 1 pear	141	83	85	1	1	—	—	—
D'Anjou, 3-in diameter (about 2 per lb with cores and stems), 1 pear	200	83	120	1	1	—	—	—
Canned, solids and liquid, heavy syrup pack, (halves or slices), 1 cup	255	80	195	1	1	—	—	—
Pineapple:								
Raw, diced, 1 cup	155	85	80	1	Tr	—	—	—
Canned, heavy syrup pack, solids and liquid:								
Crushed, chunks, tidbits, 1 cup	255	80	190	1	Tr	—	—	—
Slices and liquid:								
Large, 1 slice; 2¼ tbsp liquid	105	80	80	Tr	Tr	—	—	—
Medium, 1 slice; 1¼ tbsp liquid	58	80	45	Tr	Tr	—	—	—
Pineapple juice, unsweetened, canned, 1 cup	250	86	140	1	Tr	—	—	—

Nutrients in Indicated Quantity

For notes, see end of table.

Nutrients in Indicated Quantity

Carbohydrate (g)	Calcium (mg)	Phosophorus (mg)	Iron (mg)	Potassium (mg)	Vitamin A Value (IU)	Thiamin (mg)	Riboflavin (mg)	Niacin (mg)	Ascorbic Acid (mg)
78	61	99	.8	1308	800	.48	.06	2.3	302
26	20	32	.2	439	270	.15	.02	.7	102
14	28	22	.4	328	2450	.06	.06	.4	78
10	9	19	.5	202	1330[34]	.02	.05	1.0	7
16	15	32	.9	343	2260[34]	.03	.09	1.7	12
51	10	31	.8	333	1100	.03	.05	1.5	8
20	10	32	.7	334	1100	.02	.07	1.5	7
109	77	187	9.6	1520	6240	.02	.30	8.5	29
54	38	93	4.8	743	3050	.01	.15	3.8	5
64	11	37	1.4	352	1850	.03	.11	2.0	116[36]
57	10	33	1.3	310	1630	.03	.10	1.8	103[36]
25	13	18	.5	213	30	.03	.07	.2	7
22	11	16	.4	83	30	.03	.06	.1	6
31	16	22	.6	260	40	.04	.08	.2	8
50	13	18	.5	214	10	.03	.05	.3	3
21	26	12	.8	226	110	.14	.05	.3	26
49	28	13	.8	245	130	.20	.05	.5	18
20	12	5	.3	101	50	.06	.02	.2	7
11	6	3	.2	56	30	.05	.01	.1	4
34	38	23	.8	373	130	.13	.05	.5	80[27]

Foods, Approximate Measures, Units, and Weight	(g)	Water (%)	Food Energy (cal)	Protein (g)	Fat (g)	Fatty Acids: Saturated (total) (g)	Fatty Acids: Unsaturated: Oleic (g)	Fatty Acids: Unsaturated: Linoleic (g)
Plums:								
Raw, without pits:								
Japanese and hybrid (2⅛-in diameter, about 6½ per lb with pits)								
1 plum	66	87	30	Tr	Tr	—	—	—
Prune-type (1½-in diameter, about 15 per lb with pits), 1 plum	28	79	20	Tr	Tr	—	—	—
Canned, heavy syrup pack (Italian prunes), with pits and liquid:								
Cup, 1 cup[36]	272	77	215	1	Tr	—	—	—
Portion, 3 plums; 2¾ tbsp liquid[36]	140	77	110	1	Tr	—	—	—
Prunes, dried, "softenized," with pits:								
Uncooked, 4 extra large or 5 large prunes[36]	49	28	110	1	Tr	—	—	—
Cooked, unsweetened, all sizes, fruit and liquid, 1 cup[36]	250	66	255	2	1	—	—	—
Prune juice, canned or bottled 1 cup	256	80	195	1	Tr	—	—	—
Raisins, seedless:								
Cup, not pressed down, 1 cup	145	18	420	4	Tr	—	—	—
Packet, ½ oz (1½ tbsp), 1 packet	14	18	40	Tr	Tr	—	—	—
Raspberries, red:								
Raw, capped, whole, 1 cup	123	84	70	1	1	—	—	—
Frozen, sweetened, 10 oz container 1 container	284	74	280	2	1	—	—	—
Rhubarb, cooked, added sugar:								
From raw, 1 cup	270	63	380	1	Tr	—	—	—
From frozen, sweetened, 1 cup	270	63	385	1	1	—	—	—
Strawberries:								
Raw, whole berries, capped 1 cup	149	90	55	1	1	—	—	—
Frozen, sweetened:								
Sliced, 10 oz container 1 container	284	71	310	1	1	—	—	—
Whole, 1 lb container (about 1¾ cups), 1 container	454	76	415	2	1			
Tangerine, raw, 2⅜-in diameter, size 176, without peel (about 4 per lb with peels and seeds), 1 tangerine	86	87	40	1	Tr	—	—	—
Tangerine juice, canned, sweetened 1 cup	249	87	125	1	Tr	—	—	—
Watermelon, raw, 4 × 8 in wedge with rind and seeds (1/16 of 32⅔ lb melon, 10 × 16 in)								
1 wedge with rind and seeds	926	93	110	2	1	—	—	—

For notes, see end of table.

Nutrients in Indicated Quantity

Carbohydrate (g)	Calcium (mg)	Phosophorus (mg)	Iron (mg)	Potassium (mg)	Vitamin A Value (IU)	Thiamin (mg)	Riboflavin (mg)	Niacin (mg)	Ascorbic Acid (mg)
8	8	12	.3	112	160	.02	.02	.3	4
6	3	5	.1	48	80	.01	.01	.1	1
56	23	26	2.3	367	3130	.05	.05	1.0	5
29	12	13	1.2	189	1610	.03	.03	.5	3
29	22	34	1.7	298	690	.04	.07	.7	1
67	51	79	3.8	695	1590	.07	.15	1.5	2
49	36	51	1.8	602	—	.03	.03	1.0	5
112	90	146	5.1	1106	30	.16	.12	.7	1
11	9	14	.5	107	Tr	.02	.01	.1	Tr
17	27	27	1.1	207	160	.04	.11	1.1	31
70	37	48	1.7	284	200	.06	.17	1.7	60
97	211	41	1.6	548	220	.05	.14	.8	16
96	211	32	1.9	475	190	.05	.11	.5	16
13	31	31	1.5	244	90	.04	.10	.9	88
79	40	48	2.0	318	90	.06	.17	1.4	151
107	59	73	2.7	472	140	.09	.27	2.3	249
10	34	15	.3	108	360	.05	.02	.1	27
30	44	35	.5	440	1040	.15	.05	.2	54
27	30	43	2.1	426	2510	.13	.13	.9	30

Foods, Approximate Measures, Units, and Weight	(g)	Water (%)	Food Energy (cal)	Protein (g)	Fat (g)	Fatty Acids: Saturated (total) (g)	Unsaturated: Oleic (g)	Unsaturated: Linoleic (g)
Grain Products								
Bagel, 3-in diameter:								
Egg, 1 bagel	55	32	165	6	2	.5	.9	.8
Water, 1 bagel	55	29	165	6	1	.2	.4	.6
Barley, pearled, light, uncooked 1 cup	200	11	700	16	2	.3	.2	.8
Biscuits, baking powder, 2-in diameter (enriched flour, vegetable shortening):								
From home recipe, 1 biscuit	28	27	105	2	5	1.2	2.0	1.2
From mix, 1 biscuit	28	29	90	2	3	.6	1.1	.7
Breadcrumbs (enriched)[36]:								
Dry, grated, 1 cup	100	7	390	13	5	1.0	1.6	1.4
Soft; see White bread								
Breads:								
Boston brown bread, canned, slice, 3¼ × ½ in[36], 1 slice	45	45	95	2	1	.1	.2	.2
Cracked-wheat bread (¾ enriched wheat flour, ¼ cracked wheat)[36].								
Slice (18 per loaf), 1 slice	25	35	65	2	1	.1	.2	.2
French or Vienna bread, enriched[36] Slice:								
French (5 × 2½ × 1 in), 1 slice	35	31	100	3	1	.2	.4	.4
Vienna (4¾ × 4 × ½ in), 1 slice	25	31	75	2	1	.2	.3	.3
Italian bread enriched:								
Slice, 4½ × 3¼ × ¾ in, 1 slice	30	32	85	3	Tr	Tr	Tr	.1
Raisin bread, enriched[36]:								
Slice (18 per loaf), 1 slice	25	35	65	2	1	.2	.3	.2
Rye bread:								
American, light (⅔ enriched wheat flour, ⅓ rye flour):								
Slice (4¾ × 3¾ × 7⁄16 in), 1 slice	25	36	60	2	Tr	Tr	Tr	.1
Pumpernickel (⅔ rye flour, ⅓ enriched wheat flour):								
Slice (5 × 4 × ⅜ in), 1 slice	32	34	80	3	Tr	.1	Tr	.2
White bread, enriched[38]:								
Soft-crumb type[38]								
Slice (18 per loaf), 1 slice	25	36	70	2	1	.2	.3	.3
Slice, toasted, 1 slice	22	25	70	2	1	.2	.3	.3
Slice (22 per loaf), 1 slice	20	36	55	2	1	.2	.2	.2
Slice, toasted, 1 slice	17	25	55	2	1	.2	.2	.2
Slice (24 per loaf), 1 slice	28	36	75	2	1	.2	.3	.3
Slice, toasted, 1 slice	24	25	75	2	1	.2	.3	.3
Slice (28 per loaf), 1 slice	24	36	65	2	1	.2	.3	.2
Slice, toasted, 1 slice	21	25	65	2	1	.2	.3	.2
Cubes, 1 cup	30	36	80	3	1	.2	.3	.3
Crumbs, 1 cup	45	36	120	4	1	.3	.5	.5

For notes, see end of table.

Carbohydrate (g)	Calcium (mg)	Phosophorus (mg)	Iron (mg)	Potassium (mg)	Vitamin A Value (IU)	Thiamin (mg)	Riboflavin (mg)	Niacin (mg)	Ascorbic Acid (mg)
				Nutrients in Indicated Quantity					
28	9	43	1.2	41	30	.14	.10	1.2	0
30	8	41	1.2	42	0	.15	.11	1.4	0
158	32	378	4.0	320	0	.24	.10	6.2	0
13	34	49	.4	33	Tr	.08	.08	.7	Tr
15	19	65	.6	32	Tr	.09	.08	.8	Tr
73	122	141	3.6	152	Tr	.35	.35	4.8	Tr
21	41	72	.9	131	0[39]	.06	.04	.7	0
13	22	32	.5	34	Tr	.08	.06	.8	Tr
19	15	30	.8	32	Tr	.14	.08	1.2	Tr
14	11	21	.6	23	Tr	.10	.06	.8	Tr
17	5	23	.7	22	0	.12	.07	1.0	0
13	18	22	.6	58	Tr	.09	.06	.6	Tr
13	19	37	.5	36	0	.07	.05	.7	0
17	27	73	.8	145	0	.09	.07	.6	0
13	21	24	.6	26	Tr	.10	.06	.8	Tr
13	21	24	.6	26	Tr	.08	.06	.8	Tr
10	17	19	.5	21	Tr	.08	.05	.7	Tr
10	17	19	.5	21	Tr	.06	.05	.7	Tr
14	24	27	.7	29	Tr	.11	.07	.9	Tr
14	24	27	.7	29	Tr	.09	.07	.9	Tr
12	20	23	.6	25	Tr	.10	.06	.8	Tr
12	20	23	.6	25	Tr	.08	.06	.8	Tr
15	25	29	.8	32	Tr	.12	.07	1.0	Tr
23	38	44	1.1	47	Tr	.18	.11	1.5	Tr

Foods, Approximate Measures, Units, and Weight	(g)	Water (%)	Food Energy (cal)	Protein (g)	Fat (g)	Fatty Acids: Saturated (total) (g)	Unsaturated: Oleic (g)	Unsaturated: Linoleic (g)
Firm-crumb type[38]								
Slice (20 per loaf), 1 slice	23	35	65	2	1	.2	.3	.3
Slice, toasted, 1 slice	20	24	65	2	1	.2	.3	.3
Slice (34 per loaf), 1 slice	27	35	75	2	1	.2	.3	.3
Slice, toasted, 1 slice	23	24	75	2	1	.2	.3	.3
Whole-wheat bread:								
Soft-crumb type:								
Slice (16 per loaf), 1 slice	28	36	65	3	1	.1	.2	.2
Slice, toasted, 1 slice	24	24	65	3	1	.1	.2	.2
Firm-crumb type:								
Slice (18 per loaf), 1 slice	25	36	60	3	1	.1	.2	.3
Slice, toasted, 1 slice	21	24	60	3	1	.1	.2	.3
Breakfast cereals:								
Hot type, cooked:								
Corn (hominy) grits, degermed:								
Enriched, 1 cup	245	87	125	3	Tr	Tr	Tr	.1
Unenriched, 1 cup	245	87	125	3	Tr	Tr	Tr	.1
Farina, quick-cooking, enriched 1 cup	245	89	105	3	Tr	Tr	Tr	.1
Oatmeal or rolled oats, 1 cup	240	87	130	5	2	.4	.8	.9
Wheat, rolled, 1 cup	240	80	180	5	1	—	—	—
Wheat, whole-meal, 1 cup	245	88	110	4	1	—	—	—
Ready-to-eat:								
Bran flakes (40% bran), added sugar, salt, iron, vitamins, 1 cup	35	3	105	4	1	—	—	—
Bran flakes with raisins, added sugar, salt, 1 cup iron, vitamins, 1 cup	50	7	145	4	1	—	—	—
Corn flakes:								
Plain, added sugar, salt, iron, vitamins, 1 cup	25	4	95	2	Tr	—	—	—
Sugar-coated, added salt, iron, vitamins, 1 cup	40	2	155	2	Tr	—	—	—
Corn, oat flour, puffed, added sugar, salt, iron, vitamins, 1 cup	20	4	80	2	1	—	—	—
Corn, shredded, added sugar, salt, iron, thiamin, niacin, 1 cup	25	3	95	2	Tr	—	—	—
Oats, puffed, added sugar, salt, minerals, vitamins, 1 cup	25	3	100	3	1	—	—	—
Rice, puffed:								
Plain, added iron, thiamin, niacin, 1 cup	15	4	60	1	Tr	—	—	—
Presweetened, added salt, iron, vitamins, 1 cup	28	3	115	1	0	—	—	—

For notes, see end of table.

Nutrients in Indicated Quantity

Carbohydrate (g)	Calcium (mg)	Phosophorus (mg)	Iron (mg)	Potassium (mg)	Vitamin A Value (IU)	Thiamin (mg)	Riboflavin (mg)	Niacin (mg)	Ascorbic Acid (mg)
12	22	23	.6	28	Tr	.09	.06	.8	Tr
12	22	23	.6	28	Tr	.07	.06	.8	Tr
14	26	28	.7	33	Tr	.11	.06	.9	Tr
14	26	28	.7	33	Tr	.09	.06	.9	Tr
14	24	71	.8	72	Tr	.09	.03	.8	Tr
14	24	71	.8	72	Tr	.07	.03	.8	Tr
12	25	57	.8	68	Tr	.06	.03	.7	Tr
12	25	27	.8	68	Tr	.05	.03	.7	Tr
27	2	25	.7	27	Tr[40]	.10	.07	1.0	0
27	2	25	.2	27	Tr[40]	.05	.02	.5	0
22	147	113[41]	([42])	25	0	.12	.07	1.0	0
23	22	137	1.4	146	0	.19	.05	.2	0
41	19	182	1.7	202	0	.17	.07	2.2	0
23	17	127	1.2	118	0	.15	.05	1.5	0
28	19	125	5.6	137	1540	.46	.52	6.2	0
40	28	146	7.9	154	2200[43]	([44])	([44])	([44])	0
21	([44])	9	([44])	30	([44])	([44])	([44])	([44])	13[45]
37	1	10	([44])	27	1760	.53	.60	7.1	21[45]
16	4	18	5.7	—	880	.26	.30	3.5	11
22	1	10	.6	—	0	.33	.05	4.4	13
19	44	102	4.0	—	1100	.33	.38	4.4	13
13	3	14	.3	15	0	.07	.01	.7	0
26	3	14	([44])	43	1240[45]	([44])	([44])	([44])	15[45]

Foods, Approximate Measures, Units, and Weight	(g)	Water (%)	Food Energy (cal)	Protein (g)	Fat (g)	Fatty Acids: Saturated (total) (g)	Fatty Acids: Unsaturated Oleic (g)	Fatty Acids: Unsaturated Linoleic (g)
Wheat flakes, added sugar, salt, iron, vitamins, 1 cup	30	4	105	3	Tr	—	—	—
Wheat, puffed:								
Plain, added iron, thiamin, niacin, 1 cup	15	3	55	2	Tr	—	—	—
Presweetened, added salt, iron, vitamins, 1 cup	38	3	140	3	Tr	—	—	—
Wheat, shredded, plain, 1 oblong biscuit or ½ cup spoon-size biscuits	25	7	90	2	1	—	—	—
Wheat germ, without salt and sugar, toasted, 1 tbsp	6	4	25	2	1	—	—	—
Buckwheat flour, light, sifted, 1 cup	98	12	340	6	1	.2	.4	.4
Bulgur, canned, seasoned, 1 cup	135	56	245	8	4	—	—	—
Cake icings; see Sugars and sweets								
Cakes made from cake mixes with enriched flour[46]:								
Angelfood:								
Piece, 1/12 of cake, 1 piece	53	34	135	3	Tr	—	—	—
Coffeecake:								
Piece, 1/6 of cake, 1 piece	72	30	230	5	7	2.0	2.7	1.5
Cupcakes, made with egg, milk, 2½-in diameter:								
Without icing, 1 cupcake	25	26	90	1	3	.8	1.2	.7
With chocolate icing, 1 cupcake	36	22	130	2	5	2.0	1.6	.6
Devil's food with chocolate icing:								
Piece, 1/16 of cake, 1 piece	69	24	235	3	8	3.1	2.8	1.1
Cupcake, 2½-in diameter 1 cupcake	35	24	120	2	4	1.6	1.4	.5
Gingerbread:								
Piece, 1/9 of cake, 1 piece	63	37	175	2	4	1.1	1.8	1.1
White, 2 layer with chocolate icing:								
Piece, 1/16 of cake, 1 piece	71	21	250	3	8	2.0	2.9	1.2
Yellow, 2 layer with chocolate icing:								
Piece, 1/16 of cake, 1 piece	69	26	235	3	8	3.0	3.0	1.3
Cakes made from home recipes using enriched flour[47]:								
Boston cream pie with custard filling:								
Whole cake (8-in diameter), 1 cake	825	35	2490	41	78	23.0	30.1	15.2
Piece, 1/12 of cake, 1 piece	69	35	210	3	6	1.9	2.5	1.3
Fruitcake, dark:								
Slice, 1/30 of loaf, 1 slice	15	18	55	1	2	.5	1.1	.5
Plain, sheet cake:								
Without icing:								
Whole cake (9-in sq), 1 cake	777	25	2830	35	108	29.5	44.4	23.9
Piece, 1/9 of cake, 1 piece	86	25	315	4	12	3.3	4.9	2.6

For notes, see end of table.

Nutrients in Indicated Quantity									
Carbohydrate (g)	Calcium (mg)	Phosophorus (mg)	Iron (mg)	Potassium (mg)	Vitamin A Value (IU)	Thiamin (mg)	Riboflavin (mg)	Niacin (mg)	Ascorbic Acid (mg)
24	12	83	4.8	81	1320	.40	.45	5.3	16
12	4	48	.6	51	0	.08	.03	1.2	0
33	7	52	([44])	63	1680	.50	.57	6.7	20[45]
20	11	97	.9	87	0	.06	.03	1.1	0
3	3	70	.5	57	10	.11	.05	.3	1
78	11	86	1.0	314	0	.08	.04	.4	0
44	27	263	1.9	151	0	.06	.05	4.1	0
32	50	63	.2	32	0	.03	.08	.3	0
38	44	125	1.2	78	120	.14	.15	1.3	Tr
14	40	59	.3	21	40	.05	.05	.4	Tr
21	47	71	.4	42	60	.05	.06	.4	Tr
40	41	72	1.0	90	100	.07	.10	.6	Tr
20	21	37	.5	46	50	.03	.05	.3	Tr
32	57	63	.9	173	Tr	.09	.11	.8	Tr
45	70	127	.7	82	40	.09	.11	.8	Tr
40	63	126	.8	75	100	.08	.10	.7	Tr
412	553	833	8.2	734[48]	1730	1.04	1.27	9.6	2
34	46	70	.7	61[48]	140	.09	.11	.8	Tr
9	11	17	.4	74	20	.02	.02	.2	Tr
434	497	793	8.5	614[48]	1320	1.21	1.40	10.2	2
48	55	88	.9	68[48]	150	.13	.15	1.1	Tr

Foods, Approximate Measures, Units, and Weight	(g)	Water (%)	Food Energy (cal)	Protein (g)	Fat (g)	Fatty Acids: Saturated (total) (g)	Unsaturated: Oleic (g)	Unsaturated: Linoleic (g)
With uncooked white icing:								
Piece, ⅙ of cake, 1 piece	121	21	445	4	14	4.7	5.5	2.7
Pound[49]:								
Loaf, 8½ × 3½ × 3¼ in, 1 loaf	565	16	2725	31	170	42.9	73.1	39.6
Slice, 1/17 of loaf, 1 slice	33	16	160	2	10	2.5	4.3	2.3
Spongecake:								
Whole cake (9¾-in diameter tube cake), 1 cake	790	32	2345	60	45	13.1	15.8	5.7
Piece, 1/12 of cake, 1 piece	66	32	195	5	4	1.1	1.3	.5
Cookies made with enriched flour[50,51]:								
Brownies with nuts:								
Home-prepared, 1¾ × 1¾ × ⅞ in:								
From home recipe, 1 brownie	20	10	95	1	6	1.5	3.0	1.2
From commercial recipe, 1 brownie	20	11	85	1	4	.9	1.4	1.3
Frozen, with chocolate icing, 1½ × 1¾ × ⅞ in[52], 1 brownie	25	13	105	1	5	2.0	2.2	.7
Chocolate chip:								
Commercial, 2¼-in diameter, ⅜ in thick, 4 cookies	42	3	200	2	9	2.8	2.9	2.2
From home recipe, 2⅓-in diameter, 4 cookies	40	3	205	2	12	3.5	4.5	2.9
Fig bars, square (1⅝ × 1⅝ × ⅜ in) or rectangular (1½ × 1¾ × ½ in), 4 cookies	56	14	200	2	3	.8	1.2	.7
Gingersnaps, 2-in diameter, ¼ in thick, 4 cookies	28	3	90	2	2	.7	1.0	.6
Macaroons, 2¾-in diameter, ¼ in thick, 2 cookies	38	4	180	2	9	—	—	—
Oatmeal with raisins, 2⅝-in diameter, ¼ in thick, 4 cookies	52	3	235	3	8	2.0	3.3	2.0
Plain, prepared from commercial chilled dough, 2½-in diameter, ¼ in thick, 4 cookies	48	5	240	2	12	3.0	5.2	2.9
Sandwich type (chocolate or vanilla), 1¾-in diameter, ⅜ in thick, 4 cookies	40	2	200	2	9	2.2	3.9	2.2
Vanilla wafers, 1¾-in diameter, ¼ in thick, 10 cookies	40	3	185	2	6	—	—	—
Cornmeal								
Whole-ground, unbolted, dry form, 1 cup	122	12	435	11	5	.5	1.0	2.5
Bolted (nearly whole-grain), dry form, 1 cup	122	12	440	11	4	.5	.9	2.1

For notes, see end of table.

Nutrients in Indicated Quantity

Carbohydrate (g)	Calcium (mg)	Phosophorus (mg)	Iron (mg)	Potassium (mg)	Vitamin A Value (IU)	Thiamin (mg)	Riboflavin (mg)	Niacin (mg)	Ascorbic Acid (mg)
77	61	91	.8	74	240	.14	.16	1.1	Tr
273	107	418	7.9	345	1410	.90	.99	7.3	0
16	6	24	.5	20	80	.05	.06	.4	0
427	237	885	13.4	687	3560	1.10	1.64	7.4	0
36	20	74	1.1	57	300	.09	.14	.6	Tr
10	8	30	.4	38	40	.04	.03	.2	Tr
13	9	27	.4	34	20	.03	.02	.2	Tr
15	10	31	.4	44	50	.03	.03	.2	Tr
29	16	48	1.0	56	50	.10	.17	.9	Tr
24	14	40	.8	47	40	.06	.06	.5	Tr
42	44	34	1.0	111	60	.04	.14	.9	Tr
22	20	13	.7	129	20	.08	.06	.7	0
25	10	32	.3	176	0	.02	.06	.2	0
38	11	53	1.4	192	30	.15	.10	1.0	Tr
31	17	35	.6	23	30	.10	.06	.9	0
28	10	96	.7	15	0	.06	.10	.7	0
30	16	25	.6	29	50	.10	.09	.8	0
90	24	312	2.9	346	620[53]	.46	.13	2.4	0
91	21	272	2.2	303	590[53]	.37	.10	2.3	0

Foods, Approximate Measures, Units, and Weight	(g)	Water (%)	Food Energy (cal)	Protein (g)	Fat (g)	Fatty Acids: Saturated (total) (g)	Unsaturated: Oleic (g)	Unsaturated: Linoleic (g)
Degermed, enriched:								
Dry form, 1 cup	138	12	500	11	2	.2	.4	.9
Cooked, 1 cup	240	88	120	3	Tr	Tr	.1	.2
Degermed, unenriched:								
Dry form, 1 cup	138	12	500	11	2	.2	.4	.9
Cooked, 1 cup	240	88	120	3	Tr	Tr	.1	.2
Crackers[36]:								
Graham, plain, 2½-in square, 2 crackers	14	6	55	1	1	.3	.5	.3
Rye wafers, whole-grain, 1⅞ × 3½ in, 2 wafers	13	6	45	2	Tr	—	—	—
Saltines, made with enriched flour, 4 crackers or 1 packet	11	4	50	1	1	.3	.5	.4
Danish pastry (enriched flour), plain without fruit or nuts[54]:								
Round piece, about 4¼-in diameter × 1 in, 1 pastry	65	22	275	5	15	4.7	6.1	3.2
Ounce, 1 oz	28	22	120	2	7	2.0	2.7	1.4
Doughnuts, made with enriched flour[36]:								
Cake type, plain, 2½-in diameter, 1 in high, 1 doughnut	25	24	100	1	5	1.2	2.0	1.1
Yeast-leavened, glazed, 3¾-in diameter, 1 ¼ in high, 1 doughnut	50	26	205	3	11	3.3	5.8	3.3
Macaroni, enriched, cooked (cut lengths, elbows, shells):								
Firm stage (hot), 1 cup	130	64	190	7	1	—	—	—
Tender stage:								
Cold macaroni, 1 cup	105	73	115	4	Tr	—	—	—
Hot macaroni, 1 cup	140	73	155	5	1	—	—	—
Macaroni (enriched) and cheese[56]:								
Canned, 1 cup	240	80	230	9	10	4.2	3.1	1.4
From home recipe (served hot)[56], 1 cup	200	58	430	17	22	8.9	8.8	2.9
Muffins made with enriched flour[38]:								
From home recipe:								
Blueberry, 2⅜-in diameter, 1½ in high, 1 muffin	40	39	110	3	4	1.1	1.4	.7
Bran, 1 muffin	40	35	105	3	4	1.2	1.4	.8
Corn (enriched degermed cornmeal and flour), 2⅜-in diameter, 1½ in high, 1 muffin	40	33	125	3	4	1.2	1.6	.9
Plain, 3-in diameter, 1½ in high, 1 muffin	40	38	120	3	4	1.0	1.7	1.0
From mix, egg, milk:								
Corn, 2⅜-in diameter, 1 ½ in high[58], 1 muffin	40	30	130	3	4	1.2	1.7	.9

For notes, see end of table.

Nutrients in Indicated Quantity

Carbohydrate (g)	Calcium (mg)	Phosophorus (mg)	Iron (mg)	Potassium (mg)	Vitamin A Value (IU)	Thiamin (mg)	Riboflavin (mg)	Niacin (mg)	Ascorbic Acid (mg)
108	8	137	4.0	166	610[53]	.61	.36	4.8	0
26	2	34	1.0	38	140[53]	.14	.10	1.2	0
108	8	137	1.5	166	610[53]	.19	.07	1.4	0
26	2	34	.5	38	140[53]	.05	.02	.2	0
10	6	21	.5	55	0	.02	.08	.5	0
10	7	50	.5	78	0	.04	.03	.2	0
8	2	10	.5	13	0	.05	.05	.4	0
30	33	71	1.2	73	200	.18	.19	1.7	Tr
13	14	31	.5	32	90	.08	.08	.7	Tr
13	10	48	.4	23	20	.05	.05	.4	Tr
22	16	33	.6	34	25	.10	.10	.8	0
39	14	85	1.4	103	0	.23	.13	1.8	0
24	8	53	9	64	0	.15	.08	1.2	0
32	11	70	1.3	85	0	.20	.11	1.5	0
26	199	182	1.0	139	260	.12	.24	1.0	Tr
40	362	322	1.8	240	860	.20	.40	1.8	Tr
17	34	53	.6	46	90	.09	.10	.7	Tr
17	57	162	1.5	172	90	.07	.10	1.7	Tr
19	42	68	7	54	120[57]	.10	.10	.7	Tr
17	42	60	6	50	40	.09	.12	.9	Tr
20	96	152	.6	44	100[57]	.08	.09	.7	Tr

Foods, Approximate Measures, Units, and Weight	(g)	Water (%)	Food Energy (cal)	Protein (g)	Fat (g)	Fatty Acids: Saturated (total) (g)	Fatty Acids: Unsaturated Oleic (g)	Fatty Acids: Unsaturated Linoleic (g)
Noodles (egg noodles), enriched, cooked, 1 cup	160	71	200	7	2	—	—	—
Noodles, chow mein, canned, 1 cup	45	1	220	6	11	—	—	—
Pancakes (4-in diameter)[36]:								
Buckwheat, made from mix (with buckwheat and enriched flour), egg and milk added, 1 cake	27	58	55	2	2	.8	.9	.4
Plain:								
Made from home recipe using enriched flour, 1 cake	27	50	60	2	2	.5	.8	.5
Made from mix with enriched flour, egg and milk added, 1 cake	27	51	60	2	2	.7	.7	.3
Pies, piecrust made with enriched flour, vegetable shortening (9-in diameter):								
Apple:								
Sector, ⅐ of pie, 1 sector	135	48	345	3	15	3.9	6.4	3.6
Banana cream:								
Sector, ⅐ of pie, 1 sector	130	54	285	6	12	3.8	4.7	2.3
Blueberry:								
Sector, ⅐ of pie, 1 sector	135	51	325	3	15	3.5	6.2	3.6
Cherry:								
Sector, ⅐ of pie, 1 sector	135	47	350	4	15	4.0	6.4	3.6
Custard:								
Sector, ⅐ of pie, 1 sector	130	58	285	8	14	4.8	5.5	2.5
Lemon meringue:								
Sector, ⅐ of pie, 1 sector	120	47	305	4	12	3.7	4.8	2.3
Mince:								
Sector ⅐ of pie, 1 sector	135	43	365	3	16	4.0	6.6	3.6
Peach:								
Sector ⅐ of pie, 1 sector	135	48	345	3	14	3.5	6.2	3.6
Pecan:								
Sector ⅐ of pie, 1 sector	118	20	495	6	27	4.0	14.4	6.3
Pumpkin:								
Sector ⅐ of pie, 1 sector	130	59	275	5	15	5.4	5.4	2.4
Piecrust (home recipe) made with enriched flour vegetable shortening, baked, and 1 pie shell, 9-in diameter	180	15	900	11	60	14.8	26.1	14.9
Pizza (cheese) baked, 4¾-in sector; ⅛ of 12-in diameter pie[19], 1 sector	60	45	145	6	4	1.7	1.5	0.6
Popcorn, popped:								
Plain, large kernel, 1 cup	6	4	25	1	Tr	Tr	.1	.2
With oil (coconut) and salt added, large kernel, 1 cup	9	3	40	1	2	1.5	.2	.2
Sugar coated, 1 cup	35	4	135	2	1	.5	.2	.4

For notes, see end of table.

Nutrients in Indicated Quantity

Carbohydrate (g)	Calcium (mg)	Phosophorus (mg)	Iron (mg)	Potassium (mg)	Vitamin A Value (IU)	Thiamin (mg)	Riboflavin (mg)	Niacin (mg)	Ascorbic Acid (mg)
37	16	94	1.4	70	110	.22	.13	1.9	0
26	—	—	—	—	—	—	—	—	—
6	59	91	4	66	60	.04	.05	.2	Tr
9	27	38	.4	33	30	.06	.07	.5	Tr
9	58	70	.3	42	70	.04	.06	.2	Tr
51	11	30	.9	108	40	.15	.11	1.3	2
40	86	107	1.0	264	330	.11	.22	1.0	1
47	15	31	1.4	88	40	.15	.11	1.4	4
52	19	34	.9	142	590	.16	.12	1.4	Tr
30	125	147	1.2	178	300	.11	.27	.8	0
45	17	59	1.0	60	200	.09	.12	.7	4
56	38	51	1.9	240	Tr	.14	.12	1.4	1
52	14	39	1.2	201	990	.15	.14	2.0	4
61	55	122	3.7	145	190	.26	.14	1.0	Tr
32	66	90	1.0	208	3210	.11	.18	1.0	Tr
79	25	90	3.1	89	0	.47	.40	5.0	0
22	86	89	1.1	67	230	.16	.18	1.6	4
5	1	17	.2	—	—	—	.01	.1	0
5	1	19	.2	—	—	—	.01	.2	0
30	2	47	.5	—	—	—	.02	.4	0

Foods, Approximate Measures, Units, and Weight	(g)	Water (%)	Food Energy (cal)	Protein (g)	Fat (g)	Fatty Acids: Saturated (total) (g)	Fatty Acids: Unsaturated: Oleic (g)	Fatty Acids: Unsaturated: Linoleic (g)
Pretzels, made with enriched flour:								
Dutch, twisted, 2¾ × 2⅝ in, 1 pretzel	16	5	60	2	1	—	—	—
Thin, twisted, 3¼ × 2¼ × ¼ in, 10 pretzels	60	5	235	6	3	—	—	—
Stick, 2¼ in long 10 pretzels,	3	5	10	Tr	Tr	—	—	—
Rice, white, enriched:								
Instant, ready-to-serve, hot, 1 cup	165	73	180	4	Tr	Tr	Tr	Tr
Long grain:								
Raw, 1 cup	185	12	670	12	1	.2	.2	.2
Cooked, served hot, 1 cup	205	73	225	4	Tr	.1	.1	.1
Parboiled:								
Raw, 1 cup	185	10	685	14	1	.2	.1	.2
Cooked, served hot, 1 cup	175	73	185	4	Tr	.1	.1	.1
Rolls, enriched:								
Commercial:								
Brown-and-serve (12 per 12-oz pkg), browned, 1 roll	26	27	85	2	2	.4	.7	.5
Cloverleaf or pan, 2½-in diameter, 2 in high, 1 roll	28	31	85	2	2	.4	.6	.4
Frankfurter and hamburger (8 per 11½-oz pkg), 1 roll	40	31	120	3	2	.5	.8	.6
Hard, 3¾-in diameter, 2 in high, 1 roll	50	25	155	5	2	.4	.6	.5
Hoagie or submarine, 11½ × 3 × 2½ in, 1 roll	135	31	390	12	4	.9	1.4	1.4
From home recipe:								
Cloverleaf, 2½-in diameter, 2 in high, 1 roll	35	26	120	3	3	.8	1.1	.7
Spaghetti, enriched, cooked:								
Firm stage, "al dente," served hot, 1 cup	130	64	190	7	1	—	—	—
Tender stage, served hot, 1 cup	140	73	155	5	1	—	—	—
Spaghetti (enriched) in tomato sauce with cheese:								
From home recipe, 1 cup	250	77	260	9	9	2.0	5.4	.7
Canned, 1 cup	250	80	190	6	2	.5	.3	.4
Spaghetti (enriched) with meat balls and tomato sauce:								
From home recipe, 1 cup	248	70	330	19	12	3.3	6.3	.9
Canned, 1 cup	250	78	260	12	10	2.2	3.3	3.9
Toaster pastries, 1 pastry	50	12	200	3	6	—	—	—

Nutrients in Indicated Quantity

For notes, see end of table.

Nutrients in Indicated Quantity									
Carbohydrate (g)	Calcium (mg)	Phosophorus (mg)	Iron (mg)	Potassium (mg)	Vitamin A Value (IU)	Thiamin (mg)	Riboflavin (mg)	Niacin (mg)	Ascorbic Acid (mg)
12	4	21	.2	21	0	.05	.04	.7	0
46	13	79	.9	78	0	.20	.15	2.5	0
2	1	4	Tr	4	0	.01	.01	.1	0
40	5	31	1.3	—	0	.21	([59])	1.7	0
149	44	174	5.4	170	0	.81	.06	6.5	0
50	21	57	1.8	57	0	.23	.02	2.1	0
150	111	370	5.4	278	0	.81	.07	6.5	0
41	33	100	1.4	75	0	.19	.02	2.1	0
14	20	23	.5	25	Tr	.10	.06	.9	Tr
15	21	24	.5	27	Tr	.11	.07	.9	Tr
21	30	34	.8	38	Tr	.16	.10	1.3	Tr
30	24	46	1.2	49	Tr	.20	.12	1.7	Tr
75	58	115	3.0	122	Tr	.54	.32	4.5	Tr
20	16	36	.7	41	30	.12	.12	1.2	Tr
39	14	85	1.4	103	0	.23	.13	1.8	0
32	11	70	1.3	85	0	.20	.11	1.5	0
37	80	135	2.3	408	1080	.25	.18	2.3	13
39	40	88	2.8	303	930	.35	.28	4.5	10
39	124	236	3.7	665	1590	.25	.30	4.0	22
29	53	113	3.3	245	1000	.15	.18	2.3	5
36	54[80]	67[60]	1.9	74[60]	500	.16	.17	2.1	([60])

Foods, Approximate Measures, Units, and Weight	(g)	Water (%)	Food Energy (cal)	Protein (g)	Fat (g)	Fatty Acids: Saturated (total) (g)	Fatty Acids: Unsaturated: Oleic (g)	Fatty Acids: Unsaturated: Linoleic (g)
Waffles, made with enriched flour, 7-in diameter[38]:								
From home recipe, 1 waffle	75	41	210	7	7	2.3	2.8	1.4
From mix, egg and milk added, 1 waffle	75	42	205	7	8	2.8	2.9	1.2
Wheat flours:								
All-purpose or family flour, enriched:								
Sifted, spooned, 1 cup	115	12	420	12	1	.2	.1	0.5
Unsifted, spooned, 1 cup	125	12	455	13	1	.2	.1	.5
Cake or pastry flour, enriched, sifted, spooned, 1 cup	96	12	350	7	1	.1	.1	.3
Self-rising, enriched, unsifted, spooned, 1 cup	125	12	440	12	1	.2	.1	.5
Whole-wheat, from hard wheats, stirred, 1 cup	120	12	400	16	2	.4	.2	1.0
Legumes (Dry), Nuts, Seeds; Related Products								
Almonds, shelled:								
Chopped (about 130 almonds), 1 cup	130	5	775	24	70	5.6	47.7	12.8
Slivered, not pressed down (about 115 almonds), 1 cup	115	5	690	21	62	5.0	42.2	11.3
Beans, dry:								
Common varieties as Great Northern, navy, and others:								
Cooked, drained:								
Great Northern, 1 cup	180	69	210	14	1	—	—	—
Pea (navy), 1 cup	190	69	225	15	1	—	—	—
Canned, solids and liquid:								
White with:								
Frankfurters (sliced), 1 cup	255	71	365	19	18	—	—	—
Pork and tomato sauce, 1 cup	255	71	310	16	7	2.4	2.8	.6
Pork and sweet sauce, 1 cup	255	66	385	16	12	4.3	5.0	1.1
Red kidney, 1 cup	255	76	230	15	1	—	—	—
Lima, cooked, drained, 1 cup	190	64	260	16	1	—	—	—
Blackeye peas, dry, cooked (with residual cooking liquid), 1 cup	250	80	190	13	1	—	—	—
Brazil nuts, shelled (6-8 large kernels), 1 oz	28	5	185	4	19	4.8	6.2	7.1
Cashew nuts, roasted in oil, 1 cup	140	5	785	24	64	12.9	36.8	10.2
Coconut meat, fresh:								
Piece, about 2 × 2 × ½ in, 1 piece	45	51	155	2	16	14.0	.9	.3

For notes, see end of table.

Nutrients in Indicated Quantity

Carbohydrate (g)	Calcium (mg)	Phosophorus (mg)	Iron (mg)	Potassium (mg)	Vitamin A Value (IU)	Thiamin (mg)	Riboflavin (mg)	Niacin (mg)	Ascorbic Acid (mg)
28	85	130	1.3	109	250	.17	.23	1.4	Tr
27	179	257	1.0	146	170	.14	.22	.9	Tr
88	18	100	3.3	109	0	0.74	0.46	6.1	0
95	20	109	3.6	119	0	.80	.50	6.6	0
76	16	70	2.8	91	0	.61	.38	5.1	0
93	331	583	3.6	—	0	.80	.50	6.6	0
85	49	446	4.0	444	0	.66	.14	5.2	0
25	304	655	6.1	1005	0	.31	1.20	4.6	Tr
22	269	580	5.4	889	0	.28	1.06	4.0	Tr
38	90	266	4.9	749	0	.25	.13	1.3	0
40	95	281	5.1	790	0	.27	.13	1.3	0
32	94	303	4.8	668	330	.18	.15	3.3	Tr
48	138	235	4.6	536	330	.20	.08	1.5	5
54	161	291	5.9	—	—	.15	.10	1.3	—
42	74	278	4.6	673	10	.13	.10	1.5	—
49	55	293	5.9	1163	—	.25	.11	1.3	—
35	43	238	3.3	573	30	.40	.10	1.0	—
3	53	196	1.0	203	Tr	.27	.03	.5	—
41	53	522	5.3	650	140	.60	.35	2.5	—
4	6	43	.8	115	0	.02	.01	.2	1

Foods, Approximate Measures, Units, and Weight	(g)	Water (%)	Food Energy (cal)	Protein (g)	Fat (g)	Fatty Acids: Saturated (total) (g)	Fatty Acids: Unsaturated: Oleic (g)	Fatty Acids: Unsaturated: Linoleic (g)
Shredded or grated, not pressed down, 1 cup	80	51	275	3	28	24.8	1.6	.5
Filberts (hazelnuts), chopped (about 60 kernels), 1 cup	115	6	730	14	72	5.1	55.2	7.3
Lentils, whole, cooked, 1 cup	200	72	210	16	Tr	—	—	—
Peanuts, roasted in oil, salted (whole, halves, chopped), 1 cup	144	2	840	37	72	13.7	33.0	20.7
Peanut butter, 1 tbsp	16	2	95	4	8	1.5	3.7	2.3
Peas, split, dry, cooked, 1 cup	200	70	230	16	1	—	—	—
Pecans, chopped or pieces (about 120 large halves), 1 cup	118	3	810	11	84	7.2	50.5	20.0
Pumpkin and squash kernels, dry, hulled, 1 cup	140	4	775	41	65	11.8	23.5	27.5
Sunflower seeds, dry, hulled, 1 cup	145	5	810	35	69	8.2	13.7	43.2
Walnuts:								
Black:								
Chopped or broken kernels, 1 cup	125	3	785	26	74	6.3	13.3	45.7
Ground (finely), 1 cup	80	3	500	16	47	4.0	8.5	29.2
Persian or English, chopped (about 60 halves), 1 cup	120	4	780	18	77	8.4	11.8	42.2
Sugars and Sweets								
Cake icings:								
Boiled, white:								
Plain, 1 cup	94	18	295	1	0	0	0	—
With coconut, 1 cup	166	15	605	3	13	11.0	.9	Tr
Uncooked:								
Chocolate made with milk and butter, 1 cup	275	14	1035	9	38	23.4	11.7	1.0
Creamy fudge from mix and water, 1 cup	245	15	830	7	16	5.1	6.7	3.1
White, 1 cup	319	11	1200	2	21	12.7	5.1	.5
Candy:								
Caramels, plain or chocolate, 1 oz	28	8	115	1	3	1.6	1.1	.1
Chocolate:								
Milk, plain, 1 oz	28	1	145	2	9	5.5	3.0	.3
Semisweet, small pieces (60 per oz), 1 cup or 6-oz pkg	170	1	860	7	61	36.2	19.8	1.7
Chocolate-coated peanuts, 1 oz	28	1	160	5	12	4.0	4.7	2.1
Fondant, uncoated (mints, candy corn, other), 1 oz	28	8	105	Tr	1	.1	.3	.1
Fudge, chocolate, plain, 1 oz	28	8	115	1	3	1.3	1.4	.6
Gum drops, 1 oz	28	12	100	Tr	Tr	—	—	—

For notes, see end of table.

Nutrients in Indicated Quantity

Carbohydrate (g)	Calcium (mg)	Phosophorus (mg)	Iron (mg)	Potassium (mg)	Vitamin A Value (IU)	Thiamin (mg)	Riboflavin (mg)	Niacin (mg)	Ascorbic Acid (mg)
8	10	76	1.4	205	0	.04	.02	.4	2
19	240	388	3.9	810	—	.53	—	1.0	Tr
39	50	238	4.2	498	40	.14	.12	1.2	0
27	107	577	3.0	971	—	.46	.19	24.8	0
3	9	61	.3	100	—	.02	.02	2.4	0
42	22	178	3.4	592	80	.30	.18	1.8	—
17	86	341	2.8	712	150	1.01	.15	1.1	2
21	71	1602	15.7	1386	100	.34	.27	3.4	—
29	174	1214	10.3	1334	70	2.84	.33	7.8	—
19	Tr	713	7.5	575	380	.28	.14	.9	—
12	Tr	456	4.8	368	240	.18	.09	.6	—
19	119	456	3.7	540	40	.40	.16	1.1	2
75	2	2	Tr	17	0	Tr	0.03	Tr	0
124	10	50	.8	277	0	.02	.07	.3	0
185	165	305	3.3	536	580	.06	.28	.6	1
183	96	218	2.7	238	Tr	.05	.20	.7	Tr
260	48	38	Tr	57	860	Tr	.06	Tr	Tr
22	42	35	.4	54	Tr	.01	.05	.1	Tr
16	65	65	.3	109	80	.02	.10	.1	Tr
97	51	255	4.4	553	30	.02	.14	.9	0
11	33	84	.4	143	Tr	.10	.05	2.1	Tr
25	4	2	.3	1	0	Tr	Tr	Tr	0
21	22	24	.3	42	Tr	.01	.03	.1	Tr
25	2	Tr	.1	1	0	0	Tr	Tr	0

Foods, Approximate Measures, Units, and Weight	(g)	Water (%)	Food Energy (cal)	Protein (g)	Fat (g)	Fatty Acids: Saturated (total) (g)	Fatty Acids: Unsaturated Oleic (g)	Fatty Acids: Unsaturated Linoleic (g)
Hard, 1 oz	28	1	110	0	Tr	—	—	—
Marshmallows, 1 oz	28	17	90	1	Tr	—	—	—
Chocolate-flavored beverage powders, (about 4 heaping tsp per oz):								
With nonfat dry milk, 1 oz	28	2	100	5	1	.5	.3	Tr
Without milk, 1 oz	28	1	100	1	1	.4	.2	Tr
Honey, strained or extracted, 1 tbsp	21	17	65	Tr	0	0	0	0
Jams and preserves, 1 tbsp	20	29	55	Tr	Tr	—	—	—
1 packet	14	29	40	Tr	Tr	—	—	—
Jellies, 1 tbsp	18	29	50	Tr	Tr	—	—	—
1 packet	14	29	40	Tr	Tr	—	—	—
Syrups:								
Chocolate-flavored syrup or topping:								
Thin type, 1 fl oz or 2 tbsp	38	32	90	1	1	.5	.3	Tr
Fudge type, 1 fl oz or 2 tbsp	38	25	125	2	5	3.1	1.6	.1
Molasses, cane:								
Light (first extraction), 1 tbsp	20	24	50	—	—	—	—	—
Blackstrap (third extraction), 1 tbsp	20	24	45	—	—	—	—	—
Sorghum, 1 tbsp	21	23	55	—	—	—	—	—
Table blends, chiefly corn, light and dark, 1 tbsp	21	24	60	0	0	0	0	0
Sugars:								
Brown, pressed down, 1 cup	220	2	820	0	0	0	0	0
White:								
Granulated, 1 cup	200	1	770	0	0	0	0	0
1 tbsp	12	1	45	0	0	0	0	0
1 packet	6	1	23	0	0	0	0	0
Powdered, sifted, spooned into cup, 1 cup	100	1	385	0	0	0	0	0
Vegetable and Vegetable Products								
Asparagus, green:								
Cooked, drained:								
Cuts and tips, 1½- to 2-in lengths:								
From raw, 1 cup	145	94	30	3	Tr	—	—	—
From frozen, 1 cup	180	93	40	6	Tr	—	—	—
Spears, ½-in diameter at base:								
From raw, 4 spears	60	94	10	1	Tr	—	—	—
From frozen, 4 spears	60	92	15	2	Tr	—	—	—
Canned, spears, ½-in diameter at base, 4 spears	80	93	15	2	Tr	—	—	—

For notes, see end of table.

Nutrients in Indicated Quantity

Carbohydrate (g)	Calcium (mg)	Phosophorus (mg)	Iron (mg)	Potassium (mg)	Vitamin A Value (IU)	Thiamin (mg)	Riboflavin (mg)	Niacin (mg)	Ascorbic Acid (mg)
28	6	2	.5	1	0	0	0	0	0
23	5	2	.5	2	0	0	Tr	Tr	0
20	167	155	.5	227	10	.04	.21	.2	1
25	9	48	.6	142	—	.01	.03	.1	0
17	1	1	.1	11	0	Tr	.01	.1	Tr
14	4	2	.2	18	Tr	Tr	.01	Tr	Tr
10	3	1	.1	12	Tr	Tr	Tr	Tr	Tr
13	4	1	.3	14	Tr	Tr	.01	Tr	1
10	3	1	.2	11	Tr	Tr	Tr	Tr	1
24	6	35	.6	106	Tr	.01	.03	.2	0
20	48	60	.5	107	60	.02	.08	.2	Tr
13	33	9	.9	183	—	.01	.01	Tr	—
11	137	17	3.2	585	—	.02	.04	.4	—
14	35	5	2.6	—	—	—	.02	Tr	—
15	9	3	.8	1	0	0	0	0	0
212	187	42	7.5	757	0	.02	.7	.4	0
199	0	0	.2	6	0	0	0	0	0
12	0	0	Tr	Tr	0	0	0	0	0
6	0	0	Tr	Tr	0	0	0	0	0
100	0	0	.1	3	0	0	0	0	0
5	30	73	.9	265	1310	.23	.26	2.0	38
6	40	115	2.2	396	1530	.25	.23	1.8	41
2	13	30	.4	110	540	.10	.11	.8	16
2	13	40	.7	143	470	.10	.08	.7	16
3	15	42	1.5	133	640	.05	.08	.6	12

Foods, Approximate Measures, Units, and Weight	(g)	Water (%)	Food Energy (cal)	Protein (g)	Fat (g)	Fatty Acids: Saturated (total) (g)	Fatty Acids: Unsaturated Oleic (g)	Fatty Acids: Unsaturated Linoleic (g)
Beans:								
Lima, immature seeds, frozen, cooked, drained:								
Thick-seeded types (Fordhooks), 1 cup	170	74	170	10	Tr	—	—	—
Thin-seeded types (baby limas), 1 cup	180	69	210	13	Tr	—	—	—
Snap:								
Green:								
Cooked, drained:								
From raw (cuts and French style), 1 cup	125	92	30	2	Tr	—	—	—
From frozen:								
Cuts, 1 cup	135	92	35	2	Tr	—	—	—
French style, 1 cup	130	92	35	2	Tr	—	—	—
Canned, drained solids (cuts), 1 cup	135	92	30	2	Tr	—	—	—
Yellow or wax:								
Cooked, drained:								
From raw (cuts and French style), 1 cup	125	93	30	2	Tr	—	—	—
From frozen (cuts), 1 cup	135	92	35	2	Tr	—	—	—
Canned, drained solids (cuts), 1 cup	135	92	30	2	Tr	—	—	—
Beans, mature. See Beans, dry and Blackeye peas, dry.								
Bean sprouts (mung):								
Raw, 1 cup	105	89	35	4	Tr	—	—	—
Cooked, drained, 1 cup	125	91	35	4	Tr	—	—	—
Beets:								
Cooked, drained, peeled:								
Whole beets, 2-in diameter, 2 beets	100	91	30	1	Tr	—	—	—
Diced or sliced, 1 cup	170	91	55	2	Tr	—	—	—
Canned, drained solids:								
Whole beets, small, 1 cup	160	89	60	2	Tr	—	—	—
Diced or sliced, 1 cup	170	89	65	2	Tr	—	—	—
Beet greens, leaves and stems, cooked, drained, 1 cup	145	94	25	2	Tr	—	—	—
Blackeye peas, immature seeds, cooked and drained,								
From raw, 1 cup	165	72	180	13	1	—	—	—
From frozen, 1 cup	170	66	220	15	1	—	—	—

Nutrients in Indicated Quantity

For notes, see end of table.

Nutrients in Indicated Quantity									
Carbohydrate (g)	Calcium (mg)	Phosophorus (mg)	Iron (mg)	Potassium (mg)	Vitamin A Value (IU)	Thiamin (mg)	Riboflavin (mg)	Niacin (mg)	Ascorbic Acid (mg)
32	34	153	2.9	724	390	.12	.09	1.7	29
40	63	227	4.7	709	400	.16	.09	2.2	22
7	63	45	.8	189	680	.09	.11	.6	15
8	54	43	.9	205	780	.09	.12	.5	7
8	49	39	1.2	177	690	.08	.10	.4	9
7	61	34	2.0	128	630	.04	.07	.4	5
6	63	46	.8	189	290	.09	.11	.6	16
8	47	42	.9	221	140	.09	.11	.5	8
7	61	34	2.0	128	140	.04	.07	.4	7
7	20	67	1.4	234	20	.14	.14	.8	20
7	21	60	1.1	195	30	.11	.13	.9	8
7	14	23	.5	206	20	.03	.04	.3	6
12	24	39	.9	354	30	.05	.07	.5	10
14	30	29	1.1	267	30	.02	.05	.2	5
15	32	31	1.2	284	30	.02	.05	.2	5
5	144	36	2.8	481	7400	.10	.22	.4	22
30	40	241	3.5	625	580	.50	.18	2.3	28
40	43	286	4.8	573	290	.68	.19	2.4	15

Foods, Approximate Measures, Units, and Weight	(g)	Water (%)	Food Energy (cal)	Protein (g)	Fat (g)	Fatty Acids: Saturated (total) (g)	Fatty Acids: Unsaturated Oleic (g)	Fatty Acids: Unsaturated Linoleic (g)
Broccoli, cooked, drained:								
From raw:								
Stalk, medium size, 1 stalk	180	91	45	6	1	—	—	—
Stalks cut into ½-in pieces, 1 cup	155	91	40	5	Tr	—	—	—
From frozen:								
Stalk, 4½ to 5 in long, 1 stalk	30	91	10	1	Tr	—	—	—
Chopped, 1 cup	185	92	50	5	1	—	—	—
Brussels sprouts, cooked, drained:								
From raw, 7-8 sprouts (1¼- to 1½-in diameter), 1 cup	155	88	55	7	1	—	—	—
From frozen, 1 cup	155	89	50	5	Tr	—	—	—
Cabbage:								
Common varieties:								
Raw:								
Coarsely shredded or sliced, 1 cup	70	92	15	1	Tr	—	—	—
Finely shredded or chopped, 1 cup	90	92	20	1	Tr	—	—	—
Cooked, drained, 1 cup	145	94	30	2	Tr	—	—	—
Red, raw, coarsely shredded or sliced, 1 cup	70	90	20	1	Tr	—	—	—
Savoy, raw, coarsely shredded or sliced, 1 cup	70	92	15	2	Tr	—	—	—
Cabbage, celery (also called pe-tsai or wongbok), raw, 1-in pieces 1 cup	75	95	10	1	Tr	—	—	—
Cabbage, white mustard (also called bokchoy or pakchoy), cooked, drained, 1 cup	170	95	25	2	Tr	—	—	—
Carrots:								
Raw, without crowns and tips, scraped:								
Whole, 7½ × 1⅛ in, or strips, 2½ to 3 in long, 1 carrot or 18 strips	72	88	30	1	Tr	—	—	—
Grated, 1 cup	110	88	45	1	Tr	—	—	—
Cooked (crosswise cuts), drained, 1 cup	155	91	50	1	Tr	—	—	—
Canned:								
Sliced, drained solids, 1 cup	155	91	45	1	Tr	—	—	—
Strained or junior (baby food) 1 oz (1¾ to 2 tbsp)	28	92	10	Tr	Tr	—	—	—
Cauliflower:								
Raw, chopped, 1 cup	115	91	31	3	Tr	—	—	—
Cooked, drained:								
From raw (flower buds), 1 cup	125	93	30	3	Tr	—	—	—
From frozen (flowerets), 1 cup	180	94	30	3	Tr	—	—	—

For notes, see end of table.

Nutrients in Indicated Quantity									
Carbohydrate (g)	Calcium (mg)	Phosophorus (mg)	Iron (mg)	Potassium (mg)	Vitamin A Value (IU)	Thiamin (mg)	Riboflavin (mg)	Niacin (mg)	Ascorbic Acid (mg)
8	158	112	1.4	481	4500	.16	.36	1.4	162
7	136	96	1.2	414	3880	.14	.31	1.2	140
1	12	17	.2	66	570	.02	.03	.2	22
9	100	104	1.3	392	4810	.11	.22	.9	105
10	50	112	1.7	423	810	.12	.22	1.2	135
10	33	95	1.2	457	880	.12	.16	.9	126
4	34	20	.3	163	90	.04	.04	.2	33
5	44	26	.4	210	120	.05	.05	.3	42
6	64	29	.4	236	190	.06	.06	.4	48
5	29	25	.6	188	30	.06	.04	.3	43
3	47	38	.6	188	140	.04	.06	.2	39
2	32	30	.5	190	110	.04	.03	.5	19
4	252	56	1.0	364	5270	.07	.14	1.2	26
7	27	26	.5	246	7930	.04	.04	.4	6
11	41	40	.8	375	12,100	.07	.06	.7	9
11	51	48	.9	344	16,280	.08	.08	.8	9
10	47	34	1.1	186	23,250	.03	.05	.6	3
2	7	6	.1	51	3690	.01	.01	.1	1
6	29	64	1.3	339	70	.13	.12	.8	90
5	26	53	.9	258	80	.11	.10	.8	69
6	31	68	.9	373	50	.07	.09	.7	74

Foods, Approximate Measures, Units, and Weight	(g)	Water (%)	Food Energy (cal)	Protein (g)	Fat (g)	Fatty Acids: Saturated (total) (g)	Unsaturated: Oleic (g)	Unsaturated: Linoleic (g)
Celery, Pascal type, raw:								
Stalk, large outer, 8 × 1½ in, at rood end, 1 stalk	40	94	5	Tr	Tr	—	—	—
Pieces, diced, 1 cup	120	94	20	1	Tr	—	—	—
Collards, cooked, drained:								
From raw (leaves without stems), 1 cup	190	90	65	7	1	—	—	—
From frozen (chopped), 1 cup	170	90	50	5	1	—	—	—
Corn, sweet:								
Cooked, drained:								
From raw, ear 5 × 1¾ in, 1 ear[61]	140	74	70	2	1	—	—	—
From frozen:								
Ear, 5 in long, 1 ear[61]	229	73	120	4	1	—	—	—
Kernels, 1 cup	165	77	130	5	1	—	—	—
Canned:								
Cream style, 1 cup	256	76	210	5	2	—	—	—
Whole kernel:								
Vacuum pack, 1 cup	210	76	175	5	1	—	—	—
Wet pack, drained solids, 1 cup	165	76	140	4	1	—	—	—
Cowpeas; see Blackeye peas								
Cucumber slices, ⅛ in thick (large, 2⅛-in diameter; small, 1¾-in diameter):								
With peel, 6 large or 8 small slices	28	95	5	Tr	Tr	—	—	—
Without peel, 6½ large or 9 small pieces	28	96	5	Tr	Tr	—	—	—
Dandelion greens, cooked, drained 1 cup	105	90	35	2	1	—	—	—
Endive, curly (including escarole), raw, small pieces, 1 cup	50	93	10	1	Tr	—	—	—
Kale, cooked, drained:								
From raw (leaves without stems and midribs), 1 cup	110	88	45	5	1	—	—	—
From frozen (leaf style), 1 cup	130	91	40	4	1	—	—	—
Lettuce, raw:								
Butterhead, as Boston types:								
Head, 5-in diameter1 head[63]	220	95	25	2	Tr	—	—	—
Leaves, 1 outer or 2 inner or 3 heart leaves	15	95	Tr	Tr	Tr	—	—	—
Crisphead, as Iceberg:								
Head, 6-in diameter, 1 head[64]	567	96	70	5	1	—	—	—
Wedge, ¼ of head, 1 wedge	135	96	20	1	Tr	—	—	—
Pieces, chopped or shredded 1 cup	55	96	5	Tr	Tr	—	—	—

For notes, see end of table.

Nutrients in Indicated Quantity

Carbohydrate (g)	Calcium (mg)	Phosophorus (mg)	Iron (mg)	Potassium (mg)	Vitamin A Value (IU)	Thiamin (mg)	Riboflavin (mg)	Niacin (mg)	Ascorbic Acid (mg)
2	16	11	.1	136	110	.01	.01	.1	4
5	47	34	.4	409	320	.04	.04	.4	11
10	357	99	1.5	498	14,820	.21	.38	2.3	144
10	299	87	1.7	401	11,560	.10	.24	1.0	56
16	2	69	.5	151	310[62]	.09	.08	1.1	7
27	4	121	1.0	291	440[62]	.18	.10	2.1	9
31	5	120	1.3	304	580[62]	.15	.10	2.5	8
51	8	143	1.5	248	840[62]	.08	.13	2.6	13
43	6	153	1.1	204	740[62]	.06	.13	2.3	11
33	8	81	.8	160	580[62]	.05	.08	1.5	7
1	7	8	.3	45	70	.01	.01	.1	3
1	5	5	.1	45	Tr	.01	.01	.1	3
7	147	44	1.9	244	12,290	.14	.17	—	19
2	41	27	.9	147	1650	.04	.07	.3	5
7	206	64	1.8	243	9130	.11	.20	1.8	102
7	157	62	1.3	251	10,660	.08	.20	.9	49
4	57	42	3.3	430	1580	.10	.10	.5	13
Tr	5	4	.3	40	150	.01	.01	Tr	1
16	108	118	2.7	943	1780	.32	.32	1.6	32
4	27	30	.7	236	450	.08	.08	.4	8
2	11	12	.3	96	180	.03	.03	.2	3

Foods, Approximate Measures, Units, and Weight	(g)	Water (%)	Food Energy (cal)	Protein (g)	Fat (g)	Fatty Acids: Saturated (total) (g)	Fatty Acids: Unsaturated Oleic (g)	Fatty Acids: Unsaturated Linoleic (g)
Looseleaf (bunching varieties including romaine or cos), chopped or shredded pieces, 1 cup	55	94	10	1	Tr	—	—	—
Mushrooms, raw, sliced or chopped, 1 cup	70	90	20	2	Tr	—	—	—
Mustard greens, without stems and midribs, cooked, drained, 1 cup	140	93	30	3	1	—	—	—
Okra pods, 3 × ⅝ in, cooked, 10 pods	106	91	30	2	Tr	—	—	—
Onions:								
Mature:								
Raw:								
Chopped, 1 cup	170	89	65	3	Tr	—	—	—
Sliced, 1 cup	115	89	45	2	Tr	—	—	—
Cooked (whole or sliced), drained, 1 cup	210	92	60	3	Tr	—	—	—
Young green, bulb (⅜-in diameter) and white portion of top, 6 onions	30	88	15	Tr	Tr	—	—	—
Parsley, raw, chopped, 1 tbsp	4	85	Tr	Tr	Tr	—	—	—
Parsnips, cooked (diced or 2-in lengths), 1 cup	155	82	100	2	1	—	—	—
Peas, green:								
Canned:								
Whole, drained solids, 1 cup	170	77	150	8	1	—	—	—
Strained (baby food), 1 oz (1¾ to 2 tbsp)	28	86	15	1	Tr	—	—	—
Frozen, cooked, drained, 1 cup	160	82	110	8	Tr	—	—	—
Peppers, hot, red, without seeds, dried (ground chili powder, added seasonings), 1 tsp	2	9	5	Tr	Tr	—	—	—
Peppers, sweet (about 5 per lb, whole), stem and seeds removed:								
Raw, 1 pod	74	93	15	1	Tr	—	—	—
Cooked, boiled, drained, 1 pod	73	95	15	1	Tr	—	—	—
Potatoes, cooked:								
Baked, peeled after baking (about 2 per lb, raw), 1 potato	156	75	145	4	Tr	—	—	—
Boiled (about 3 per lb, raw):								
Peeled after boiling, 1 potato	137	80	105	3	Tr	—	—	—
Peeled before boiling, 1 potato	135	83	90	3	Tr	—	—	—
French-fried, strip, 2 to 3½ in long:								
Prepared from raw, 10 strips	50	45	135	2	7	1.7	1.2	3.3
Frozen, oven heated, 10 strips	50	53	110	2	4	1.1	.8	2.1
Hashed brown, prepared from frozen, 1 cup	155	56	345	3	18	4.6	3.2	9.0

For notes, see end of table.

Nutrients in Indicated Quantity

Carbohydrate (g)	Calcium (mg)	Phosophorus (mg)	Iron (mg)	Potassium (mg)	Vitamin A Value (IU)	Thiamin (mg)	Riboflavin (mg)	Niacin (mg)	Ascorbic Acid (mg)
2	37	14	.8	145	1050	.03	.04	.2	10
3	4	81	.6	290	Tr	.07	.32	2.9	2
6	193	45	2.5	308	8120	.11	.20	.8	67
6	98	43	.5	184	520	.14	.19	1.0	21
15	46	61	.9	267	Tr[65]	.05	.07	.3	17
10	31	41	.6	181	Tr[65]	.03	.05	.2	12
14	50	61	.8	231	Tr[65]	.06	.06	.4	15
3	12	12	.2	69	Tr[65]	.02	.01	.1	8
Tr	7	2	.2	25	300	Tr	.01	Tr	6
23	70	96	.9	587	50	.11	.12	.2	16
29	44	129	3.2	163	1170	.15	.10	1.4	14
3	3	18	.3	28	140	.02	.03	.3	3
19	30	138	3.0	216	960	.43	.14	2.7	21
1	5	4	.3	20	1300	Tr	.02	.2	Tr
4	7	16	.5	157	310	.06	.06	.4	94
3	7	12	.4	109	310	.05	.05	.4	70
33	14	101	1.1	782	Tr	.15	.07	2.7	31
23	10	72	.8	556	Tr	.12	.05	2.0	22
20	8	57	.7	385	Tr	.12	.05	1.6	22
18	8	56	.7	427	Tr	.07	.04	1.6	11
17	5	43	.9	326	Tr	.07	.01	1.3	11
45	28	78	1.9	439	Tr	.11	.03	1.6	12

Foods, Approximate Measures, Units, and Weight	(g)	Water (%)	Food Energy (cal)	Protein (g)	Fat (g)	Fatty Acids: Saturated (total) (g)	Unsaturated: Oleic (g)	Unsaturated: Linoleic (g)
Mashed, prepared from:								
Raw:								
Milk added, 1 cup	210	83	135	4	2	.7	.4	Tr
Milk and butter added, 1 cup	210	80	195	4	9	5.6	2.3	0.2
Dehydrated flakes (without milk), water, milk, butter, and salt added, 1 cup	210	79	195	4	7	3.6	2.1	.2
Potato chips, 1¾ × 2½-in oval cross section, 10 chips	20	2	115	1	8	2.1	1.4	4.0
Potato salad, made with cooked salad dressing, 1 cup	250	76	250	7	7	2.0	2.7	1.3
Pumpkin, canned, 1 cup	245	90	80	2	1	—	—	—
Radishes, raw (prepackaged) stem ends, rootlets cut off, 4 radishes	18	95	5	Tr	Tr	—	—	—
Sauerkraut, canned, solids and liquid 1 cup	235	93	40	2	Tr	—	—	—
Southern peas; see Blackeye peas								
Spinach:								
Raw, chopped, 1 cup	55	91	15	2	Tr	—	—	—
Cooked, drained:								
From raw, 1 cup	180	92	40	5	1	—	—	—
From frozen:								
Chopped, 1 cup	205	92	45	6	1	—	—	—
Leaf, 1 cup	190	92	45	6	1	—	—	—
Canned, drained solids, 1 cup	205	91	50	6	1	—	—	—
Squash, cooked:								
Summer (all varieties), diced, drained, 1 cup	210	96	30	2	Tr	—	—	—
Winter (all varieties), baked, mashed, 1 cup	205	81	130	4	1	—	—	—
Sweet potatoes:								
Cooked (raw, 5 × 2 in; about 2½ per lb):								
Baked in skin, peeled, 1 potato	114	64	160	2	1	—	—	—
Broiled in skin, peeled, 1 potato	151	71	170	3	1	—	—	—
Candied, 2½ × 2-in piece, 1 piece	105	60	175	1	3	2.0	.8	.1
Canned:								
Solid pack (mashed), 1 cup	255	72	275	5	1	—	—	—
Vacuum pack, piece 2¾ × 1 in, 1 piece	40	72	45	1	Tr	—	—	—
Tomatoes:								
Raw, 2⅗-in diameter (3 per 12 oz pkg), 1 tomato[66]	135	94	25	1	Tr	—	—	—
Canned, solids and liquid, 1 cup	241	94	50	2	Tr	—	—	—

For notes, see end of table.

Nutrients in Indicated Quantity									
Carbohydrate (g)	Calcium (mg)	Phosophorus (mg)	Iron (mg)	Potassium (mg)	Vitamin A Value (IU)	Thiamin (mg)	Riboflavin (mg)	Niacin (mg)	Ascorbic Acid (mg)
27	50	103	.8	548	40	.17	.11	2.1	21
26	50	101	.8	525	360	.17	.11	2.1	19
30	65	99	.6	601	270	.08	.08	1.9	11
10	8	28	.4	226	Tr	.04	.01	1.0	3
41	80	160	1.5	798	350	.20	.18	2.8	28
19	61	64	1.0	588	15,680	.07	.12	1.5	12
1	5	6	.2	58	Tr	.01	.01	.1	5
9	85	42	1.2	329	120	.07	.09	.5	33
2	51	28	1.7	259	4460	.06	.11	.3	28
6	167	68	4.0	583	14,580	.13	.25	.9	50
8	232	90	4.3	683	16,200	.14	.31	.8	39
7	200	84	4.8	688	15,390	.15	.27	1.0	53
7	242	53	5.3	513	16,400	.04	.25	.6	29
7	53	53	.8	296	820	.11	.17	1.7	21
32	57	98	1.6	945	8610	.10	.27	1.4	27
37	46	66	1.0	342	9230	.10	.08	.8	25
40	48	71	1.1	367	11,940	.14	.09	.9	26
36	39	45	.9	200	6620	.06	.04	.4	11
63	64	105	2.0	510	19,890	.13	.10	1.5	36
10	10	16	.3	80	3120	.02	.02	.2	6
6	16	33	.6	300	1110	.07	.05	.9	28[67]
10	14[68]	46	1.2	523	2170	.12	.07	1.7	41

Foods, Approximate Measures, Units, and Weight	(g)	Water (%)	Food Energy (cal)	Protein (g)	Fat (g)	Fatty Acids: Saturated (total) (g)	Fatty Acids: Unsaturated Oleic (g)	Fatty Acids: Unsaturated Linoleic (g)
Tomato catsup, 1 cup	273	69	290	5	1	—	—	—
1 tbsp	15	69	15	Tr	Tr	—	—	—
Tomato juice, canned:								
Cup, 1 cup	243	94	45	2	Tr	—	—	—
Glass (6 fl oz), 1 glass	182	94	35	2	Tr	—	—	—
Turnips, cooked, diced, 1 cup	155	35	35	1	Tr	—	—	—
Turnip greens, cooked, drained:								
From raw (leaves and stems), 1 cup	145	94	30	3	Tr	—	—	—
From frozen (chopped), 1 cup	165	93	40	4	Tr	—	—	—
Vegetables, mixed, frozen, cooked, 1 cup	182	83	115	6	1	—	—	—
Miscellaneous Items								
Baking powders for home use:								
Sodium aluminum sulfate:								
With monocalcium phosphate monohydrate, 1 tsp	3.0	2	5	Tr	Tr	0	0	0
With monocalcium phosphate monohydrate, calcium sulfate, 1 tsp	2.9	1	5	Tr	Tr	0	0	0
Straight phosphate, 1 tsp	3.8	2	5	Tr	Tr	0	0	0
Low sodium, 1 tsp	4.3	2	5	Tr	Tr	0	0	0
Barbecue sauce, 1 cup	250	81	230	4	17	2.2	4.3	10.0
Beverages, alcoholic:								
Beer, 12 fl oz	360	92	150	1	0	0	0	0
Gin, rum, vodka, whisky:								
80 proof, 1½ fl oz jigger	42	67	95	—	—	0	0	0
86 proof, 1½ fl oz jigger	42	64	105	—	—	0	0	0
90 proof, 1½ fl oz jigger	42	62	110	—	—	0	0	0
Wines:								
Dessert, 3½ fl oz glass	103	77	140	Tr	0	0	0	0
Table, 3½ fl oz glass	102	86	85	Tr	0	0	0	0
Beverages, carbonated, sweetened, nonalcoholic:								
Carbonated water, 12 fl oz	366	92	115	0	0	0	0	0
Cola type, 12 fl oz	369	90	145	0	0	0	0	0
Fruit-flavored sodas and Tom Collins mixer, 12 fl oz	372	88	170	0	0	0	0	0
Ginger ale, 12 fl oz	366	92	115	0	0	0	0	0
Root beer, 12 fl oz	370	90	150	0	0	0	0	0
Chili powder; see Peppers, hot, red								
Chocolate:								
Bitter or baking, 1 oz	28	2	145	3	15	8.9	4.9	.4
Semisweet; see Candy, chocolate								

For notes, see end of table.

Nutrients in Indicated Quantity									
Carbohydrate (g)	Calcium (mg)	Phosophorus (mg)	Iron (mg)	Potassium (mg)	Vitamin A Value (IU)	Thiamin (mg)	Riboflavin (mg)	Niacin (mg)	Ascorbic Acid (mg)
69	60	137	2.2	991	3820	.25	.19	4.4	41
4	3	8	.1	54	210	.01	.01	.2	2
10	17	44	2.2	552	1940	.12	.07	1.9	39
8	13	33	1.6	413	1460	.09	.05	1.5	29
8	54	34	.6	291	Tr	.06	.08	.5	34
5	252	49	1.5	—	8270	.15	.33	.7	68
6	195	64	2.6	246	11,390	.08	.15	.7	31
24	46	115	2.4	348	9010	.22	.13	2.0	15
1	58	87	—	5	0	0	0	0	0
1	183	45	—	—	0	0	0	0	0
239	359	—	6	0	0	0	0	0	
2	207	314	—	471	0	0	0	0	0
20	53	50	2.0	435	900	.03	.03	.8	13
14	18	108	Tr	90	—	.01	.11	2.2	—
Tr	—	—	—	1	—	—	—	—	—
Tr	—	—	—	1	—	—	—	—	—
Tr	—	—	—	1	—	—	—	—	—
8	8	—	—	77	—	.01	.02	.2	—
4	9	10	.4	94	—	Tr	.01	.1	—
29	—	—	—	—	0	0	0	0	0
37	—	—	—	—	0	0	0	0	0
45	—	—	—	—	0	0	0	0	0
29	—	—	—	0	0	0	0	0	0
39	—	—	—	0	0	0	0	0	0
8	22	109	1.9	235	20	.01	.07	.4	0

Foods, Approximate Measures, Units, and Weight	(g)	Water (%)	Food Energy (cal)	Protein (g)	Fat (g)	Fatty Acids: Saturated (total) (g)	Fatty Acids: Unsaturated Oleic (g)	Fatty Acids: Unsaturated Linoleic (g)
Gelatin, dry, 1 7 g envelope	7	13	25	6	Tr	0	0	0
Gelatin dessert prepared with gelatin dessert powder and water,1 cup	240	84	140	4	0	0	0	0
Mustard, prepared, yellow, 1 tsp or individual serving pouch or cup	5	80	5	Tr	Tr	—	—	—
Olives, pickled, canned:								
Green, 4 medium or 3 extra large or 2 giant[69]	16	78	15	Tr	2	.2	1.2	.1
Ripe, Mission3 small or 2 large[69]	10	73	15	Tr	2	.2	1.2	.1
Pickles, cucumber:								
Dill, medium, whole, 3¾ in long, 1¼-in diameter, 1 pickle	65	93	5	Tr	Tr	—	—	—
Fresh-pack, slices 1½-in diameter, ¼ in thick, 2 slices	15	79	10	Tr	Tr	—	—	—
Sweet gherkin, small, whole, about 2½ in long, ¾-in diameter, 1 pickle	15	61	20	Tr	Tr	—	—	—
Relish, finely chopped, sweet, 1 tbsp	15	63	20	Tr	Tr	—	—	—
Popsicle, 3 fl oz size, 1 popsicle	95	80	70	0	0	0	0	0
Soups:								
Canned, condensed:								
Prepared with equal volume of milk:								
Cream of chicken, 1 cup	245	85	180	7	10	4.2	3.6	1.3
Cream of mushroom, 1 cup	245	83	215	7	14	5.4	2.9	4.6
Tomato, 1 cup	250	84	175	7	7	3.4	1.7	1.0
Prepared with equal volume of water:								
Bean with pork, 1 cup	250	84	170	8	6	1.2	1.8	2.4
Beef broth, bouillon, consomme, 1 cup	240	96	30	5	0	0	0	0
Beef noodle, 1 cup	240	93	65	4	3	.6	.7	.8
Clam chowder, Manhattan type (with tomatoes, without milk), 1 cup	245	92	80	2	3	.5	.4	1.3
Cream of chicken, 1 cup	240	92	95	3	6	1.6	2.3	1.1
Cream of mushroom, 1 cup	240	90	135	2	10	2.6	1.7	4.5
Minestrone, 1 cup	245	90	105	5	3	.7	.9	1.3
Split pea, 1 cup	245	85	145	9	3	1.1	1.2	.4
Tomato, 1 cup	245	91	90	2	3	.5	.5	1.0
Vegetable beef, 1 cup	245	92	80	5	2	—	—	—
Vegetarian, 1 cup	245	92	80	2	2	—	—	—

For notes, see end of table.

Nutrients in Indicated Quantity

Carbohydrate (g)	Calcium (mg)	Phosophorus (mg)	Iron (mg)	Potassium (mg)	Vitamin A Value (IU)	Thiamin (mg)	Riboflavin (mg)	Niacin (mg)	Ascorbic Acid (mg)
0	—	—	—	—	—	—	—	—	—
34	—	—	—	—	—	—	—	—	—
Tr	4	4	.1	7	—	—	—	—	—
Tr	8	2	.2	7	40	—	—	—	—
Tr	9	1	.1	2	10	Tr	Tr	—	—
1	17	14	.7	130	70	Tr	.01	Tr	4
3	5	4	.3	—	20	Tr	Tr	Tr	1
5	2	2	.2	—	10	Tr	Tr	Tr	1
5	3	2	.1	—	—	—	—	—	—
18	0	—	Tr	—	0	0	0	0	0
15	172	152	0.5	260	610	0.05	0.27	0.7	2
16	191	169	.5	279	250	.05	.34	.7	1
23	168	155	.8	418	1200	.10	.25	1.3	15
22	63	128	2.3	395	650	.13	.08	1.0	3
3	Tr	31	.5	130	Tr	Tr	.02	1.2	—
7	7	48	1.0	77	50	.05	.07	1.0	Tr
12	34	47	1.0	184	880	.02	.02	1.0	—
8	24	34	.5	79	410	.02	.05	.5	Tr
10	41	50	.5	98	70	.02	.12	.7	Tr
14	37	59	1.0	314	2350	.07	.05	1.0	—
21	29	149	1.5	270	440	.25	.15	1.5	1
16	15	34	.7	230	1000	.05	.05	1.2	12
10	12	49	.7	162	2700	.05	.05	1.0	—
13	20	39	1.0	172	2940	.05	.05	1.0	—

Foods, Approximate Measures, Units, and Weight	(g)	Water (%)	Food Energy (cal)	Protein (g)	Fat (g)	Fatty Acids: Saturated (total) (g)	Fatty Acids: Unsaturated Oleic (g)	Fatty Acids: Unsaturated Linoleic (g)
Dehydrated:								
Bouillon cube, ½ in, 1 cube	4	4	5	1	Tr	—	—	—
Mixes:								
Unprepared:								
Onion, 1½ oz pkg	43	3	150	6	5	1.1	2.3	1.0
Prepared with water:								
Chicken noodle, 1 cup	240	95	55	2	1	—	—	—
Onion, 1 cup	240	96	35	1	1	—	—	—
Tomato vegetable with noodles, 1 cup	240	93	65	1	1	—	—	—
Vinegar, cider, 1 tbsp	15	94	Tr	Tr	0	0	0	0
White sauce, medium, with enriched flour, 1 cup	250	73	405	10	31	19.3	7.8	.8
Yeast:								
Baker's dry, active, 1 pkg	7	5	20	3	Tr	—	—	—
Brewer's, dry, 1 tbsp	8	5	25	3	Tr	—	—	—

[1]Vitamin A value is largely from beta-carotene used for coloring. Riboflavin value for powdered sweet creamers applies to products with added riboflavin.
[2]Applies to product without added vitamin A. With added vitamin A, value is 500 IU.
[3]Applies to product without vitamin A added.
[4]Applies to product with added vitamin A. Without added vitamin A, value is 20 IU.
[5]Yields 1 qt of fluid milk when reconstituted according to package directions.
[6]Applies to product with added vitamin A.
[7]Weight applies to product with label claim on 1⅓ cups equal 3.2 oz.
[8]Applies to products made from thick shake mixes and that do not contain added ice cream. Products made from milk shake mixes are higher in fat and usually contain added ice cream.
[9]Content of fat, vitamin A, and carbohydrate varies. Consult the label when precise values are needed for special diets.
[10]Applies to product made with milk containing no added vitamin A.
[11]Based on year-round average.
[12]Based on average vitamin A content of fortified margarine. Federal specifications for fortified margarine require a minimum of 15,000 IU of vitamin A per pound.
[13]Fatty acid values apply to product made with regular-type margarine.
[14]Dipped in egg, milk, or water, and breadcrumbs; fried in vegetable shortening.
[15]If bones are discarded, value for calcium will be greatly reduced.
[16]Dipped in egg, breadcrumbs, and flour or batter.
[17]Prepared with tuna, celery, salad dressing (mayonnaise type), pickle, onion, and egg.
[18]Outer layer of fat on the cut was removed to within approximately ½ in of the lean. Deposits of fat within the cut were not removed.
[19]Crust made with vegetable shortening and enriched flour.
[20]Regular-type margarine used.
[21]Value varies widely.
[22]About one fourth of the outer layer of fat on the cut was removed. Deposits of fat within the cut were not removed.
[23]Vegetable shortening used.
[24]Also applies to pasteurized apple cider.
[25]Applies to product without added ascorbic acid. For value of product with added ascorbic acid, refer to label.

Nutrients in Indicated Quantity									
Carbohydrate (g)	Calcium (mg)	Phosphorus (mg)	Iron (mg)	Potassium (mg)	Vitamin A Value (IU)	Thiamin (mg)	Riboflavin (mg)	Niacin (mg)	Ascorbic Acid (mg)
Tr	—	—	—	4	—	—	—	—	—
23	42	49	.6	238	30	.05	.03	.3	6
8	7	19	.2	19	50	.07	.05	.5	Tr
6	10	12	.2	58	Tr	Tr	Tr	Tr	2
12	7	19	.2	29	480	.05	.02	.5	5
1	1	1	.1	15	—	—	—	—	—
22	288	233	.5	348	1150	.12	.43	.7	2
3	3	90	1.1	140	Tr	.16	.38	2.6	Tr
3	17[70]	140	1.4	152	Tr	1.25	.34	3.0	Tr

[26]Based on product with label claim of 45% of U.S. RDA in 6 fl oz.
[27]Based on product with label claim of 100% of U.S. RDA in 6 fl oz.
[28]Weight includes peel and membranes between sections. Without these parts, the weight of the edible portion is 123 g for ½ pink or red grapefruit and 118 g for ½ white grapefruit.
[29]For white-fleshed varieties, value is about 20 IU per cup; for red-fleshed varieties, 1080 IU.
[30]Weight includes seeds. Without seeds, weight of the edible portion is 57 g.
[31]Applies to product without added ascorbic acid. With added ascorbic acid, based on claim that 6 fl oz of reconstituted juice contains 45% or 50% of the U.S. RDA, value in milligrams is 106 or 120 for a 6 fl oz can (undiluted, frozen concentrate grape juice), 36 or 40 for 1 cup of diluted juice (diluted frozen concentrate grape juice.)
[32]For products with added thiamin and riboflavin but without added ascorbic acid, values in milligrams would be .60 for thiamin, .80 for riboflavin, and Tr for ascorbic acid. For products with only ascorbic acid added, valued varies with the brand. Consult the label.
[33]Weight includes rind. Without rind, the weight of the edible portion is 272 g for cantaloup and 149 g for honeydew melon.
[34]Represents yellow-fleshed varieties. For white-fleshed varieties, value is 50 IU for 1 peach, 90 IU for 1 cup of slices.
[35]Value represents products with added ascorbic acid. For products without added ascorbic acid, value in milligrams is 116 for a 10 oz container, 103 for 1 cup.
[36]Weight includes pits. After removal of the pits, the weight of the edible portion is 258 g for 1 cup plums in heavy syrup, 133 g for 3 plums in heavy syrup, 43 g for 4 dried prunes, and 213 g for 1 cup cooked, unsweetened prunes.
[37]Weight includes rind and seeds. Without rind and seeds, weight of the edible portion is 426 g.
[38]Made with vegetable shortening.
[39]Applies to product made with white cornmeal. With yellow cornmeal, value is 30 IU.
[40]Applies to white varieties. For yellow varieties, value is 150 IU.
[41]Applies to products that do not contain disodium phosphate. If disodium phosphate is an ingredient, value is 162 mg.
[42]Value may range from less than 1 mg to about 8 mg, depending on the brand. Consult the label.
[43]Applies to product with added nutrient. Without added nutrient, value is trace.
[44]Value varies with the brand. Consult the label.
[45]Applies to product with added nutrient. Without added nutrient, value is trace.
[46]Excepting angelfood cake, cakes were made from mixes containing vegetable shortening; icings, with butter.

[47]Excepting sponge cake, vegetable shortening used for cake portion; butter, for icing. If butter or margarine used for cake portion, vitamin A values would be higher.
[48]Applies to product made with a sodium aluminum-sulfate type of baking powder. With a low-sodium type of baking powder containing potassium, value would be about twice the amount shown.
[49]Equal weights of flour, sugar, eggs, and vegetable shortening.
[50]Products are commercial unless otherwise specified.
[51]Made with enriched flour and vegetable shortening except for macaroons, which do not contain flour or shortening.
[52]Icing made with butter.
[53]Applies to yellow varieties; white varieties contain only a trace.
[54]Contains vegetable shortening and butter.
[55]Made with corn oil.
[56]Made with regular margarine.
[57]Applies to product made with yellow cornmeal.
[58]Made with enriched degermed cornmeal and enriched flour.
[59]Product may or may not be enriched with riboflavin. Consult the label.
[60]Value varies with the brand. Consult the label.
[61]Weight includes cob. Without cob, weight is 77 g for 1 ear cooked, drained sweet corn, 126 g for 1 frozen 5-in ear.
[62]Based on yellow varieties. For white varieties, value is trace.
[63]Weight includes refuse of outer leaves and core. Without these parts, weight is 163 g.
[64]Weight includes core. Without core, weight is 539 g.
[65]Value based on white-fleshed varieties. For yellow-fleshed varieties, values in IU is 70 for 1 cup chopped raw onions, 50 for 1 cup sliced raw onions, and 80 for 1 cup cooked onions.
[66]Weight includes cores and stem ends. Without these parts, weight is 123 g.
[67]Based on year-round average. For tomatoes marketed from November through May, value is about 12 mg; from June through October, 32 mg.
[68]Applies to product without calcium salts added. Value for products with calcium salts added may be as much as 63 mg for whole tomatoes, 241 mg for cut forms.
[69]Weight includes pits. Without pits, weight is 13 g for 4 medium (or 3 extra large or 2 giant) green pickled olives, 9 g for 3 small (or 2 large) ripe pickled olives.
[70]Values may vary from 6 to 60 mg.

APPENDIX M

National Center for Health Statistics Growth Charts

From Ross Laboratories, Columbus, Ohio.

GIRLS: BIRTH TO 36 MONTHS PHYSICAL GROWTH NCHS PERCENTILES*

NAME ____________________ RECORD # ____________

AGE (MONTHS)

LENGTH

WEIGHT

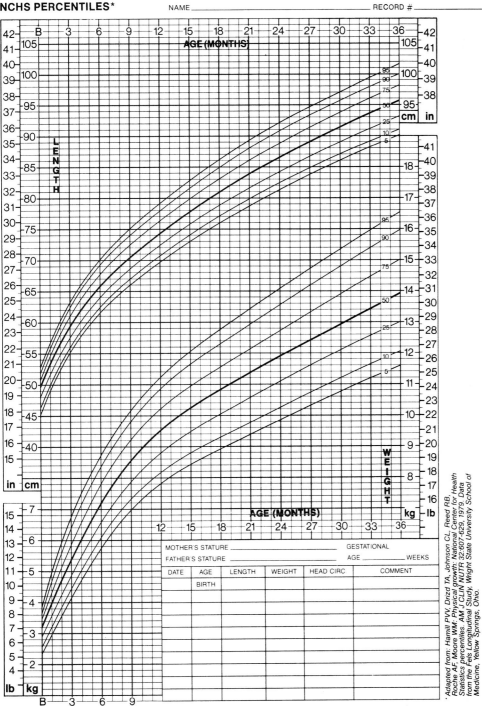

MOTHER'S STATURE ____________ GESTATIONAL AGE ________ WEEKS

FATHER'S STATURE ____________

DATE	AGE	LENGTH	WEIGHT	HEAD CIRC	COMMENT
	BIRTH				

* Adapted from: Hamill PVV, Drizd TA, Johnson CL, Reed RB, Roche AF, Moore WM: Physical growth: National Center for Health Statistics percentiles. AM J CLIN NUTR 32:607-629, 1979. Data from the Fels Longitudinal Study, Wright State University School of Medicine, Yellow Springs, Ohio.

GIRLS: BIRTH TO 36 MONTHS PHYSICAL GROWTH NCHS PERCENTILES*

NAME ______________________ RECORD # ____________

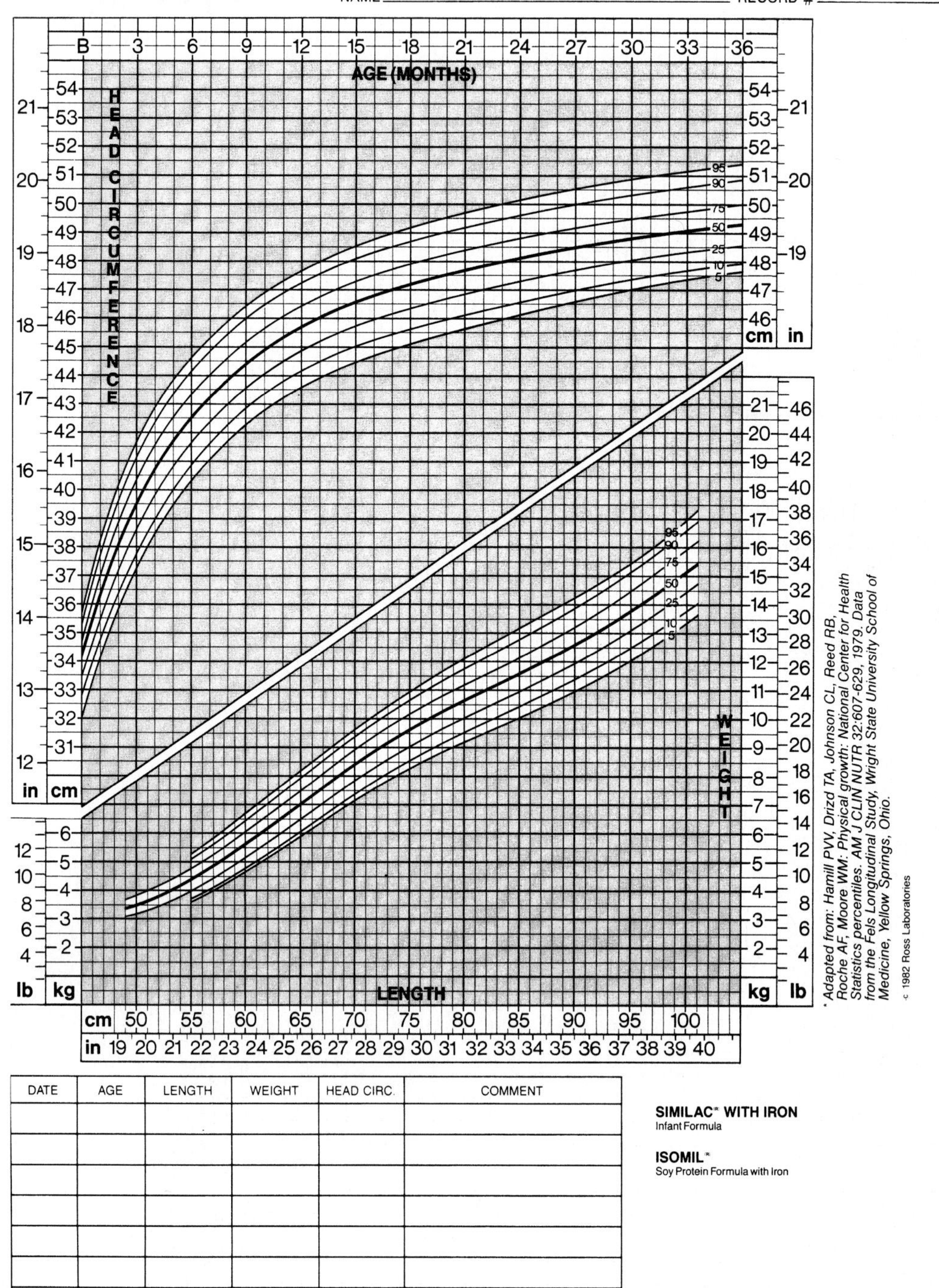

DATE	AGE	LENGTH	WEIGHT	HEAD CIRC.	COMMENT

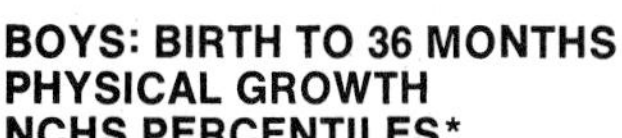

BOYS: BIRTH TO 36 MONTHS
PHYSICAL GROWTH
NCHS PERCENTILES*

NAME ____________________ RECORD # ____________

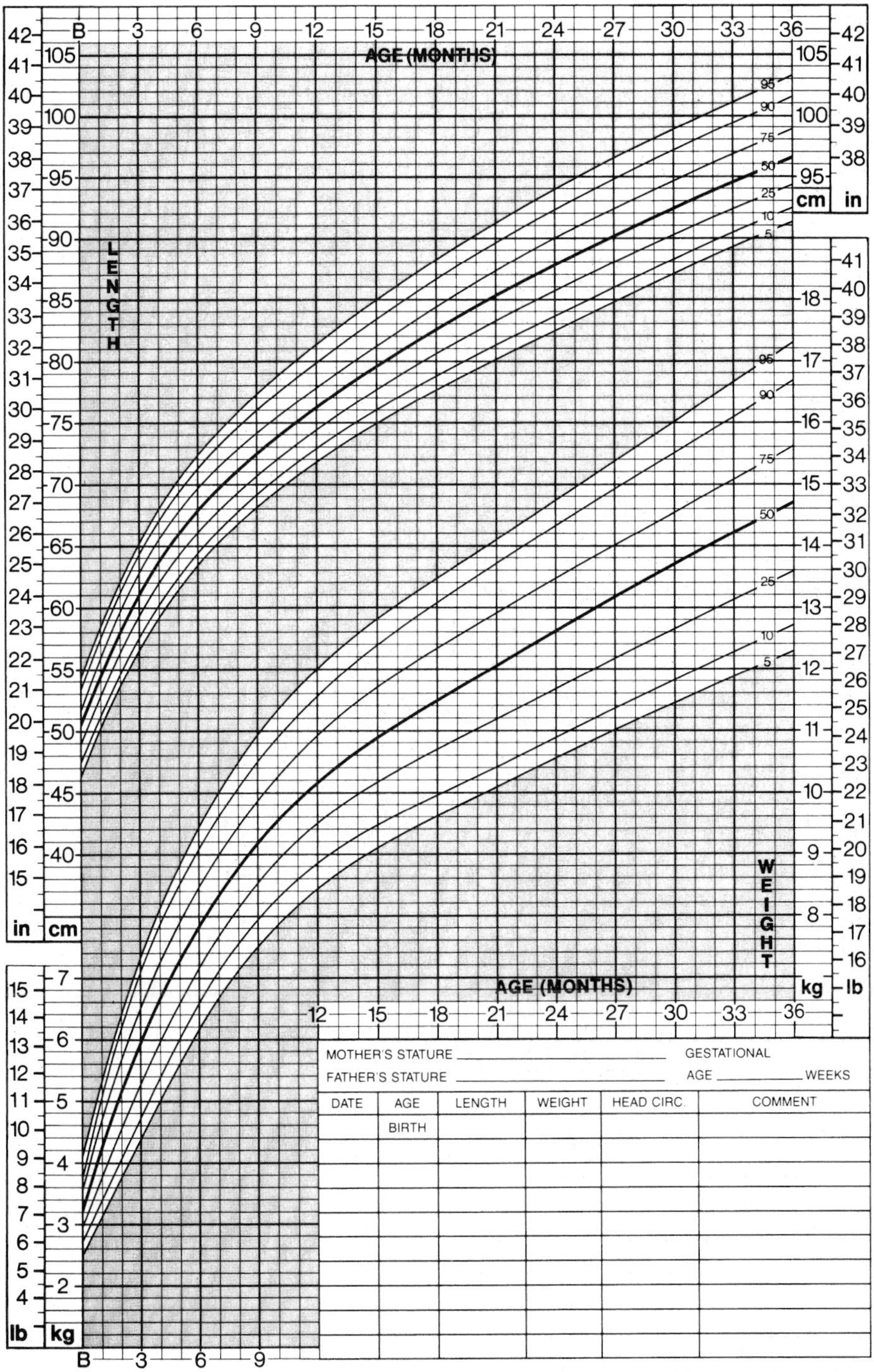

AGE (MONTHS)

B 3 6 9 12 15 18 21 24 27 30 33 36

LENGTH (in / cm) — WEIGHT (kg / lb)

Percentiles: 95, 90, 75, 50, 25, 10, 5

MOTHER'S STATURE ____________ GESTATIONAL

FATHER'S STATURE ____________ AGE ________ WEEKS

DATE	AGE	LENGTH	WEIGHT	HEAD CIRC.	COMMENT
	BIRTH				

*Adapted from: Hamill PVV, Drizd TA, Johnson CL, Reed RB, Roche AF, Moore WM: Physical growth: National Center for Health Statistics percentiles. AM J CLIN NUTR 32:607-629, 1979. Data from the Fels Longitudinal Study, Wright State University School of Medicine, Yellow Springs, Ohio.

BOYS: BIRTH TO 36 MONTHS PHYSICAL GROWTH NCHS PERCENTILES*

NAME ____________________ RECORD # ____________

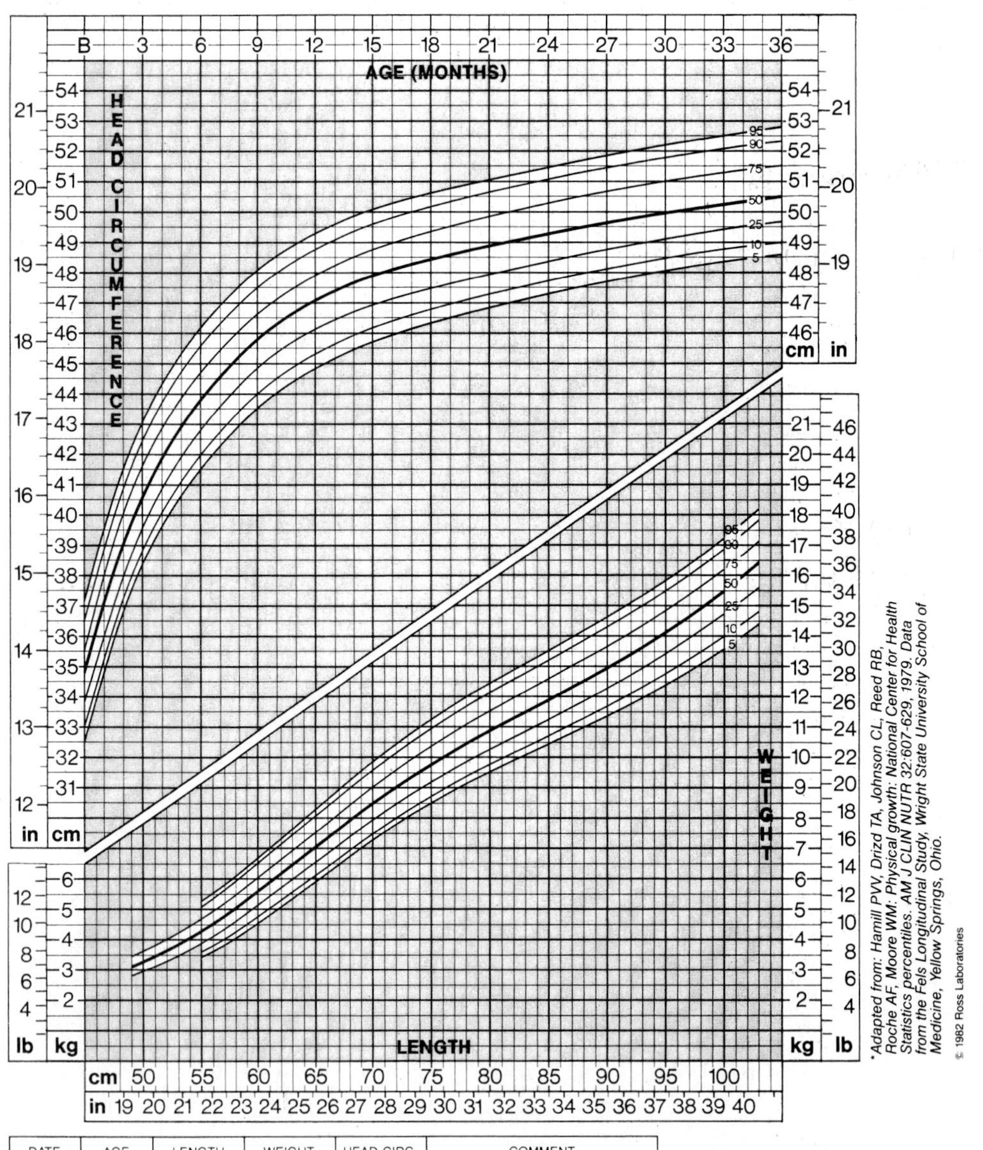

DATE	AGE	LENGTH	WEIGHT	HEAD CIRC.	COMMENT

SIMILAC® WITH IRON
Infant Formula

ISOMIL®
Soy Protein Formula with Iron

Reprinted with permission of Ross Laboratories

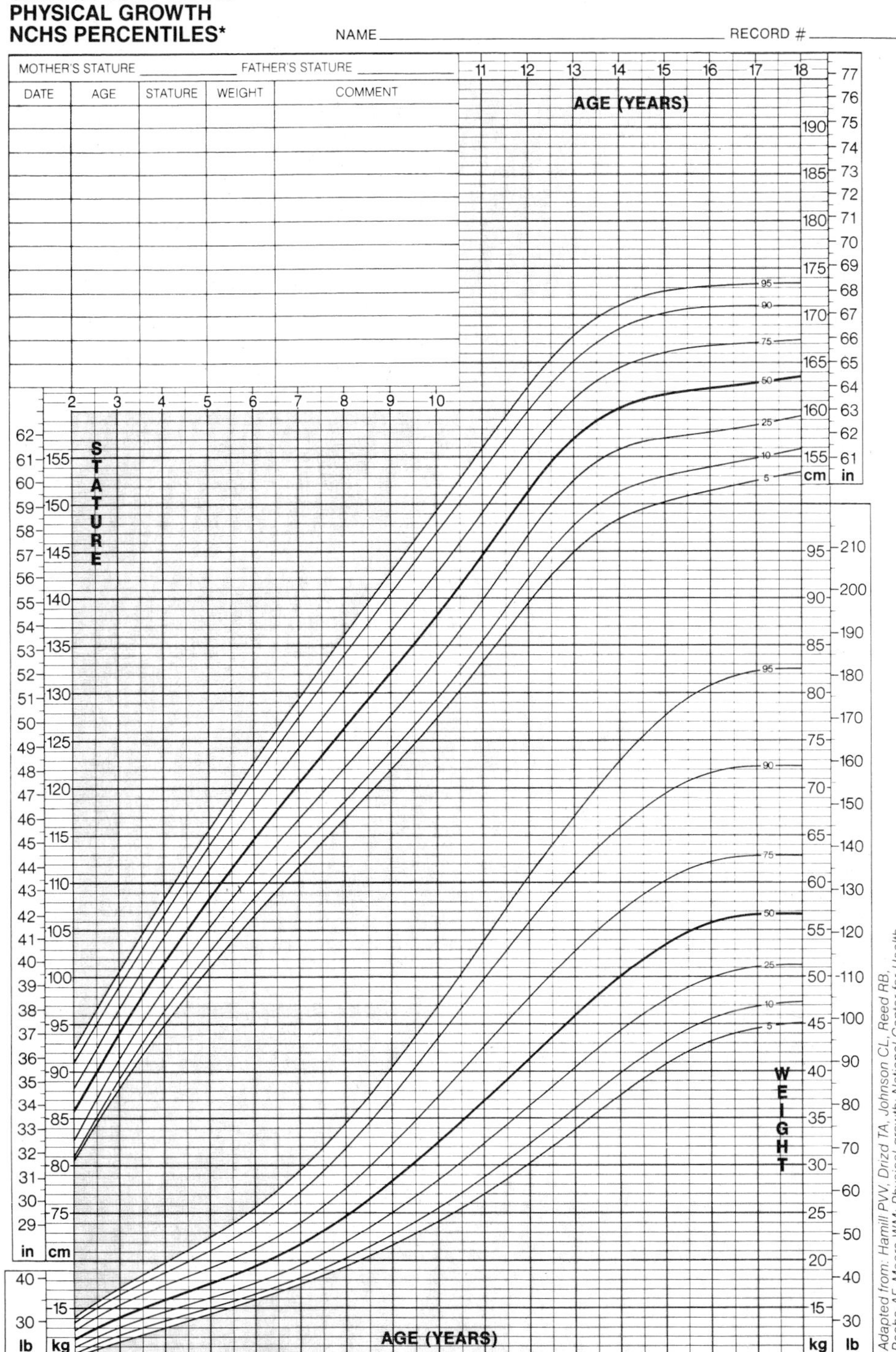

*Adapted from: Hamill PVV, Drizd TA, Johnson CL, Reed RB, Roche AF, Moore WM: Physical growth: National Center for Health Statistics percentiles. AM J CLIN NUTR 32:607-629, 1979. Data from the National Center for Health Statistics (NCHS), Hyattsville, Maryland.

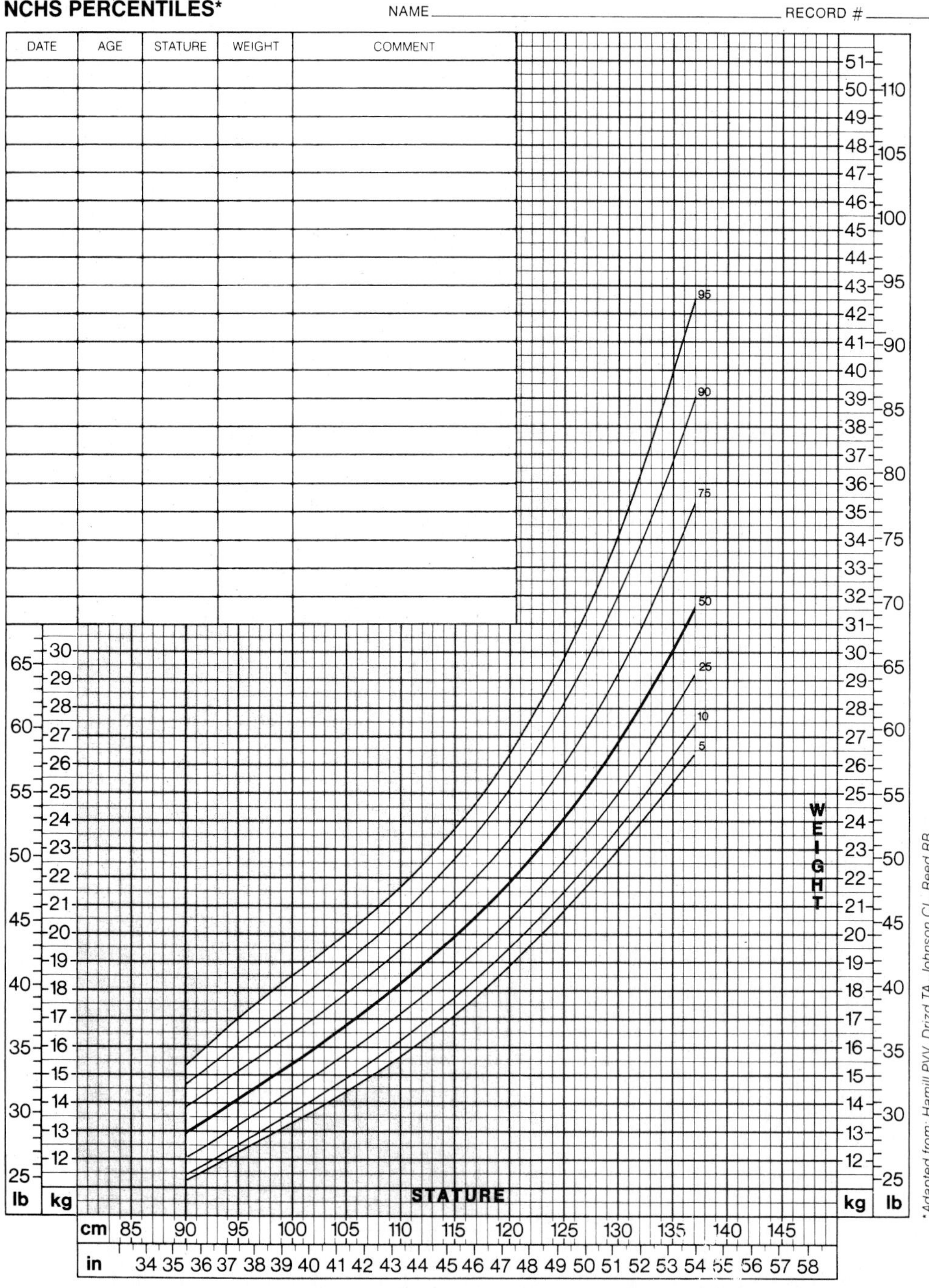

Reprinted with permission of Ross Laboratories

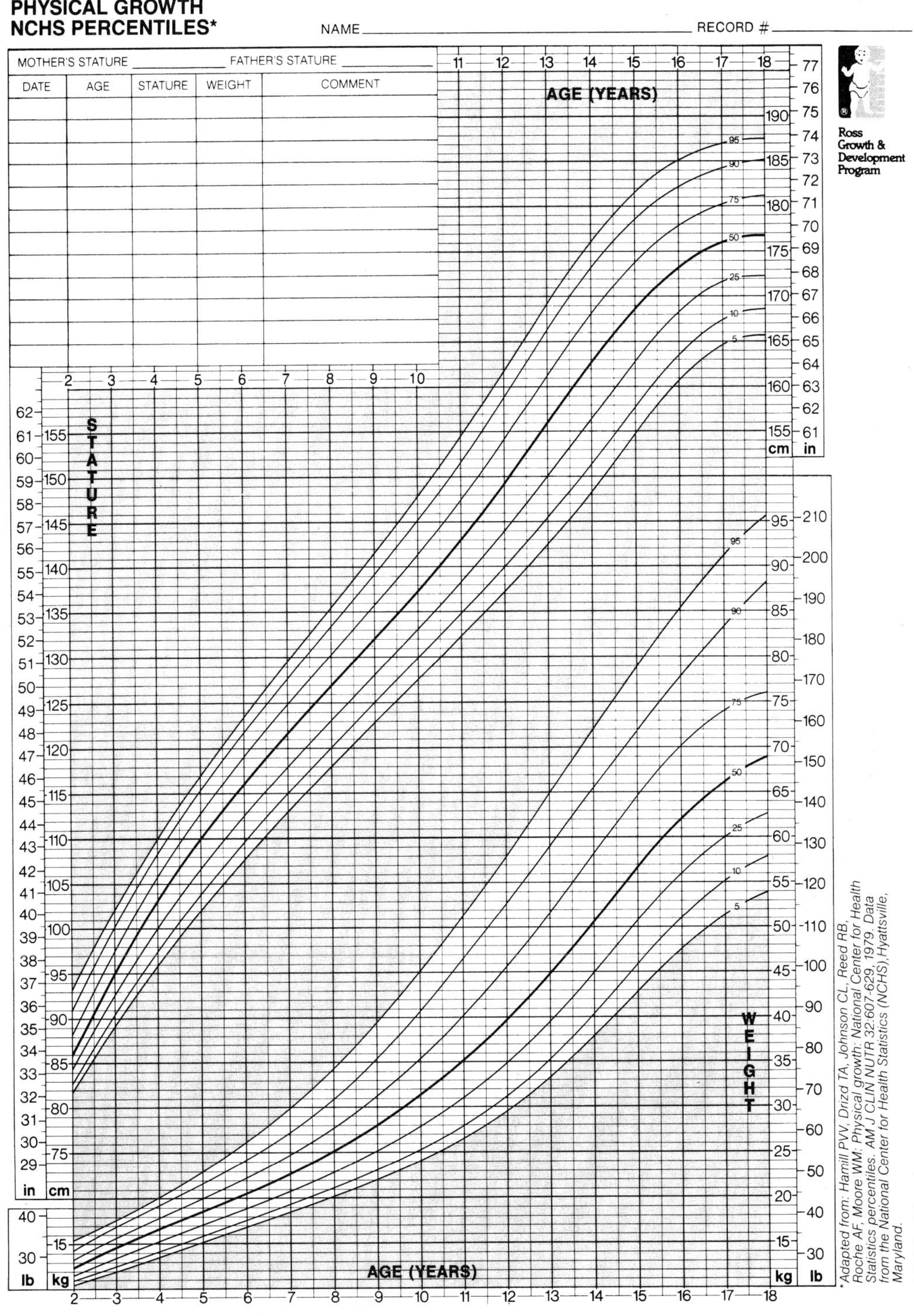
BOYS: 2 TO 18 YEARS
PHYSICAL GROWTH
NCHS PERCENTILES*
NAME
RECORD #
MOTHER'S STATURE
FATHER'S STATURE
DATE
AGE
STATURE
WEIGHT
COMMENT
AGE (YEARS)
STATURE
WEIGHT
cm
in
kg
lb
Ross Growth & Development Program
*Adapted from: Hamill PVV, Drizd TA, Johnson CL, Reed RB, Roche AF, Moore WM: Physical growth: National Center for Health Statistics percentiles. AM J CLIN NUTR 32:607-629, 1979. Data from the National Center for Health Statistics (NCHS), Hyattsville, Maryland.
© 1982 Ross Laboratories

BOYS: PREPUBESCENT PHYSICAL GROWTH NCHS PERCENTILES*

NAME ______________________ RECORD # ____________

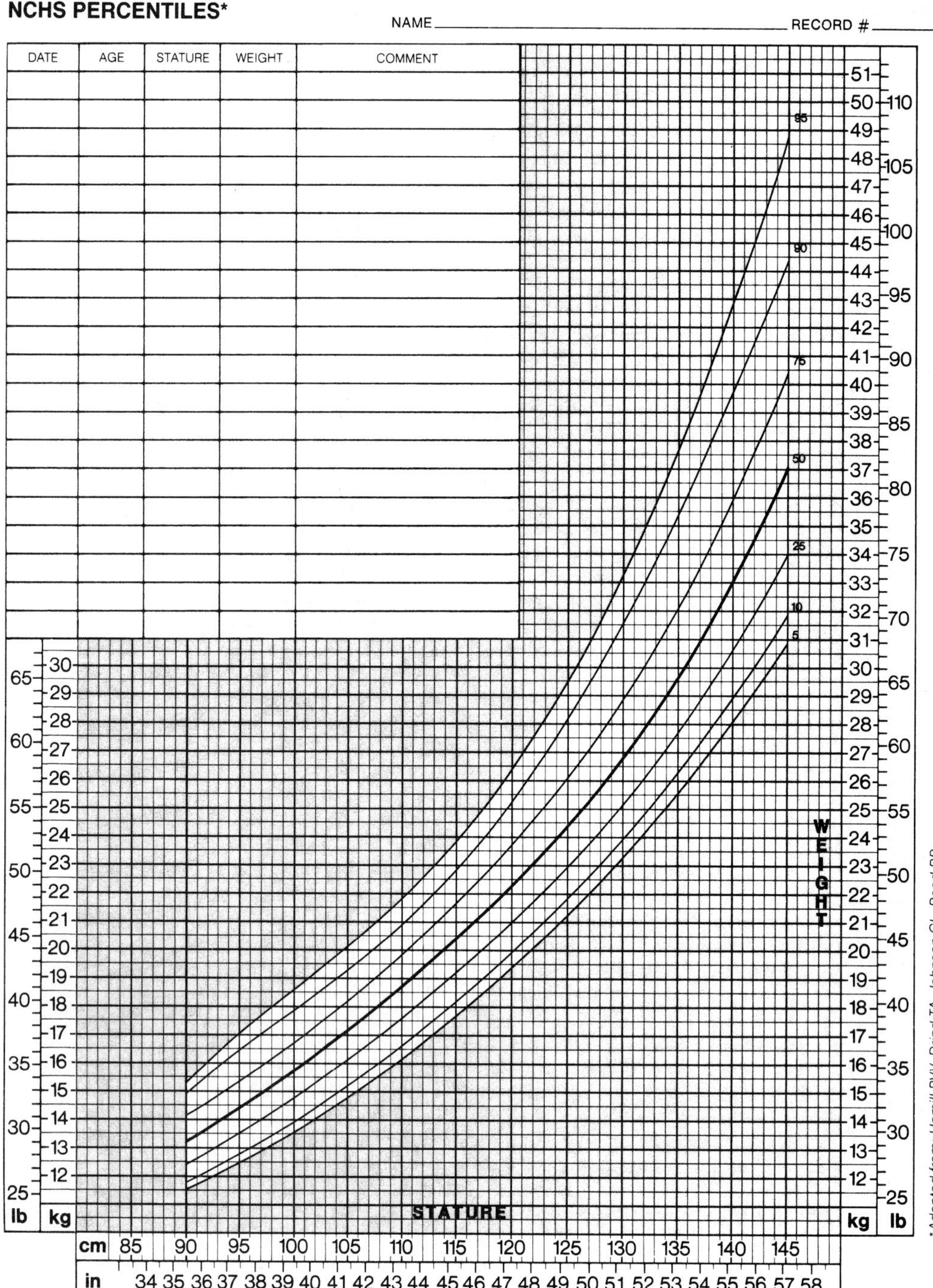

*Adapted from: Hamill PVV, Drizd TA, Johnson CL, Reed RB, Roche AF, Moore WM: Physical growth: National Center for Health Statistics percentiles. AM J CLIN NUTR 32:607-629, 1979. Data from the National Center for Health Statistics (NCHS), Hyattsville, Maryland.

Reprinted with permission of Ross Laboratories

**GIRLS: 2 TO 5 YEARS
PHYSICAL GROWTH
NCHS PERCENTILES***

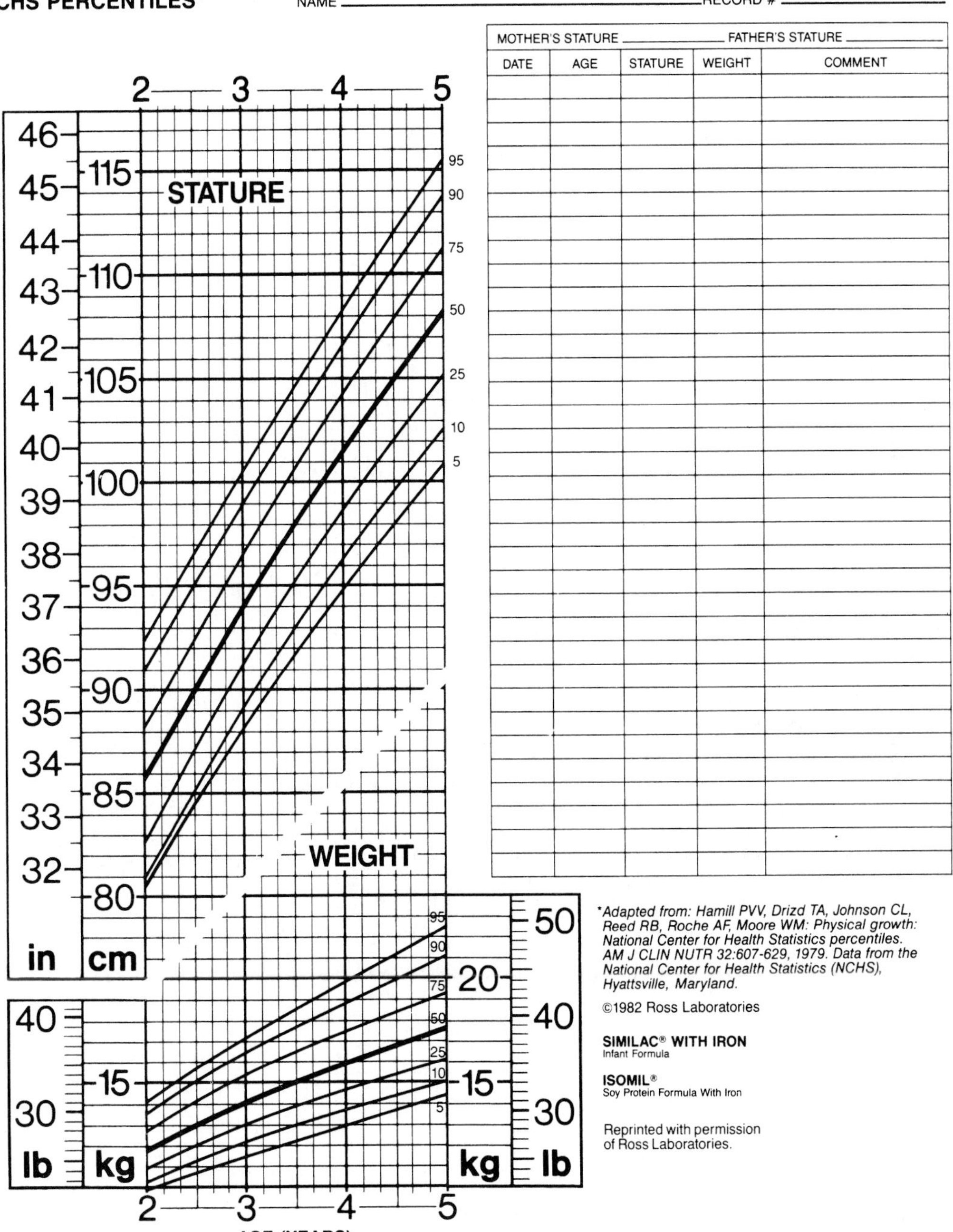

*Adapted from: Hamill PVV, Drizd TA, Johnson CL, Reed RB, Roche AF, Moore WM: Physical growth: National Center for Health Statistics percentiles. AM J CLIN NUTR 32:607-629, 1979. Data from the National Center for Health Statistics (NCHS), Hyattsville, Maryland.

Reprinted with permission of Ross Laboratories.

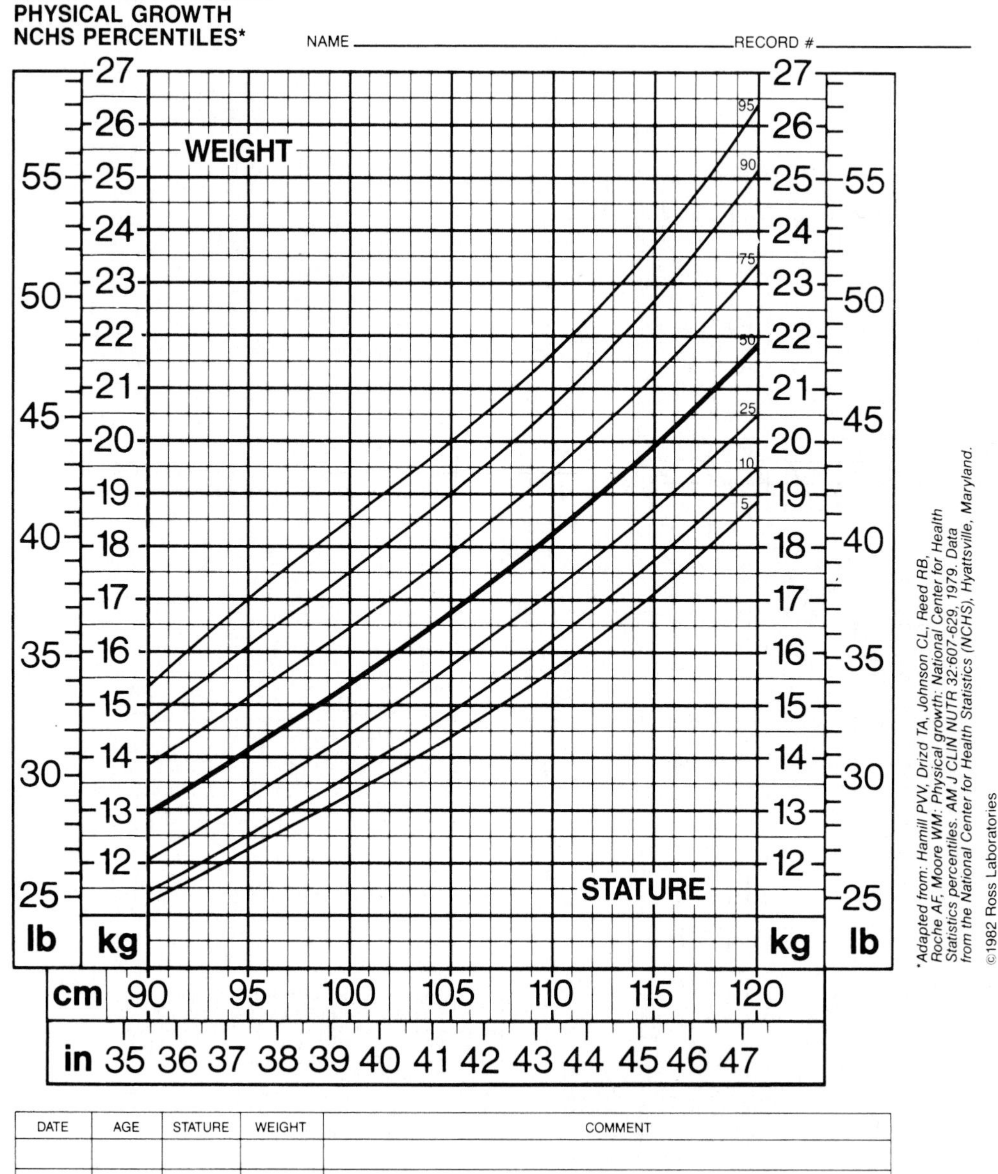
GIRLS: PREPUBESCENT
PHYSICAL GROWTH
NCHS PERCENTILES*
NAME
RECORD #
WEIGHT
STATURE
95
90
75
50
25
10
5
lb
kg
cm 90 95 100 105 110 115 120
in 35 36 37 38 39 40 41 42 43 44 45 46 47
kg 12 13 14 15 16 17 18 19 20 21 22 23 24 25 26 27
lb 25 30 35 40 45 50 55
*Adapted from: Hamill PVV, Drizd TA, Johnson CL, Reed RB, Roche AF, Moore WM: Physical growth: National Center for Health Statistics percentiles. AM J CLIN NUTR 32:607-629, 1979. Data from the National Center for Health Statistics (NCHS), Hyattsville, Maryland.
©1982 Ross Laboratories

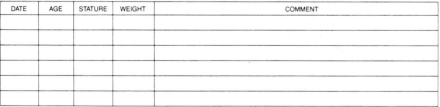

DATE	AGE	STATURE	WEIGHT	COMMENT

BOYS: 2 TO 5 YEARS
PHYSICAL GROWTH
NCHS PERCENTILES*

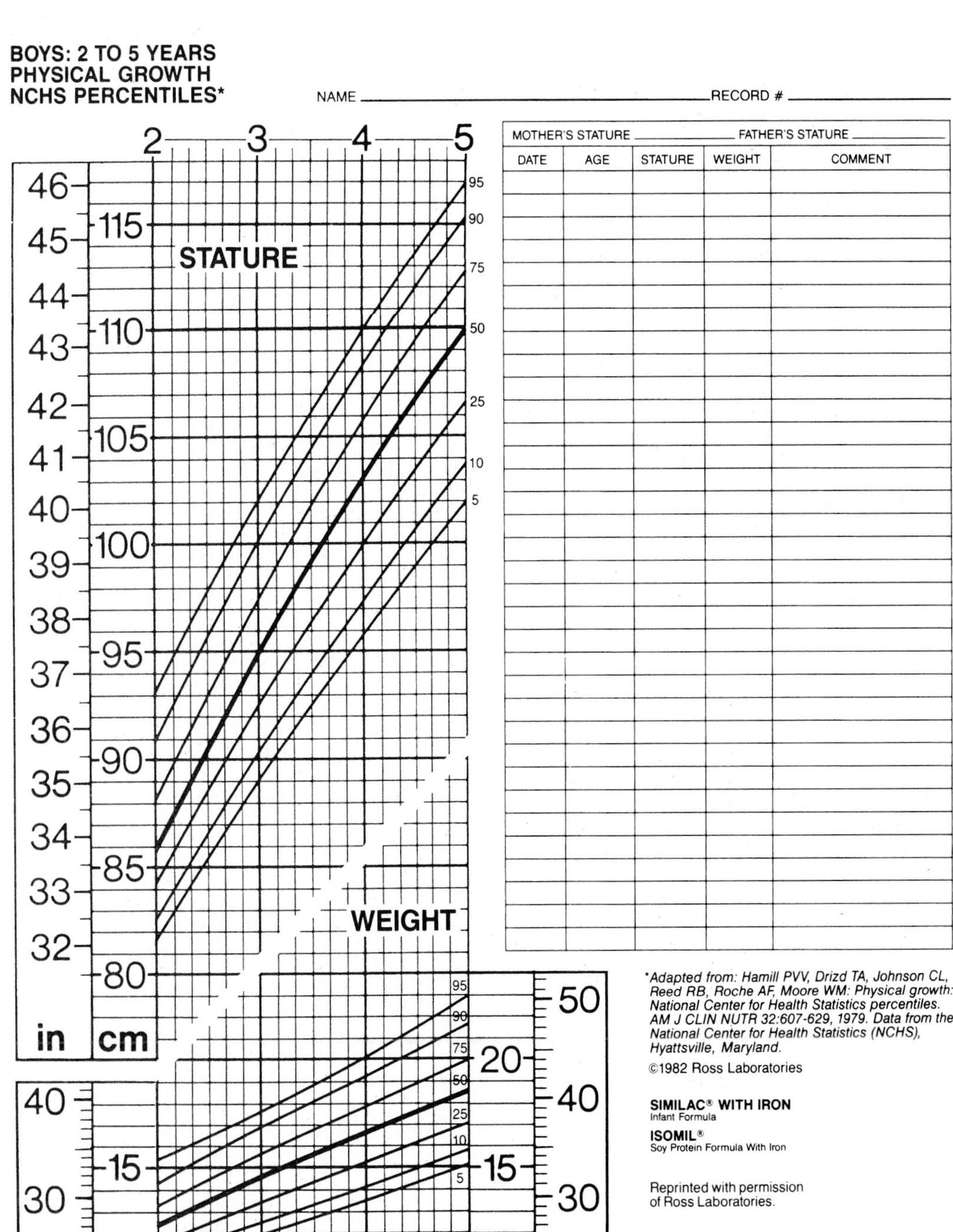

*Adapted from: Hamill PVV, Drizd TA, Johnson CL, Reed RB, Roche AF, Moore WM: Physical growth: National Center for Health Statistics percentiles. AM J CLIN NUTR 32:607-629, 1979. Data from the National Center for Health Statistics (NCHS), Hyattsville, Maryland.

SIMILAC® WITH IRON
Infant Formula

ISOMIL®
Soy Protein Formula With Iron

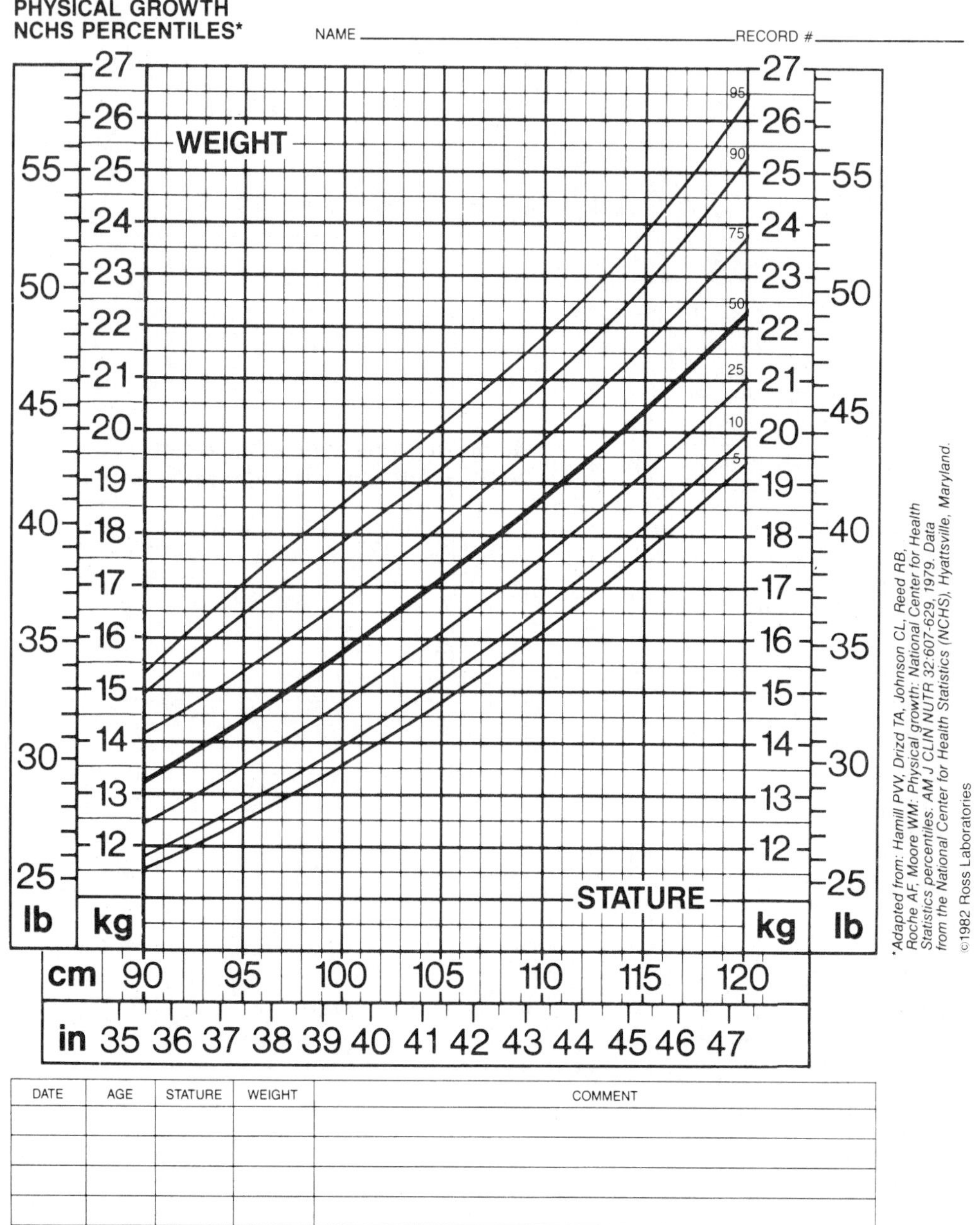

DATE	AGE	STATURE	WEIGHT	COMMENT

APPENDIX N

SUPPLIERS OF NUTRITIONAL ASSESSMENT EQUIPMENT

Suppliers

Throughout the Achievement Center
916 Sixth Avenue
Box 176
Worthington, Minnesota 56187–0176
507–376–3168

Beta Technology (formerly Cambridge Scientific)
151 Harvey West Blvd.
Santa Cruz, California 95060
408–426–0882
800–638–9566
408–423–4573 (fax)

Cardinal-Detecto
P.O. Box 151
Webb City, Missouri 64870
417–673–4631
417–673–5001 (fax)

Country Technology, Inc.
P.O. Box 87
Gays Mills, Wisconsin 54631
608–735–4718
608–735–4859 (fax)

Creative Health Products, Inc.
5148 Saddle Ridge Road
Plymouth, Michigan 48170
313–996–5900
800–742–4478

Fat Control, Inc.
Box 10117
Towson, Maryland 21285
717–993–3550

Health Products
2126 Ridge
Ann Arbor, Michigan 48104
313–996–0953

Illinois Department of Public Health
Division of Health Promotion and Screening
Nutrition Services Section
535 West Jefferson Street
Springfield, Illinois 62761

ITAC Corporation
P.O. Box 1742
Silver Spring, Maryland 20915
301–593–8007

Lafayette Instrument
P.O. Box 5729
Lafayette, Indiana 47903
317–423–1505
800–428–7545

Metropolitan Life Insurance Company
Health and Safety Education Division
MetLife Healthy Living[sm] Program
One Madison Avenue
New York, New York 10010–3690

Novel Products, Inc.
P.O. Box 408
3266 Yale Bridge Road
Rockton, Illinois 61072
815–624–4888
800–323–5143
815–624–4866 (fax)

Ralph's Wood Crafts
3875 East Brookstown Drive
Baton Rouge, Louisiana 70805
504–357–3932

RJL Systems, Inc.
33955 Harper Avenue
Clinton Township, Michigan 48035
810–790–0200

Ross Laboratories
625 Cleveland Avenue
Columbus, Ohio 43216

Seca Corporation
8920 A Route 108
Oakland Center
Columbia, Maryland 21045
410–964–3858
800–542–7322

Seritex, Inc.
450 Barell Avenue
Carlstadt, New Jersey 07072
201–939–4606

Valhalla Scientific, Inc.
7576 Trade Street
San Diego, California 92121
800–395–4565

VWR Scientific Company
P.O. Box 6016
Cerritos, California 90702
800–932–5000

Products

Anthropometric Tapes

Country Technology
Creative Health Products
Lafayette Instrument
Novel Products
Seritex

Bioelectrical Impedance Instruments

RJL Systems
Valhalla Scientific

Elbow Breadth Gauges

Creative Health Products
Health Products
Metropolitan Life Insurance Company
Seritex

Recumbent Length Measurement Equipment

The Achievement Center
Ralph's Wood Crafts
Seritex

Skinfold Calipers

Beta Technology
Country Technology
Creative Health Products
Fat Control
Lafayette Instrument
Novel Products
Seritex

Sliding Calipers

Seritex

Stadiometers

The Achievement Center
Creative Health Products
Illinois Department of Public Health (blueprints)
Novel Products
Ralph's Wood Crafts
Seritex

Weighing Scales

Cardinal-Detecto
Country Technology
Creative Health Products
ITAC Corporation
Novel Products
Seca
VWR Scientific

APPENDIX O

TRICEPS SKINFOLD NORMS FROM NHANES II

From National Center for Health Statistics. 1987. Anthropometric reference data and prevalence of overweight, United States, 1976–80. Vital and Health Statistics Series 11, No. 238. U.S. Department of Health and Human Services: National Center for Health Statistics, Centers for Disease Control, Public Health Service.
Data from the National Center for Health Statistics.

Triceps skinfold in millimeters for persons 6 months to 19 years of age—United States, 1976–1980

Sex and age	Number of examined persons	Mean	Standard deviation	Percentile 5th	10th	15th	25th	50th	75th	85th	90th	95th
Male												
6–11 months	179	10.4	3.1	6.5	7.0	7.0	8.0	10.0	12.0	14.0	15.0	16.0
1 year	370	10.4	2.7	6.5	7.0	7.5	8.5	10.0	12.0	13.0	14.0	15.5
2 years	375	10.2	2.9	6.0	7.0	7.0	8.0	10.0	12.0	13.0	14.5	15.0
3 years	418	10.0	2.6	6.5	7.0	7.5	8.0	9.5	11.5	12.5	13.0	15.0
4 years	404	9.6	3.0	6.0	6.5	7.0	7.5	9.0	11.0	12.0	13.0	15.0
5 years	397	8.9	2.9	5.5	6.0	6.5	7.0	8.0	10.5	11.5	12.5	14.5
6 years	133	9.3	4.4	5.0	5.5	6.0	6.5	8.0	10.5	12.0	13.0	17.5
7 years	148	9.2	4.0	5.0	5.5	6.0	6.5	8.5	11.0	12.0	15.0	17.5
8 years	147	10.5	4.9	5.5	6.0	6.0	7.0	9.0	12.0	16.5	17.0	22.0
9 years	145	10.6	5.7	5.0	5.0	6.0	7.0	9.0	12.5	16.0	19.0	23.0
10 years	157	12.6	6.6	5.0	6.0	6.5	7.5	11.0	16.5	20.0	22.0	26.0
11 years	155	13.3	7.7	4.5	5.5	6.0	7.5	10.5	17.0	22.0	25.0	30.0
12 years	145	12.4	6.4	5.0	6.0	6.0	8.0	11.0	15.0	18.0	21.5	26.5
13 years	173	11.2	7.0	5.0	5.5	6.0	7.0	9.0	12.5	16.5	20.5	22.5
14 years	186	10.4	5.8	4.0	5.0	5.5	6.0	9.0	13.0	15.0	17.0	23.0
15 years	184	10.1	7.2	5.0	5.0	6.0	6.0	7.5	11.0	14.5	18.0	22.0
16 years	178	10.9	6.6	4.5	5.0	5.5	6.5	8.0	13.0	18.5	20.5	25.5
17 years	173	8.5	4.6	4.0	4.5	5.0	5.5	7.0	10.5	12.5	15.0	18.0
18 years	164	11.1	6.6	4.0	5.0	5.0	6.0	9.5	14.5	17.5	19.0	22.5
19 years	148	10.9	6.1	5.0	5.5	6.0	6.5	9.0	13.0	16.0	18.5	23.0
Female												
6–11 months	177	9.9	2.6	6.5	7.0	7.0	8.0	10.0	11.5	12.5	13.0	14.5
1 year	336	10.6	3.3	6.0	7.0	7.5	8.0	10.5	12.0	13.5	15.0	16.5
2 years	336	10.6	3.0	6.0	7.0	7.5	8.0	10.5	12.5	13.5	15.0	16.0
3 years	366	10.3	2.9	6.0	7.0	7.0	8.0	10.0	12.0	12.5	13.5	16.5
4 years	396	10.4	3.1	6.0	6.5	7.5	8.0	10.0	12.0	13.0	14.0	15.5
5 years	364	10.6	3.2	6.0	7.0	7.5	8.5	10.5	12.5	14.0	14.5	16.0
6 years	135	11.0	3.9	6.0	7.0	7.5	8.0	10.0	12.0	14.5	16.0	18.5
7 years	157	11.5	4.5	6.0	7.0	7.5	9.0	10.5	13.0	15.0	18.0	20.0
8 years	123	11.9	5.2	6.0	6.5	7.0	8.5	11.0	14.0	16.0	18.0	21.0
9 years	149	14.3	6.5	7.0	7.5	8.5	10.0	13.0	16.0	20.0	23.0	27.0
10 years	136	14.5	5.9	7.0	8.0	8.0	10.0	13.5	18.0	21.0	22.5	24.5
11 years	140	15.7	6.9	8.0	8.5	9.0	11.0	14.0	19.5	21.5	23.0	29.5
12 years	147	15.1	6.0	7.5	8.0	9.0	11.5	13.5	18.5	21.5	23.0	27.0
13 years	162	15.9	7.9	6.0	7.5	9.0	10.5	15.0	19.0	22.0	25.0	30.0
14 years	178	17.6	7.5	8.0	10.0	10.5	12.0	17.0	21.5	25.0	29.5	32.0
15 years	145	17.1	7.1	8.5	9.5	10.0	11.5	16.5	20.5	24.5	26.0	32.1
16 years	170	19.5	7.2	11.0	11.5	12.0	14.0	18.0	23.0	27.0	30.5	33.1
17 years	134	19.8	7.8	9.5	11.0	11.5	14.0	20.0	24.5	26.5	28.5	34.5
18 years	170	19.9	7.6	11.0	12.0	12.5	14.0	18.0	23.5	27.0	32.5	35.0
19 years	158	20.4	7.6	10.5	11.5	13.0	15.0	19.0	25.0	28.0	30.0	33.5

Triceps skinfold in millimeters for males 18–74 years of age—United States, 1976–1980

Race and age	Number of examined persons	Mean	Standard deviation	Percentile								
				5th	10th	15th	25th	50th	75th	85th	90th	95th
All races*												
18–74 years	5916	12.9	6.7	5.0	6.0	6.5	8.0	12.0	16.0	19.5	22.0	25.5
18–24 years	988	11.6	6.5	4.5	5.0	6.0	6.5	10.0	15.0	17.5	20.0	24.5
25–34 years	1067	12.9	7.0	4.5	5.5	6.5	7.5	11.5	16.5	20.0	23.0	26.0
35–44 years	745	13.8	7.1	5.0	6.0	7.0	9.0	12.5	17.0	20.0	23.0	27.0
45–54 years	690	13.5	6.7	5.5	6.5	7.0	9.0	12.0	16.5	20.0	22.0	25.5
55–64 years	1227	13.2	6.3	5.0	6.0	7.5	9.0	12.0	16.0	19.5	21.5	25.5
65–74 years	1199	12.7	6.1	5.0	6.0	7.0	8.0	11.5	16.0	18.5	21.0	25.0
White												
18–74 years	5148	13.0	6.6	5.0	6.0	7.0	8.0	12.0	16.0	19.5	22.0	25.5
18–24 years	846	11.9	6.5	4.5	5.0	6.0	7.0	10.0	15.0	18.0	20.0	25.0
25–34 years	901	13.1	6.9	5.0	6.0	7.0	8.0	12.0	16.5	20.0	22.5	26.0
35–44 years	653	13.9	7.0	5.5	6.5	7.0	9.0	12.5	17.0	21.0	23.0	27.0
45–54 years	617	13.4	6.5	5.5	6.5	7.5	9.0	12.0	16.5	20.0	21.0	25.0
55–64 years	1086	13.1	5.9	5.5	6.5	7.5	9.0	12.0	16.0	19.0	21.0	24.5
65–74 years	1045	12.9	6.0	5.0	6.5	7.0	8.0	12.0	16.0	19.0	21.0	25.0
Black												
18–74 years	649	12.1	7.8	4.0	4.5	5.0	6.5	10.0	16.0	19.0	23.0	27.0
18–24 years	121	9.7	6.4	4.0	4.0	4.5	5.0	7.5	13.0	15.0	18.5	21.5
25–34 years	139	11.5	7.5	3.5	4.0	5.0	6.0	10.0	15.5	19.0	23.0	24.5
35–44 years	70	13.0	8.1	—	5.0	6.5	9.0	11.0	16.0	18.5	20.0	—
45–54 years	62	15.0	8.7	—	5.5	6.0	9.0	13.0	18.0	25.5	27.5	—
55–64 years	129	12.9	7.8	3.5	4.5	5.5	7.0	10.5	17.5	22.0	25.0	29.0
65–74 years	128	11.6	6.7	4.0	4.5	5.5	7.0	10.0	14.5	16.0	19.5	27.5

*Includes all other races not shown as separate categories.

Triceps skinfold in millimeters for females 18–74 years of age—United States, 1976–1980

Race and age	Number of examined persons	Mean	Standard deviation	Percentile 5th	10th	15th	25th	50th	75th	85th	90th	95th
All races*												
18–74 years	6588	24.9	9.8	11.0	13.0	15.0	17.5	24.0	31.0	35.1	38.0	43.0
18–24 years	1066	20.7	8.6	10.0	11.5	12.5	15.0	19.0	25.0	29.5	32.0	37.0
25–34 years	1170	23.6	9.9	10.0	13.0	14.0	16.5	22.0	29.0	33.5	36.6	43.5
35–44 years	844	26.3	9.8	12.0	14.5	16.5	19.5	25.0	32.6	37.0	40.5	44.5
45–54 years	763	27.5	9.7	12.5	15.0	17.0	20.5	27.0	34.0	38.0	40.5	45.0
55–64 years	1329	27.2	9.5	12.0	15.0	17.5	21.0	26.5	33.0	37.0	40.0	43.6
65–74 years	1416	25.7	9.0	12.0	14.5	16.5	19.0	25.0	31.0	35.0	37.6	42.0
White												
18–74 years	5686	24.7	9.5	11.5	13.5	15.0	17.5	23.5	30.5	35.0	37.5	42.5
18–24 years	892	20.8	8.5	10.5	11.5	13.0	15.0	19.0	25.0	29.0	32.0	37.1
25–34 years	1000	23.3	9.4	10.5	13.0	14.0	16.5	22.0	28.5	33.0	36.0	42.1
35–44 years	726	26.1	9.6	12.0	14.5	16.0	19.0	24.5	32.0	36.5	40.0	44.0
45–54 years	647	27.2	9.4	13.0	15.0	16.5	20.5	27.0	33.0	37.0	40.0	43.1
55–64 years	1176	27.0	9.4	12.5	15.0	17.5	21.0	26.0	32.6	36.5	39.1	43.1
65–74 years	1245	25.5	8.8	12.0	14.5	16.5	19.0	25.0	30.5	34.0	37.0	41.1
Black												
18–74 years	782	26.6	11.6	10.0	12.0	14.0	17.5	25.5	35.0	39.0	42.5	48.0
18–24 years	147	20.6	8.8	8.0	10.0	11.0	14.0	19.0	27.0	31.0	35.0	37.0
25–34 years	145	25.5	12.2	8.0	11.0	13.0	16.0	24.0	32.0	37.0	47.0	49.5
35–44 years	103	28.7	11.4	9.0	14.0	15.5	20.5	29.5	36.6	40.5	45.0	48.0
45–54 years	100	31.6	11.8	10.5	16.0	20.0	23.5	31.5	40.0	43.5	48.5	53.1
55–64 years	135	29.5	10.8	12.0	14.0	18.0	22.0	28.5	38.5	42.0	43.0	46.0
65–74 years	152	29.0	10.5	11.5	14.5	17.0	21.5	29.0	37.0	38.6	44.0	47.5

*Includes all other races not shown as separate categories.

APPENDIX P

SUBSCAPULAR SKINFOLD NORMS FROM NHANES II

From National Center for Health Statistics. 1987. Anthropometric reference data and prevalence of overweight, United States, 1976–80. Vital and Health Statistics Series 11, No. 238. U.S. Department of Health and Human Services: National Center for Health Statistics, Centers for Disease Control, Public Health Service.

Subscapular skinfold in millimeters for persons 6 months–19 years of age—United States, 1976–1980

Sex and age	Number of examined persons	Mean	Standard deviation	Percentile 5th	10th	15th	25th	50th	75th	85th	90th	95th
Male												
6–11 months	179	6.5	1.9	4.0	5.0	5.0	5.5	6.0	7.5	8.0	8.5	9.0
1 year	370	6.6	1.9	4.0	4.5	5.0	5.0	6.5	7.5	8.0	9.0	10.5
2 years	375	6.1	2.2	3.5	4.0	4.0	5.0	5.5	7.0	7.5	9.0	10.0
3 years	418	5.7	1.6	4.0	4.0	4.0	4.5	5.5	6.5	7.0	7.5	9.0
4 years	404	5.5	2.2	3.5	3.5	4.0	4.0	5.0	6.0	7.0	7.5	9.0
5 years	397	5.3	2.4	3.0	3.5	4.0	4.0	5.0	6.0	6.5	7.0	8.0
6 years	133	6.0	3.9	3.5	3.5	4.0	4.0	5.0	6.0	8.0	10.0	16.0
7 years	148	5.8	3.1	3.5	4.0	4.0	4.0	5.0	6.0	7.0	7.5	11.5
8 years	147	6.7	4.9	3.5	4.0	4.0	4.5	5.0	6.5	8.0	11.0	21.0
9 years	145	7.0	5.0	3.5	4.0	4.0	4.5	6.0	7.0	10.0	12.0	15.0
10 years	157	8.6	6.6	4.0	4.0	4.5	5.0	6.0	9.5	11.5	17.0	22.0
11 years	155	10.0	8.5	4.0	4.0	4.5	5.0	6.5	10.0	17.5	25.0	31.0
12 years	145	9.2	6.8	4.0	4.5	4.5	5.0	6.5	10.0	15.5	19.0	22.5
13 years	173	9.1	7.3	4.0	4.5	5.0	5.0	7.0	9.0	13.0	15.0	24.0
14 years	186	8.9	5.3	4.5	5.0	5.5	6.0	7.0	9.0	12.0	13.5	20.0
15 years	184	10.0	8.2	5.0	5.5	6.0	6.0	7.5	10.0	12.0	16.0	24.5
16 years	178	10.8	6.4	5.0	6.0	6.5	6.5	9.0	12.5	14.5	21.5	25.0
17 years	173	10.1	5.3	5.5	6.0	6.5	7.0	8.5	11.5	14.0	17.0	20.5
18 years	164	11.9	6.7	6.0	7.0	7.0	8.0	10.0	14.0	16.0	18.0	24.0
19 years	148	12.5	6.9	7.0	7.0	7.5	8.0	10.5	13.5	16.5	22.0	29.0
Female												
6–11 months	177	6.7	1.7	4.5	5.0	5.0	5.5	6.5	7.5	8.0	9.0	10.0
1 year	336	6.7	2.0	4.0	4.0	5.0	5.0	6.5	8.0	8.5	9.5	10.5
2 years	336	6.5	2.2	4.0	4.5	4.5	5.0	6.0	7.5	8.5	9.5	11.0
3 years	366	6.3	2.2	3.5	4.0	4.5	5.0	6.0	7.0	8.0	9.0	11.0
4 years	396	6.2	2.2	3.5	4.0	4.5	5.0	5.5	7.0	8.0	9.0	10.5
5 years	364	6.5	3.5	4.0	4.0	4.5	5.0	5.5	7.0	8.0	10.0	12.0
6 years	135	6.8	3.8	4.0	4.0	4.0	5.0	6.0	7.5	9.0	10.5	14.0
7 years	157	7.0	3.7	3.5	4.0	4.0	4.5	6.0	7.5	9.0	12.0	16.5
8 years	123	7.4	4.9	3.5	4.0	4.5	5.0	6.0	8.0	10.5	12.0	15.0
9 years	149	9.6	7.5	4.0	5.0	5.0	5.5	7.0	9.5	13.0	21.0	29.0
10 years	136	10.4	6.6	4.5	5.0	5.0	6.0	8.0	13.5	18.0	19.5	23.0
11 years	140	11.4	8.1	4.5	5.0	5.5	6.5	8.0	12.0	17.0	22.0	29.0
12 years	147	11.5	7.5	5.0	5.5	6.0	6.5	9.0	13.0	17.0	22.0	29.0
13 years	162	11.9	8.5	4.5	5.5	6.0	7.0	9.5	14.0	17.5	20.0	29.0
14 years	178	13.2	7.7	6.0	6.5	7.0	7.5	10.5	16.0	22.0	26.0	31.0
15 years	145	13.1	6.9	6.0	7.0	7.5	8.5	10.5	16.0	20.5	22.5	27.5
16 years	170	15.2	9.2	6.5	7.5	8.5	9.5	12.0	16.5	23.5	26.0	36.6
17 years	134	15.9	9.2	6.5	7.0	8.0	9.5	13.0	19.5	27.0	29.0	37.0
18 years	170	15.3	8.6	7.0	7.5	8.0	10.0	13.0	18.5	22.0	27.5	34.5
19 years	158	16.0	9.5	7.0	7.5	8.5	9.5	13.0	18.5	23.5	26.5	35.5

Subscapular skinfold in millimeters for males 18–74 years of age—United States, 1976–1980

Race and age	Number of examined persons	Mean	Standard deviation	Percentile								
				5th	10th	15th	25th	50th	75th	85th	90th	95th
All races*												
18–74 years	5916	17.4	8.8	7.0	8.0	9.0	10.5	15.0	22.5	26.0	30.0	34.6
18–24 years	988	13.7	7.5	6.5	7.0	7.5	8.5	11.5	16.0	20.0	23.0	30.0
25–34 years	1067	16.9	8.6	7.0	8.0	9.0	10.0	15.0	22.0	25.5	29.0	34.0
35–44 years	745	18.7	9.2	7.0	8.5	10.0	12.0	17.0	24.0	28.0	30.5	37.0
45–54 years	690	19.4	8.9	7.5	9.0	10.0	12.5	18.0	25.0	29.0	31.0	36.0
55–64 years	1227	18.9	8.4	7.5	9.0	10.0	12.5	18.0	24.0	27.0	30.0	34.5
65–74 years	1199	17.9	8.7	7.0	8.0	9.5	11.0	16.0	23.0	27.5	30.5	35.1
White												
18–74 years	5148	17.3	8.5	7.0	8.0	9.0	11.0	15.5	22.0	26.0	29.5	34.0
18–24 years	846	13.8	7.5	6.5	7.0	7.5	8.5	11.5	16.5	20.5	24.0	30.0
25–34 years	901	16.9	8.3	7.0	8.0	9.0	10.5	15.0	22.0	25.5	29.0	32.5
35–44 years	653	18.5	8.7	7.0	9.0	10.0	12.0	17.0	23.5	27.0	30.0	35.0
45–54 years	617	19.1	8.6	8.0	9.0	10.0	12.5	17.5	24.0	28.5	30.5	35.1
55–64 years	1086	18.9	8.3	7.5	9.5	10.5	12.5	18.0	24.0	27.0	29.5	34.0
65–74 years	1045	18.0	8.5	7.0	8.0	9.5	11.5	16.0	23.0	27.5	30.0	35.0
Black												
18–74 years	649	17.8	10.5	6.5	7.5	8.5	10.0	14.0	24.0	30.0	32.1	38.1
18–24 years	121	12.6	6.6	6.5	7.5	8.0	9.0	10.5	14.5	16.5	19.5	25.0
25–34 years	139	17.2	10.1	7.0	8.0	8.5	9.0	13.0	23.0	27.0	34.0	38.0
35–44 years	70	20.3	12.2	—	8.5	9.5	11.0	17.0	26.0	35.0	40.0	—
45–54 years	62	22.8	11.1	—	8.0	10.0	13.0	21.5	30.0	37.0	37.0	—
55–64 years	129	18.7	9.9	6.0	7.0	8.0	9.5	18.0	26.0	30.0	32.1	37.0
65–74 years	128	18.4	10.4	5.5	7.0	8.0	10.0	15.0	26.5	30.5	33.0	37.0

*Includes all other races not shown as separate categories.

Subscapular skinfold in millimeters for females 18–74 years of age—United States, 1976–1980

Race and age	Number of examined persons	Mean	Standard deviation	Percentile 5th	10th	15th	25th	50th	75th	85th	90th	95th
All races*												
18–74 years	6588	21.2	12.0	7.0	8.0	9.5	11.5	18.0	29.0	35.0	38.5	45.0
18–24 years	1066	16.6	9.9	7.0	7.5	8.0	10.0	13.0	20.5	26.0	31.0	38.0
25–34 years	1170	20.0	12.2	7.0	8.0	8.5	10.5	16.0	27.0	33.5	38.0	45.0
35–44 years	844	22.3	12.4	7.0	8.5	10.0	12.0	19.0	31.0	36.6	40.1	46.5
45–54 years	763	24.1	12.2	7.0	10.0	11.0	14.5	22.0	32.5	37.5	40.5	47.6
55–64 years	1329	23.7	12.3	7.5	9.0	11.0	13.5	22.0	32.0	37.0	41.0	47.0
65–74 years	1416	22.3	11.1	7.0	8.5	10.0	13.0	21.0	30.0	35.0	37.1	43.0
White												
18–74 years	5686	20.5	11.7	7.0	8.0	9.0	11.0	17.0	27.5	34.0	37.5	43.5
18–24 years	892	16.1	9.6	7.0	7.5	8.0	10.0	13.0	19.0	25.0	29.5	37.5
25–34 years	1000	19.1	11.7	7.0	7.5	8.5	10.5	15.0	25.0	32.0	36.0	43.0
35–44 years	726	21.4	12.1	7.0	8.0	9.5	11.5	17.5	30.0	36.0	39.5	46.0
45–54 years	647	23.1	11.8	7.0	9.5	11.0	14.0	20.5	31.0	36.6	40.0	45.0
55–64 years	1176	23.0	12.0	7.0	9.0	11.0	13.0	21.5	31.0	36.0	39.5	45.6
65–74 years	1245	21.8	10.9	6.5	8.5	10.0	13.0	20.5	29.5	34.0	36.1	41.1
Black												
18–74 years	782	26.1	13.3	8.0	9.5	11.0	14.0	25.0	35.5	40.6	45.0	50.0
18–24 years	147	19.1	10.6	7.0	8.0	9.0	11.0	15.0	26.0	31.0	34.0	37.0
25–34 years	145	25.4	13.3	8.5	9.5	11.0	14.0	22.5	35.5	40.6	44.5	48.1
35–44 years	103	27.9	13.0	7.0	10.5	12.0	17.0	28.0	36.5	42.5	46.5	52.0
45–54 years	100	32.0	13.1	11.0	15.0	17.0	22.5	30.5	39.5	45.6	50.5	56.0
55–64 years	135	30.0	13.5	8.0	12.5	13.0	19.5	31.0	40.6	45.0	47.5	50.5
65–74 years	152	27.1	12.1	7.5	9.5	12.0	18.0	27.0	35.5	41.0	44.5	47.0

*Includes all other races not shown as separate categories.

APPENDIX Q

Means, Standard Deviations, and Percentiles of Sum of Skinfold Thickness (mm) by Age for Males and Females of 1 to 74 Years. See Table 7-2 for Interpretation Guidelines.

Means, standard deviations, and percentiles of sum of skinfold thickness (mm) by age for males and females of 1 to 74 years

Age (yrs)	N	Mean	SD	Percentile								
				5th	10th	15th	25th	50th	75th	85th	90th	95th
Males												
1.0–1.9	681	16.8	4.1	11.0	12.0	12.5	14.0	16.5	19.0	21.0	22.0	24.0
2.0–2.9	677	16.0	4.3	10.0	11.0	12.0	13.0	15.5	18.0	20.0	21.5	24.0
3.0–3.9	716	15.4	4.1	10.5	11.0	12.0	13.0	14.5	17.5	19.0	20.5	23.0
4.0–4.9	707	14.5	4.2	9.5	10.5	11.0	12.0	14.0	16.5	18.0	19.0	21.5
5.0–5.9	677	14.2	5.0	9.0	10.0	10.0	11.0	13.0	16.0	18.0	19.0	22.0
6.0–6.9	298	14.3	6.7	8.0	9.0	10.0	10.5	13.0	15.2	18.0	20.0	28.0
7.0–7.9	312	14.8	6.9	8.5	9.0	9.5	10.5	13.0	16.0	19.5	23.0	26.6
8.0–8.9	296	15.6	7.8	8.5	9.0	10.0	11.0	13.5	17.0	20.0	24.5	30.5
9.0–9.9	322	17.0	9.4	8.5	9.5	10.0	11.0	14.0	19.0	24.0	29.0	34.0
10.0–10.9	334	19.1	10.6	9.0	10.0	11.0	12.0	15.5	22.0	27.0	33.5	42.0
11.0–11.9	324	21.4	13.9	9.0	10.0	11.0	12.5	16.5	25.0	33.0	40.0	53.5
12.0–12.9	348	21.0	13.2	9.0	10.0	11.0	12.5	17.0	24.0	34.0	40.5	53.0
13.0–13.9	350	19.8	13.3	8.5	10.5	11.0	12.5	15.0	21.0	29.0	37.0	48.0
14.0–14.9	358	19.4	12.6	9.0	10.0	11.0	12.0	15.0	22.0	27.0	33.0	45.0
15.0–15.9	356	19.3	12.8	10.0	10.5	11.0	12.0	15.0	21.0	27.0	32.5	43.0
16.0–16.9	349	20.0	11.4	10.0	11.5	12.0	13.0	16.0	22.5	27.5	33.5	44.0
17.0–17.9	337	19.1	10.8	10.0	11.0	12.0	13.0	16.0	22.0	27.0	31.5	41.0
18.0–24.9	1748	24.6	13.1	11.0	12.0	13.5	15.0	21.0	30.0	37.0	41.5	50.5
25.0–29.9	1246	27.6	13.9	11.5	13.0	14.0	17.0	24.5	35.0	41.0	46.0	54.5
30.0–34.9	938	30.4	14.1	12.0	14.5	16.5	20.0	28.0	38.0	44.0	49.0	58.0
35.0–39.9	829	30.3	13.3	12.0	14.5	16.5	21.0	29.0	37.0	42.4	47.0	54.5
40.0–44.9	816	30.1	13.3	13.0	15.0	16.5	20.5	28.5	37.0	42.5	47.5	55.0
45.0–49.9	856	30.9	13.6	12.5	15.0	17.5	20.5	29.0	39.0	44.0	48.0	55.0
50.0–54.9	872	30.1	13.1	13.0	15.0	17.0	20.5	28.0	37.5	43.0	48.0	55.5
55.0–59.9	802	29.9	12.7	12.0	15.0	17.0	21.0	28.5	37.0	43.0	47.0	53.5
60.0–64.9	1250	30.5	13.1	13.0	15.5	17.5	21.0	29.0	37.5	43.0	47.0	55.5
65.0–69.9	1770	28.9	13.1	11.0	13.5	16.0	19.5	27.0	36.0	42.0	46.5	53.5
70.0–74.9	1247	28.2	12.4	11.5	14.0	16.0	19.0	26.0	35.0	41.0	45.0	51.0

Age (yrs)	N	Mean	SD	Percentile								
				5th	10th	15th	25th	50th	75th	85th	90th	95th
Females												
1.0–1.9	622	16.9	4.5	10.5	12.0	12.0	13.5	16.5	19.5	21.0	23.0	25.0
2.0–2.9	614	16.9	4.5	11.0	12.0	12.5	14.0	16.0	19.0	21.5	23.5	25.5
3.0–3.9	652	16.5	4.5	10.5	11.5	12.0	13.5	16.0	18.5	20.5	21.5	25.0
4.0–4.9	681	16.3	4.7	10.0	11.0	12.0	13.0	15.5	18.5	20.5	22.5	24.5
5.0–5.9	672	16.5	5.9	10.0	11.0	11.5	12.5	15.0	18.5	21.0	24.0	28.5
6.0–6.9	296	16.7	6.5	10.0	10.5	11.0	12.5	15.5	18.5	21.0	23.5	28.0
7.0–7.9	330	17.8	7.1	10.0	11.0	12.0	13.5	16.0	20.0	23.0	26.0	32.5
8.0–8.9	276	20.0	10.7	10.5	11.0	12.0	13.0	17.0	22.5	28.5	31.0	41.5
9.0–9.9	322	22.4	11.8	11.0	12.0	12.5	14.5	19.0	25.5	30.0	39.0	48.9
10.0–10.9	329	23.6	12.1	12.0	12.5	13.0	15.0	20.0	28.5	34.5	40.5	51.0
11.0–11.9	300	25.5	13.6	12.0	13.5	14.5	16.0	22.0	30.0	37.0	42.0	55.0
12.0–12.9	323	26.6	13.3	13.0	14.0	15.0	18.0	23.0	31.0	37.0	44.0	57.0
13.0–13.9	360	28.7	14.6	12.5	14.0	15.5	18.5	24.5	35.5	43.0	47.5	56.5
14.0–14.9	370	30.1	14.3	14.5	16.0	17.5	20.0	26.0	37.0	44.5	48.5	62.0
15.0–15.9	308	30.1	14.1	15.0	17.0	18.0	20.5	26.5	34.5	42.5	48.5	62.5
16.0–16.9	343	33.9	14.9	17.5	20.0	21.5	24.0	30.0	39.5	47.0	53.5	69.5
17.0–17.9	291	34.5	16.2	16.5	18.5	20.0	23.0	31.0	42.0	49.0	55.5	67.4
18.0–24.9	2586	36.1	16.6	16.7	19.0	21.0	24.0	32.0	44.0	52.0	58.5	70.0
25.0–29.9	1907	39.0	18.0	17.5	20.0	22.0	25.5	35.0	48.5	58.0	64.5	73.9
30.0–34.9	1613	43.3	19.8	18.0	22.0	24.5	28.5	39.0	55.0	64.0	71.0	83.0
35.0–39.9	1443	45.2	19.5	19.0	22.5	25.5	30.0	42.0	57.5	66.0	72.2	82.5
40.0–44.9	1378	45.8	18.9	20.0	23.5	27.0	31.0	43.0	58.0	67.0	73.0	80.0
45.0–49.9	953	47.7	19.2	21.0	24.0	27.5	33.5	45.0	59.5	69.0	74.5	81.0
50.0–54.9	992	49.3	18.9	21.0	26.0	30.0	35.5	47.0	61.0	70.0	75.3	83.5
55.0–59.9	868	49.5	19.5	21.0	26.0	29.0	35.0	47.5	62.0	69.5	75.0	85.0
60.0–64.9	1374	49.2	18.6	22.0	27.0	30.0	35.5	48.0	61.0	68.0	74.0	83.5
65.0–69.9	1930	46.3	17.6	21.0	25.0	28.5	34.0	44.0	57.0	64.0	70.0	78.0
70.0–74.9	1458	44.5	17.1	19.0	23.5	27.0	32.0	43.0	56.0	62.0	67.0	75.5

N = number of persons in each age/sex category.

SD = standard deviation.

Skinfold thickness values are in millimeters.

APPENDIX R

MEANS, STANDARD DEVIATIONS, AND PERCENTILES OF UPPER ARM MUSCLE AREA (cm^2) BY AGE FOR MALES AND FEMALES OF 1 TO 74 YEARS. SEE TABLE 7-6 FOR INTERPRETATION GUIDELINES.

Means, standard deviations, and percentiles of upper arm muscle area (cm^2) by age for males and females of 1 to 74 years

				Percentile								
Age (yrs)	N	Mean	SD	5th	10th	15th	25th	50th	75th	85th	90th	95th
							Males					
1.0–1.9	681	13.2	2.3	9.7	10.4	10.8	11.6	13.0	14.6	15.4	16.3	17.2
2.0–2.9	672	14.1	3.2	10.1	10.9	11.3	12.4	13.9	15.6	16.4	16.9	18.4
3.0–3.9	715	15.2	3.1	11.2	12.0	12.6	13.5	15.0	16.4	17.4	18.3	19.5
4.0–4.9	707	16.3	2.7	12.0	12.9	13.5	14.5	16.2	17.9	18.8	19.8	20.9
5.0–5.9	676	17.8	3.7	13.2	14.2	14.7	15.7	17.6	19.5	20.7	21.7	23.2
6.0–6.9	298	19.3	4.0	14.4	15.3	15.8	16.8	18.7	21.3	22.9	23.8	25.7
7.0–7.9	312	21.0	4.5	15.1	16.2	17.0	18.5	20.6	22.6	24.5	25.2	28.6
8.0–8.9	296	22.1	4.2	16.3	17.8	18.5	19.5	21.6	24.0	25.5	26.6	29.0
9.0–9.9	322	24.5	5.1	18.2	19.3	20.3	21.7	23.5	26.7	28.7	30.4	32.9
10.0–10.9	333	26.7	5.9	19.6	20.7	21.6	23.0	25.7	29.0	32.2	34.0	37.1
11.0–11.9	324	28.8	6.7	21.0	22.0	23.0	24.8	27.7	31.6	33.6	36.1	40.3
12.0–12.9	348	31.9	7.4	22.6	24.1	25.3	26.9	30.4	35.9	39.3	40.9	44.9
13.0–13.9	350	36.8	9.0	24.5	26.7	28.1	30.4	35.7	41.3	45.3	48.1	52.5
14.0–14.9	358	42.4	9.1	28.3	31.3	33.1	36.1	41.9	47.4	51.3	54.0	57.5
15.0–15.9	356	46.8	9.6	31.9	34.9	36.9	40.3	46.3	53.1	56.3	57.7	63.0
16.0–16.9	350	52.6	10.0	37.0	40.9	42.4	45.9	51.9	57.8	63.6	66.2	70.5
17.0–17.9	337	54.7	10.5	39.6	42.6	44.8	48.0	53.4	60.4	64.3	67.9	73.1
18.0–24.9	1752	50.5	11.6	34.2	37.3	39.6	42.7	49.4	57.1	61.8	65.0	72.0
25.0–29.9	1250	54.1	11.9	36.6	39.9	42.4	46.0	53.0	61.4	66.1	68.9	74.5
30.0–34.9	940	55.6	12.1	37.9	40.9	43.4	47.3	54.4	63.2	67.6	70.8	76.1
35.0–39.9	832	56.5	12.4	38.5	42.6	44.6	47.9	55.3	64.0	69.1	72.7	77.6
40.0–44.9	828	56.6	11.7	38.4	42.1	45.1	48.7	56.0	64.0	68.5	71.6	77.0
45.0–49.9	867	55.9	12.3	37.7	41.3	43.7	47.9	55.2	63.3	68.4	72.2	76.2
50.0–54.9	879	55.0	12.5	36.0	40.0	42.7	46.6	54.0	62.7	67.0	70.4	77.4
55.0–59.9	807	54.7	11.8	36.5	40.8	42.7	46.7	54.3	61.9	66.4	69.6	75.1
60.0–64.9	1259	52.8	11.7	34.5	38.7	41.2	44.9	52.1	60.0	64.8	67.5	71.6
65.0–69.9	1773	49.8	11.6	31.4	35.8	38.4	42.3	49.1	57.3	61.2	64.3	69.4
70.0–74.9	1250	47.8	11.5	29.7	33.8	36.1	40.2	47.0	54.6	59.1	62.1	67.3

Age (yrs)	N	Mean	SD	Percentile								
				5th	10th	15th	25th	50th	75th	85th	90th	95th
				Females								
1.0–1.9	622	12.3	2.3	8.9	9.7	10.1	10.8	12.3	13.8	14.6	15.3	16.2
2.0–2.9	614	13.3	2.3	10.1	10.6	10.9	11.8	13.2	14.7	15.6	16.4	17.3
3.0–3.9	651	14.3	2.4	10.8	11.4	11.8	12.6	14.3	15.8	16.7	17.4	18.8
4.0–4.9	680	15.4	2.8	11.2	12.2	12.7	13.6	15.3	17.0	18.0	18.6	19.8
5.0–5.9	672	16.7	3.1	12.4	13.2	13.9	14.8	16.4	18.3	19.4	20.6	22.1
6.0–6.9	296	18.0	3.9	13.5	14.1	14.6	15.6	17.4	19.5	21.0	22.0	24.2
7.0–7.9	329	19.3	4.0	14.4	15.2	15.8	16.7	18.9	21.2	22.6	23.9	25.3
8.0–8.9	275	21.1	4.7	15.2	16.0	16.8	18.2	20.8	23.2	24.6	26.5	28.0
9.0–9.9	321	22.9	4.6	17.0	17.9	18.7	19.8	21.9	25.4	27.2	28.3	31.1
10.0–10.9	329	24.3	5.5	17.6	18.5	19.3	20.9	23.8	27.0	29.1	31.0	33.1
11.0–11.9	302	27.6	6.7	19.5	21.0	21.7	23.2	26.4	30.7	33.5	35.7	39.2
12.0–12.9	323	29.7	6.5	20.4	21.8	23.1	25.5	29.0	33.2	36.3	37.8	40.5
13.0–13.9	360	31.9	7.4	22.8	24.5	25.4	27.1	30.8	35.3	38.1	39.6	43.7
14.0–14.9	370	33.9	7.7	24.0	26.2	27.1	29.0	32.8	36.9	39.8	42.3	47.5
15.0–15.9	309	33.8	7.0	24.4	25.8	27.5	29.2	33.0	37.3	40.2	41.7	45.9
16.0–16.9	343	34.8	8.0	25.2	26.8	28.2	30.0	33.6	38.0	40.2	43.7	48.3
17.0–17.9	291	36.1	8.8	25.9	27.5	28.9	30.7	34.3	39.6	43.4	46.2	50.8
18.0–24.9	2588	29.8	8.4	19.5	21.5	22.8	24.5	28.3	33.1	36.4	39.0	44.2
25.0–29.9	1921	31.1	9.1	20.5	21.9	23.1	25.2	29.4	34.9	38.5	41.9	47.8
30.0–34.9	1619	32.8	10.4	21.1	23.0	24.2	26.3	30.9	36.8	41.2	44.7	51.3
35.0–39.9	1453	34.2	11.5	21.1	23.4	24.7	27.3	31.8	38.7	43.1	46.1	54.2
40.0–44.9	1390	35.2	13.3	21.3	23.4	25.5	27.5	32.3	39.8	45.8	49.5	55.8
45.0–49.9	961	34.9	11.8	21.6	23.1	24.8	27.4	32.5	39.5	44.7	48.4	56.1
50.0–54.9	1004	35.6	11.0	22.2	24.6	25.7	28.3	33.4	40.4	46.1	49.6	55.6
55.0–59.9	879	37.1	13.3	22.8	24.8	26.5	28.7	34.7	42.3	47.3	52.1	58.8
60.0–64.9	1389	36.3	11.3	22.4	24.5	26.3	29.2	34.5	41.1	45.6	49.1	55.1
65.0–69.9	1946	36.3	11.3	21.9	24.5	26.2	28.9	34.6	41.6	46.3	49.6	56.5
70.0–74.9	1463	36.0	10.8	22.2	24.4	26.0	28.8	34.3	41.8	46.4	49.2	54.6

N = number of persons in each age/sex category.

SD = standard deviation.

Values are in cm^2.

Note: Values for males and females age 18 years and older have been adjusted for bone area by subtracting 10.0 cm^2 and 6.5 cm^2, respectively, from the calculated mid-upper-arm muscle area.

APPENDIX S

REFERENCE VALUES FOR SERUM LIPID AND LIPOPROTEIN LEVELS FOR U.S. ADULTS, 1981–1991

From National Cholesterol Education Program. 1993. *Second Report of the Expert Panel on Detection, Evaluation, and Treatment of High Blood Cholesterol in Adults*. Bethesda, MD: U.S. Department of Health and Human Services: Public Health Service; National Institutes of Health; National Heart, Lung, and Blood Institute.

Total serum cholesterol levels in milligrams per deciliter (mg/dl) for persons 20 years of age and older by race/ethnicity, sex, and age—United States, 1988–1991

Race/ethnicity, sex, and age	Number of examined persons	Mean	Selected percentile								
			5th	10th	15th	25th	50th	75th	85th	90th	95th
Men											
20 years and older	3953	205	143	153	162	176	201	231	247	260	276
20–34 years	1186	189	134	145	151	162	186	211	225	236	260
35–44 years	653	207	144	155	167	182	205	231	245	258	269
45–54 years	508	218	152	170	180	191	215	242	257	268	283
55–64 years	535	221	154	169	180	195	221	245	264	274	285
65–74 years	557	218	157	173	179	190	214	241	256	270	286
75 and older	514	205	145	156	164	175	202	232	248	257	275
Women											
20 years and older	3885	207	143	154	162	175	202	233	252	269	287
20–34 years	1777	185	134	143	150	160	182	204	218	229	254
35–44 years	709	195	142	152	159	170	193	215	232	242	254
45–54 years	464	217	158	165	171	187	212	240	264	279	297
55–64 years	503	237	168	184	191	204	228	264	280	291	323
65–74 years	493	234	168	180	186	205	232	261	278	290	308
75 and older	539	230	163	175	184	198	227	263	279	287	316
Mexican Americans											
Men	1092	202	140	151	159	172	199	225	245	257	277
Women	1046	200	139	149	158	169	195	224	241	258	279
Non-Hispanic black											
Men	992	199	136	149	156	170	195	224	242	252	276
Women	985	203	137	150	159	172	200	227	248	262	286
Non-Hispanic white											
Men	1816	206	144	154	163	177	203	232	247	260	276
Women	1734	208	144	155	163	176	202	234	254	271	288

Low-density-lipoprotein cholesterol (LDL-C) in milligrams per deciliter (mg/dl) for persons 20 years of age and older by race/ethnicity, sex, and age—United States, 1988–1991

Race/ethnicity, sex, and age	Number of examined persons	Mean	Selected percentile								
			5th	10th	15th	25th	50th	75th	85th	90th	95th
Men 20 years and older	1669	131	75	87	95	106	129	154	167	179	194
20–34 years	487	120	67	78	86	97	121	139	152	165	186
35–44 years	274	134	85	92	98	111	131	156	166	176	192
45–54 years	224	138	78	91	100	118	136	163	174	187	195
55–64 years	228	142	78	90	104	117	143	165	175	194	205
65–74 years	259	141	93	104	109	119	134	163	177	185	199
75 and older	197	132	83	88	93	106	130	154	170	186	196
Women 20 years and older	1673	126	69	81	88	99	122	150	165	175	191
20–34 years	525	110	59	70	75	88	108	129	142	155	173
35–44 years	316	117	67	85	88	97	116	138	146	155	165
45–54 years	214	132	70	87	93	107	130	157	173	182	198
55–64 years	213	145	79	90	101	122	145	170	184	189	209
65–74 years	202	147	92	97	109	119	148	169	185	192	206
75 and older	203	147	90	102	109	121	143	168	189	197	209
Mexican Americans											
Men	448	124	70	77	85	96	120	148	161	172	188
Women	471	122	67	80	86	95	118	144	158	166	189
Non-Hispanic black											
Men	393	126	69	76	82	96	123	146	168	186	206
Women	422	126	67	76	86	100	124	147	162	174	192
Non-Hispanic white											
Men	773	132	76	88	97	108	129	154	168	179	194
Women	729	126	69	82	89	99	122	151	166	176	192

From National Cholesterol Education Program. 1993. *Second Report of the Expert Panel on Detection, Evaluation, and Treatment of High Blood Cholesterol in Adults.* Bethesda, MD: U.S. Department of Health and Human Services: Public Health Service; National Institutes of Health; National Heart, Lung, and Blood Institute.

High-density-lipoprotein cholesterol (HDL-C) in milligrams per deciliter (mg/dl) for persons 20 years of age and older by race/ethnicity, sex, and age—United States, 1988–1991

Race/ethnicity, sex, and age	Number of examined persons	Mean	Selected percentile								
			5th	10th	15th	25th	50th	75th	85th	90th	95th
Men											
20 years and older	3920	46.5	28.0	31.0	34.0	37.0	44.1	53.1	59.1	64.0	73.0
20–34 years	1178	47.1	30.0	34.0	35.1	38.0	46.0	54.0	60.1	64.0	71.0
35–44 years	642	46.3	28.0	30.0	33.0	37.0	44.0	53.0	58.1	63.0	73.0
45–54 years	502	46.6	28.0	30.0	33.0	36.0	43.1	53.0	61.0	66.1	77.1
55–64 years	533	45.6	29.0	31.0	33.0	36.1	43.0	53.0	59.0	62.0	72.0
65–74 years	553	45.3	28.0	31.0	32.0	36.0	43.0	53.0	58.0	62.1	71.0
75 and older	512	47.2	28.0	32.0	34.0	38.0	45.0	54.0	62.0	67.0	75.1
Women											
20 years and older	3855	55.7	34.0	38.0	41.0	44.1	54.0	65.0	71.0	76.1	83.0
20–34 years	1167	55.7	34.0	38.0	41.0	44.1	54.0	64.1	70.1	75.1	83.1
35–44 years	701	54.3	33.0	37.0	40.0	44.0	53.0	64.1	69.1	72.1	79.0
45–54 years	459	56.7	37.0	38.1	41.0	46.0	56.0	65.0	72.1	77.1	84.1
55–64 years	500	56.1	33.0	37.0	40.0	44.0	53.0	66.0	73.0	79.0	87.1
65–74 years	492	55.7	34.0	37.0	40.0	44.1	54.0	65.1	73.0	78.0	83.1
75 and older	536	57.1	33.0	39.0	41.0	44.1	56.0	66.1	73.1	78.1	87.0
Mexican Americans											
Men	1077	46.9	30.0	33.0	34.1	38.0	45.0	54.0	59.0	64.0	69.0
Women	1040	53.3	34.0	37.0	40.0	44.0	52.0	61.0	68.0	72.1	78.0
Non-Hispanic black											
Men	918	53.3	30.0	35.0	38.0	42.0	51.0	62.0	69.1	75.1	86.1
Women	978	57.8	37.0	40.0	43.0	47.0	55.1	67.1	74.0	78.1	86.0
Non-Hispanic white											
Men	1803	45.5	28.0	30.0	33.1	36.1	44.0	52.1	58.0	62.0	71.1
Women	1717	55.7	33.1	37.0	40.0	44.0	54.0	65.1	71.1	77.0	83.1

From National Cholesterol Education Program. 1993. *Second Report of the Expert Panel on Detection, Evaluation, and Treatment of High Blood Cholesterol in Adults.* Bethesda, MD: U.S. Department of Health and Human Services: Public Health Service; National Institutes of Health; National Heart, Lung, and Blood Institute.

Serum total cholesterol levels in U.S. children and adolescents (mg/dl)*

Age (years)	Number	Overall mean	Percentiles 5	10	25	50	75	90	95
Males									
0–4	238	159	117	129	141	156	176	192	209
5–9	1253	165	125	134	147	164	180	197	209
10–14	2278	162	123	131	144	160	178	196	208
15–19	1980	154	116	124	136	150	170	188	203
Females									
0–4	186	161	115	124	143	161	177	195	206
5–9	1118	169	130	138	150	168	184	201	211
10–14	2087	164	128	135	148	163	179	196	207
15–19	2079	162	124	131	144	160	177	197	209

*All values have been converted from plasma to serum. Plasma value × 1.03 = serum value.

Reprinted from the *Report of the Expert Panel on Blood Cholesterol Levels in Children and Adolescents*. Courtesy of the National Cholesterol Education Program.

Serum LDL-C levels in U.S. children and adolescents (mg/dl)*

Age (years)	Number	Overall mean	Percentiles 5	10	25	50	75	90	95
White males									
5–9	131	95	65	71	82	93	106	121	133
10–14	284	99	66	74	83	97	112	126	136
15–19	298	97	64	70	82	96	112	127	134
White females									
5–9	114	103	70	75	91	101	118	129	144
10–14	244	100	70	75	83	97	113	130	140
15–19	294	99	61	67	80	96	114	133	141

*All values have been converted from plasma to serum. Plasma value × 1.03 = serum value.

Note: The number of children ages 0–4 who had LDL-C and HDL-C measured was too small to allow calculation of percentiles in this age group. However, note that the percentiles for total cholesterol for ages 0–4 and 5–9 are similar.

Reprinted from the *Report of the Expert Panel on Blood Cholesterol Levels in Children and Adolescents*. Courtesy of the National Cholesterol Education Program.

Serum HDL-C levels in U.S. children and adolescents (mg/dl)*

Age (years)	Number	Overall mean	Percentiles 5	10	25	50	75	90	95
White males									
5–9	142	57	39	43	50	56	65	72	76
10–14	296	57	38	41	47	57	63	73	76
15–19	299	48	31	35	40	47	54	61	65
White females									
5–9	124	55	37	39	48	54	63	69	75
10–14	247	54	38	41	46	54	60	66	72
15–19	295	54	36	39	44	53	63	70	76

*All values have been converted from plasma to serum. Plasma value × 1.03 = serum value.

Note: The number of children ages 0–4 who had LDL-C and HDL-C measured was too small to allow calculation of percentiles in this age group. However, note that the percentiles for total cholesterol for ages 0–4 and 5–9 are similar.

Reprinted from the *Report of the Expert Panel on Blood Cholesterol Levels in Children and Adolescents*. Courtesy of the National Cholesterol Education Program.

Serum triglyceride levels in U.S. children and adolescents (mg/dl)*

Age (years)	Number	Overall mean	Percentiles 5	10	25	50	75	90	95
Males									
0–4	238	58	30	34	41	53	69	87	102
5–9	1253	30	31	34	41	53	67	88	104
10–14	2278	68	33	38	46	61	80	105	129
15–19	1980	80	38	44	56	71	94	124	152
Females									
0–4	186	66	35	39	46	61	79	99	115
5–9	1118	30	33	37	45	57	73	93	108
10–14	2087	78	38	45	56	72	93	117	135
15–19	2079	78	40	45	55	70	90	117	136

*All values have been converted from plasma to serum. Plasma value × 1.03 = serum value.

Reprinted from the *Report of the Expert Panel on Blood Cholesterol Levels in Children and Adolescents*. Courtesy of the National Cholesterol Education Program.

APPENDIX T

An Example of a Form That Can Be Used for Self-Monitoring Eating Behavior

Food Record

Name ________________________ Day of week ______________ Date ______________

Time	Time Spent	Food Eaten—How Prepared	Amount	Place, Person(s) with Whom Food Was Eaten, Other Activities, Mood/Feelings

Remember: Do not alter your normal diet while keeping this record. For the requested information, provide responses that are as accurate as possible.

APPENDIX U

COMPENTENCY CHECKLIST FOR NUTRITION COUNSELORS

This can be used by counselors to identify the competencies they already possess and those they want to develop.

From Raab C, and Tillotson JL. 1985. *Heart to heart: A manual on nutrition counseling for the reduction of cardiovascular disease risk factors*. Bethesda, MD: U.S. Department of Health and Human Services: Public Health Service; National Institutes of Health.

Nutrition Information for Particular Patient	Performance Objectives	Needs More Work	Not Attempted Yet	Good
1. Counselor knows the essential elements and rationale behind patient's prescribed diet (e.g., low-fat, low-sodium, etc.)	1a. Is familiar with all the food categories of the diet.	______	______	______
	1b. Is comfortable with substitutions and rationale for selection of food.	______	______	______
	1c. Is prepared to help patient adapt diet to his or her needs.	______	______	______
2. Counselor has knowledge of local eating patterns.	2a. Has some grasp of regional customs and of what foods are available in area.	______	______	______
	2b. Is familiar with frequently patronized restaurants and food chains and will ask patient his or her favorites.	______	______	______
3. At the outset, counselor makes reasonably sure that patient's knowledge of prescribed diet is adequate.	3a. Takes a history to find out patient's dietary background.	______	______	______
	3b. At first session, discusses long-term goals and explains diet thoroughly, making sure patient understands.	______	______	______
	3c. Eliminates patient's knowledge gaps (by discussing diet further, giving examples, using visuals, etc.) so following sessions can concentrate on goal-setting.	______	______	______
	3d. Initially, asks patient for food diary. Analyzes with patient to assess current diet and eating behavior.	______	______	______

Nutrition Information for Particular Patient	Performance Objectives	Needs More Work	Not Attempted Yet	Good
Communication Skills				
4. Counselor sets appropriate tone for counseling sessions through preparation, manner, and physical setting.	4a. Makes appointment with patient, allowing enough time for comfortable, thorough discussion.	______	______	______
	4b. Arranges for private, quiet setting.	______	______	______
	4c. Establishes patient's ability to see and to read and speak English. Adapts counseling if necessary.	______	______	______
	4d. Shows interest in patient as an individual, looks for his or her particular needs and preferences.	______	______	______
	4e. Maintains relaxed, comfortable manner. Makes patient feel at ease.	______	______	______
	4f. Indicates intentions to talk and to listen.	______	______	______
5. Counselor prepares self and patient for continuing relationship over a specified period.	5a. Explains initially the necessity of follow-up over time.	______	______	______
	5b. Outlines plans for working with patient—a certain number of sessions over a certain period of time with occasional contact by phone and mail.	______	______	______
6. Counselor uses principles of good communication.	6a. Uses primarily open-ended questions (rather than those answered by yes or no).	______	______	______
	6b. Guards against doing most of the talking. Shows ability to listen.	______	______	______
	6c. Is able to tolerate periods of silence.	______	______	______
	6d. Shows nonjudgmental, noncritical attitude toward patient's eating pattern and chosen lifestyle.	______	______	______
	6e. Uses words the patient can understand.	______	______	______

Nutrition Information for Particular Patient	Performance Objectives	Needs More Work	Not Attempted Yet	Good
Communication Skills—*Cont'd*				
7. Counselor communicates interest and confidence both nonverbally and verbally.	7a. Shows poise and interest through posture and "body language."			
	7b. Has frequent eye contact with patient.			
	7c. Uses gestures and words to encourage patient to communicate freely, without putting words in patient's mouth.			
Counseling Approaches				
8. Counselor is aware that the change process is the responsibility of the patient.	8a. Does not assume responsibility for changes or consequences.			
	8b. Does not become too ego-involved in the patient's eventual success or failure.			
9. Counselor is aware of need for patient to recognize manageable goals.	9a. Helps patient choose initial goal that is easily achieved.			
	9b. Helps patient set specific and short-term goals that are progressively more challenging.			
	9c. Is able to help patient evaluate goals.			
	9d. Helps patient avoid failure through too large or too may goals.			
10. Counselor is able to help patient set up record keeping and/or tally systems.	10a. Can help patient verbalize a method appropriate to the task.			
	10b. Can suggest alternate methods for patient's consideration without dictating choice.			
	10c. Emphasizes need for accurate records.			
	10d. Is able to help the patient review food records.			

Nutrition Information for Particular Patient	Performance Objectives	Needs More Work	Not Attempted Yet	Good
Counseling Approaches—*Cont'd*				
11. Counselor is aware of the need to examine and anticipate obstacles that will interfere with progress.	11a. Can review with patient potential obstacles in social, personal, and physical environments.	______	______	______
	11b. Can help patient identify actual or potential problems and deal with these by encouraging the patient to restructure environment and by role-playing problem situations with him or her.	______	______	______
	11c. Discusses how patient will deal with possible failure.	______	______	______
12. Counselor is able to define own role in giving support and feedback.	12a. Can avoid taking the major responsibility.	______	______	______
	12b. Can place the responsibility for change on the patient.	______	______	______
	12c. Is aware of own biases and belief systems, and is able to ignore them.	______	______	______
13. Counselor is able to evaluate progress toward the stated goal.	13a. Is able to give patient feedback about progress.	______	______	______
	13b. Keeps notes in sufficient detail to depict patient's responsibilities and progress.	______	______	______
	13c. Measures progress by a combination of biologic measures, food intake evaluation, and subjective judgments, with an emphasis on changing *behavior*.	______	______	______

Nutrition Information for Particular Patient	Performance Objectives	Needs More Work	Not Attempted Yet	Good
Counseling Approaches—*Cont'd*				
14. Counselor encourages patient to get family and friends involved.	14a. Helps patient recognize their strong influence on him or her; suggests that patient ask openly for their support.	______	______	______
	14b. Suggests that patient ask them to participate in some way: sharing new tastes and habits, helping with food selection, limiting inappropriate foods.	______	______	______
	14c. Can help patient cope with negative feedback through anticipating and rehearsing problem situations.	______	______	______
	14d. Can evaluate whether they are potentially supportive or destructive.	______	______	______
	14e. Can utilize them as a support without losing sight of the primary responsibility resting with patient.	______	______	______
15. Counselor is able to understand that his or her role is not simply that of information-giver or instructor.	15a. Acts as facilitator for patient.	______	______	______
	15b. Is appropriately assertive.	______	______	______
	15c. Is able to resist "lecturing."	______	______	______
16. Counselor is aware of the need to keep the patient task-oriented.	16a. Recognizes delaying tactics and distractions.	______	______	______
	16b. Is able to redirect the session toward specifics.	______	______	______
	16c. Responds pleasantly but professionally to patient's attempts at humor.	______	______	______

GLOSSARY

acromion process The spine of the scapula (shoulder blade) extending toward the outside of the body. The acromion process or tip is used as an anatomic landmark in arm anthropometric measurements (e.g., midarm circumference and triceps skinfold measurement).

actuarial data Statistical information relating to life expectancy, collected by the insurance industry and used, for example, to develop height-weight charts.

age-adjusted death rate The number of deaths in a specific age group for a given calendar year, divided by the population of the same age group as of July 1 of that year. (The quotient being multiplied by 1000.) Also known as "age-specific" death rate.

albumin A serum protein produced by the liver used as an indicator of nutritional status.

anabolism The process by which body cells convert simple biologic substances into more complex compounds.

android obesity Excess body fat that is predominantly within the abdomen and upper body as opposed to the hips and thighs. This is the typical pattern of male obesity.

anemia A hemoglobin level below the normal reference range for individuals of the same sex and age.

anergy A less than expected or absent immune reaction in response to the injection of antigens within the skin.

angina pectoris Chest pain caused by lack of oxygen supply (known as ischemia) within the heart muscle or myocardium.

anorexia nervosa A condition of disturbed or disordered eating behavior characterized by a refusal to maintain a minimally normal body weight, an intense fear of gaining weight (not alleviated by losing weight), and a distorted perception of body shape or size in which a person feels overweight (either globally or in certain body areas) despite being markedly underweight.

antecedent A preceding event, condition, or cause. Behaviorists regard an action as being preceded by an antecedent. Behavior modification theory states holds that when antecedents to behaviors are recognized, the antecedents can be modified or controlled to decrease the occurrence of negative behaviors and increase the occurrence of positive behaviors. This is referred to as stimulus control.

anthropometry Measurement of the body (stature, weight, circumferences, and skinfold thickness).

apoproteins Special proteins found in lipoproteins that control the interaction and metabolic fate of lipoproteins. Apoproteins activate enzymes that modify the composition and structure of lipoproteins, are involved in the binding and ingestion of lipoproteins by cells, and participate in the exchange of lipids between lipoproteins of different classes.

appendicular skeleton The portion of the skeleton that contains the bones of the limbs, pelvis, clavicles, and scapulae.

Archimedes' principle The fact that an object's volume, when submerged in water, equals the volume of water the object displaces. Thus, if the mass and the volume of a body are known, the density of that body can be calculated. This principle is used to determine whole-body density in hydrostatic weighing.

arm muscle area An indicator of total body muscle calculated from the triceps skinfold thickness and midarm circumference.

arteriography A radiographic study of an artery or arterial system in which contrast medium is injected into an artery to determine the condition of the artery (e.g. narrowing due to atherosclerosis).

atherogenic Atherosclerosis-producing.

atherosclerosis A progressive disorder beginning in childhood with the appearance of lesions in the form of fatty streaks in the lining of the coronary arteries or aorta. These may eventually progress to fatty and fibrous plaques or even larger, more complicated lesions. As the lesions develop, the progressive narrowing of the vessels reduces blood flow to the tissues supplied by the affected vessels.

attenuated Becoming weakened or thinned. For example, x-ray beams are attenuated by passing through body tissue.

axial skeleton The part of the skeleton composed of the skull, vertebral column, sternum, and ribs.

balance sheet approach The most common method of estimating per capita food availability at the national level. Food exports, nonfood use (e.g. livestock feed, seed, and industrial use), and year-end inventories are subtracted from data on beginning-year inventories, total food production, and imports to arrive at an estimate of per capita food availability.

balloon angioplasty A surgical procedure in which a balloon catheter is inserted through the skin into a narrowed blood vessel and inflated to enlarge its interior opening, or lumen, in order to increase blood flow through the affected vessel.

basal metabolic rate (BMR) An individual's energy expenditure measured in the postabsorptive state, (no food consumed during the previous 12 hours) after resting quietly for 30 minutes in a thermally neutral environment. (Room temperature is perceived as neither hot nor cold.)

beriberi A disease resulting from thiamine deficiency and characterized by nervous tingling throughout the body, poor arm-leg coordination, deep calf muscle pain, heart enlargement, and occasional edema.

bias A measure of inaccuracy or departure from accuracy.

bioelectrical impedance The measure of resistance to an alternating current in an organism. Used to estimate total body water from which the percent of body fat and lean body mass can be calculated using various equations.

biopsy The removal and examination of tissue samples to determine the presence or concentration of certain nutrients (or the presence or absence of disease).

BMI Body mass index.

body cell mass The metabolically active, energy-requiring mass of the body.

body density The mass of the body per unit volume, generally measured by hydrostatic weighing. Percentage of body fat can then be estimated from body density using the Siri or Brozek equations.

body mass index *See* Quetelet's index.

bypass surgery A surgical procedure creating an auxiliary flow, shunt, or pathway around a diseased or malfunctioning body area to restore normal or nearnormal body function (e.g., coronary bypass, intestinal bypass).

cachexia Profound physical wasting and malnutrition usually associated with chronic disease, advanced acquired immunodeficiency syndrome, alcoholism, or drug abuse.

cadaver A dead body used for anatomic, anthropometric, or other study. Only by analyzing cadavers can direct measurement of human body composition be made.

calorie count Calculation of the energy and nutrient value of foods eaten by a subject such as a hospitalized patient.

calorimetry Measurement of a subject's energy expenditure.

cancer A group of diseases characterized by abnormal growth of cells that, when uncontrolled, invade other tissues or organs, interfering with their normal function and nutrition.

cardiovascular disease A variety of pathological processes pertaining to the heart and blood vessels (coronary artery disease and hypertension).

case-control study Comparison of current disease status with the level of past exposure to some factor of interest (e.g. some nutrient or dietary component) in two groups of subjects, (cases and controls) in an attempt to determine how past exposure to the factor relates to currently existing disease.

catabolism The breaking down of more complex compounds into simple biological substances, generally resulting in energy release.

cerebrovascular disease A group of disorders, characterized by decreased blood supply to the brain, resulting from hemorrhage of or atherosclerosis within the cerebral arteries.

CHD Coronary heart disease.

CHI Creatinine-height index.

cholesterol A fatlike sterol found in animal products and normally produced by the body. It serves as a precursor for bile acids and steroid hormones and is an essential component of the plasma membrane and the myelin sheaths of nerves. Serum cholesterol levels are causally related to risk of coronary artery disease.

chronic disease A disease progressing over a long period of time, such as coronary heart disease, certain cancers, stroke, diabetes mellitus, and atherosclerosis.
chylomicrons Lipoproteins synthesized in the small intestine that transport dietary triglycerides from the small intestine to adipose tissue, muscle, and the liver. They are 90% triglyceride by weight and are naturally found in serum shortly after meals, but are not normally present in fasting serum.
cirrhosis Inflammation of an organ's interstitial tissue, especially the liver.
closed questions Questions that are restrictive in nature and allow an interviewer to control answers and ask for specific information. They are often answered by a simple "yes" or "no" response.
coefficient of variation (CV) A measure of precision calculated by dividing the standard deviation by the mean and multiplying by 100 (CV = SD ÷ mean × 100).
cognitive restructuring Elimination of negative, irrational thoughts through increasing awareness of one's self-talk, disputing and changing negative self-talk, and by using cognitive rehearsal and thought stopping.
cohort studies See longitudinal studies.
computed tomography (CT) An imaging technique producing highly detailed cross-sectional body images from computerized processing of x-ray beam transmission through body tissues of differing density.
computer hardware The physical components of a computer (e.g., the monitor, disc drives, central processing unit, and keyboard).
conjunctival impression cytology Microscopic examination of the conjunctival epithelial cells used to detect early morphologic changes indicative of vitamin A deficiency.
consequences Events that follow and are causally linked to certain behaviors. Consequences reinforce or reward the behavior they follow, and they may be positive, negative, or neutral. When consequences are positive, behavior is more likely to be repeated. Behavior followed by negative consequences is less likely to be repeated.
Continuing Survey of Food Intakes by Individuals (CSFII) A national survey of individual dietary intake intended to be conducted annually by the USDA (except when the Nationwide Food Consumption Survey is in progress).
coronary heart disease (CHD) A disease of the heart resulting from inadequate circulation of blood to local areas of the heart muscle. The disease is almost always a consequence of focal narrowing of the coronary arteries by atherosclerosis and is also known as ischemic heart disease or coronary artery disease.
correlational study A research design in which the occupance of one variable is compared with the occupance of another variable within the same population. The study is useful for generating hypotheses regarding the associations between suspected risk factors and disease risk.
creatine A nitrogen-containing compound, 98% of which is found in muscle in the form of creatine phosphate. Creatine spontaneously dehydrates to form creatinine that is then excreted unaltered in the urine.
creatinine The end product of creatine metabolism. Twenty-four-hour urinary creatinine excretion is used as an index of body muscle mass.
creatinine-height index (CHI) An index or ratio sometimes used to assess body protein status. CHI = 24-hour urinary creatinine excretion ÷ expected creatinine excretion of a reference adult of the same sex and stature × 100.
cross-sectional survey A study design in which disease and various factors of interest are simultaneously examined in groups at a specific period of time.
CSFII Continuing Survey of Food Intakes by Individuals.
CT Computed tomography.
CV Coefficient of variation.

Daily Value (DV) A dietary reference value appearing on the nutrition labels of foods regulated by the FDA and the USDA as part of the Nutrition Labeling and Education Act of 1990. It is derived from the Daily Reference Values (DRVs) and the Reference Daily Intakes (RDIs). The daily value on food labels shows the percent of the DRVs or RDIs that a serving of food provides.
Daily Reference Value (DRV) A dietary reference value serving as a basis for the Daily Values. DRVs are for nutrients (e.g. total fat, cholesterol, total carbohydrate, and dietary fiber) for which no set of standards existed before passage of the Nutrition Labeling and Education Act of 1990.
deciliter (dl) A unit of volume in the metric system. One deciliter equals 10^{-1} liter, 1/10 of a liter or 100 milliliters.

deficiency diseases Diseases caused by a lack of adequate dietary nutrients, vitamins, or minerals (e.g., rickets, pellagra, beriberi, xerophthalmia, and goiter).
densitometry Measurement of body density.
density See body density.
deuterium A radioactive hydrogen isotope having twice the mass of common light hydrogen atoms. Known as "heavy hydrogen."
deuterium oxide "Heavy water" composed of oxygen and deuterium (D20 or 2H20). Used in the determination of total body water.
DEXA Dual-energy x-ray absorptiometry.
DHHS United States Department of Health and Human Services.
diabetes mellitus A metabolic disorder characterized by inadequate insulin secretion by the pancreas or the inability of certain cells to use insulin and resulting in abnormally high serum glucose levels. Diabetes mellitus can be classified as type I or insulin-dependent diabetes mellitus (IDDM), type II, or noninsulin dependent diabetes mellitus (NIDDM), or gestational diabetes mellitus (GDM).
Dietary Goals for the United States Seven dietary goals established by the U.S. senate select committee on nutrition and human needs in 1977 for improving the quality of the American diet.
diet history An approach to assessing an individual's usual dietary intake over an extended period of time (e.g., past month, or year). This typically involves Burke's four assessment-steps: collecting general information about the subject's health habits, questioning the subject about his or her usual eating pattern, performing a "cross check" on the data given in step two, and having the subject complete a 3 day food record.
dilution techniques An approach to indirectly measure total body water (TBW). A known concentration and volume of a tracer is given to a subject orally or parenterally, time is allowed for the tracer to equilibrate with the subject's body water, and the concentration of the tracer is analyzed in a sample of the subject's blood, urine, or saliva.
direct calorimetry Measurement of the body's heat output using an airtight, thermally insulated living chamber.
distal Away from the center of the body.
distribution See normal distribution.
diurnal variations Cyclical changes occurring throughout the day.
dL Deciliter.
DPA Dual-photon absorptiometry.
DRV Daily reference value.
dual-energy x-ray absorptiometry (DEXA) An approach for measuring bone mineral content in the appendicular skeleton, axial skeleton, or whole body using an x-ray source operating at two energy levels.
dual-photon absorptiometry (DPA) An approach for measuring bone mineral content using photons at two different energy levels derived from a radioisotopic source (gadolinium-153).
duplicate food collections A direct method of calculating nutrient intake in which subjects place an identical portion of all foods and beverages consumed during a specified period in collection containers. This is then chemically analyzed at a laboratory for nutrient content, which provides a potentially more accurate determination of actual nutrient intake, and is compared with calculations based on food composition data.
DV Daily value.

electrolyte An electrically charged particle (anion or cation) present in solution within the body that is capable of conducting an electrical charge. Sodium, chloride, potassium, and bicarbonate are electrolytes commonly found in the body.
enrichment The replacement of certain nutrients lost in food during processing according to some standard stipulated by law.
enteral nutrition The delivery of food or nutrients into the esophagus, stomach, or small intestine through tubes to improve nutritional status.
erythrocyte Red blood cell or RBC.
ESADDI Estimated Safe and Adequate Daily Dietary Intakes.
essential lipid The small amount of lipid (constituting about 1.5% to 3% of lean body weight) serving as a structural component of cell membranes and the nervous system that is necessary for life.
estimated food record A method of recording individual food intake in which the amounts and types of all food and beverages are recorded for a specific period of time, usually ranging from 1 to 7 days. Portion sizes are estimated using household measures (such as cups, tablespoons, teaspoons), a ruler, or containers (such as coffee cups, bowls, glasses). Certain items (eggs, apples, or 12 ounce cans of soda) are counted as units.

Estimated Safe and Adequate Daily Dietary Intakes (ESADDI) An estimated range of intake that is considered adequate for health without being excessive in certain essential nutrients because data are unavailable to establish a Recommended Dietary Allowance.
etiology The study of the causes of disease.

false negative Nutrient intake misclassified as adequate when it is actually inadequate.
false positive Nutrient intake misclassified as inadequate when it is actually adequate.
fatty streak The initial step of atherosclerosis, usually beginning in childhood, in which lipids (primarily cholesterol and its esters) become deposited in macrophages and smooth muscle cells within the inner lining of large elastic and muscular arteries.
FDA Food and Drug Administration.
femtoliter (fL) A unit of volume in the metric system. One femtoliter equals 10^{-15} liter.
ferritin The combination of the protein apoferritin and iron that functions as the primary storage form for body iron. It is primarily found in the liver, spleen, and bone marrow.
ferritin model A model for assessing the prevalence of iron deficiency, requiring abnormal values for at least two of the following measurements: serum ferritin level, transferrin saturation, or erythrocyte protoporphyrin level.
fibrous plaque A collection of lipids within the arterial walls during adolescence and early adulthood, creating a projection into the channel or lumen of the artery, thus resulting in impaired blood flow and oxygen delivery to a tissue or organ.
fl Femoliter.
food balance sheet *See* balance sheet approach.
food exchange system A meal planning method originally developed for the diabetic diet that simplifies control of energy consumption, helps insure adequate nutrient intake, and allows considerable variety in food selection.
food frequency questionnaire A questionnaire listing foods on which individuals indicate how often they consume each listed item during certain time intervals (daily, weekly, or monthly). Standard portion sizes are used and an estimate of nutrient intake is provided on the questionnaire. Sometimes referred to as the semi-quantitative food frequency or list-based diet history approach.
food inventory record An approach to household food consumption measurement in which total household food use is calculated by subtracting food on hand at the end of the survey period (ending inventory) from the sum of food on hand at the start of the survey period (beginning inventory) and food brought into the household during the survey.
food list-recall approach A method of measuring household food consumption in which an interviewer, using a detailed listing of foods, asks the respondent to recall the amount of food used by the household during the preceding week and the amount paid for purchased items. This approach has been used in the Nationwide Food Consumption Survey (NFCS).
fortification Addition of nutrients to food at a nutrient concentration greater than originally present, and/or addition of nutrients not initially existing in food.
four-compartment model A body composition model viewing the body as being composed of four chemical groups: water, protein, mineral, and fat.
Frankfort horizontal plane An imaginary plane intersecting the lowest point on the margin of the orbit (the bony socket of the eye) and the tragion (the notch above the tragus, the cartilaginous projection just anterior to the external opening of the ear). This plane should be horizontal with the head and in line with the spine.

g Gram.
generalized equations Regression equations for estimating body density or percentage of body fat from anthropometric measures that are applicable to population groups varying widely in adiposity and age.
goiter Thyroid gland enlargement caused by dietary iodine deficiency.
gram A unit of mass in the metric system. One gram equals 10^{-3} kilogram, 1 pound equals 453.5924 grams, and 1 ounce equals 28.350 grams.
gynoid obesity Excess body fat that is predominantly within the hips and thighs as opposed to within the abdomen and upper body. This is the usual pattern of female obesity.

HANES Health and Nutrition Examination Survey.
HDL High-density lipoprotein.
height-weight indices Various ratios or indices expressing body weight in terms of height. Among these are Quetelet's index and Benn's index.

hemoglobin The iron-containing protein pigment of red blood cells that carries oxygen to body cells. Blood hemoglobin levels can reflect iron status (e.g. abnormally low hemoglobin may mean anemia).

HHANES Hispanic Health and Nutrition Examination Survey.

high-density lipoprotein (HDL) A serum lipoprotein synthesized by the liver and intestine that transports cholesterol within the blood stream. As the serum level of HDL increases, risk of coronary artery disease decreases.

HNIS Human Nutrition Information Service of the USDA.

hydrostatic weighing Underwater weighing. The most widely used technique of determining whole-body density, based on Archimedes' principle.

hydroxyapatite Calcium and phosphate crystals providing rigidity to teeth and bones.

hyperlipidemia Excessively high levels of lipids in the blood.

hypermetabolism Increased rate of energy and protein metabolism accompanying trauma, infection, burns, or surgery.

hypertension Persistently elevated arterial blood pressure.

hypervitaminosis A Excessive consumption of vitamin A.

IDDM Insulin-dependent diabetes mellitus.

IDL Intermediate-density lipoproteins

iliac crest The crest, or top, of the ilium (the largest of three bones making up the outer half of the pelvis). The crest is the bony spine located just below the "waist." Used as an anatomic landmark in skinfold measurement sites.

impedance The opposition to an alternating current, composed of two elements: resistance and reactance.

imputed data Data used by compilers of food composition tables when certain nutrient data are unavailable. This data is obtained from similar foods or ingredients for which data are more complete.

incidence The number of new events or cases of a disease in a defined population, within a specified time period.

index of nutritional quality (INQ) A concept related to nutrient density that allows the quantity of a nutrient per 1,000 kcal in a food, meal, or diet to be compared with a nutrient standard.

in vivo neutron activation analysis *See* neutron activation analysis.

indirect calorimetry Determination of energy expenditure by measuring the body's oxygen consumption and carbon dioxide production.

infarct Death of local tissues fed by an obstructed artery or occluded venous drainage because of insufficient blood supply.

infectious disease Any disease caused by the invasion and multiplication of microorganisms such as bacteria, fungi, or virus.

infrared interactance When infrared light is projected through the skin, some of the energy is reflected from the skin and underlying tissues. Estimates of body composition are made by analyzing certain characteristics of this reflected energy.

insulin-dependent diabetes mellitus (IDDM) *See* diabetes mellitus.

intermediate-density lipoproteins (IDL) Lipoprotein particles created by the removal of triglycerides from VLDL. IDL is a midway product in the conversion of VLDL to LDL.

International Unit (IU) An amount defined by the International Conference for Unification of Formulae and used to express the quantity of certain substances.

intraindividual variability Change in an individual's nutrient intake from day-to-day.

INQ Index of nutritional quality.

iron deficiency The depletion of body iron stores, corresponding to the second and third stages in the development of iron deficiency.

iron deficiency anemia A low hemoglobin value found in association with iron deficiency. Theoretically, anemia corresponds to the third stage of iron deficiency.

iron overload Excessive accumulation of iron storage in tissues.

ischemia Impaired blood flow causing oxygen-nutrition deprivation to associated tissues, resulting in pain (e.g. angina pectoris) or, if severe enough, tissue death as in heart attack.

IU International Unit.

joule A unit of work or energy in the metric system. The amount of work done by a force of 1 newton acting over the distance of 1 meter. *See also kilojoule.*

kat/L The SI unit of enzyme activity. One katal per liter is the amount of enzyme necessary to catalyze a reaction at the rate of 1 mole of substrate per second per liter ($mol \cdot s^{-1} \cdot L^{-1}$).

kg Kilogram.
kilocalorie (kcal) The amount of energy required to raise the temperature of 1 liter of water 1° C. A unit of heat equal to 1,000 calories. Also known as a large calorie. One kcal equals 0.239 kilojoule.
kilogram (kg) A unit of mass in the metric system. One kilogram equals 1,000 grams or 2.2046 pounds.
kilojoule (kj) A unit of work or energy in the metric system. A kilojoule equals 1,000 joules. A kilojoule is equivalent to 4.18 kcal. *See also* joule.
kj Kilojoule.
kcal Kilocalorie.
kwashiorkor A protein deficiency, generally seen in children, characterized by edema, growth failure, and muscle wasting.

lapse A single or temporary recurrence of an unwanted habit or behavior that one has, overcome or turned from for a period of time.
LDL Low-density lipoprotein.
LDL receptors Molecules on the surface of plasma membranes of hepatic and peripheral cells that recognize and remove low-density lipoprotein from the blood.
leading question A question that contains an implicit or explicit suggestion about the expected or desired answer.
lipoproteins Spherical macromolecular complexes of lipids (triglycerides, cholesterol, cholesterol esters, and phospholipids) and special proteins known as apoproteins that transport lipids from sites of absorption or synthesis to sites of storage or metabolism via the blood. They include chylomicrons, LDL, IDL, VLDL, and HDL.
list-based diet history *See* food frequency questionnaire.
longitudinal study Cohort study. A study design comparing future exposure to various factors in a group (cohort) of subjects in an attempt to determine how exposure with the factors relates to diseases that may develop.
low-density lipoprotein (LDL) A serum lipoprotein whose primary role is transporting cholesterol to the various cells of the body. LDL contains approximately 70% of the serum's total cholesterol, is considered the most atherogenic (atherosclerosis-producing) lipoprotein, and is the prime target of attempts to lower serum cholesterol. Low serum levels of LDL cholesterol are desirable.

μ The Greek letter mu used as a prefix in such instances as μg (microgram) and μL (microliter) where it indicates 10^{-6} or one-millionth.
m Meter.
magnetic resonance imaging (MRI) A technology allowing both imaging of the body and *in vivo* chemical analysis without radiation hazard to the subject.
malnutrition This may mean any nutrition disorder, but usually refers to failing health caused by to long-term nutritional inadequacies.
marasmus Predominantly an energy (kilocalorie) deficiency presenting with significant loss of body weight, skeletal muscle, and adipose tissue mass, but with serum protein concentrations relatively intact.
marasmic kwashiorkor A combination of chronic energy deficiency and chronic or acute protein deficiency.
MCV Mean corpuscular (red blood cell) volume.
MCV model A model for assessing the prevalence of iron deficiency that requires abnormal values for at least two of the following measurements: mean corpuscular volume, transferrin saturation, or erythrocyte protoporphyrin level.
mean The measure of central tendency (average) calculated by adding all individual values and dividing by the number of values.
median The value that divides a distribution of values into two equal parts, with 50% of the values above and 50% of the values below this point. Also known as the 50th percentile.
meter (m) A unit of distance in the metric system. One meter equals 100 centimeters, 1,000 millimeters, or 39.37 inches.
menopause Cessation of monthly menses.
Metropolitan relative weight An individual's actual body weight divided by the midpoint value of weight range for a given height (obtained from a Metropolitan Life Insurance Company-height-weight table) and then multiplied by 100. *See also* relative weight.
mg Milligram.
MI Myocardial infarction.
milligram (mg) A unit of mass in the metric system. 10^{-3} gram or one-thousandth of a gram.
midaxillary line An imaginary line running vertically through the middle of the axilla used as an anatomic landmark in skinfold measurements.
millimeter (mm) A unit of distance in the metric system. 10^{-3} meter or 1/1,000 of a meter.

millimole (mmol) 10^{-3} mole or one-thousandth of a gram.
missing foods Foods eaten but not reported by participants of nutritional surveys.
mm Millimeter.
mmol Millimole.
modeling Observational learning or imitation. A learning process in behavior modification in which observers learn new behaviors by watching the actions of a model.
morbidity Illness or sickness.
morphology The study of the shape and structure of organisms, organs, or parts.
mortality Death.
myocardial infarction (MI) Heart attack. Death of an area of heart tissue caused by blockage of the coronary artery feeding that area.
myocardium Heart muscle.

National Health and Nutrition Examination Survey (NHANES) A cross-sectional survey conducted by the U.S. Department of Health and Human Services that assesses food intake, height, weight, blood pressure, vitamin and mineral levels, and a number of other health parameters in a statistically selected group of Americans. Conducted every 10 years.
National Nutrition Monitoring System (NNMS) A congressionally mandated system in which the USDA and USDHHS are to work cooperatively in collecting data relating to health and nutrition status measurements, food composition measurements, dietary knowledge, attitude assessment, and surveillance of the food supply.
Nationwide Food Consumption Survey (NFCS) A survey of food consumption at the household and individual levels, conducted by the USDA.
NCEP National Cholesterol Education Program.
NCHS National Center for Health Statistics.
negative nitrogen balance A condition in which nitrogen loss from the body exceeds nitrogen intake. Negative nitrogen balance is often seen in the case of illness, trauma, burns, and recovery from major surgery.
negative reinforcer An unpleasant consequence of a behavior that maintains and strengthens the behavior by the negative reinforcer being removed from the situation.
neutral questions Questions that allow a client to respond without pressure or direction from the interviewer.
neutron activation analysis A technology allowing in vivo measurement of the body's content of calcium, iodine, hydrogen, sodium, chloride, phosphorus, carbon and other elements. A neutron beam is directed to the subject and the response of various elements within the body allows estimation of the quantities of these elements.
NFCS Nationwide Food Consumption Survey.
NHANES National Nutritional Monitoring System.
NHANES I First National Health and Nutrition Examination Survey.
NHANES II Second National Health and Nutrition Examination Survey.
NHANES III Third National Health and Nutrition Examination Survey.
NHES National Health Examination Survey.
NIDDM Non-insulin dependent diabetes mellitus.
nitrogen balance A condition in which nitrogen losses from the body are equal to nitrogen intake. Nitrogen balance is the expected state of the healthy adult.
NLEA Nutrition Labeling and Education Act.
NMR Nuclear magnetic resonance.
nomogram A graphic device with several vertical scales allowing calculation of certain values when a straightedge is connected between two scales and the desired value is read from a third scale.
nonambulatory Unable to walk (ambulate).
non-insulin dependent diabetes mellitus (NIDDM) *See* diabetes mellitus.
non-quantitative food frequency questionnaire A food frequency questionnaire assessing frequency of food consumption but not the size of food servings.
nuclear magnetic resonance (NMR) Earlier name for magnetic resonance imaging (MRI).
nutrient data base A compilation of data on the nutrient content of various foods. The data base may exist in book form or as an electronic file accessible by computer.
nutrient density The nutritional composition of foods expressed in terms of nutrient quantity per 1,000 kcal. If the quantity of nutrients per 1,000 kcal is great enough, then the nutrient needs of a person will be met when his or her energy needs are met.
Nutrition Labeling and Education Act (NLEA) A law passed by the U.S. congress in 1990 mandating nutrition labeling for virtually all processed foods regulated by the U.S. Food and Drug Administration,

authorizing appropriate health claims on food labels, and calling for activities to educate consumers about food labels.

nutrition monitoring The assessment of dietary or nutritional status at intermittent times with the aim of detecting changes in the dietary or nutritional status of a population.

nutritional assessment The measurement of indicators of dietary status and nutrition-related health status of individuals or populations to identify the possible occurrence, nature, and extent of impaired nutritional status (ranging from deficiency to toxicity).

nutritional epidemiology The application of epidemiologic principles to study how diet and nutrition influence the occurrence of disease.

nutritional screening The process of identifying characteristics known to be associated with nutrition problems in order to pinpoint individuals who are malnourished or at risk of malnutrition.

nutritional surveillance Continuous assessment of nutritional status for the purpose of detecting changes in trend or distribution in order to initiate corrective measures.

obesity Excessive accumulation of body fat.

observational standards A dietary standard based on clinical observation as opposed to scientific measurement of actual need.

olecranon process The bony projection of the distal ulna at the elbow. Used as an anatomic landmark in upper arm anthropometric measurements.

open questions Questions providing individuals with considerable freedom in deciding the amount and type of information to give in answering an interviewer's questions.

osteoporosis A condition in which bone mineral content is decreased, resulting in greater susceptibility to bone fracture, deformity, and pain.

overnutrition The condition resulting from the excessive intake of foods in general or particular food components.

overweight Body weight in excess of a particular standard and sometimes used as an index of obesity.

parallax The apparent difference in the reading of a measurement scale (e.g., a skinfold caliper's needle) when viewed from various points not in a straight line with the eye.

parenteral nutrition The process of administering nutrients directly into veins to improve nutritional status.

pellagra A niacin deficiency syndrome characterized by inflamed mucous membranes, mental deterioration, diarrhea, and eruptions in skin areas exposed to light or injury.

PEM Protein-energy malnutrition.

percentiles Divisions of a distribution into equal, ordered subgroups of hundredths. The 50th percentile is the median. The 90th percentile, for example, is an observation whose value exceeds 90% of the set of observations and is exceeded by only 10%.

peripheral vascular disease Atherosclerotic changes within the aorta and iliac and femoral arteries affecting blood flow in the body's periphery.

pg Picograms.

phantom foods Foods not eaten but reported as having been eaten by participants of nutrition surveys.

picograms (pg) A unit of mass in the metric system. One picogram equals 10^{-12} gram or one-trillionth of a gram.

plethysmograph A device for measuring volume without requiring the subject to be totally immersed in water. Generally, the volume measurement is then used to calculate body density and percentage of body fat.

population-specific equations Regression equations for estimating body density or percentage of body fat from anthropometric measures that can only be applied to population groups sharing certain common features such as sex, age, and adiposity.

positive nitrogen balance When nitrogen intake exceeds nitrogen loss from the body. This is commonly seen in growth, pregnancy, and during recovery from trauma, surgery, or illness.

positive reinforcer Any consequence (reward) that maintains and strengthens behavior by its presence. (The positive reinforcer makes the behavior more likely to recur.)

postprandial After a meal.

power-type indices Indices such as Quetelet's index and Benn's index.

prevalence The existing cases of a disease or other condition in a given population at a designated time.

protein-energy malnutrition (PEM) Inadequate consumption of protein and energy resulting in a gradual body wasting and increased susceptibility to infection.

provisional tables Provisional data supplied by the United States Department of Agriculture for special nutrients or foods such as dietary fiber, bakery foods, vitamin K, fatty acids, sugar, etc. that are often released years before more complete data are available.

proximal Toward the center of the body.

QCT Quantitative computed tomography.

quantitative food frequency questionnaire *See* semi-quantitative food frequency questionnaire.

quantitative computed tomography (QCT) An imaging technique consisting of an array of x-ray sources and radiation detectors aligned opposite each other. As the x-ray beams pass through the subject, they are weakened or attenuated by the body's tissues and eventually picked up by the detectors. Data from the detectors are then transmitted to a computer that reconstructs the subject's cross-sectional anatomy utilizing mathematic equations adapted for computer processing.

Quetelet's index Weight in kilograms divided by height in meters squared (W/H^2). The most widely used weight-height or power type index.

rational-emotive therapy (RET) A counseling approach based on the premise that emotional disturbances are a product of irrational thinking. RET holds that emotions are primarily the result of our beliefs, evaluations, interpretations, and reactions to life situations, which in turn determine one's behavior. Behavior is altered by correcting the thought process using methods such as cognitive restructuring, language changing, cognitive rehearsal, and thought stopping.

RDA Recommended Dietary Allowance.

RDIs Reference Daily Intakes

reality therapy A therapy based primarily on the work of psychiatrist William Glasser and his premise that every person's behavior is an attempt to fulfill his or her basic human needs (behavior driven completely from within). Emphasis is placed on individual responsibility for actions and client participation in decision making.

Recommended Dietary Allowances Suggested levels of intake for 29 nutrients and energy established by the Food and Nutrition Board of the National Research Council.

recumbent The position of lying down. Recumbent length, for example, is obtained with the subject lying down and is generally reserved for children less than 24 months of age or for children between 24 and 36 months who cannot stand erect without assistance.

REE Resting energy expenditure.

Reference Daily Intakes (RDIs) A set of dietary references that serve as the basis for the Daily Values and are based on the Recommended Dietary Allowances (RDAs) for essential vitamins and minerals and, in selected groups, protein. The RDIs replace the U.S. Recommended Daily Allowances (U.S. RDAs).

regression equations Equations developed by comparing a variety of anthropometric measures with measurements of body density (usually by hydrostatic weighing) to see which anthropometric measures are best at predicting body density. A statistical process called multiple-regression analysis is used to develop the equations.

relapse Resumption of an unwanted habit or behavior that one has, for a period of time, overcome or turned from.

relative weight A subject's actual body weight divided by the midpoint value of weight range for a given height and then multiplied by 100. *See also* Metropolitan relative weight.

reliability *See* reproducibility.

remodeling The dynamic process of skeletal change in which bones are constantly undergoing resorption and reformation.

reproducibility Also known as reliability. The ability of a method to yield the same measurement value on two or more different occasions, assuming that nothing has changed in the interim.

resting energy expenditure (REE) Also known as resting metabolic rate. This term is used for metabolic rate or energy expenditure in the awake, resting, and postabsorptive individual.

RET Rationalemotive therapy.

rickets A condition especially found in infants and children characterized by malformed bones, delayed fontanel closure, and muscle pain, due to a deficiency of vitamin D.

scurvy An ascorbic acid (vitamin C) deficiency disease characterized by anemia, spongy and bleeding gums, and capillary hemorrhages.

self-contract An agreement an individual makes with himself or herself to help build commitment to behavior change.

semi-quantitative food frequency Food frequency questionnaire that assesses both frequency and portion size of food consumption. *See also* food frequency questionnaire.

sensitivity A test's ability to indicate an abnormality where there is one.

serum proteins Proteins present in serum (the liquid portion of clotted blood) that are often regarded as indicators of the body's visceral protein status (e.g. albumin).
shortfall nutrients Nutrients whose intakes are below recommended levels among a significant part of the population.
SI Système International.
signs Observations made by a qualified examiner during a physical examination.
single-photon absorptiometry (SPA) An approach for measuring bone mineral content using photons at a single energy level derived from a radioisotopic source (iodine-125).
skinfold thickness A double fold of skin that is measured with skinfold calipers at various body sites.
software program The entire set of programs, procedures, and related documentation associated with computer programs. The list of program commands that operate a particular program on the computer.
somatic protein Protein contained in the body's skeletal muscles.
SPA Single-photon absorptiometry.
specificity A test's ability to indicate normalcy where there is no abnormality.
standard deviation A measure of how much a frequency distribution varies from the mean.
stadiometer A device capable of measuring stature in children over 2 years of age and in adults. This measure is taken in a standing position.
stature Standing height.
stimulus control A behavior modification technique in which behavioral antecedents are recognized and modified or controlled to decrease the occurrence of negative behaviors and increase the occurrence of positive behaviors.
stroke Blockage or rupture of a blood vessel supplying the brain with resulting loss of consciousness, paralysis, or other symptoms.
supine The position in which one is lying on his or her back.
surrogate source A source of information about a subject's behavior (e.g. dietary practices) from a source other than the subject. Typical surrogate sources include a spouse, child, close relative, or friend of the subject.
symptoms Disease manifestations that the patient is usually aware of and often complains of.
Système International (SI) An international system of measurement units allowing interchangeability of information between nations and disciplines.

TEF Thermal effect of food.
thermic effect of exercise Energy expenditure resulting from physical activity.
thermic effect of food (TEF) Also known as diet induced thermogenesis or the specific dynamic action of food. TEF is the increased energy expenditure following food consumption or administration of parenteral or enteral nutrition caused by absorption and metabolism of food and nutrients.
TOBEC Total body electrical conductivity.
total body electrical conductivity (TOBEC) A method of assessing body composition in which a subject is placed in an electromagnetic field (EMF). Since electrolytes within the fat-free mass are capable of conducting electricity, the degree to which the EMF is disrupted is related to the amount of fat-free mass within the subject's body.
transferrin The form in which iron is transported within the blood.
tritium An isotope of hydrogen having three times the mass of ordinary hydrogen. It is commonly used as a tracer in the determination of total body water.
twenty-four hour recall A method of dietary recall in which a trained interviewer asks the subject to remember in detail all foods and beverages consumed during the past 24 hours. This information is recorded by the interviewer for later coding and analysis.
two-compartment model A body composition model that views the body as being composed of two compartments: fat mass and fat-free mass, or, according to an alternative approach, into adipose tissue and lean body mass.

ulna The larger, inner bone of the forearm. Used as an anatomic landmark in arm anthropometry.
ultrasound A diagnostic method used for imaging internal organs and estimating the thickness of subcutaneous adipose tissue. High frequency sound waves are transmitted into the body from a transducer (sound transmitter) applied to the skin surface. As ultrasound strikes the interface between two tissues differing in density (e.g. adipose tissue and muscle), some of it is reflected back and received by the transducer. Alterations between the signal as it is transmitted and received are used to image internal organs and to determine subcutaneous tissue thickness.

undernutrition A condition resulting from the inadequate intake of food in general or particular food components.
underwater weighing *See* hydrostatic weighing.
USDA United States Department of Agriculture.
USRDA U.S. Recommended Daily Allowances.
U.S. Recommended Daily Allowances (USRDA) A set of nutrition standards developed by the FDA for use in regulating the nutritional labeling of food. They replaced the Minimum Daily Requirement (MDR) and should not be confused with the RDA's established by the National Research Council.

validity The ability of an instrument to measure what it is intended to measure. Validating a method of measuring dietary intake, for example, involves comparing measurements of intake obtained by that method with intake measurements obtained by some other accepted approach.
very-low-density lipoprotein (VLDL) A lipoprotein present in blood that is synthesized by the liver and primarily carries triglyceride to cells for storage and metabolism.
viscera Organs of the body (such as liver, kidneys, heart).
visceral protein Protein found in the body's organs or viscera, as well as that in the serum and in blood cells.
VLDL Very low-density lipoprotein.

waist-to-hip ratio The waist or abdominal circumference divided by the hip or gluteal circumference. This is used as an index for assessing the regional body fat distribution and its attendant health risks.
weighed food record A method of recording individual food intake in which the amounts and types of all food and beverages are recorded for a specific period of time, usually ranging from 1 to 7 days. Portion sizes are determined by accurate weighing.
weight-height indices See height-weight indices.
WIC Special Supplemental Food Program for Women, Infants, and Children.

xerophthalmia An eye disease caused by vitamin A deficiency in which the conjunctiva and cornea dry and thicken, in part because of decreased mucus production. If not treated in earlier stages with vitamin A supplements, permanent damage may ensue, with softening of the cornea and subsequent blindness.

PHOTO CREDITS

Chapter 1
Fig. 1-1, Prints and Photograph Division, Library of Congress. Photo: Walker Evans.

Chapter 2
Fig. 2-3, Courtesy of Kellogg Corporation.

Chapter 3
Fig. 3-5, Courtesy of Dr. M. Kretsch, USDA, Agricultural Research Service, San Francisco, Cal.

Chapter 4
Fig. 4-3, Courtesy of the National Center for Health Statistics, US Department of Health and Human Services.
Fig. 4-5, Courtesy of the National Center for Health Statistics, US Department of Health and Human Services.

Chapter 6
Fig. 6-18, 6-20, 6-22, 6-24, 6-26, 6-28, 6-29, 6-31, 6-32, 6-37, 6-39, Nieman, DC: *Fitness and Sports Medicine: An Introduction*. Bull Publishing Company, Palo Alto, Cal, 1990.
Fig. 6-40, Courtesy of RJL Systems, Mt. Clemens, Mich.

Chapter 7
Fig. 7-16, Courtesy of Dr. James L. Seale, US Department of Agriculture, Agriculture Research Service, Beltsville Human Nutrition Research Center, Energy and Protein Nutrition Laboratory, Beltsville, Md.
Fig. 7-17, Courtesy of SensorMedics Corporation, DeltaTrac II Metabolic Monitor, Yorba Linda, Cal.

Chapter 8
Fig. 8-18, Dempster DW, Shane E, Horbert W, Lindsay R. 1986. Journal of Bone and Mineral Research 1:15–21. 1986.
Fig. 8-20, Courtesy of Bayer Corporation, Diagnostics Division.

Chapter 10
Fig. 10-2, 10-3, 10-4, Journal of the American Medical Association.
Fig. 10-6, 10-7, 10-9, 10-11, 10-12, McLaren DD: A Color Atlas and Text of Diet-Related Disorders, 2e, Mosby-Wolfe, 1993.
Fig. 10-10, Courtesy Sycamore Hospital, a division of Kettering Medical Center, Dayton, OH.

INDEX

A

D

E

F

G

H

I

N

O

P

Q

R

W

X

Y

Z